APHASIOLOGY

DISORDERS AND CLINICAL PRACTICE

SECOND EDITION

G. ALBYN DAVIS

University of Massachusetts at Amherst

Boston ■ New York ■ San Francisco
Mexico City ■ Montreal ■ Toronto ■ London ■ Madrid ■ Munich ■ Paris
Hong Kong ■ Singapore ■ Tokyo ■ Cape Town ■ Sydney

Executive Editor and Publisher: Stephen D. Dragin
Series Editorial Assistant: Katie Heimsoth
Marketing Manager: Kris Ellis-Levy
Production Editor: Gregory Erb
Editorial-Production Service: Omegatype Typography, Inc.
Manufacturing Buyer: Linda Morris
Composition and Prepress Buyer: Linda Cox
Cover Coordinator: Kristina Mose-Libon
Electronic Composition: Omegatype Typography, Inc.

For related titles and support materials, visit our online catalog at www.ablongman.com.

Between the time website information is gathered and then published, it is not unusual for some sites to have closed. Also, the transcription of URLs can result in typographical errors. The publisher would appreciate notification where these errors occur so that they may be corrected in subsequent editions.

Many of the designations used by manufacturers and sellers to distinguish their products are claimed as trademarks. Where those designations appear in this book, and Allyn and Bacon was aware of a trademark claim, the designations have been printed in initial or all caps.

Library of Congress Cataloging-in-Publication Data

Davis, G. Albyn (George Albyn)
    Aphasiology : disorders and clinical practice / G. Albyn Davis.—2nd ed.
       p.   cm.
    Includes bibliographical references and index.
    ISBN 0-205-48099-3 (alk. paper)
    1. Aphasia. 2. Language disorders. I. Title.
    [DNLM: 1. Aphasia. WL 340.5 D261a 2007]
  RC425.D379   2007
  618.85'52—dc22

                       2006048577

Printed in the United States of America

10   9   8   7   6   5   4   3   2   1   RRD-VA   11   10   09   08   07   06

Contents

PREFACE

Although 12 of the original 13 chapters are preserved, *Aphasiology: Disorders and Clinical Practice* has undergone numerous modifications. A new organization groups together 10 chapters on stroke-related aphasia, which are then followed by three chapters on other cognitive-communication disorders. Six of the chapters on aphasia contain basic information (Chapters 1–2, 4–7). The other four chapters on aphasia (3, 8–10) explicitly present rehabilitative activities. Many may argue that all of the chapters support rehabilitation, because understanding the disorders supports clinical thinking. Similarly, research predicts some of our clinical future, because experimental methodology often becomes new assessments and treatments.

What is new? Most obvious is the final chapter that pulls together information about dementia. *Aphasiology* also now includes more on managed care, life participation, and outcome measurements. I updated functional considerations with introductions to conversational analysis and quality of life measures. The three chapters on cognitive-communication disorders conclude with new surveys of rehabilitation. Some new details include information about medical records, data banks, and the study of verbs. There is also an example of daily patient contact notes. Most chapters end with a matching quiz. Answers to the quizzes are not provided, and the quizzes should promote recollection, review, and discussion.

Aphasiology is intended to supplement classroom presentations by providing a current and comprehensive education. The text should be challenging but readable for students and should be relatively light in the backpack. The examples that are provided should clarify lessons about psycholinguistic theory and language impairments. The absence of glamorous photos, baffling diagrams, and fuzzy radiology is intentional. Simple figures, even those of 25 years ago, still get the idea across, and students know better than I that instructive illustrations can be found by doing a Google search.

My strategy is to emphasize fundamentals. As a result, I sometimes present an earlier study containing the basics rather than a more recent study that is burdened with complexity. I trimmed away some psycholinguistic esoterica, and devoted more space to clinical realities and patients' stories. I relied mainly on (a) primary expertise as sources, (b) peer-reviewed research for quality control, and (c) published works so the accuracy of my renditions can be checked. I searched through our knowledge stores, closets, and trunks for sources, holding on to what looks good and what will most likely endure. One of my goals has been to maximize the conceptual logic that goes into making a diagnosis and targeting a particular treatment. Some of my instruction may seem like personal opinion. Occasionally I could not tell the difference myself, and I hope that this will encourage constructive debate in the classroom.

I gratefully acknowledge the patience and understanding of my family and of colleagues and students at the University of Massachusetts, especially our department chair, Dr. Jane Baran. Mary Sutherland, a speech-language pathologist, reintroduced me to clinical realities, and I want to further extend my appreciation for the good will of the staff at Weldon Rehabilitation Hospital in Springfield, Massachusetts. Courtney Lippe, a graduate student, helped pull together my references. At Allyn and Bacon, Steve Dragin and Meaghan Minnick put up with my angst and gave me plenty of room. At Omegatype Typography, Dawn McIlvain made necessary repairs. Thanks also should be conveyed to the reviewers of this edition, namely, Kelly Ingram, Arizona State University, and Frances S. Smith, Valdosta State University. Again, I want to thank Lyn Serper for inspiring the not-so-contrived story of Martin Exeter that weaves throughout the book. Betsy Elias reprised her job as "the whip" to keep me going. She cheerfully did most of the dirty work and heroically preserved my sanity. When this edition was finished, we got married.

G. Albyn Davis

CHAPTER 1

INTRODUCTION TO ACQUIRED LANGUAGE DISORDERS

Not long ago, Professor Martin Exeter was home practicing an important lecture when he suddenly stopped, stared at his wife Jackie, and dropped to the floor. An ambulance rushed him to the hospital. He did not recognize Jackie at first, was not quite sure where he was, and could not talk. She tried to get him to write, but he had to hold the pen with his left hand and just threw it at his feet. "I can't . . . talk" was all he could say. He looked frightened, and she was scared to death. The doctor told her that her husband probably had suffered a stroke. A couple days later she remembered the doctor also mentioned something called "aphasia." She thought she knew what a stroke was, but she had never heard of aphasia before.

The doctor also told Jackie of someone at the hospital who was trained to help people with aphasia. This has not been a common situation for very long. In 1925 in the United States, the field of speech-language pathology was established mainly to provide "speech correction" in public schools. However, the great wars left many young adults to struggle with long-lasting language disorders. Neurologists, psychologists, and speech pathologists created rehabilitation programs in military hospitals throughout the world. Therapies were quickly borrowed from speech correction, classroom teaching, and psychotherapy. Since then, veterans have been living longer, and pathologies of aging have challenged the health care system. In addition, aphasia is now understood to be a unique communicative disorder.

This introductory chapter has two main goals. One is to help the reader acquire a good idea of what aphasia is. The other goal is to help the reader acquire a foundation of thought that under-

lies the study of aphasia. **Clinical aphasiology** is an evolving discipline that includes (a) research intended to help us identify and explain aphasia and (b) rehabilitation intended to help patients and their families tackle their challenges.

Throughout this text, we shall occasionally check in on Martin Exeter and his family. We shall look into his recovery, language therapy, and adjustments to a new life. Toward the end of the first day after his stroke, Jackie was asking a lot of questions and wondering how their lives were going to change: "When can he come home? How soon will he walk again? How soon will he get his speech back? Marty talks for a living."

DIAGNOSING APHASIA

The physician's first task is to preserve a patient's life. Once survival is assured, the doctor starts considering a plan for discharge from acute care. This plan includes rehabilitation. When there is paralysis, a patient is referred to a physical therapist. When a patient is likely to have communication problems, the patient is referred to a speech-language pathologist. A written request for services is conveyed on a *consultation* or *referral* form. The form includes a provisional diagnosis, the patient's location in the hospital, and perhaps some medical history. The clinician's first responsibilities are to evaluate oral motor function and communicative capacity. The clinician also determines whether the patient has aphasia.

At the Mayo Clinic several years ago, Frederic Darley pointed out the fundamental diagnostic features of aphasia in a relatively long definition that reads as follows:

Impairment, as a result of brain damage, of the capacity for interpretation and formulation of language symbols; multimodality loss or reduction in efficiency of the ability to decode and encode conventional meaningful linguistic elements (morphemes and larger syntactic units); disproportionate to impairment of other intellective functions; not attributable to dementia, confusion, sensory loss, or motor dysfunction; and manifested in reduced availability of vocabulary, reduced efficiency in application of syntactic rules, reduced auditory attention span, and impaired efficiency in input and output channel selection. (Darley, 1982, p. 42)

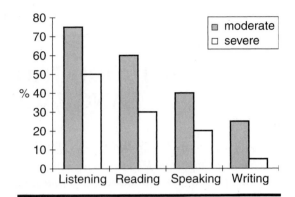

FIGURE 1.1   General pattern of aphasia at two severity levels, when comparing performance among the language modalities.

This expansive definition includes the cause of aphasia, some linguistic elaboration, and some indication of what is *not* aphasia. We need much of this information to make a diagnosis, but we do not need all of it to define aphasia. Let us think about what is tricky about defining aphasia later. For now, we shall focus on the key distinguishing elements that Darley noted, namely:

- multimodality deficit in the communicative modalities of speaking, writing, listening, and reading
- greater impairment of language than "other intellective" or mental functions

Multimodality Deficit

When someone's name is on the tips of our tongues, it is also on the tips of our fingers. Finding words is the most common problem with aphasia, and it is manifested through writing as well as speech. The same patient has problems comprehending when reading as well as when listening. Moreover, the modalities are not impaired equally, and there is a typical pattern of comparative deficit. Aphasic people nearly always comprehend better than they talk or write, and reading-writing skills are usually more impaired than auditory-speech skills (e.g., Duffy and Ulrich, 1976). When language skills in each modality are measured, the results look like the graph in Figure 1.1.

How does a clinical aphasiologist measure language skill in each modality? Martin Exeter

was evaluated for possible aphasia with a test structured like the one shown in Table 1.1. The clinician administers tasks involving language at different levels of difficulty. The patient deals with words in some tasks, sentences in others, and paragraph-length material in the most difficult tasks. A common result is that the fewest errors are made at the word level and the most errors are made at the paragraph level. The measure in Figure 1.1 is the percentage of correct responses in each modality. No matter the severity of aphasia, a patient usually displays the pattern in Figure 1.1.

Jackie did not need a test to tell her that her husband had difficulty talking, but the test was informative with respect to subtle pockets of expressive ability displayed in a controlled situation. The test was particularly informative regarding level of comprehension, which is difficult to ascertain when a patient is not talking much in conversation. The clinician also uses the test to support a diagnosis of aphasia as opposed to impairment of a specific sensory or motor channel. Let us review some of the modality-specific disorders that were not part of Martin's aphasia.

Martin's doctor did not find sensory problems in the initial evaluation. Aphasia per se does not include **sensory disorders** involving channels for transmitting information to the brain, such as hearing, sight, or touch. When someone has only

TABLE 1.1   A model of assessment for aphasia consisting of tasks at different levels of language in each modality. The level of multiple sentences is represented by discourse (spoken) and text (written).

LEVEL	COMPREHENSION		PRODUCTION	
	Listening	*Reading*	*Speaking*	*Writing*
Word	Listen to a word, then point to an object	Read a word, then point to an object	Name objects	Write names of objects
Sentence	Follow simple command	Follow simple instruction	Describe simple actions	Describe action
Discourse/Text	Listen to a story, answer questions about it	Read a paragraph, then answer questions	Describe a complex picture	Write a letter

aphasia, he or she hears speech and sees print as well as before the stroke. Nevertheless, once Martin started going to a speech-language clinic, he received a hearing test anyway. When someone with aphasia does have a severe hearing loss, the graph in Figure 1.1 is likely to look quite different. The listening score may be well below the reading score, an exception to the aphasic pattern.

Another general category of modality-specific disorders is somewhat enigmatic. **Agnosia** is the impairment of the ability to recognize a stimulus even though sensory transmission is intact. With *visual agnosia,* an object can be seen but it is unfamiliar. With *auditory agnosia,* a person hears a common sound, such as a hissing teapot, but does not turn off the stove because of failure to recognize what the sound is. *Tactile agnosia,* also called astereognosis, is the inability to recognize an object by touch even though the patient senses pain, texture, and temperature. Although agnosias are not inherent features of aphasia, they still present the following challenges for clinical diagnosis:

- whether a patient has aphasia *or* an agnosia (or sensory deficit)
- whether a patient has aphasia *and* an agnosia (or sensory deficit)

In either case, the multimodality test pattern would differ from the one shown in Figure 1.1. The affected input modality would be distinctly depressed relative to the other input modality.

An aphasic individual often speaks easily. Aphasia does not include muscle weakness or other neuromuscular abnormalities such as rigidity or uncontrollable movement. One type of motor speech disorder is the **dysarthrias,** which are impairments of the ability to execute movement with the muscles used for speaking. With dysarthria, speech may be slowed or slurred; and the patient may also have difficulty chewing and swallowing food (i.e., dysphagia). Dysarthria accounted for 46 percent of around 3,400 cases of neurogenic communicative disorders evaluated at the Mayo Clinic between 1987 and 1990 (Duffy, 1995). Aphasia accounted for 27 percent. Duffy indicated that aphasia may constitute a larger proportion of the caseload in a long-term rehabilitation setting.

Another motor disorder is called **apraxia of speech** (AOS), which is a little like the agnosias because of intact peripheral transmission. AOS is an impaired programming of movement for the purpose of speaking *without* neuromuscular deficit. Someone with this disorder is quite likely to have no difficulty chewing and swallowing.

Like the diagnostic challenges for sensory deficits, one person can have aphasia, another person can have a motor speech disorder, and someone else can have aphasia *and* a motor speech disorder. Although a referring neurologist examines a patient for these problems, it is the job of a speech-language pathologist to make a definitive diagnosis. Many aphasic patients also have apraxia of speech. When dysarthria accompanies aphasia, it is usually fairly mild; and a swallowing problem, if there is one, does not last long.

As a multimodality disorder, aphasia is not simply the sum of separate auditory, visual, speaking, and writing disorders. The damage causing aphasia is in one location in the brain, not four locations. Aphasia is often called a **central disorder,** suggesting that language functions are somewhat independent of each of the transmissive or peripheral functions of the nervous system (Table 1.2). Centralized functions have been identified historically with linguistic components, because word-meaning relationships are the same whether we are listening or reading. We do not learn one grammar for talking and another one for writing.

Language Disorder

When Jackie first met the speech-language pathologist (SLP), she remarked that "Marty doesn't talk but his mind is OK." This is what Darley (1982) meant when he wrote that aphasic language impairment is "disproportionate to impairment of other intellective functions." Both statements characterize a pattern of impaired and retained mental faculties across the range of everyday things people do such as dressing, cooking, and driving as well as reading, writing, and conversing. With aphasia, many of the so-called nonverbal skills may be downright preserved. A day or two after a stroke, people with aphasia are not forgetting who everyone is; or, when able to move about, they are not getting lost in the maze of hospital corridors. They simply have trouble with names for people, places, and things. When these skills are measured in a clinic, the pattern of results is roughly low marks for linguistic tasks and high marks for nonverbal tasks such as drawing a flower or putting a puzzle together.

Brain damage can cause other patterns of difficulty and success. Let us go back to where Darley wrote that the language problems of aphasia are "not attributable to dementia, confusion . . ." and so on. Let us consider **confusion.** Robert Wertz (1985) wrote about the "language of confusion" in which discourse can be twisted by disorientation, inability to sustain attention, failures of recollection, and extreme impatience and irritation. A patient may be said to be incoherent. Many of these problems are associated with the intellective functions of attention and memory.

In particular, we may be familiar with theatrical portrayals of *amnesia,* which is a problem with remembering people, places, and events. Distinguishing amnesia from aphasia may help in making a diagnostic distinction that can be subtle for the layperson. Brain damage has shown that retrieving a memory of a person or event is different from retrieving their names. That is, an amnesic person may be unable to recognize a friend or remember a birthday party, whereas an aphasic person recognizes the friend and remembers the party but has difficulty retrieving the words *Mar-*

TABLE 1.2 Differentiation of aphasia from modality-specific communicative impairments, similar to Wepman and Van Pelt's (1955) historic construct.

	INPUT TRANSMISSION		CENTRAL PROCESSES	OUTPUT TRANSMISSION	
Function	Sensation	Recognition	Language	Programming	Execution
Dysfunction	Hearing loss	Agnosia	Aphasia	Apraxia	Dysarthria

sha or *birthday party.* An aphasic person often expresses frustration when saying, "I know what I want to say, but I cannot think of the words."

Dementias are somewhat similar to confusion because of their involvement of varied intellectual skills, but the two terms are commonly associated with (but not necessarily tied to) different causes. Confusion is associated with traumatic brain injury. Irreversible dementias are associated with insidious onset and relentlessly progressive deterioration over months or years (although progression is not necessary for a diagnosis of dementia). Alzheimer's disease is one well-known progressive neuropathology. Patients with confusion or dementia tend to have substantially reduced performance on clinical tests beyond the tests for language. The pattern of deficit is often uneven with some retained strengths as well as multiple deficiencies.

Besides language skills, visuospatial or musical skills can be uniquely impaired by stroke. These functions contribute to artistic expression as well as orientation to everyday sights and sounds. A music lover may no longer tolerate listening to the radio due to a problem called *amusia,* a difficulty or inability recognizing melodies. The general pattern of performance is the opposite of the pattern with aphasia, namely, deficits of nonverbal functions with verbal functions relatively spared. For a long time, physicians did not refer persons with **nonverbal dysfunctions** to SLPs, because these patients exhibit impressive word-finding and grammatical abilities. Nevertheless, communicating with some of these individuals can be disconcerting. For example, they do not get the punch line of jokes, or they randomly stray from the point of a conversation. Researchers have been studying the question of whether nonverbal dysfunctions or a more elusive dysfunction leads to this occasionally bizarre language use.

In addition to comparing speech and language abilities, the initial evaluation is structured broadly around a comparison between verbal and nonverbal abilities. However, the SLP's training is still mainly for dealing with speech and language disorders. The clinical aphasiologist may rely on information from a **clinical neuropsychologist** who conducts a comprehensive evaluation of attention, perception, memory, and reasoning. Many of these specialists, who were trained as clinical psychologists, employ familiar IQ tests that balance examination of certain verbal and nonverbal skills.

Propositional Use of Language

Jackie was amazed when the SLP got Martin to count to ten. The clinician had to prod him a little, but counting came out much easier than any talking Martin had been attempting. Fluent counting illustrates one fundamental feature of aphasia that is absent from Darley's definition. Aphasic people tend to retain so-called *subpropositional* forms, which "come 'ready made' or preformulated for the speaker" (Eisenson, 1984, p. 6). These speaking acts include counting to ten, singing a song, or producing routine greetings like "How are you?" or "I'm fine." Also, usually silent patients may curse uncharacteristically when frustrated. Jackie did not know enough about aphasia to be relieved that Martin was not hurling profanities across the room.

Aphasic impairment concentrates on the *propositional* language that we use for normal conversation. Eisenson defined it as "a creative formulation of words with specific and appropriate regard to the situation" (p. 6). Propositional deficit distinguishes aphasia from dysarthria. That is, dysarthrias diminish all levels of verbal expression, whereas aphasia is manifested mainly in the propositional mode of language formulation. Fluent counting or reciting a daily prayer is proof that an aphasic person's neuromuscular mechanism for speaking is intact.

Acquired Disorder

The term *aphasia* is also applied to language-specific disorders in childhood, and this double usage can lead to some confusion. Consumers of speech-language services may wonder if the adult and child verisons are the same disorder, which may lead to the same expectations for recovery and rehabilitation. "Aphasia in adults" is said to be an acquired disorder because its onset occurs after a substantial or completed period of normal language development. **Developmental language disorders** of childhood are diagnosed at an early age, and the cause often appears to have germinated prior to birth. One major classification of developmental delay in childhood is broadly consistent with Darley's definition but is not called aphasia. This disorder is known as specific language impairment (SLI) (Leonard, 1998).

There is a crucial overlap between the broad categories of acquired and developmental disorder such that we should not identify them strictly with adulthood and childhood, respectively. Young children who were normal at birth can acquire aphasia, sometimes by stroke. Also, when developmentally delayed children start to go to school, they may be diagnosed as having a learning disability; and they may carry the learning disability with them into adolescence and adulthood (Reed, 2005). The key distinction is not the age at which aphasia is diagnosed. It is whether the developmental process is compromised.

DESCRIBING APHASIA

The grist for our clinical mill is a patient's behavior. It is what we can observe for evaluation and manipulate for rehabilitation. Different types of behavior arise because of the effects of brain damage. For his best-selling book about "the man who mistook his wife for a hat and other clinical tales," Oliver Sacks (1985) organized chapters around two kinds of abnormality, namely, *loss* of function (e.g., not talking enough) and *excess* of function (e.g., talking too much). Also, some behaviors are the effect of the damage, and other behaviors are the product of intact brain tissue. A broad classification of symptoms is indicated with the following:

- negative symptoms (indicative of impaired processing)
- positive symptoms (indicative of processes remaining intact)
- symptoms of omission (units of language that are missing)
- symptoms of commission (language that was not normally present before the brain injury)

A linguistic sensitivity enhances our precision in looking for symptoms of omission and commission in expressive language. We analyze utterances with respect to units at the sound level, word level, and sentence level.

Word Finding

As mentioned earlier, many aphasic individuals get to the point of saying things like, "I know what I want to say, I just can't think of the words." Each of us has experienced having a word on the tip of our tongue, but for someone with aphasia, saying any word at any time can be like reaching for the distant fruit on a tree. **Anomia** (also, *dysnomia*) is a broad term for the problem of finding words, and it is the most consistent feature of aphasia. A patient may be just unusually slow coming up with intended words. When unable to find a word, some patients talk around it saying, "I wear it right here, and I tell time with it. Mine goes tick, tick." This positive symptom is called **circumlocution,** which tells us that a patient has found a concept without the word for it.

Another possibility is that an aphasic person says "clock" when thinking about a watch. Word substitution errors are a symptom of commission and are called **paraphasias.** Paraphasias are produced unintentionally, and patients may be surprised when hearing these mistakes. Paraphasias differ according to the linguistic relationship between the intended word and the error. Without a circumlocution or clear context, the patient's target can be difficult to identify during conversation. Types of paraphasia are revealed best when a clinician already knows the targeted word. Therefore, we ask patients to name objects, repeat words, or read words aloud (Table 1.3).

TABLE 1.3 A basic and incomplete classification of paraphasias, including examples in Spanish (Cuetos, Aguado, Izura et al., 2002). Here, no distinction is made between word and nonword errors (see Chapter 5 on conduction aphasia).

	ENGLISH		SPANISH	
Paraphasia	*Target*	*Error*	*Target*	*Error*
Phonemic	tiger	kiger	tigre	trigo
Semantic	tiger	lion	tigre	león
Mixed semantic and phonemic	telephone	telegraph	cuchillo	cuchara
Unrelated	tiger	flag	tigre	bandera
Neologistic	tiger	floosis		

Sentence Production

Aphasic people tend to differ according to two styles of spontaneous verbal production. Right after his stroke, Martin Exeter's utterances were similar to **nonfluent aphasia,** in which patients produce fewer words than normal. Although Martin's words tended to be accurate, getting each word or phrase out was hard work. Jackie felt like she was waiting forever for the next word to come. His remarks about not being able to talk were islands of fluency amidst exhausting struggle. A listener has to be patient, which is something Jackie had to learn.

Labored nonfluent aphasias often contain a problem with grammar. The behavior is usually a symptom of omission called **agrammatism,** in which certain types of linguistic units tend to drop out of utterances. When asked to tell what happened before coming to the hospital, a patient might say one of the following:

- "Bathroom . . . shave."
- "Sleeping . . . get up . . . bathroom . . . fall down . . . um . . . wife . . . um . . . ambulance."
- "I was standing mirror . . . shave . . . the . . . uh . . . fall on floor . . . and I did, too . . . I could not talk."

Knowing the situation, these fragments make sense. They represent different degrees of grammatical deficit. The omitted units are what linguists call *grammatical morphemes,* including inflectional word endings such as *-ing* and closed-class or function words (e.g., *the, is, on*). The agrammatic patient produces mainly open-class or content words or what has been called "telegramese" (Gardner, 1974). In severe agrammatism, just one or two nouns are produced. It should be noted that the words in the examples are not necessarily simple to pronounce, which is indicative of language disorder rather than a mechanical speech disorder.

The other general style is called **fluent aphasia,** in which patients talk with an easy flow of complete sentences. The main problem is with selection of words. Patients either have trouble finding a word they want to use, or they make many word-finding errors. With mild forms of fluent aphasia, patients communicate fairly well. They have problems finding common words from time to time. When a word does not come to them, they often resort to vague wording or circumlocution. In the following example, an auto mechanic explains how to drive a car:

> *When you get into the car, close your door. Put your feet on those two things on the floor. So, all I have to do is pull . . . I have to put my . . . You just put your thing which I know of which I cannot say right now, but I can make a picture of it . . . you put it in . . . on your . . . inside the thing that turns the car on. You put your foot on the thing that makes the stuff come on. It's called the, uh . . .*

TABLE 1.4   Traditional contrasting features of agrammatism (nonfluent) and jargon (fluent).

	AGRAMMATISM	JARGON
Utterance length	Reduced	Normal or increased
Content words	On target	Paraphasic substitutions
Grammatical morphemes	Omissions or errors	Occasional substitutions
Initiation and flow	Hesitant, slow	Smooth
Prosody	Reduced	Seemingly normal

Another type of fluent production, **jargon,** makes little sense. Talking has the sound of normal statements and questions, but it is peppered with paraphasias that transform utterances into pervasive nonsense. A listener is likely to be amazed and sometimes a bit amused at what is depicted informally as word salad or jibberish. It is nearly the opposite of agrammatism (Table 1.4). Two kinds of jargon are recognized based on the type of paraphasias dominating utterances. Mostly semantic paraphasias is called *semantic jargon,* sounding like a confused version of the speaker's language. When neologisms dominate, *neologistic jargon* sounds like a strange language invented by the patient. Semantic jargon is thought to be a less severe deficit because it contains mostly real words.

In his popular book about brain dysfunction, Howard Gardner (1974) reported asking a patient to talk about what brought him to the hospital. The following reply is mainly semantic jargon with one neologism tossed in:

> "Oh sure, go ahead, any old think you want. If I could I would. Oh, I'm taking the word the wrong way to say, all of the barbers here whenever they stop you it's going around and around, if you know what I mean, that is tying and tying for repucer, repuceration, well, we were trying the best that we could while another time it was with the beds over there the same thing . . ." (p. 68)

Recurring or Stereotypic Utterance

Some people with severe aphasia are unable to say anything except some repeated involuntary and seemingly subpropositional utterances. These **stereotypic utterances** occur at the onset of aphasia and tend to persist for months. They may appear in any attempt to respond, as if they were the only language forms available. A patient may produce a recurrent syllable called iterative stereotype (e.g., "dee, dee, dee") or a jargonized or neologistic stereotype. A neologistic version was heard by Hughlings Jackson, a nineteenth-century neurologist, during a boyhood seaside holiday:

> . . . he lodged at a house where the landlady—as he discovered to his wonderment and awe—could say nothing but "watty." This unlikely disyllable was articulated with such a range of cadence that it could express a variety of emotions. Her laugh was merry and ringing, and when anything amused her she would say: "Watty, watty, watty." (Critchley, 1960, p. 8)

When stereotypy consists of dictionary words, a common example is the use of *yes* and *no* (often incorrectly) as the only verbalization. Another example is a phrase, such as "down the hatch." Ask the patient how he is doing, and he will say, "Down the hatch."

EXPLAINING APHASIA

Why does one aphasic person speak in fragmented sentences, whereas another speaks in fluent jargon? The explanation of these behaviors lies hidden inside a patient's head. Figure 1.2 represents the internal processes of propositional speaking as encoding an idea or message into sounds and the process of listening as decoding the message from sounds. These notions are certainly vague. They will not help us to understand why one patient does one thing, and another does something else. There are two types of explanation of human behavior, and they originate in an ancient philosophical conundrum called the "mind-body problem."

The Mind-Body Problem

Aphasiologists differ in their orientation to the internal processes of communication. Many focus on the concrete wiring of the brain, speaking of *neural* processes that encode and decode messages. Others are more "psychological," which is to say that they speak of *mental* processes that encode and decode messages. To be psychological is to speak of ideas or memories instead of cerebral convolutions or neurons. Aphasiology was born with a neurologi-

cal orientation over a hundred years ago, whereas a truly scientific approach to the mind has been emerging only since the early 1970s. The brain and the mind are not usually treated as alternative versions of the truth. The brain is the physical mechanism responsible for mentalistic things like memory and comprehension.

For centuries, philosophers have been contemplating the nature of the mind, arguing over whether it exists or where it lives. In medieval times, the clergy was the government. Laws were based on such beliefs as the Earth being the center of the universe, and material and spiritual worlds being unable to cohabitate. Anatomic dissection was frowned on in medical schools, and dissection of sex organs and the brain was forbidden. Drawings by Leonardo da Vinci provide evidence of a belief that the mind or soul inhabits little spaces inside the brain. During the 1600s, the Age of

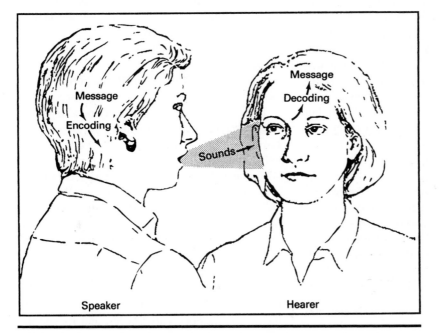

FIGURE 1.2   A simplified indication of psychological or "mental" mechanisms of communication.

Reprinted by permission from Akmajian, A., Demers, R. A., & Harnish, R. M., *Linguistics: An introduction to language and communication* (Second Edition). Cambridge, Ma: MIT Press, 1984, p. 393.

Reason, René Descartes was one of the first to speculate that memory and thought are managed in a material part of the brain. This was about as upsetting as Copernicus having the nerve to claim that the sun is the center of the universe.

Now, experimental psychologists speak of the mind as cognition. **Cognition** is "the collection of mental processes and activities used in perceiving, remembering, thinking, and understanding" (Ashcraft, 1994, p. 12). Cognitive science was born when these processes could be measured in the fractions of a second in which they occur. Just as archaeologists build models of Pompeii based on tiny fragments of its remains, cognitive scientists construct the most likely "functional architecture" of the mind from bits and pieces of behavior (e.g., Anderson, 1983).

Although most psychologists believe that cognition represents the jobs performed by the brain, they approach their work as if "the mind can be studied independently from the brain" (Johnson-Laird, 1983). Johnson-Laird added: "Once you know the way in which a computer program works, your understanding of it is in no way improved by learning about the particular machine on which it runs" (p. 9). At one time, texts on cognitive psychology contained almost nothing about the brain (e.g., Ashcraft, 1989; Solso, 1988), but the 1990s saw inclusions of at least a chapter on brain studies (e.g., Ashcraft, 1994; Solso, 1991).

The ensuing instruction is managed by attending to neurological and cognitive orientations as independent entities. This separation is not entirely artificial. A neuroscientist learns important things from studying pathologic brain tissue under a mircroscope without any knowledge of the patient's cognitive or communicative dysfunction. An SLP can evaluate a patient's language abilities without attending to what went on in the patient's brain.

Neurological Explanation

The importance of neurological explanation was advanced by Brookshire (1997) from the start of his text, where he wrote that "features and severity of neurogenic communication disorders depend on location and magnitude of the damage . . . clinicians who wish to understand these communication disorders must have a rudimentary understanding of the human nervous system and what can go wrong with it" (p. 1). The nervous system is divided into central and peripheral components. The peripheral modalities are wired for transmissive input to and transmissive output from the central nervous system. The brain is the principal integrating device in the central nervous system.

Distribution of faculties in the brain was contemplated when even the appearance of materialistic explanation of the human spirit was rejected by church-guided authorities. Early in the 1800s, Franz Gall traveled to a tolerant Paris to escape the Austrian Kaiser's wrath, because Gall was relating traits such as pugnacity and love of wine to areas of the brain. People with a quarrelsome disposition were assumed to have a large pugnacity cortex. Based on a "science" called phrenology, Gall would detect wine lovers or those with strong "alimentariness" by feeling bumps on their skulls. Physicians, however, were looking forward to serious proof that human faculties could be localized in cerebral matter.

Reported in 1861, Paul Broca performed an autopsy on a patient with a dissociated speech disorder and discovered a lesion in a frontal region of the left cerebral cortex (Broca, 1960). Broca's discovery was enthusiastically received by the medical community. In 1874, Carl Wernicke wrote of someone with a severe comprehension deficit and a lesion in the left temporal cortex (Wernicke, 1977). Medical journals filled with descriptions of specific disorders linked to sites of damaged brain. Physicians were convinced that these relationships indicated sites of normal functions.

Aphasiologists are most familiar with the topographical view of the brain or **cerebrum** depicted in the upper left of Figure 1.3. The brain has two halves or **hemispheres,** and we see the left cerebral hemisphere in the figure. Also, we see the gross geography of the cerebral **cortex,** which is formed by a 2 to 2½ square foot sheet folded into wormy convolutions so that it can fit within the skull. The cortex is actually a layered sheet that is less than two typewriter spaces thick, consisting of 30 billion delicately networked neurons (Calvin and Ojemann, 1980). The thin spaces between convolutions provide important boundaries for regions of the cortex. The central sulcus, for example, divides each half of the brain into what are known as anterior and posterior regions.

Figure 1.3 also illustrates Russian neuropsychologist A. R. Luria's (1970a) division of the central nervous system (CNS) into three functional levels. The first level has something to do with general awareness and distribution of sensory input. It includes deep cerebral nuclei (e.g., thalamus) and the reticular formation running through the brainstem. The **reticular activating system** (RAS) distributes nerve impulses to all areas of the cortex. The second level is the posterior cortex, which perceives, recognizes, and integrates sensory information. The third level is the anterior cortex, which generates volitional response.

Returning to the upper left of the figure, four main **lobes** provide a frame of reference for identifying more specific locations of the cerebral cortex. The frontal lobe coincides with the ante-

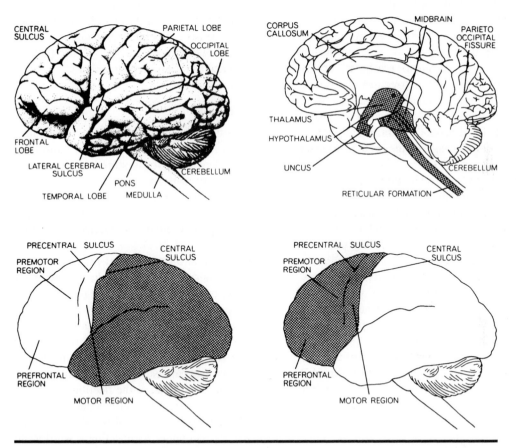

FIGURE 1.3 Gross anatomy of the brain is depicted in the upper left (lateral view) and upper right (medial view). The shaded regions represent Luria's three functional levels or "blocks": reticular formation, posterior cortex, and anterior cortex.

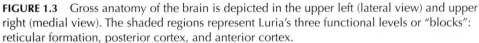

Reprinted by permission of Lorelle Raboni from Luria, A. R., The functional organization of the brain. *Scientific American, 222*(3), 66–78, 1970. Copyright © 1970 by Scientific American, Inc. All rights reserved.

rior cortex, and a part of this region serves motor functions. Posterior cortex receives auditory input in the temporal lobe, visual input in the occipital lobe, and tactile input in the parietal lobe. To summarize simply, posterior cortex receives a stimulus, and anterior cortex makes a response.

Now, let us turn to the vocabulary of pathology. Damaged tissue is called a *lesion.* Aphasia is thought to be most clearly caused by a lesion in the cerebral cortex. A few neuropathologies can destroy a small part of the brain, and such localized damage is called a **focal lesion.** Focal lesions are a typical result of disrupted blood flow or *stroke.* However, stroke is not the only cause of focal lesions. A region of the cortex can gradually shrink (called atrophy) for mysterious reasons. Small parts of the brain can be scraped during life-saving surgery. Surgeons are quite serious about avoiding the areas for speech and language. A person may also accumulate multiple lesions by suffering several little strokes through the years, called a **multifocal lesion** pattern. Finally, damage spread evenly throughout the brain is referred to as being "diffuse."

We learned a great deal about the effects of focal lesions from extensive studies of soldiers who fought in the world wars decades ago. From his studies, Luria (1970b) characterized *traumatic brain injury* (TBI) as "a cleanly punched out defect in a cerebrum." Yet, contemporary life can inflict damage that is more varied or complex depending on whether the damage was caused by modern firearms, motor vehicle accidents, or other forms of violence. To put it simply for now, TBI can be multifocal and diffuse.

The anterior and posterior regions of the cortex serve the same peripheral sensory and motor functions in each hemisphere. However, the left and right hemispheres have different intellectual functions. When one hemisphere is damaged, its functional specialty is impaired and the other hemisphere's expertise is relatively preserved. For most people, the left hemisphere is specialized for language functions, and the right hemisphere is specialized for fundamental nonverbal functions. Within the left hemisphere, lesions in an anterior

region produce nonfluent aphasia, and posteriorly located lesions produce fluent aphasias. When taking a neurological perspective, some researchers speak materially of anterior aphasia and posterior aphasia.

The objective of neurological diagnosis is to figure out what has happened to the brain. For example, an observation of fluent aphasia indicates that the posterior left hemisphere is damaged. However, it is still hard to tell in neurological terms why someone names objects slowly, why someone else produces more neologisms than semantic paraphasias, or why someone else omits certain kinds of grammatical morphemes. To understand fully why a particular lesion causes aphasias, we need a better understanding of the functional significance of fairly specific parts of the brain and how they work together.

Cognitive Explanation

A mechanism for encoding and decoding messages can also be understood as a relationship between ideas and words stored in our heads. Encoding starts with an idea that is connected to a word. Decoding starts with a word that is connected to an idea. This is the start of characterizing a "cognitive chain" of events, or "central processes" (Table 1.2).

There are two fundamental features of cognition. One is our relatively stable storage of information, or our fund of **knowledge.** It includes knowledge of the world and knowledge of the language we speak. When referring to mental "architecture," authors often use spatial metaphors to characterize knowledge. Our mental vocabulary is said to have form and structure. The other feature of cognition is **process,** or the fleeting activity of the mind. A cognitive process is not only a complex act of problem solving. It is also a simple mental response to a stimulus. Connecting a word to an idea is a type of mental process. Processes are temporal. In principal, their duration can be measured.

A fundamental question in cognitive sciences applies to both knowledge and process. How is information in our heads represented? What form does it take? The form of information in our heads differs from the form of a stimulus. This inner form is called a **mental representation.** Information is represented either in permanent storage or in a transient state. A theory of the neural representation of a new memory can appeal to concrete tissues and chemicals. Characterizing a memory in functional terms, however, is more problematic. Again, scientists use analogies or metaphors. For example, a mental image may be like a photograph. Characteristics of the brain are invoked to depict the mind, such as talking about knowledge as being stored like a "network" or talking about a representation as being "activated."

All cognitive functions are carried on the shoulders of **memory.** Ashcraft (1989) wrote that cognition is "the coordinated operation of active mental processes within a multicomponent memory system" (p. 39). All sorts of notions about memory exist. The basic nature of memory is that it is the retention of information in the mind beyond the life of an external stimulus. Thus, a stimulus is represented and retained. A memory can last just a small fraction of a second. The ability to hold information in our heads is fundamental to the mind's (or brain's) ability to perform various functions, including simple ones like perception and recognition.

Let us take a moment to become familiar with the overall organization of the memory system. Figure 1.4 is a traditional model, which is still helpful for identifying different kinds of memory deficits in cognitive disorders such as dementia. This information management system is much like a library. A library system stores books, acquires new ones, and has procedures for efficient access to the books on the shelves. In the mind, knowledge is shelved in **long-term memory** (LTM). The store of books in a library is organized so we do not have to wander around all day looking for a particular book. Cognitive scientists test theories of lexical organization by determining which theory predicts the speed of finding words. In this way, structure has an influence on process.

Also like a library, LTM contains different types of information. Knowledge may have a verbal format, like novels, and a photographic format, like picture books. The following types of knowledge were identified by Tulving (1972) and Anderson (1983):

- **episodic memory** for individually experienced events (also, *autobiographical memory*)
- **semantic memory** for common knowledge of the world
- **procedural memory** for knowledge of skills, such as swinging a golf club
- **lexical memory** for words and information about words

Aphasia provides evidence for the notion that words and world knowledge are kept in different stores. That is, an aphasic person knows what he or she wants to convey but cannot access the words. In general, the validity of memory stores is supported by many case studies showing that neuropathologies can impair access to one type of memory but not others (Schacter, 1996).

Now, let us turn to cognitive processing. Our processing system has a limited capacity for doing work. That is, the mind can do only so much at one time. The short-term memory in Figure 1.4 is now called **working memory** (WM), which is the "work space" for any cognitive activity. It constrains our capacity for keeping information active and for processing information, just as computers have a limited capacity for the number of programs that can run at the same time. Asking someone to do two things at once is one way of assessing WM capacity. In addition to being informed by the external environment, WM is informed by the **activation** of information in long-term storage.

Short-term memory (STM) is now considered to be one component of working memory. The memory span test of STM tells us the amount of a stimulus that can be represented in working memory. Although some researchers have tried, STM span cannot be used to represent working memory in general.

Are we aware of information activated in working memory? We are aware of some information, but "intellective" activity is more than our conscious thoughts. Cognitive processing occurs at both

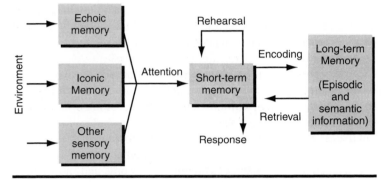

FIGURE 1.4 Three levels of memory have implications for language function. Processing for comprehension and production takes place within the capacity and time constraints of short-term memory, also called working memory. The knowledge base for communication is housed in long-term memory.

Reprinted by permission from Smith, A.D., and Fullerton, A. M., Age differences in episodic semantic memory: Implications for language and cognition. In D. S. Beasley and G. A. Davis, (Eds.), *Aging: Communication Processes and Disorders.* New York: Grune & Stratton, 1981.

subconscious and conscious levels of awareness. Subconscious processing is said to be automatic. Scientists use so-called *fast tasks* and millisecond timers to measure automatic activity, such as comprehending a common word. **Automatic processing** has the following characteristics:

- it is subconscious or beneath our awareness
- it is obligatory (i.e., mandatory)
- it takes up little or no room in working memory

In the presence of a stimulus, the brain does not just sit there waiting for our conscious commands. It responds or activates on its own. Fundamental decoding and encoding for communication is automatic and obligatory. When we hear an utterance, comprehension happens whether we want it to or not.

Clinical aphasiologists are most experienced with assessment and treatment of **controlled processing,** which has the following features:

- it can be conscious or in our awareness
- it can be intentional and, therefore, optional
- it is effortful and takes up room in working memory

Also known as strategic or attentional processing, controlled processing is studied with *slow tasks* that allow enough time for decision making or planning to occur. Unlike automatic processes, strategic processes clog the system. When a patient scans picture choices in a typical comprehension task, there is time for all sorts of controlled processing to occur, and a pointing response is the result of both automatic and controlled processing. Language processes become particularly effortful in metalinguistic tasks, such as sorting words into categories or editing a manuscript (see Table 12.7 for similar terminology).

In sum, language functions operate within a cognitive framework. Language processing is constrained by the capacity of working memory and draws from knowledge stored in long-term memory. Language processing operates at automatic and controlled levels.

Moreover, the constructs of cognition coincide with common explanations of aphasia. For example, Martin Exeter would explain that he knows what he wants to say but cannot find the words. Focusing on language, Schuell's (1969) clinical experience led her to believe that the "language storage system" is at least relatively intact. Most aphasiologists consider aphasia to be an impairment of processing rather than an erasure of linguistic knowledge. In this way, cognitive constructs help us to put into words what we think aphasia is. They provide a framework for functionally locating a disorder in the human information processing system.

Implications for Basic Terminology

It is hoped that this temporary separation of neurological and cognitive domains helps to put some basic concepts in their proper place. Problems with terminology are reflected in a mixing of neurological and functional terms. For example, this book refers to aphasia for some chapter titles and to traumatic brain injury and the right hemisphere for other titles. Thus, some titles refer to the brain, whereas most others refer to dysfunction. Table 1.5 shows a logical alignment of terms. For example, *stroke* refers to something that happens to the brain. *Aphasia* is a dysfunction caused by stroke and, therefore, is logically parallel to other dysfunctions like amnesia.

We should recognize that clinical diagnosis is a process of using behavioral clues to diagnose a disorder that exists in someone's brain or mind. Neurologists use clinical evaluation to make an initial guess about what literally happened to the

TABLE 1.5 Basic terminology and classification of function, neuropathology, and dysfunction.

FUNCTION	NEUROPATHOLOGY (CAUSE)	DYSFUNCTION (EFFECT)
Language	Stroke	Aphasia
Music	Stroke	Amusia
Memory	Traumatic brain injury	Amnesia

brain. A stroke can cause sudden changes in language comprehension and word finding, both of which happen in the brain. Clinical evaluation of behavior is employed to support a diagnosis of aphasia or something else, and it has been suggested here that aphasic disorder is specified in terms of the jobs performed by the brain (i.e., cognition).

Defining Aphasia

It is possible that what we thought 30 years ago may need some minor adjustments. After all, the cognitive science of language functioning did not get underway until around 1970, and clinical practice has yet to incorporate the fast tasks that measure automatic obligatory processes. To modernize a bit, a reconsideration of Darley's definition of aphasia may be worthwhile.

So, let us consider another definition: *Aphasia is a selective impairment of the cognitive system specialized for comprehending and formulating language, leaving other cognitive capacities relatively intact.* Besides its brevity, this definition differs from Darley's by omitting any reference to etiology, because a logical sorting of concepts suggests that the cause of a dysfunction does not comprise the dysfunction, and by stating in cognitive terms the idea that aphasia is impairment of the language processing system. By speaking of aphasia as a cognitive impairment, it does not necessarily become something that is different from what Darley thought. The new wording is problematic only if we continue to believe that language is one thing and cognition is something else.

Of course, neither Martin nor Jackie Exeter were interested in our problems with terminology. They did want a correct diagnosis of Martin's communicative difficulties, however. A diagnosis of aphasia leads to recommending a particular plan of rehabilitation that is conducted at great cost of time and energy as well as money. In this sense, our understanding of what aphasia is becomes important for clinical practice.

TREATING APHASIA

Aphasia rehabilitation is conducted initially within a medical environment and eventually just about anywhere with the help of family members. A speech-language pathologist (SLP) follows broad guidelines for health care and specific guidelines for aphasia developed by professional organizations. This section gives an overview of the health care environment and provides a framework for discussions of clinical practice throughout this text.

Health Care Delivery

Between World War II and the mid-1970s, physicians and speech-language pathologists in the United States provided services without much interference. During this period, most of our major clinical tests and many treatment strategies were developed in government-supported Veterans Administration medical centers. In the 1980s, health care costs skyrocketed along with double-digit inflation. **Managed care** became the collective term for new approaches to the delivery of health care, approaches that would improve quality as well as contain costs.

The delivery of health care is determined partly by payment method. In theory, payment can be provided by the first party (patient) or by the second party (service provider). Yet, because the expense is usually too great for either party, health care is supported by **third-party payers,** who cover the cost on behalf of patients. A third-party payer can be public (i.e., the government) or private (i.e., insurance). In many countries, the third party is exclusively the government, which leads to some variation in rehabilitation programs around the world.

The first party receives services in different settings, depending partly on the stage of recovery. **Acute care** commences upon admission to a hospital; these hospital stays are as brief as medically reasonable (Table 1.6). **Subacute care** (or postacute care) is a category that was established by the managed care industry to focus as soon as possible on rehabilitation. It is thought to be a bridge between acute hospitalization and independence at home. **Chronic care** is provided for long-term residual impairments such as aphasia. An *inpatient* resides in the facility providing service, whereas an *outpatient* comes to the facility during the day and returns home. Currently, stroke survivors leave the hospital as soon as possible and receive therapies at a rehabilitation center or at home.

Health care delivery is different in countries where professional direct treatment is possible for months. One example is Belgium, where every citizen is covered by a federal social security program (European Observatory on Health Care Systems, 2000). Patients at the Brussels Neuropsychological Rehabilitation Unit sign a contract for a maximum 6-month period (Seron and de Partz, 1993). This contract specifies treatment objectives and a schedule for therapy. Initial evaluation and diagnosis may take one to two months,

TABLE 1.6   General categories of health care and typical settings in the United States.

CATEGORY	DEFINITION	SETTING
Acute	Immediate and short-term (e.g., stroke unit)	Acute care hospital
Subacute	Transition between acute hospitalization and independence at home	Rehabilitation hospital (inpatient or outpatient)
Chronic	Long-term for persistent diseases or conditions; living with permanent residual impairment	Rehabilitation center (outpatient) Home health care University clinic Nursing home

and this assessment often overlaps with early therapy. Therapy can be renewed for up to four contract periods (or two years).

This is not to say that innovative and comprehensive treatment programs are easily funded outside the United States. The Pat Arato Aphasia Centre in Canada provides group therapies and activities with a great deal of help from volunteers (see Chapter 10). After an initial seven years of relying on donations and bake sales, the Centre began to receive partial support from the Ontario Ministry of Health. Fund-raising is still necessary to keep such programs going (Kagan and Cohen-Schneider, 1999).

Health Care Services

Since 1980, the World Health Organization (WHO) has been developing a framework for evaluation and treatment of all medical conditions. This framework has contributed to conceptualization of rehabilitation for aphasia and other communicative disorders, and it has been explained and dissected so often that Claire Penn (2005) of the University of Witwatersrand in South Africa declared, "Who's tired of the WHO? I am for one" (p. 875).

There have been two major revisions. WHO began with the classification of medical conditions into levels of "impairment, disability, and handicap." After some complaints, a revision expanded definitions with more neutral terminology of "impairment, activity limitation, and participation limitation" (World Health Organization, 1997). A third and more complex classification emerged a few years later, now called the *International Classification of Functioning, Disability and Health* with the short moniker **WHO ICF** (World Health Organization, 2001; see Ross and Wertz, 2005). However, the simpler three-level classification still has some merit for organizing our thoughts about rehabilitation, and it is referred to from time to time throughout this text (see Table 1.7).

Historically, aphasia rehabilitation has emphasized evaluation and treatment of language impairment. Attention to the levels of activity limitation and participation limitation increases the likelihood of caring for the "whole patient." The overall objectives of poststroke rehabilitation are as follows:

- to improve linguistic and communicative abilities
- to maximize functional independence
- to restore a quality of life

Improving linguistic and communicative abilities contributes to functional independence and quality of life. Accomplishing these broad objectives efficiently is the challenge that managed care presents to patients and speech-language pathologists (SLPs).

TABLE 1.7 The first two frameworks from the World Health Organization known as the International Classification of Impairment, Disabilities, and Handicaps (ICIDH-1 and ICIDH-2).

1980 ICIDH-1	ORIGINAL DEFINITIONS	1997 ICIDH-2	FURTHER DEFINITIONS	APHASIA
Impairment	Disordered system			Language disorder
Disability	Functional consequences of impairment	Activity limitation	Reduction of personal activities	Communicative difficulties
Handicap	Social consequences of disability	Participation limitation	Reduced involvement in life situations	Loss of employment; social isolation

SUMMARY AND CONCLUSIONS

This chapter had two principal goals. One was to help the reader acquire a general idea of what aphasia is. Aphasia is an acquired disruption of the cognitive system responsible for language comprehension and production. It is usually caused by a stroke, which leaves other cognitive functions relatively intact. It is a problem with words, not ideas. An aphasic person knows what he or she wants to say but just cannot come up with the words.

The other goal of this chapter was to help the reader acquire a foundation of thought that underlies clinical decision making as well as the study of aphasia. The main point is that poststroke behavior is symptomatic of an internal dysfunction, one that we cannot observe directly. For clinical purposes, dysfunction is characterized in cognitive terms. Speech-language pathologists think about general processes involved in attaching meaning to sounds and putting thoughts into words. Clarity about what we can observe and what we cannot observe contributes to the validity of claims about cause and effect (e.g., Did our language therapy literally remodel someone's brain?).

Many patients with aphasia have other problems, such as a motor speech disorder or a problem with attention. With some aphasias, finding nouns is harder than producing sentences. With others, producing sentences is harder than retrieving nouns. Such observations lead to decisions about targeting treatment of impairment and, thus, making the best use of time.

Meanwhile, we know that Martin Exeter suffered a stroke while practicing an important lecture. He had been invited to speak about psycholinguistics at a conference on aphasia in Brussels. He was going to take Jackie with him, and it would have been their first trip to Europe. After the conference they were going to see London, Paris, and Rome. Martin wanted to sip espresso at a Left Bank cafe like Hemingway, and Jackie wanted to reminisce about her high school Latin teacher while walking through the Roman Forum. While in the hospital, paralysis and aphasia seemed to have destroyed these dreams; but Martin and Jackie later learned that a lot is possible with rehabilitation. We shall see.

CHAPTER 2

CAUSES OF THE APHASIAS

The ambulance arrived at Martin Exeter's home a few minutes after he collapsed. In another 20 minutes, he was in the emergency room of the hospital. He was conscious but could not move his right side. The doctor had been informed of what had happened, and, on preliminary evaluation, he suspected that a stroke was a strong possibility. His main objectives were to preserve life and stabilize the patient's vital functions. Martin was hooked up for electrocardiogram monitoring and blood pressure readings. The doctor asked him questions. Do you know your name? Do you know where you are? Martin nodded inconsistently and could not speak.

Meanwhile, Jackie Exeter had been separated from her husband. She paced around the waiting area as the ER team decided whether to admit Martin to the hospital. After about 15 minutes and while she was starting to fill out admission forms, the doctor appeared and told her his preliminary diagnosis. Martin would be taken to the Stroke Unit for specialized intensive care. He asked about Martin's primary care physician at the university health center, who in managed care is called the "gatekeeper physician." Jackie recalled that their insurance plan allowed 48 hours to contact the gatekeeper in case of emergencies, and the ER physician said that he would take care of it the next day.

STROKE

A stroke, or cerebrovascular accident (CVA), disrupts blood flow to the brain. It is the third most common cause of death over age 45 in the United States. The National Stroke Association reported that the number of strokes had increased to about 730,000 in the mid-1990s (www.stroke.org). The National Stroke Association also reported a Gallup survey stating that 40 percent of the American public does not know that a stroke occurs in the brain.

To understand what happens in the brain, we should have some knowledge of the cerebral circulatory system. Like other tissue in the body, neurons thrive on the process of **metabolism,** or the exchange of nutrients and waste products between the circulatory system and neurons. Arteries transport nutrients in the bloodstream, including oxygen and glucose, from the heart to the brain. The brain's large appetite is indicated by its use of 15 to 20 percent of the body's blood while taking up only 2 percent of body weight. The nutrients pass through the capillary membrane at the end of arteries, cross a space, and then pass through the neural membrane. The nerve cell transforms the nutrients into waste products that are carried away through veins. The effectiveness of medications depends on the permeability of the capillary membrane, which is impermeable to many substances (i.e., *blood-brain barrier*).

Two mechanisms can disrupt metabolism. One is an **ischemic stroke** (or ischemia), which is a blockage or occlusion of an arterial vessel. The occlusion keeps blood from getting to an area of the brain. The other general type of stroke is a **hemorrhage,** which is a bursting artery causing blood to accumulate around nearby brain tissue. Ischemic stroke is much more common than hemorrhage. Different patterns of deficit are related to site of occlusion or hemorrhage in the circulatory system. Marler (2005), in his *Stroke for Dummies,* refers to ischemia as "white stroke" and hemorrhage as "red stroke."

The blood supply to the brain has three structural levels: arteries in the neck that transport blood from the heart to the base of the brain, interconnecting arteries in the base of the brain, and cerebral arteries on the surface of the cortex. In the neck, the left and right common carotid arteries course upward and divide near the larynx. The left and right **internal carotid arteries** proceed to the interconnecting arteries at the base of the brain. Behind the carotid arteries, the left and right *vertebral arteries* are held in place along the vertebral column. The vertebral arteries join to become the *basilar artery* at the level of the medulla in the brainstem. Branches of the basilar artery supply the brainstem and cerebellum.

Three cerebral arteries supply the cortical surface for each hemisphere, and their locations are sketched in Figure 2.1 in relation to key speech and language areas of the left hemisphere. The main vessel of the **middle cerebral artery (MCA)** runs along the Sylvian fissure and branches to most of the lateral cortical convexity. Figure 2.1a shows the left hemisphere's middle cerebral artery (or **LMCA**) supplying key language areas including Broca's area, Wernicke's area, and the ideational speech area. It is continuous with the internal carotid artery and, thus, can suffer effects of occlusion in the carotid. The *anterior cerebral artery* (ACA) is distributed mostly throughout medial frontal and parietal regions (Figure 2.1b). The *posterior cerebral artery* (PCA) covers the medial surface of the occipital lobe and the base of the temporal lobe. In Figure 2.1a, it can be seen reaching around the posterior portion of the occipital region.

The cerebral arteries originate in the *communicating arteries* at the base of the brain, which collectively form the *Circle of Willis*. This polygon of small arteries is one **collateral system** in which some compensation may occur for occlusion in a carotid artery below. For example, the anterior communicating artery allows for collateral flow between the left and right anterior cerebral arteries. If flow in the left ACA is reduced by left carotid occlusion, the right carotid can be an alternative source through the communicating artery. This possibility is often prohibited in persons with communicating arteries narrowed by vascular disease.

Also in the lateral view (Figure 2.1a), we see areas in which the cerebral arteries approach each other, almost touching. These are called **watershed areas** or zones. For example, end-branches of the MCA and ACA meet anteriorly in the frontal lobe. An occlusion in one artery may not cause damage to neural tissue in a watershed area if collateral circulation from the other artery is effective.

ISCHEMIC STROKE

As indicated earlier, an ischemic stroke is an occlusion of an artery that keeps the bloodstream from reaching areas of the brain. The most common cause of occlusion is *atherosclerosis,* which is a proliferation of cells (i.e., blood platelets) along arterial walls and an accumulation of fatty substances (i.e., lipid) within associated connective tissue. Another factor that could lead to ischemic stroke is high cholesterol or too much fat in the blood. Atherosclerosis is an untreatable risk factor, whereas high cholesterol is a treatable risk factor.

Types of Ischemic Stroke

Two types of ischemic stroke produce similar clinical characteristics but result from different processes. Most strokes are a **thrombosis,** which occurs from accumulation of atherosclerotic platelets and fatty plaque on the vessel wall at the site of occlusion. Thrombus formation may take minutes or weeks to clog an artery. Dysfunction arises suddenly and increases in severity over minutes, hours, or even days during the final stages of accumulation. This *stroke-in-evolution* (or "progressing stroke") may proceed in a stepwise fashion, and maximum deficit is referred to as *completed stroke.* There is higher incidence of thrombosis among people with diabetes mellitus and hypertension (or high blood pressure) than in the general population.

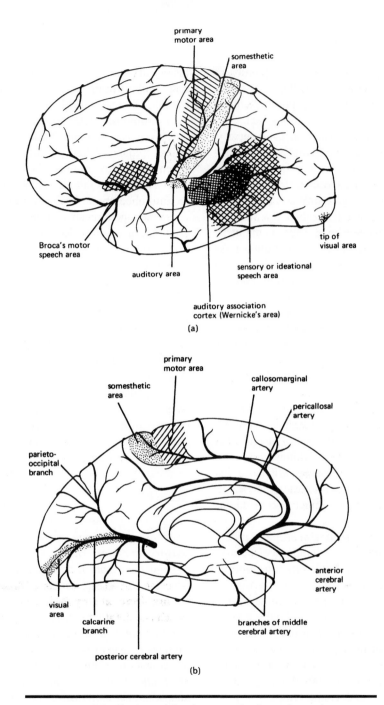

FIGURE 2.1 Distribution of the three cerebral arteries to the (a) lateral and (b) medial surfaces of the brain are shown relative to functional areas for speech and language (also see Figure 3.1). The lateral view primarily depicts the middle cerebral artery.

Reprinted by permission from Barr, M. L., *The human nervous system.* Hagerstown, Md.: Harper & Row, 1974.

A frequent signal of impending thrombosis is the *transient ischemic attack* (TIA), or "little stroke." TIAs are temporary disruptions of blood flow. They produce transient neurological signs indicating that platelet formation is underway, generally in the internal carotid artery. The neurological signs include blurring of vision, numbness or weakness on one side, speech difficulty, imbalance or unsteadiness of gait, or a combination of these. The event frequently lasts a few minutes and usually less than an hour. There is about 20 percent chance of suffering a stroke during the first year after TIAs begin and a 30 to 60 percent chance in five years (Mlcoch and Metter, 2001).

A TIA's warning may be heeded with medication or surgery in order to prevent a stroke. Medication is aimed at preventing thrombus formation. *Anticoagulants,* such as heparin, improve blood flow and prevent clotting. *Antiplatelets* inhibit platelet adhesion (e.g., aspirin, clopidigrel, or Plavix). Ticlopidine reduces risk of stroke in patients who are intolerant to aspirin (Wilson, Shannon, and Stang, 2006). High blood pressure (hypertension) is treated with *diuretics* that increase salt excreted by the kidneys and *beta blockers* that reduce pulse rate. *Vasodilators* relax the smooth muscles of arterial walls. The vasodilator minoxidil, such as Rogaine, also promotes hair growth.

Carotid endarterectomy is a surgical procedure that entails inserting a temporary shunt to keep blood flowing while the surgeon removes the thrombotic material. This procedure is usually performed in the neck where the common carotid divides into the left and right internal carotids. The field of **interventional radiology** has been exploring the application of angioplasty to clearing arteries in the neck. The physician threads a balloon-tipped catheter into the blocked artery and inflates the tube to open the vessel.

Whereas the sites of origin and occlusion are the same in thrombosis, these sites differ with an **embolism.** Platelets and fatty plaque break off a vessel wall and then travel until they become stuck in a smaller cerebral artery. The heart is the most common source of embolic material, and medical history of a patient is likely to include cardiac disease. Embolism may also be a secondary effect of trauma. Clinical onset is quicker or more abrupt than thrombosis. Time to maximum deficit takes only seconds or minutes. Thus, stroke-in-evolution is less frequent. There are usually no warnings. Often physicians are unable to determine whether an ischemia is thrombotic or embolic and may refer to "thromboembolic CVA" in a medical report.

When metabolism is prohibited for about two minutes, the result is death (or necrosis) of neural tissue. The necrotic tissue is called an **infarction.** A physician may report that a patient has suffered a "thromboembolic infarct." Over time the damaged tissue softens and liquifies. This waste is removed by a process called *gliosis* because of the assistance of star-shaped astroglial cells (astrocytes) that hold neurons in place. Gliosis leaves a cavity on the surface of cortex that looks like a crater on the moon.

Technically, ischemia refers to the occlusion in an artery, whereas infarction is the resultant necrosis of brain tissue. However, in medical reports, we may see the terms used interchangeably when identifying type of stroke.

Acute Phase

The doctor informed Jackie Exeter that Martin has weakness on only one side of his body and intact sensory functions. The doctor added, "It is hard to know the extent of damage until some pictures can be taken of Martin's brain, and he gets past his confusion. This bewilderment is common and temporary in most cases." Stroke is unlike more familiar medical conditions with specific treatments and recuperation periods. It took a few days to know more about what happened in Martin's head, and it took a few days more to have some idea about the more lasting outcome.

Caution about prognosis is prompted by **diaschisis,** which is a temporary suspension of functions that depend on structures remote from an infarct. Upon infarction or other injury to the brain, a swelling of surrounding tissue develops due to accumulation of water called **edema.** It takes two or three days to peak and one or two more weeks to subside. Sometimes edema extends throughout the brain. In addition, a reduction of blood flow extends to both hemispheres following a single occlusion. Flow to the uninfarcted side improves dramatically within two or three weeks after onset. Edema and reduced blood flow are likely to cause temporary generalized deficits for most patients.

In a hospital's Stroke Unit, a physician's main concern is the patient's survival. The patient is confined to bed with feet slightly elevated to avoid rapid lowering of blood pressure during stroke-in-evolution. Patients with low levels of consciousness are nourished with intravenous fluids. Within two or three days after a completed stroke, physical exercises may be started a few times per day to prevent muscle contractures. Self-care activities are started for psychological and physical well-being.

A target of acute medical treatment is a zone surrounding an infarction known as the ischemic **penumbra,** a term defined in the dictionary as the grayish margin of a sunspot. Blood flow to this margin is reduced, but the tissue is still intact. The zone of penumbra may either recover or progress to more infarction. **Thrombolysis** is a general term for treatments that break up blood clots to minimize the extent of damage. A "clot buster" known as *tissue plasminogen activator* (tPA, TPA) activates a natural substance in the body that dissolves blood clots. Approved in 1996 by the U.S. Food and Drug Administration, tPA must be administered promptly within three hours after an ischemic stroke (Mlcoch and Metter, 2001). Candidacy for tPA treatment, however, is very stringent; and the patient must be monitored very closely.

Another medication, called nimodipine, may minimize damage when administered within the first six hours after an episode. It is a *calcium channel blocker,* which inhibits muscle contraction in blood vessels and is selective for cerebral arteries compared with other arteries in the body. It is used particularly following subarachnoid hemorrhage (Wilson et al., 2006).

Traditional approaches to poststroke treatment include surgery and medication mainly to prevent further ischemia (Table 2.1). Carotid endarterectomy considerably reduces the chance of a second stroke. Medication includes antiplatelets such as aspirin or abciximab. Antiplatelets can be "clot dissolving." A few hospitals now have a

TABLE 2.1   Medications given for stroke prevention and acute treatment of stroke (Mlcoch and Metter, 2001; Wilson, Shannon, and Stang, 2006).

TYPE	DRUG	TRADE NAME	PREVENTION	ACUTE THERAPY
Anticoagulant	heparin	Hepalean	x	x
	warfarin	Coumadin	x	x
Antiplatelet	aspirin		x	
	ticlopidine	Ticlid	x	
	clopidigrel	Plavix	x	
	abciximab	ReoPro	x	x
Vasodilator	hydralazine	Alazine	x	
	minoxidil	Loniten	x	
Neuroprotective	nimodipine	Nimotop		x

neurointensive care unit (NICU), and studies have shown that this mix of traditional and experimental care shortens the length of acute hospitalization for ischemic stroke and hemorrhages. This neurointensive care may be extended for patients who are unconscious for a period of time. However, NICUs are also controversial, and many physicians fear that they foster unrealistic expectations for recovery.

Using sophisticated measures of blood flow introduced later in this chapter, Hillis and Heidler (2002) found that recovery of auditory word comprehension in the first three days after stroke is associated with restoration of the flow of blood to Wernicke's area (Figure 2.1). This restoration occurred spontaneously in some patients and with medical treatment in others.

Chronic Phase

Five days after admission to the Stroke Unit, Martin was transferred to the Rehabilitation Unit of the same facility for subacute care. Patients in smaller acute care hospitals may be discharged to a freestanding rehabilitation center or even to home. For Martin, diaschisis had not completely subsided. It generally takes two or three weeks before edema has largely cleared and the pattern of dysfunction attributable to the infarct emerges.

Because neural tissue in the cortex does not regenerate, infarction presents a permanent neurological condition. Speech-language pathologists often delay full examination two or three weeks after onset, until medical stability is established and the specific disorder is manifested. In Martin's situation, he was examined briefly at bedside while in the Stroke Unit, and the clinician explained his aphasia to Jackie. Once in the Rehab Unit, he was immediately evaluated by the rehabilitation team for overall functional status as an initial baseline before therapy began.

For a long time, chronic dysfunction was thought to be caused solely by the size and location of infarction. However, studies of cerebral metabolism support a more complex picture of pathophysiology because of **remote effects** some

distance from infarction. For years beyond the period of diaschisis, a patient may still have a reduction of blood flow. Such reduction of blood flow is called *hypoperfusion,* a term mainly associated with inadequate cardiac function. The restoration of blood flow described previously is called *reperfusion.*

The diminished blood flow reduces metabolism (called *hypometabolism*). The research shows that, with an infarct in left language areas, hypometabolism occurs in adjacent and distant cortex of the same hemisphere and in some subcortical regions. Over half of aphasic patients showed hypometabolism in the left prefrontal region, anterior to Broca's area, but one-fifth had structural damage in that region. In general, a chronic symptom pattern may be attributed to tissue damage and these remote effects. Frontal remote effects may also be indicative of the brain's attempt to adjust to infarction in language areas (Mlcoch and Metter, 2001).

HEMORRHAGE

> *Dr. K. begins to talk, I hear almost nothing after the words "brain hemorrhage" . . . My mouth hangs open, and my respiration comes in percussive bursts, like a cap gun. Each breath pokes the fingertip of this new danger into my ribs, and hurts. My eyes work the shadows, I can't meet Dr. K.'s gaze . . . I imagine a navy-blue baseball jacket with a gold team patch, the one I wore as a clumsy teen to make me feel pride. This isn't like me to be so sick . . . (Fishman, 1988, pp. 65–66)*

While in a hotel lobby in Nicaragua, journalist Steve Fishman's vision suddenly became fuzzy and undulating, and then an arcing pain pounded in his head with each heartbeat. He wrote a book about his experiences, including neurological evaluations and neurosurgery. A hemorrhage is a bursting artery causing blood to flood the brain's surface or invade brain tissue. The accumulation, called a **hematoma,** is a rapidly expanding mass that displaces and compresses adjacent structures. Common initial symptoms of this sudden "space-occupying lesion" include excruciating headache, nausea, and vomiting. A hemorrhage can be caused by naturally weakened vessel walls or by tearing of arteries during traumatic brain injury.

Hemorrhages are classified with respect to location. Mostly occurring in patients with high blood pressure, an **intracerebral hemorrhage** invades deep regions of the thalamus, internal capsule, and lenticular nuclei or basal ganglia (Figure 2.2). About half of these cases lose consciousness in minutes to hours after rupture, which may be precipitated by a sudden increase of blood pressure during physical activity or emotional stress. Branches of the Circle of Willis and basilar artery are most susceptible. Medication reduces edema and blood pressure, and surgical evacuation of the hematoma is possible from some areas.

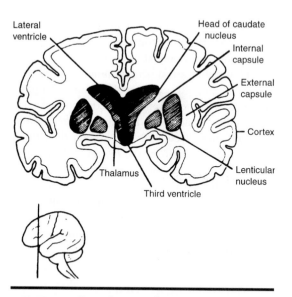

FIGURE 2.2 Frontal (coronal) section of the cerebrum shows location of the layer of cortex and certain interior structures.

From Willard R. Zemlin, *SPEECH AND HEARING SCIENCE: Anatomy and Physiology*, © 1968, pp. 466, 469. Reprinted by permission of Prentice-Hall, Inc., Englewood Cliffs, N. J.

Subarachnoid hemorrhage occurs in the pia-arachnoid space surrounding the brain and can be caused by a ruptured aneurysm near the Circle of Willis. An *aneurysm* is a dilated blood vessel from the size of a pea to an orange, stretching and weakening the vessel wall (Chusid, 1979). Rupture of an aneurysm may be provoked by sudden physical exertion but can be prevented by surgery when the dilation is accessible. Procedures include trapping the reservoir by applying clips on both sides, clipping the neck of the bulge, or packing muscle around the aneurysm. Plastics may be sprayed on the dilation and surrounding vessels.

Arterial walls are also weakened in the condition of *arteriovenous malformation* (AVM), in which the capillary network between arteries and veins is absent. Vessels are twisted and tangled. It may occupy a tiny area or an entire hemisphere. Presumably a congenital condition, presence of AVM may not be signaled until hemorrhage or seizures occur in adulthood. Bleeding occurs in the subarachnoid space. A hemorrhaging AVM is usually less damaging than a bursting aneurysm.

TUMOR

A tumor (or neoplasm) is an abnormal mass of tissue caused by an increased rate in the reproduction of cells. A neoplasm is a space-occupying lesion that presses against adjacent tissue and obstructs circulation. *Benign* tumors do not spread to other parts of the body and are not recurrent. However, in the brain they can grow large enough to be dangerous. *Malignant* or cancerous tumors expand uncontrollably and are resistent to treatment. They may spread to other parts of the body via the bloodstream (called *metastasis*).

Medical Diagnosis

Early symptoms of malignant neoplasms usually are quite general reductions of function. Like hemorrhage, space-occupying pressure causes headache, nausea, and vomiting. Sensory impairments and dulled mental function may occur; and, if the tumor is allowed to enlarge, impairment may evolve to stupor and coma. Specific dysfunctions depend on location and may include loss of vision or hearing when there is pressure on the optic or acoustic cranial nerves.

To determine whether a tumor is benign or malignant, a pathologist performs a *biopsy* in which tissue or cells are removed from the body with a needle for examination under a microscope. Cells of a benign tumor are very much like their tissue origin. Cells of a malignant tumor are less recognizable. For areas that are difficult to reach, a guided biopsy can be performed with the aid of neuroimaging techniques such as CT or ultrasound scanning that help the physician follow progress of the needle (discussed later in this chapter). Another advance is the use of very fine needles, called stereotactic biopsy.

A study was done to determine if CT-guided stereotactic biopsy in the left hemisphere causes deterioration of language functions. Language was assessed with standard aphasia tests before and after a biopsy sample was obtained. Results showed that the particular biopsy procedure carries a 9 percent risk of impairing language functions if the patient is not aphasic preoperatively. If the patient is aphasic preoperatively, there is a high risk of aggravating the aphasia (Thomson, Taylor, Fraser, and Whittle, 1997a).

Life-saving surgery for brain tumors may result in aphasia. For example, patient JO was 48 years old when a neoplasm was removed from her left temporal-parietal area. Right paralysis and severe language impairments appeared following the surgery and radiation treatment (Buchanan, McEwan, Westbury, and Libben, 2003).

Classification

Neoplasms are named according to their tissue origin. A common source is supportive cells throughout the central nervous system called glial cells. For example, an **astrocytoma** originates in the housekeeping astroglia mentioned earlier with respect to infarction. Several grades of malignancy can be determined based on rate of cell growth, differentiation of cell types, and number of abnormal cells.

Astrocytoma grades 3–4 (also, *glioblastoma multiforme* or malignant glioma) is the most common primary brain tumor in adults. It is a rapidly growing mass likely to infiltrate both hemispheres through the commissures. George Gershwin, composer of "Porgy and Bess," suffered the earliest signs of a temporal lobe glioblastoma multiforme while conducting the Los Angeles Philharmonic Orchestra at age 38. Preferred treatment is surgery, which consists of craniotomy (i.e., opening the skull) followed by resection of tissue. Surgeons may report "gross total removal" of the tumor, but it usually recurs in months (Weiss, 1982). Survival averages about one year. Gershwin died two days after his surgery (Rolak, 1993).

Astrocytoma grades 1–2 (low-grade astrocytoma) is much less common but has a more favorable prognosis. It expands slowly, and symptoms may appear years before the tumor is discovered. Complete removal is seldom accomplished, but repeated surgery can be beneficial when the neoplasm is accessible. Prognosis after surgery has been reported variably at three to six years.

Meningioma is a benign tumor arising from the arachnoid tissue covering the brain. After glioblastoma, it is the second most common primary brain tumor in adulthood. Unlike other tumors, it occurs more frequently in women than men. Fifty percent occur over the lateral surfaces, and 40 percent occur at the base of the brain. They grow slowly and usually do not invade the cortex. Complete removal is often possible, with prolonged survival being a frequent outcome of surgery. Recurrence is possible in a small proportion of cases.

FOCAL CORTICAL ATROPHY

Some debate has swirled around whether other neuropathologies, especially progressive ones, cause aphasia. The traditional position in speech-language pathology is reflected in Rosenbek and others' (1989) declaration that "aphasia in adults does not creep, it erupts" (p. 53). This is based on the pronounced language-specificity of aphasia subsequent to erupting strokes and a traditional association of progressive diseases with diffuse damage and generalized intellectual impairment (e.g., Wertz, 1985). However, with some intense study of progressive diseases, a significant revelation is that damage can be more localized than we once thought. A fairly specific impairment may emerge from progressive disease. This type of discovery is one reason for not including a specific causation in the definition of aphasia.

Primary progressive aphasia (PPA) or "aphasia without dementia" is an isolated language deterioration with relative preservation of other cognitive abilities. Mesulam's (1982) report of six cases led to widespread recognition of the syndrome. Westbury and Bub (1997) reviewed 119 cases appearing in the literature since Mesulam's report. The reviewers found the case studies to be unsystematic, relying on a wide variety of neuropsychological instruments. "These limitations have made it difficult to place the published reports into a coherent theoretical structure" (p. 381).

PPA usually starts as a difficulty with a particular language function, and then it spreads to other language functions. The most common early deficit is misnaming. By the third year after initial appearance of symptoms, cases are quite heterogeneous. About 45 percent have a severe naming deficit, 30 percent still have a mild deficit, and most of the rest have no naming deficit. Many have no comprehension deficit in the first two years. Reading deficits are rarely seen before the fourth or fifth year. Thus, the classic multimodality deficit does not necessarily factor into diagnosis of aphasia in early stages.

Some investigators suggest that isolated language deficit may last at least two years, before dementia begins to develop. Kertesz and Munoz (1997) noted that the aphasia may be nonfluent leading to mutism (i.e., frontal lobe degeneration) or it may be fluent (i.e., temporal lobe degeneration). Some researchers in Great Britain considered PPA to be nonfluent (e.g., Croot, Patterson, and Hodges, 1998). They used the term "semantic dementia" for a fluent aphasia caused by predominantly left anterior temporal degeneration.

These specific deficits are possible because progressive pathologies can be localized to a region the size of an infarction. The pathologies may be referred to as **non-Alzheimer lobar degeneration.** Damage can be bilateral but with one side more impaired than the other. In neuroimaging, degeneration shows up as *atrophy* or shrinkage of a portion of the brain. Interior spaces or ventricles are enlarged because of the decreased mass of adjacent brain matter. Atrophy is also viewed as enlarged sulci or spaces between cerebral convolutions.

With PPA, damage is concentrated in the perisylvian region of the left hemisphere. The existence of focal progressive neuropathologies suggests that aphasia and other specific cognitive disorders may indeed creep occasionally.

CLINICAL NEUROLOGICAL EXAMINATION

A *neurologist* is the specialist responsible for evaluation and treatment of persons with brain damage. Neurologists are able to examine the basic status of sensory, motor, and cognitive systems in about thirty minutes. In addition to determining if deficits are caused by neurological dysfunction, the physician wants to know the nature and site of damage. Radiological tests confirm and elaborate preliminary diagnosis based on clinical examination. With the accuracy and availability of brain imaging technology, the neurologist no longer has to rely on clinical examination to localize lesion. This specialist relates clinical findings to radiological findings and orders referrals to rehabilitative specialists so that impairments can be evaluated more thoroughly.

Clinical examination begins the instant the physician first sees a patient. Alertness indicates the status of the reticular activating system in the brain stem (see Figure 1.3). The doctor presses a stethoscope lightly to each temple to listen for unusual rushing sounds in the cerebral bloodstream called *bruits.* This examination is called *auscultation.* An initial interview yields clues about cognition, including language. The doctor may carry a brief screening test such as the *Mini-Mental State Examination* (Folstein, Folstein, and McHugh, 1975).

Systematic examination begins with motor and sensory systems to assess the peripheral and central nervous systems. Simple reflexes are tapped from head to toe, with hypoactivity indicating peripheral damage and hyperactivity indicating central damage. Balance and coordination are indicative of cerebellar function. Loss of sensation on one side is called *hemianesthesia,* and paralysis on one side is called *hemiplegia.* Left and right sides are compared with the normal side being a standard for estimating severity of unilateral impairment in the aphasic individual. Motor and/or sensory impairment of one side signify damage to the contralateral cerebral hemisphere, and deficits of specific body parts reflect damage to particular locations along pre- and postcentral gyri.

Visual deficits are particularly informative regarding the site of neuropathology. The visual system is not a directly contralateral connection between the eyes and the occipital lobes. Instead, contralaterality exists between *fields of vision* and the cerebral hemispheres. When we look straight ahead, we see objects to the left and right of the center. Moreover, we can see to the left and right of center with each eye. The right occipital lobe receives what we see in the left visual field (LVF), and the left occipital lobe receives vision in the right field (RVF). The left and right optic nerves make these connections by crossing only partially at the base of the brain. Neurology books have a diagram that displays this crossing point, called the optic chiasm.

Specific visual deficits are indicative of location of a tumor or other pathology, especially relative to the optic chiasm. Damage between the optic chiasm and one eye produces blindness of that eye, but a patient can still see each field with the other eye. Because of the unique structure of the optic tracts (i.e., partial crossing), damage between the optic chiasm and the left occipital lobe causes blindness for the RVF, which is a problem for each eye. The loss of a field of vision is called

homonomous hemianopia. A "right field cut" can occur with aphasia, because the optic nerve radiates through the parietal and temporal lobes on its way to the occipital lobe. The speech-language pathologist should ask a patient to look straight ahead and then should present objects to the left or right in order to determine if visual field matters in responding to visual stimuli.

CLINICAL BRAIN IMAGING

Scientists are inventing increasingly safe, efficient, and accurate means of viewing the living brain. Some newer or more expensive procedures are currently used to observe normal brain function for basic research. There are two general types. One is spatial or *structural neuroimaging,* which produces a static picture of brain anatomy. The other is temporal or *functional neuroimaging* which is sensitive to neural activity that may be associated with cognitive processes. Researchers are discovering pathologies with these procedures, such as focal cortical atrophies, that had been only hypothesized or even denied a few decades ago.

Procedures in either category can be *invasive,* with a foreign substance (e.g., contrast medium) injected in the body so that structures can seen more clearly, or they can be *noninvasive,* with no substance introduced. Because injecting any foreign substance into the circulatory system increases risks in a procedure, research is partly devoted to decreasing or eliminating the invasiveness of imaging procedures.

Structural Neuroimaging

Cerebral **angiography,** or **arteriography,** is an X-ray procedure for observing arteries in the head and neck. As an invasive approach, an iodinated opaque fluid is injected, usually in a carotid artery, so the cerebral arteries can be seen on X-ray film. With ischemia, vessels cannot be seen beyond the point of an occlusion. Tumors or other space-occupying lesions are inferred from distortion of the arterial pattern. *Digital-subtraction angiography* is a recent development based on computer computation that improves image quality and reduces the amount of contrast medium injected in the blood stream.

Computerized tomography (CT scan) permits detailed imaging of cerebral structures through computerized reconstruction. Scanners have undergone stages or generations of development, and a fourth-generation scanner is sketched in Figure 2.3. CT scan uses narrow beams of X rays on a scanner that rotates around the head. Intensity of the X rays is detected and sent to a computer that transforms the data into absorption coefficients indicative of tissue densities. Results are displayed as tiny blocks of tissue, which is a "reconstruction" of structures in a particular plane of the cerebrum.

Images of several planes are obtained in about 30 minutes. Figure 2.4 shows locations of

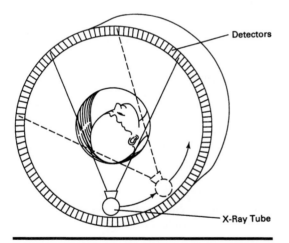

FIGURE 2.3 Schematic representative of a fourth generation CT scanner. An X-ray tube revolves around the body while emitting a beam wide enough to encompass the width of a patient. Stationary detectors measure the activity penetrating the body.

Reprinted by permission from Patronas, N. J., Deveikis, J. P., & Schellinger, D., The use of computer tomography in studying the brain. In H. G. Mueller & V. C. Geoffrey (Eds.), *Communication disorders in aging: Assessment and management.* Washington, D.C.: Gallaudet University Press, 1987, p. 110.

infarction as they might be found in a horizontal plane: anterior to the central sulcus (including the insula), deep in lenticular nuclei, medial (including posterior insula), and posterior invading the occipital lobe. Simple anterior-posterior classification may put the medial infarction in the posterior category.

An advantage of the CT scan lies in power of resolution of a lesion and detection of long-standing CVAs. Pathology is indicated by alterations in the normally expected densities of brain structures. Infarct is shown as decreased tissue density, and hemorrhage is shown as increased density. Identifying an infarction can be improved with injection of a contrast material. CT scan is particularly good at distinguishing between infarct and intracerebral hemorrhage. The main concern with this procedure is its exposure of radiation to the patient.

A much sharper image without radiation exposure is achieved with **magnetic resonance imaging** (MRI). This noninvasive procedure capitalizes on areas of high water density. It is based on the "spin" of molecules within the nucleus of an atom. First, the body is placed in an area surrounded by a large electromagnet (persons with metallic implants cannot be assessed). The magnet manipulates the spin of hydrogen molecules with the magnetic field and radio waves. Then, a computer creates a picture of the brain from the electromagnetic signals generated by this manipulation.

MRIs produce clear images of bone and soft tissue, and they contrast gray and white matter in the brain. They are superior to CT scans in their sensitivity to subtle neuropathologies and their early detection of diseases involving physiological changes. Because the procedure is noninvasive, it may be used repeatedly on the same patient and, therefore, is well suited for longitudinal studies. Brookshire (1997) noted that "MRI scans take a long time, and the patient must remain motionless in a noisy, confining space, sometimes leading to claustrophobia and blurring the MRI image because of patient movement" (p. 67).

Two advances in the MRI technique provide valuable information about hyperacute stroke,

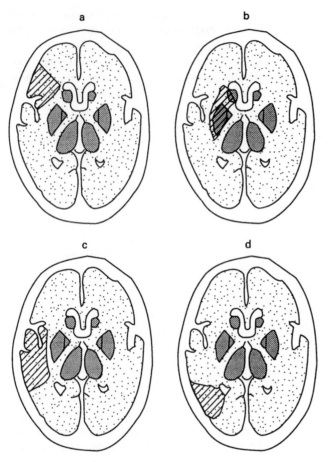

a   b

c   d

FIGURE 2.4   Four areas of infarction within the territory of the middle cerebral artery: (a) anterior, (b) deep, (c) medial, and (d) posterior.

Reprinted by permission from Habib, M., Ali-Cherif, A., Poncet, M., & Salamon, G., Age-related changes in aphasia type and stroke location. Brain and Language, 31, 1987, p. 247. Academic Press, publisher.

the first 24 hours after the onset of symptoms (Fridriksson, Holland, Coull et al., 2002; Hillis and Heidler, 2002; Hillis, Wang, Barker et al., 2000; Love, Swinney, Wong et al. 2002). The first method is called **diffusion weighted imaging** (DWI) and is based on the relative flow of water across cell membranes. It is sensitive to the extent of the acute infarction. The other method is called **perfusion-weighted imaging** (PWI) or also magnetic resonance perfusion imaging (MRPI). Based on the first passage of contrast material through the brain, PWI detects hypoperfusion or brain tissue that is currently dysfunctional but salvageable if the flow of blood is restored to that area. A combination of both procedures can detect the region

of penumbra, regions of brain tissue still alive but not functioning, and therefore, can aid prognosis for the recovery of language related to the region of penumbra.

Another noninvasive procedure is the application of **ultrasound scanning,** which has been commonly employed in obstetrics for obtaining pictures of a fetus about 16 to 18 weeks into a pregnancy. For obtaining pictures of the brain, inaudible high frequency sound waves are transmitted into the head, and reflected echoes are detected and analyzed with a computer. Ultrasound is used to scan the brain of a newborn child for diagnosing hemorrhage or tumors. As indicated earlier, it is being used to guide stereotactic biopsy.

Functional Neuroimaging

Two aspects of neurophysiology are measured in functional neuroimaging. One is the electrical activity of neurons, called electrophysiological neuroimaging. The other approach, called metabolic neuroimaging, is a little less direct and measures blood flow and metabolism. Because of their experimental use, Martin Exeter did not receive any of these procedures.

Perhaps the first method for detecting cerebral pathology in a living patient is **electroencephalography** (EEG). It records the electrical activity of the brain from the placement of electrodes at different locations on the scalp. The site of focal lesion is estimated by comparing graphic representations of brain waves detected from these locations in each lobe of each hemisphere. A lesion is indicated by electrical activity in one location that differs from regular patterns detected at other regions. Although EEG is crude for localizing pathology, it is still useful for distinguishing subcortical from cortical lesions and for estimating severity of damage when a patient is in a coma.

Because EEG is a safe procedure, it has been used extensively in the investigation of normal brain function. A refinement, called the *evoked potential* (EP) or event-related potential (ERP), has some clinical usefulness but also has provided an "exquisite" resolution of the temporal nature of cortical events (Springer and Deutsch, 1998). A computer is used to tease specific neural responses to stimuli out of the complexity of EEG activity. The neural or evoked response appears as a positive or negative spike in the computed wave. Several studies have used the EP to correlate neural responses to hypothesized cognitive stages in word and sentence processing (e.g., Kaan and Swaab, 2003).

Metabolic imaging is used to observe regional activity of the cortex while a person is performing a particular task. **Regional cerebral blood flow** (rCBF) is an indirect measure of metabolism. The procedure capitalizes on an increase of neural activity in a cortical region that causes an increased demand for nourishment and, thus, increased metabolic activity. Blood flow rate increases to satisfy this increased demand. A radioactive compound is injected in the bloodstream or inhaled as a gas. A scanner detects variations in blood flow rate over different regions. The procedure is used to look for activity that may be compensating for infarction.

Single-photon emission computed tomography (SPECT) is a relatively inexpensive procedure that produces a three-dimensional representation of cerebral blood flow. Employing a radioactive tracer nicknamed Tc-99m, investigators can "lock in" brain activity at the time of injection and view that localized activity later. This capability is advantageous for locating epileptic seizure activity as it happens and for detecting neural activity as a patient is performing a cognitive task. However, SPECT has not been used extensively for diagnosis because it is insensitive to specific etiologies such as differentiating ischemia from neoplasm. "The future role of SPECT might lie in its ability to predict recovery" (Mlcoch and Metter, 2001, p. 45).

Studies of hypometabolism mentioned earlier were conducted with **positron emission tomography** (PET). The PET scan is a direct measure of metabolism and is more responsive to rapid variations of activity than rCBF studies. Radioactive tracers, called positron-emitting isotopes, are combined either with oxygen or glucose and injected into arteries. After 50 minutes, a rotating scanner detects the rate at which tissue utilizes radioactive nutrients. Thus, PET scanning is more expensive than SPECT because PET requires that a cyclotron be available for producing the radioisotope. Both SPECT and PET detect areas of reduced blood flow, such as the frontal lobe hypometabolism mentioned earlier, that are remote from the infarction identified on CT or MRI scans (Mlcoch and Metter, 2001).

Functional magnetic resonance imaging (fMRI) can detect different oxygen levels in the brain because magnetic properties of oxygenated blood are different from deoxygenated blood. By taking a series of MRI scans, an investigator can identify regions activated while someone is performing a cognitive activity. Springer and Deutsch

(1998) reported that fMRI "has revolutionized the study of activated brain function in normal subjects because it can provide data with a temporal resolution of several seconds, can scan activation during any task multiple times, and/or can provide almost continuous information about cerebral activity occurring during changing study conditions" (p. 73).

Unlike direct measures of cerebral metabolism, fMRI does not require injection of a contrast medium and, thus, is more likely to be repeated on an individual. Other advantages are that it has better spatial resolution and is less expensive than PET. Disadvantages are its sensitivity to a patient's motion and difficulty of imaging certain areas of the brain. Like evoked potentials, the method has been used to study normal neural processing of sentences (e.g., Mason, Just, Keller et al., 2003). As shown in Chapter 7, fMRI has become important in the study of neural mechanisms underlying the recovery of language and the effects of treatment (Thompson, 2005).

Transcranial Doppler ultrasound (TDU) is a modified version of ultrasound scanning that examines moving objects such as blood pressure and flow in a cerebral artery. While a patient is reclining in a chair or on an examining table, gel is applied to an area of the head where the bone is thin enough to allow the Doppler signal to enter and be detected (called the transcranial window). A technician directs the signal toward the artery being studied and records detected rates. High flow rates indicate the narrowing of a blood vessel or an arteriovenous malformation. The procedure may also determine if a secondary route of blood flow exists prior to surgery for diseased vessels.

LOCALIZATION AND DISSOCIATION

A specific cognitive dysfunction such as aphasia is possible because the brain is organized into functionally specialized regions and certain neuropathologies can damage one of these regions while sparing others. Our knowledge of regional specialization comes mainly from studies that relate specific dysfunctions to sites of lesion. These studies began in the 1800s, relying on an autopsy to find the damage causing language difficulties. This is called the *lesion-deficit method* for determining the functional responsibilities of areas of the brain. Through the 1970s, the lesion-deficit method was modernized with improved imaging of lesions that can be identified near the time of more comprehensive and standardized evaluation of behavior.

The study of deficits for localizing functions requires the identification of patients with a single impairment. The common term is **dissociation,** which is a pronounced deficit in one task (or a set of tasks) while other performances remain intact or are clearly less impaired. It is as if one function is separated from others. With deficits primarily on language tasks, aphasia is said to be a dissociation of language functions from other abilities. Damage to the left hemispere is suggestive of a left hemisphere role in normal language function. A cognitive neuropsychologist would say that the dissociation indicates that the particular impairment signifies a distinct cognitive process.

There are problems with this simple lesion-deficit approach for inferring the jobs performed by an area of the cortex. One problem is that finding one deficit-lesion relationship does not rule out the possibility that other locations also have a role in the impaired function. For example, discovering that left hemisphere damage causes reading but not drawing deficits does not by itself rule out the possibility that the right hemisphere is also involved in reading. What if right hemisphere damage also causes difficulty with reading tasks?

One solution to this problem is for an investigator to compare the effects of damage in two areas, such as the left and right hemispheres, before concluding that one area is responsible for one function. Continuing with the same example, groups with left and right hemisphere infarcts would be given tests of reading and drawing. If the left damaged group shows the same dissociation but the right damaged group shows good reading and impaired drawing, then we have less ambiguous evidence of a left hemisphere role in reading. Conversely, we would also have evidence that the right brain has a specific role in drawing. This is called a **double dissociation,** which is shown when one patient or group of patients produces a deficit in one task or set of tasks along with no deficit in another task or set of tasks, while another patient or group produces the opposite pattern.

CLINICAL SYNDROMES OF APHASIA

Aphasic patients are observed to have specific dissociations with respect to linguistic features of language production. For example, some patients have more difficulty finding words (i.e., anomia) than forming sentences (i.e., agrammatism), whereas other patients have more difficulty with sentences than with words. Researchers interested in dividing up the functional responsibilities of the left hemisphere have taken such double dissociations to mean that one part of the left brain deals with word finding and another part deals with sentence structuring. In either case, a patient displays a particular pattern of deficit, and in this section we shall examine relationships between a pattern of aphasic deficit and site of lesion.

A *syndrome* is a recurring pattern of symptoms. The history of aphasiology is cluttered with systems for labeling different patterns of aphasia. Chapter 1 introduced a broad distinction between nonfluent and fluent aphasias. Nonfluent aphasias tend to be caused by damage in the anterior region, whereas fluent aphasias tend to be caused by damage to posterior regions (Mazzochi and Vignolo, 1979; Naeser and Hayward, 1978).

In the most common classification system, the main syndromes are differentiated according to three key areas:

- severity of *comprehension* deficit
- linguistic features of *spontaneous verbal expression*
- *repetition* ability compared to spontaneous expression

A key symptom may alert a clinician to the likelihood that a patient has a particular syndrome of aphasia. In fact, researchers who are uncomfortable with common classification may classify patients according to the key symptom (e.g., agrammatic aphasia). The syndromes are introduced here to illustrate dissociations within language, show how aphasia varies beyond the nonfluent–fluent dichotomy, and identify most likely sites of damage underlying different types of aphasia (Table 2.2).

Broca's Aphasia

Broca's aphasia is named for a nineteenth century French physician who drew attention to localization of function in the brain. It used to be associated with "expressive aphasia." Agrammatism is the dominant feature, and word finding is preserved better than sentence formulation. Auditory comprehension is slightly or moderately impaired. The clumsiness of apraxia of speech is likely to show up in the production of words, especially words that are difficult to articulate. The patient is often a good communicator, because the few words produced represent some of the message accurately. Also, our guesses as listeners are within the patient's comprehension ability.

Broca's area is also known as area 44 in the Brodmann numerical system that is used to identify cortical regions objectively or without attributing functional significance to them. Area 44 is located in the third frontal convolution anterior to the pre-central gyrus which distributes impulses to the muscles (see Figure 2.1). Because of this proximity to the primary motor strip, agrammatism is usually accompanied by right hemiplegia and a mild right facial weakness. It has been common to attribute Broca's aphasia to damage only to Broca's area.

However, chronic agrammatic aphasia is produced by lesions extending from Broca's area to the anterior insula and neighboring anterior temporal and inferior parietal areas. Damage to deeper structures also seems necessary to produce this aphasia, including the posterior internal capsule of tracts between the thalamas and basal ganglia (Levine and Sweet, 1983). Lesions restricted to area 44 can cause an acute Broca's aphasia that

TABLE 2.2   Summary of the contemporary clinical syndromes of aphasia.

GENERAL CATEGORY	SYNDROME	KEY SYMPTOMS	SITE OF LESION
Nonfluent/anterior	Broca's	Agrammatic production	Around and including Broca's area
	Transcortical motor	Like Broca's aphasia but with preserved repetition	Varied frontal lobe locations
	Global	Poor comprehension, minimal production	Posterior and frontal perisylvian language region
Fluent/posterior	Wernicke's	Poor comprehension, jargon, press for speech	Wernicke's area (posterior portion of superior temporal gyrus)
	Conduction	Surprisingly impaired repetition	Temporo-parietal boundary (supramarginal gyrus)
	Anomic	Word-finding deficit, empty speech	Posterior temporo-parietal boundary (angular gyrus)
	Transcortical sensory	Like Wernicke's aphasia but with preserved repetition	Inferior temporo-occipital border area (perhaps PCA occlusion)
	Transcortical mixed	Like global aphasia but with preserved repetition	Diffuse or multifocal damage in frontal and parietal lobes

may resolve quickly into something else (Kertesz, Harlock, and Coates, 1979). Such smaller lesions produce apraxia of speech or "Broca's area infarction syndrome" (Mohr, Pessin, Finkelstein et al., 1978). Kertesz (1979) stated "there is a spectrum of syndromes produced by Broca's area infarct . . . the larger lesions produce the full-blown symptom complex of Broca's aphasia" (p. 187). The absence of a clear relationship between Broca's area and Broca's aphasia indicates that "there is still some controversy about the anatomical underpinnings of Broca's aphasia" (Damasio, 2001, p. 25).

Global Aphasia

Global aphasia is a severe depression of language ability in all modalities. Some patients may speak noncommunicatively with verbal stereotypes (see Chapter 1). Yet, patients can be alert and aware of their surroundings, and they often express feelings and thoughts through facial, vocal, and manual gestures. The gloomy diagnosis of global aphasia should be reserved for when it can be determined that a patient has very poor language comprehension as well as an inability to speak and write.

The following problems may mask language abilities and give only the appearance of a comprehensive aphasia:

- motor impairments that make it difficult to determine comprehension
- extremely low level of arousal
- extreme disorientation or confusion
- depression or lack of motivation to communicate

The presence of these problems may lead a clinician to conclude correctly that the severity of aphasia is unknown. A diagnosis of global aphasia should be reported after careful consideration, because it can diminish the likelihood of support for speech-language treatment. Clinicians generally keep in mind that diagnosis of any aphasia pertains to how a patient deals with *language,* as opposed to processing other types of stimuli or making other types of responses.

CT scans usually expose lesions covering the entire perisylvian region including Broca's and Wernicke's areas (Kertesz, Lesk, and McCabe, 1977; Mazzocchi and Vignolo, 1979; Naeser and Hayward, 1978). Lesions may also reach deep into white matter beneath the cortex. A few cases have lesions confined to deep structures including the insula, lenticular nuclei, and internal capsule. An exception to pervasive perisylvian damage is an occasional global aphasia with Wernicke's area spared (Basso, Lecours, Maraschini, and Vanier, 1985; Vignolo, Boccardi, and Caverni, 1986). When damage is mainly frontal, a patient may present with Wernicke's aphasia in the acute phase and later resolve to a severe Broca's aphasia. Global aphasia may also arise from two separate strokes such as ischemia in anterior and posterior branches of the left middle cerebral artery, instead of a single ischemic blockage in the main trunk of the LMCA (Damasio, 2001).

Wernicke's Aphasia

The most severe form of fluent aphasia is known by other names, such as sensory aphasia, receptive aphasia, and jargon aphasia. The patient with Wernicke's aphasia has poor language comprehension, produces jargon, and often lacks awareness of semantic or neologistic paraphasias. The fluent jargon has recognizable sentence structure, indicative of a dissociation of word finding from fundamental syntactic construction. A patient may continue talking when it is his turn to listen, known as *press for speech*. Sparks (1978) described people with Wernicke's aphasia as having poor therapeutic set, because they do not realize why they are in the presence of a speech-language pathologist.

The syndrome of severe comprehension deficit and fluent jargon can be found with damage to Wernicke's area (posterior area 22) and neighboring temporal and parietal regions (Kertesz, 1979; Naeser and Hayward, 1978). On a CT scan, damage may look like the medial or posterior lesions of Figure 2.4 (Kirshner, Casey, Henson,

and Heinrich, 1989). Often the posterior insula is involved (Mazzocchi and Vignolo, 1979), and in a small percentage of many cases, some frontal lobe damage made the lesions look like they should have caused global aphasia (Basso et al., 1985; Kirshner et al., 1989). However, relative to Broca's aphasia, there has been little controversy regarding the site of damage that causes typical Wernicke's aphasia (Damasio, 2001).

Some researchers have tried to distinguish among the expressive symptoms that may dominate in the different manifestations of Wernicke's aphasia. A predominance of fluent phonemic paraphasias was related to infarction in Wernicke's area and the inferior parietal area above, whereas lexical (or verbal) paraphasias were related to infarcts in the more posterior angular gyrus and the adjacent occipital area (Cappa, Cavalotti, and Vignolo, 1981). Lesions causing neologistic jargon extended more posteriorly than lesions producing semantic jargon (Kertesz, 1982).

Conduction Aphasia

Conversation with someone who has conduction aphasia can go smoothly. We can be surprised during formal testing when the patient's verbal expression deteriorates precipitously when repeating phrases of increasing length and complexity. The identifying characteristic of this disorder is a disruption of *repetition* that is disproportionately severe relative to comprehension ability and spontaneous speech. Free verbal expression is hampered by word-finding problems and, especially, by occasional phonemic paraphasias. These patients are aware of their errors and "produce repetitive self-corrections, known as *conduite d'approche*" (Bartha and Benke, 2003, p. 93).

This aphasia is an example of a "disconnection syndrome," meaning that a dysfunction is caused by an impaired connection between structurally intact centers (Geschwind, 1965). These connections, or association tracts, are white axonal fibers running beneath the cortex and connecting one cortical region to another within a hemisphere. The *arcuate fasciculus* is an association tract beneath the left parieto-temporal juncture, and it carries impulses from Wernicke's area for listening to Broca's area for speaking. This connection enables us to repeat and is thought to be damaged in conduction aphasia.

CT scans of individuals with this repetition disorder show anticipated damage to the posterior superior temporal cortex and inferior parietal cortex along with infarction of deep white matter below (Damasio and Damasio, 1980). As predicted by disconnection theory, posterior temporal damage has been found to spare Wernicke's area (Naeser and Hayward, 1978). Mendez and Benson (1985) noted exceptions in three patients who were without lesions beneath the cortex. Kertesz and his colleagues (1977) speculated that two forms of conduction aphasia may arise depending on whether the lesion is more anterior (a less fluent "efferent conduction aphasia") or more posterior (a more fluent "afferent conduction aphasia"). Damasio (2001) centered the typical lesion in the area of the supramarginal gyrus or boundary of the parietal and temporal lobes but added that "conduction aphasia can result from somewhat different lesion patterns" (p. 27). The arcuate fasciculus need not be damaged for the symptoms of this aphasia to occur (Anderson, Gilmore, Roper et al., 1999).

Anomic Aphasia

Anomic aphasia (or "amnesic aphasia") is often the mildest form of aphasia. It consists of slightly impaired comprehension and fluent, syntactically coherent utterances that are weakened communicatively by a word retrieval deficit. Utterances are vacuous, filled with "generic terms" (indefinite nouns and pronouns) filling the void of concept-bearing content words. An example is the description of how to drive a car in Chapter 1.

Ambiguities can be resolved with situational context and knowledge of the topic. When naming objects, patients retrieve some words quickly or engage in elaborate circumlocution while trying to think of names for other objects. Although comprehension is quite good, word recognition difficulties can be detected. The patient may retrieve a word and then for a moment fail to recognize that the word is correct. It might be helpful to keep in mind that all aphasic persons have "anomia" of some kind (the symptom), whereas only some have "anomic aphasia" (the syndrome).

A specific site of damage responsible for anomic aphasia has been somewhat elusive. The syndrome has been associated with damage to the posterior parieto-temporal juncture (i.e., angular gyrus). A fairly comprehensive structural and metabolic study of 12 patients with mild "anomic aphasia" was conducted by Illes, Metter, Dennings and colleagues (1989). All patients had structural damage in the posterior superior temporal gyrus, but the researchers found two subgroups. The most fluent group had good metabolism in both frontal lobes, but a slightly less fluent group had left prefrontal hypometabolism as well as deep damage in addition to the temporal damage. Illes concluded that "an interplay between frontal cortex and neostriatal regions is essential for fluent and well-formed spontaneous language production" (p. 527).

Transcortical Aphasias

The rare transcortical aphasias are distinctive in that *repetition* is much better than would be expected from comprehension and spontaneous speech. Transcortical motor aphasia (TMA) is similar to Broca's aphasia. A patient struggles to answer a question but can repeat a fifteen-word sentence without missing a beat. Lesions are generally located in the frontal lobe, superior and anterior to Broca's area (Berthier, 1999).

Similarly, transcortical sensory aphasia (TSA) seems like Wernicke's aphasia. Ability to repeat is remarkable, because repetition is nearly impossible in Wernicke's aphasia. Echolalia, in which a person repeats a question instead of answering it, is a prominent feature. Lesions are usually posterior to the common language area. The damage has been picked up with CT imaging at the temporo-occipital border or the watershed area between middle and posterior cerebral arteries.

A mixed transcortical aphasia (MTA) is sort of a combination of TMA and TSA. Language disorder is severe with poor comprehension and meaningless stereotypic utterances. Yet, repetition can be compulsive. MTA is a global aphasia with ability to repeat. It is as if intact mechanisms of speech recognition and production are "isolated" from intentions and meanings generated in the rest of the brain. The literature is inconsistent on the presence of damage in the perisylvian language region. However, diffuse or multifocal pathologies do produce MTA with frontal and parietal damage while sparing the language area. Cimino-Knight, Hollingsworth, and Gonzalez Rothi (2005) reviewed evidence that the spared right hemisphere contributes to the preserved repetition ability.

EXCEPTIONAL APHASIAS

As noted previously, traditional diagnosis of aphasia has tied this disorder to etiologies that erupt and damage to the left perisylvian region of the cortex. Chapter 1 removed neurologic causation from the definition of dysfunction, which opens up the possibility of finding aphasias that creep. There are always going to be exceptions to traditional views as long as neuroimaging technology improves and clinical thinking continues to be inconsistent. "Exceptional aphasias" are those that are simply unusual and those that could, in some instances, be questionable because of inconsistent definition of dysfunction.

Crossed Aphasia

One unusual aphasia occurs because of individual variation in functional organization of the brain. A few people appear to have a reversed asymmetry with language functions in the right hemisphere and nonverbal functions in the left. Less than four percent of aphasic patients have crossed aphasia, in which right-handed individuals have suffered a stroke in the right hemisphere. Researchers want to study cognitive deficits carefully in these cases, wondering if they are indicative of a mirror asymmetry or pure reversal of the norm or are indicative of a more mixed or unusual functional

organization (Coppens, Hungerford, Yamaguchi, and Yamadori, 2002).

One review of reported cases indicated that 70 percent of crossed aphasias are a mirror image of typical left hemisphere profiles. Most classical syndromes are possible. Anomalous profiles occur in the remaining 30 percent. The anomalous cases tend to have large right perisylvian lesions but minimal aphasia along with absence of typical right hemisphere dysfunctions. Language deficits focus on phonological processes or lexical-semantic processes (Alexander, Fischette, and Fischer, 1989). Cases of specific aphasia syndromes have been reported (Bartha, Mariën, Poewe, and Benke, 2004; Sheehy and Haines, 2004).

Subcortical Aphasias

In the review of syndromes, it was noted that cortical damage can be accompanied by subcortical damage (Mazzocchi and Vignolo, 1979). This is due to infarctions that have depth as well as width. "Subcortical aphasias," however, are diagnosed when damage is primarily beneath the cortex in the left hemisphere. Reports of these disorders have raised eyebrows with respect to their implications for neural mechanisms of language as well as for the nature of aphasia.

The key subcortical locations are presented in Figure 2.2. The *internal capsule* is a passage of white motor and sensory fiber tracts squeezed between the thalamus and lenticular nuclei. The *lenticular nuclei* consist of the caudate nucleus and putamen, and both may be referred to collectively as the striatum. These nuclei comprise a substantial part of the basal ganglia in the extrapyramidal motor system. In the literature on subcortical aphasia, an infarct may be identified generally in the basal ganglia or specifically in the putamen or in the capsulostriatum, which includes the internal capsule, the caudate, and putamen.

The *thalamus* is the most central nucleus in the cerebrum, consisting of several parts with connections to motor, sensory, and association areas of cortex. Of particular importance are the white fiber connections between the thalamus and prefrontal regions of the cortex (see Figure 1.3), called the thalamofrontal gating system. This system may be responsible for focusing attention.

Kirk and Kertesz (1994) compared cortical and subcortical aphasias and found similarities with respect to scores on a standard aphasia test given 7 to 40 days after onset. All subcortical patients were classifiable into aphasia syndromes, but subcortical damage caused more motor and sensory impairments. In general, there is some disagreement over whether forms of subcortical language disturbance are genuine aphasia syndromes or are merely similar to these syndromes. Kennedy and Murdoch (1994) have argued strongly that subcortical damage can produce the same classical syndromes, but they also recognized reservations in using standard clinical tests to establish the true nature of a language disorder. Kirk and Kertesz noted that subcortical language deficits "change dramatically over time," so that diagnosis may be quite different even three months after a stroke.

Researchers divide subcortical language disturbances with respect to thalamic and nonthalamic lesions, mainly because these are somewhat distinct neural mechanisms. With a **thalamic lesion,** a patient is likely to have good comprehension and fluent semantic paraphasias and neologisms. Some cases have a transcortical-like sparing of repetition. In one report, two patients with left thalamic infarction demonstrated impairment limited to word retrieval difficulties in spontaneous language and structured naming tasks (Raymer, Moberg, Crosson et al., 1997). Lesions including the thalamus caused category-specific naming deficits for medical terms and names of celebrities (Crosson, Moberg, Boone et al., 1997; Lucchelli, Muggia, and Spinnler, 1997).

Nonthalamic lesions are also classified as "striatocapsular" or "capsulostriatal" lesions and include the basal ganglia. Researchers in Boston identified syndromes called anterior, posterior, and global capsular/putaminal aphasias (Helm-Estabrooks and Albert, 1991). Anterior aphasias are like Broca's aphasia because of "slow, poorly-articulated speech output" but are unlike Broca's aphasia because of "intact grammatical form" (Naeser, 1988, p. 365). The posterior syndrome is much like Wernicke's aphasia.

One problematic feature of the predominantly neurologically oriented studies of subcortical aphasia is that often no definition of *aphasia* is provided so that we know the criteria for diagnosing symptoms and selecting published cases for review (e.g., Nadeau and Crosson, 1997). It is as if we should assume that everyone agrees on what aphasia is. One reason for skepticism is the apparent interpretation of speech disturbances, especially with damage to the basal ganglia. For example, Alexander and others (1987) looked for "components of aphasic syndromes" that include "ease of speech initiation, articulation, and voice volume" (p. 961). Thus, there is the risk of suspecting that researchers are finding aphasias in apraxia of speech or voice disorders, or in any reduced test score.

Several neural mechanisms might explain how language disturbance could arise from subcortical lesions. Let us consider two general possibilities. One explanation supposes that the thalamus and parts of the basal ganglia have a direct role in language functioning so that a lesion impairs that role (e.g., Robin and Schienberg, 1990).

Another explanation need not assume a direct role of subcortical structures in language. Studies of blood flow and metabolism indicate that subcortical lesion is accompanied by remote hypoperfusion for the left perisylvian cortical regions that are directly responsible for language functions. Return of blood to the cortex may be responsible for the dramatic recoveries observed by Kirk and Kertesz. In general, diagnosis of communicative deficits depends on the time of assessment. This is one reason for considering site of lesion when suggesting a diagnosis and prognosis to a patient's family (Hillis, Barker, Wityk et al., 2004; Radanovic and Scaff, 2003).

SUMMARY AND CONCLUSIONS

Aphasia occurs because of neuropathologies that can strike regions of the brain responsible for language functions. It is not necessary that the left perisylvian region be the only site of damage for a patient to have aphasia. However, aphasia appears in its clearest form when the left perisylvian region is the only area of damage. Focal neuropathologies include ischemic and hemorrhagic stroke, tumors, and progressive focal atrophies.

Family members, who were likely in a state of shock when the doctor explained what happened, may question the speech-language pathologist about why a particular severity or pattern of language deficit occurred. Armed with knowledge of anatomy and neuropathology, we can help family members and patients understand the effects of size and location of lesion. We may anticipate residual capacities based on our knowledge of intact regions. Several books are available for helping patients and families cope with stroke, such as Stein's (2004) *Stroke and the Family* and Hutton's (2005) *After a Stroke: 300 Tips for Making Life Easier.*

Advances in neuroimaging technology reduce the use of clinical evaluation for diagnosing neuropathology. These advances also force revisions in neurological explanation of dysfunction. At one time, the diagnosis of aphasia syndromes was thought to help the neurologist diagnose site of lesion. Currently, the various syndromes simply alert us to the existence of different kinds of acquired language disorders. This individual variation indicates that goals of language treatment can vary from patient to patient.

By the way, Charles Dickens suffered a fatal left hemisphere stroke before completing "The Mystery of Edwin Drood" and revealing the solution. It became a Broadway play in which audiences voted on the ending (Rolak, 1993). Martin Exeter's stroke also left some projects unfinished.

MATCHING REVIEW

For reviewing chapters 1 and 2, select an item in the right column to go with an item in the left column. Do not use a right-side item twice.

____	1. paraphasia	a. astrocytoma
____	2. agrammatism	b. occlusion
____	3. Broca's aphasia	c. functional neuroimaging
____	4. neologisms	d. any word-finding error
____	5. Wernicke's aphasia	e. neologistic jargon
____	6. ischemic stroke	f. agrammatism
____	7. hemorrhage	g. grammatical morphemes missing
____	8. tumor	h. structural neuroimaging
____	9. MRI	i. nonword paraphasia
____	10. fMRI	j. hematoma

d-1.
g-2.
f-3.
i-4.
e-5.
b-6.
j-7.
a-8.
h-9.
c-10.

CHAPTER 3

CLINICAL ASSESSMENT AND DIAGNOSIS

Complete evaluation of an aphasic patient considers the World Health Organization's levels introduced at the end of Chapter 1. Historically, assessment has been aimed at diagnosing and measuring *impairment*. The evaluation of *disability* and *handicap* had been relegated to informal interviewing and recording basic vocational and social information on a form that might accompany a test of impairment. The emphasis of this chapter is the assessment of language impairment.

With shifts in rehabilitation settings and reimbursement plans, managed care has also focused the goals of formal evaluation and influenced the time devoted to diagnosing and assessing impairment. For example, when a patient is seen in temporary acute care, goals are tied to survival, such as determining if the patient has swallowing problems and needs for communicative assistance. Differentiating speech and language disorders is helpful for discharge planning. A somewhat more detailed analysis of language impairments can be done once a patient is transferred to a rehabilitation unit or center.

This chapter spotlights major aphasia batteries and a few supplemental tests. In between, it presents some strategies for quick initial evaluation. In covering the comprehensive batteries, the chapter presents what clinicians believe to be the observations that are important for assessing aphasia.

THE FIRST VISIT

Initially, after receiving a referral, the clinician reviews the patient's **medical history** at the nurse's station. The chart contains an admission summary with the neurologist's initial diagnosis and possibly some early radiologic findings from brain imagery. A social worker may also have obtained some family and vocational history. For her first visit with a patient, the speech-language pathologist (SLP) is armed with the following information:

- date of the cerebral incident
- medical history, including possible complicating conditions
- current medications
- family or potential caretakers

The SLP visited Martin Exeter in his hospital room. She introduced herself, asked him how he was feeling, and told him that she was there to evaluate his speech. She noticed a weakened right-handed grip. He nodded, smiled, and indicated that he does not talk very well. She sensed that Martin could comprehend and inquired if it is OK to ask him a few more questions. Do you know what happened to you? Do you know where you are? The SLP wondered if Martin could be stimulated to say a little more. Pointing to the clock, she asked if he could say its name. She pointed to the TV hanging over his bed. He said "T-V." He was able to count to ten more easily. He was particularly encouraged when she said calmly, "You know what you want to say, but just have trouble finding the words." She understood his problem. She noted that he is speaking well so soon after a stroke and said she would be seeing him again.

The first meeting takes 5 to 15 minutes depending on the patient's medical condition. The SLP may return later to do a more complete bedside evaluation following the framework for aphasia assessment introduced in Table 1.1. All that is needed is the common objects in a hospital room, a pen, and some paper (Table 3.1). The patient

TABLE 3.1 A possible bedside examination illustrating the minimal ingredients of an aphasia evaluation.

COMPREHENSION		PRODUCTION	
Listening	*Reading*	*Speaking*	*Writing*
Is your name [Fred]? (No)	Point to the object on this card.	Count to ten.	Write your name.
Point to the [window]. (lamp, etc.)	Do what it says on this card. (e.g., point to your nose)	Say Methodist Episcopal.	Write down some things you see in this room.
Point to the table and ceiling.		What day is today?	
Is Washington D.C. the capital of France?		What do you call this? (e.g., clock, pillow)	
		Tell me what happened to you.	

answers some yes/no questions, points to things, and names and describes some other things. If the patient cannot converse, the SLP wants to see if he or she can count or recite the days of the week. For standardized testing, the second edition of the *Bedside Evaluation Screening Test* (BEST-2) is intended to be used in the acute period (Fitch West, Sands, Ross-Swain, 1998), and it is presented along with other brief tests later in this chapter.

DIAGNOSTIC DECISIONS

Clinicians answer the following fundamental questions:

- Does the patient have a communicative disorder?
- If so, is the disorder aphasia?
- If so, what kind of aphasic disorder does the patient have?
- Does the patient have other disorders besides aphasia?

Communicative disorder is determined in two ways. One is by comparing a patient's test score to normative standards. The other basis for diagnosing deficit is to compare an individual patient's poststroke performance with some indication of prestroke performance. To increase the likelihood that a deficient score represents a language disorder, tests are constructed to minimize the influence of extraneous factors such as education level, cultural variation, or reasoning skill. For example, we would not evaluate language comprehension by asking a question about who was President of the United States during the Civil War. This is more a test of education than of basic language skill. If a test does not formally consider these factors, a clinician does when interpreting results.

Along with determining whether there is a language deficit, we want to determine whether the deficit represents aphasia. Tests contain features that consider the definitive characteristics of aphasia as we have understood them. For example, aphasia tests are constructed to evaluate language skills in the four major modalities (see Table 1.1). Each modality is tested independently so that nonaphasic, modality-specific impairments can be exposed.

The syndromes introduced in Chapter 2 suggest areas of test construction that might help us diagnose types of aphasia. As indicated by the key features distinguishing syndromes, we would be sure to evaluate comprehension at different levels, examine linguistic characteristics of spontaneous verbal expression, and thoroughly examine repetition ability. However, the main clinical purpose of testing repetition is to determine if a nonverbal patient is stimulable with this task.

STANDARD TESTING

The inconsistency of informal testing makes it difficult to measure progress reliably. Henry Head, a British physician, was one of the first to standardize aphasia assessment. He was particularly vexed by one problem. "An inconsistent response is one of the most striking results produced by a lesion of the cerebral cortex" (Head, 1920, p. 89). A patient names an object one moment and fails to name it the next. If we tested naming just once, we might misdiagnose a patient as having severe impairment or no impairment. Head decided that a response had to be observed at least three or four times in what he called "serial tests." He would place a set of common objects (e.g., knife, key, matches) on a table and would ask a patient to point to them by name and then try to name the objects. Head did the same thing for each patient and recorded exactly what was said.

In the 1930s, physicians developed the *Halstead-Wepman-Reitan Aphasia Screening Test* as a quick evaluation of patients at bedside (Halstead and Wepman, 1949). Two hundred were distributed to military neurologists and neurosurgeons during World War II. One version, Form M, could be carried in a shirt pocket; another version was absorbed into the more comprehensive Halstead-Reitan neuropsychological battery (Reitan and Wolfson, 1993). Other tests in our history include Eisenson's (1954) *Examining for Aphasia* and Wepman and Jones's (1961) *Language Modalities Test for Aphasia* (LMTA).

Hildred Schuell's *Minnesota Test for Differential Diagnosis of Aphasia* (MTDDA) may have been the most widely administered test in the United States and Great Britain in the 1960s and 70s. It could take from two to six hours. It evolved from seven revisions over 17 years, beginning with the first version in the summer of 1948 (Brown and Schuell, 1950). The sixth form

was made available to clinics in 1955 on a limited basis for experimental use. The marketed form in 1965 was the eighth version, indicative of the care with which the MTDDA was developed. After Schuell's death in 1970, the test and manual were revised slightly by Sefer (Schuell, 1973).

Schuell's full test is quite lengthy. It covers the four language modalities with 46 subtests. To shorten the test time, she suggested establishing a **baseline** and **ceiling** within each section of the full MTDDA (Schuell, 1966). For each modality, a clinician establishes a baseline by starting with a subtest on which the patient should make a maximum of one error. To establish a ceiling, the clinician should stop testing on the subtest producing 90 percent failure and, thus, not spend time on subtests most likely to show severe deficiency. Thompson and Enderby (1979) decided to create a short form by determining the subtests and items that are too easy or too difficult. Their version has only 5 items per subtest, contrasting with the original 20 to 32 items.

Some legal questions call for a standardized basis for identifying and measuring impairment. Questions of **competency** consider whether patients are able to function in their own best interest or in the best interests of those for whom they have been responsible (Porch and Porec, 1977). What is the patient's capacity to stand trial, assume parental responsibilities, live independently, conduct business and personal affairs? Ability to understand one's will, called testamentary capacity, is indicated by assessment of receptive language (Ferguson, Worrall, McPhee et al., 2003). These issues are important in a specialty of the legal profession called *elder law.*

A second issue deals with **compensation,** which entails determining how much impairment has been sustained. A patient may be seeking compensation from an employer or the government or may be suing a physician or hospital because of a surgical accident. In this case, we are called on for our expertise and data in determining if someone is *malingering*. People pretending to have aphasia make about the same number of errors on both easy and difficult tasks, instead of the aphasic pattern of errors following a hierarchy of task difficulty (Porec and Porch, 1977). Malingerers might show unusual patterns, such as agrammatism without accompanying paralysis or overdoing a particular symptom such as a type of naming error.

PSYCHOMETRIC CONSTRAINTS: THE PICA

Bruce Porch was disturbed by flexible test administration and vague scoring methods when he embarked on his doctoral dissertation in the late 1950s. He wanted to corral inconsistency by applying psychometric principles that were becoming the rule in educational and clinical psychology. In particular, he wanted to achieve *reliability* for the purposes of measuring progress and comparing patients. After the *Porch Index of Communicative Ability* (PICA) was published in 1967, it became an important tool for the study of recovery.

However, many speech-language pathologists were initially wary about the test's rigidity of administration and reliance on cold numbers for describing patients. Also, it was startling that a 40-hour workshop was needed to learn the complex scoring system. It took a while for clinicians to be comfortable with the PICA's unique methodology. The test has the following salient features:

- relatively small number of subtests
- emphasis on reliability, with very restrictive rules for administration
- complex multidimensional scoring requiring extensive training

The PICA does not appear to be used as much as other current batteries (Roberts, Code, and McNeil, 2003), but it has a prominent place in clinical research literature and provides an informative perspective on aphasia assessment.

Description and Administration

The PICA contains 18 subtests of the four language modalities and other functions. Similar to Henry Head's serial tests, each subtest utilizes 10 common objects arranged neatly on a table (i.e.,

cigarette, comb, fork, key, knife, matches, pen, pencil, quarter, and toothbrush). The order of subtests is unusual. Auditory, reading, and speech tasks are mixed together in subtests I through XII. Writing subtests are together at the end.

At first glance, order of subtests seems to proceed from difficult to easy, in contrast to other batteries that start with the easiest tasks in each modality. This organization is a product of the use of the same 10 objects across subtests so that functions can be compared without changes in content. Tasks are ordered to minimize a learning effect that may come from repeated use of the same objects. That is, if word comprehension were to come before naming, as in other batteries, a patient would have heard the word before the naming test. Thus, minimal linguistic information about objects is given early, and maximum information is deferred. As a result, the sequence does not follow a strict hierarchy of difficulty. Actually, some earlier subtests are likely to be easier than later subtests for many aphasic patients.

Explicit prescriptions for administration apply to the physical conditions of testing as well as what a clinician is to say and do for each subtest. It takes an average of one hour for a well-trained clinician to give the PICA, but it often takes about 90 minutes. Each of 180 responses is assigned a score based on the multidimensional scoring system shown in Table 3.2. The scale points reflect degrees of correctness and incorrectness, and there are subtle variations among subtests in the definition of scale points. The ability to assign scores quickly is learned in the 40-hour PICA workshops. Diacritical markings provide additional notation for characterizing a response.

Standardization and Interpretation

Whereas an average of one hour is needed for most aphasic patients to take the PICA, 130 neurologically intact adults breezed through in about 30 minutes (Duffy, Keith, Shane, and Podraza, 1976). Normal adults had some difficulty in areas that can be influenced by education. Ninety-five percent averaged 12.95 on the graphic

TABLE 3.2   Multidimensional scoring system of the PICA.

SCORE	LEVEL	DESCRIPTION OF RESPONSE
16	Complex	Accurate, complex, and elaborate
15	Complete	Accurate and complete
14	Distorted	Accurate, complete, but with reduced facility
13	Complete-delayed	Accurate, complete, but slow or delayed
12	Incomplete	Accurate but incomplete
11	Incomplete-delayed	Accurate, incomplete, slow or delayed
10	Corrected	Accurate after self-correction of error
9	Repetition	Accurate after repetition of instruction
8	Cued	Accurate after specified cue
7	Related	Inaccurate but related to correct response
6	Error	Inaccurate
5	Intelligible	Intelligible but not related to test item
4	Unintelligible	Unintelligible, differentiated
3	Minimal	Unintelligible, not differentiated
2	Attention	Attention to item but no response
1	No response	No awareness of test item

Adapted by permission from Porch, B. E., *Porch Index of Communicative Ability: Theory and Development, Volume 1,* Palo Alto, Calif.: Consulting Psychologists Press, 1967.

subtests, with a mean of 9.63 on writing sentences. Averages for the entire sample are shown in Table 3.3, compared to samples with left hemisphere lesions and probable aphasia.

Reliability is not worth much if a test is not valid regarding what it is purported to measure. The PICA has strong criterion-related validity with respect to other standardized tests but falls short of reflecting natural communicative abilities in daily life (Holland, 1980a; Keenan and Brassell, 1975; Sanders and Davis, 1978). For reliability, Porch (1967) reported interexaminer and test–retest correlations in the manual. The broader a score's coverage, the more stable the retest two weeks after initial testing.

Mean scores are used for documenting and interpreting performance. The most specific summary score is the individual subtest mean. An average such as 12.25 is called a *response level.* At one time, subtests were grouped according to functions shown in Table 3.3. The average for all

180 scores is called the **overall score.** To improve communication of results, response level scores can be translated into **percentiles** relative to a large sample of aphasic patients. The overall score is more reliable than subtest scores.

A score of 15 or 16 indicates a level defined by the test and does not necessarily indicate normality (see Table 3.3). Aphasia at the 95th percentile includes scores of 14.44 overall, 15.00 for auditory and reading comprehension, 14.62 for verbal subtests, and 13.46 for written language. These scores are similar to normal, leaving diagnosis of mild aphasia to clinical judgment.

Data summary forms are provided to help a clinician identify patterns of performance and to facilitate meaningful documentation. Modality-specific conditions, such as motor speech deficits or illiteracy, are revealed by depressions of speech or reading modalities beyond what would be expected with respect to the typical aphasia pattern among modalities.

TABLE 3.3 Normal adults (Duffy et al., 1976) and aphasic adults (Porch, 1971a, 1981) compared according to classification available when the normals were studied. Aphasia scores illustrate the impact of sample expansion between 1971 ($N = 280$) and ($N = 357$).

	OVERALL	GESTURAL	VERBAL	GRAPHIC
Normal Adults				
Range	13.40–14.99	13.73–15.00	13.48–15.03	11.18–15.03
Average	14.46	14.66	14.55	14.12
Left-Hemisphere Damage				
95th percentile (1981)	14.44	14.74	14.62	13.91
50th percentile (1981)	10.89	12.96	10.77	8.22
50th percentile (1971)	10.64	12.73	11.20	7.50

In the studies of reliability, shifts between first and second testing showed a mean improvement of around 0.38 points. This indicates that a subtest shift of 0.40 or more is needed to represent real change as opposed to normal between-test variation. Reliable change scores (i.e., differences between a test and retest) can be determined for general and specific abilities. A 10 percent increase in the overall score is considered to be a reasonable treatment goal, whereas a 5 percent change "has a limited effect on communicative ability" (Porch, 1981, p. 105).

Shortened PICA

It may be useful to know whether an overall score from a shortened PICA is equivalent to an overall score obtained from the complete test. A regression analysis determined that 10 subtests and 5 objects per subtest produce an equivalent overall score (DiSimoni, Keith, Holt, and Darley, 1975). Another short PICA, called the *SPICA,* had similar results (Holtzapple, Pohlman, LaPointe, and Graham, 1989). Only subtests I, VI, VII, and D are presented with the 10 objects; but the overall score from the SPICA is significantly different from the overall obtained with the PICA. Another SPICA with five objects was reliable but had less sensitivity to recovery over four weeks than the complete test (Lincoln

and Ells, 1980; Phillips and Halpin, 1978). A shortened PICA may be good for a single assessment but may not be the best means of measuring change.

DIAGNOSING SYNDROMES: THE BOSTON EXAM

Harold Goodglass and Edith Kaplan started developing the "Boston Exam" in the 1960s. The complete *Boston Diagnostic Aphasia Examination* (BDAE) was first published in 1972, and a revised royal blue edition appeared ten years later (Goodglass and Kaplan, 1983). A third edition provided extensive revisions and additions (Goodglass, Kaplan, and Barresi, 2001). A short form and "extended testing" were added.

The BDAE-3 has been used as a basis for documenting syndrome diagnosis. It lies between the PICA and the Minnesota test in length, and time of administration can be up to three hours. The Boston Exam has the following salient features:

- classification of aphasias into syndromes according to symptom patterns
- analysis of spontaneous verbalization
- the Short Form
- extended testing

Description and Scoring

The Boston Exam consists of four major sections, each focusing on a language modality. Auditory and spoken modalities are presented before reading and writing (Table 3.4). The battery is particularly distinctive with its assessment of conversational and expository utterance prior to systematic testing. Conversation is elicited with an interview and discussion of familiar topics. Then a patient is asked to describe the Cookie Theft picture: a kitchen setting in which a child, perched on a tilting stool, is reaching for a cookie jar in a cupboard while a woman, appearing unaware of the crime, is washing dishes over a sink with water running over onto the floor. The picture-description task is now supplemented with cartoons for eliciting narratives. Analysis of the discourse samples consists of noting empty utterances, utterance completeness, and utterance complexity.

Some of the changes in the third edition were cosmetic, such as replacing the section name of Understanding Written Language with Reading.

Other features of the original test were rearranged or removed. Goodglass eliminated the body-part identification subtest and inserted a few of these items into the word comprehension section. He removed the test of "animal naming" (i.e., word fluency) and inserted the *Boston Naming Test,* which is presented later in this chapter as a supplement. Also, he moved oral word and sentence reading from the oral expression section to the reading section.

Noting that "aphasia assessment has been under pressure to change from a number of directions" (Goodglass et al., 2001, p. vi), the authors modified formal testing in two opposite directions. One direction provides for shortened testing time mainly with the original battery (discussed later). The other direction extends testing options beyond the original battery with the application of neurolinguistic or cognitive neuropsychological research. This extended testing includes the following:

- narrative discourse elicited by cartoons (see Chapter 6)

TABLE 3.4 Most of the sections and subtests of the *Boston Diagnostic Aphasia Examination* (third edition). Examples of extended testing are noted in **boldface**.

AUDITORY-ORAL			WRITTEN LANGUAGE	
I. Conversational and Expository Speech	II. Auditory Comprehension	III. Oral Expression	IV. Reading	V. Writing
Interview	Point to body parts, objects, actions, letters, numbers	Oral and verbal agility	Identify letters and numbers	Mechanics
Conversation		Automized sequences and melodies	Word–picture matching	Alphabet and numbers
Cookie Theft description	**Word categories**		Lexical decision	Write to dictation
Cartoon narratives	Commands	Repeat words and sentences	**Grammatical morphemes**	Written naming
	Complex material (short stories)	Answer questions	Oral word and sentence reading	Cookie Theft description
	Syntactic processing	Boston Naming Test	Sentence–paragraph comprehension	
		Naming in categories		

- word comprehension by semantic categories such as foods and animals (see Chapters 4 and 13)
- comprehension of syntax (see Chapters 4 and 5)
- word reading (see Chapter 5)

More specifically, the syntactic processing extension examines reversible possessives (e.g., *ship's captain* vs. *captain's ship*) and embedded sentences (e.g., *The child calling her mother has dark hair*).

Standardization and Interpretation

A revised normative sample of aphasic patients was assessed between 1976 and 1982. This sample was used to relate raw scores to percentiles. Then standardization samples of 85 aphasic individuals and 15 elderly normal volunteers were obtained to support the third edition. The data mainly consist of internal agreements among items in each subtest.

Because of its lack of summary scores, it has been difficult to compare the BDAE to other tests statistically. Comparison to other tests that also classify syndromes is reviewed later in the chapter. There has been some study of the relationship between test patterns and site of lesion. Naeser and Hayward (1978) found agreement between independent classification with the test and predicted site of damage determined with CT scans for 19 patients.

Diagnosis of syndrome is facilitated by examining the pattern of results on a rating of speech characteristics and a subtest summary profile. The manual provides examples and ranges of performance that are typically seen in cases of Broca's, Wernicke's, anomic, and conduction aphasias. The profile of speech characteristics is a convenient guide for classification (Figure 3.1). The profile describes expression according to the telltale signs of the syndromes. Seven dimensions of extended utterance are compared with auditory comprehension deficit determined during formal testing. Figure 3.1 shows the range around mean performance for one fluent aphasia. An additional profile provides a summary of performance on the extended subtests.

BDAE Short Form

According to Goodglass and his colleagues (2001), the Short Form "offers a brief, no frills assessment, but one that still documents the performances that are essential for diagnostic classification and quantitative assessment" (p. vi). It consists of most of the original subtests but only a few of the items from each subtest. The following is a list of some of the subtest reductions:

- word discrimination from 37 to 16 items
- following commands from 5 to 3 commands
- repetition of sentences from 10 to 2 items
- responsive naming (e.g., *What do you do with soap?*) from 10 to 5 items
- the *Boston Naming Test* from 60 to 15 items
- word reading comprehension from 10 to 4 items

The selected items are in boldface in the scoring booklet for the full test, but the Short Form has its own record booklet and set of stimulus cards extracted from the full test. The authors computed correlations between the Short Form and the Standard Form for each subtest. Most of the correlations were in the 90s. The relatively low correlations in the 70s were for word discrimination and matching numbers.

NUMERICAL CLASSIFICATION: THE WAB

At the University of Western Ontario, Andrew Kertesz introduced the ***Western Aphasia Battery*** (WAB) as a modification of the BDAE (Kertesz and Poole, 1974). The complete test was published in 1982 for widespread clinical use, following several earlier appearances in studies of recovery and aphasia classification (Kertesz, 1979; Kertesz and McCabe, 1977; Kertesz and Phipps, 1977). Roberts, Code, and McNeil (2003) reviewed 100 studies published in 2001 and 2002, and they found that selection of aphasic participants was documented most often with the WAB (i.e., 23 studies). The Boston Exam followed with 14

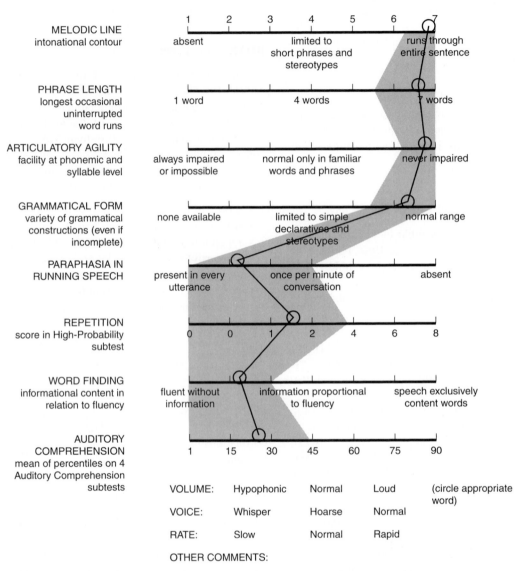

RATING SCALE PROFILE OF SPEECH CHARACTERISTICS

FIGURE 3.1 The Boston Exam's rating scale profiles of speech characteristics for Wernicke's aphasia.
Reprinted by permission from Goodglass, H., & Kaplan, F., *The Assessment of Aphasia and Language Disorders*. Chicago: Riverside, 1983, p. 81, 85.

studies. A new edition, called the Western Aphasia Battery-Enhanced (WAB-E), has been announced for the summer of 2006.

Kertesz perceived a problem with definitions of syndromes by different authors. He believed that consistency is possible "only if aphasia types are objectively defined, and classification criteria used in different centers are objectively compared" (Ferro and Kertesz, 1987, p. 374). The Western specifies ranges of test scores for key language functions as the basis for classifying aphasias. To this end, the WAB has the following salient features:

- content and administration similar to the Boston Exam
- summary scores including an overall score
- ranges of scores for classifying aphasias into syndromes

Among many changes, a new edition includes objects for manipulation, a modernized assessment of word reading, and a 15-minute Bedside WAB-E (Kertesz, 2006).

Description and Scoring

The basic battery examines oral language abilities that include auditory comprehension and spoken expression. Visual language and other subtests form an additional section consisting of (V) Reading, (VI) Writing, (VII) Apraxia, and (VIII) Constructional, Visuospatial, and Calculation tasks. The entire test could take as long as the MTDDA, and Kertesz (1982) recommended dividing it into segments across sessions. Organization of the oral and graphic sections is summarized in Table 3.5.

Calculations from test performance and summary scores set this test apart from the Boston Exam. Scores are obtained for the four sections of the oral language test. The spontaneous speech section is rated with two 10-point scales, one for information content and another for fluency. The fluency scale is used in classification. For example, 0 to 4 represents levels of nonfluency, and 5 to 10 depicts levels of fluency. The following summary scores have been calculated (see also Figure 3.2):

- *Aphasia Quotient* (AQ): Used with the test since 1974, the AQ is the summary score for auditory-spoken language. Forty percent of the score is derived from the spontaneous speech rating scales. Possible score is 100 (see Shewan and Kertesz, 1980).
- *Language Quotient* (LQ): The LQ is a composite of all language sections, including reading and writing (Shewan and Kertesz, 1984).
- *Performance Quotient* (PQ): For a while, reading, writing, apraxia, and construction tasks were combined into this score (Kertesz, 1979; Appell, Kertesz, and Fisman, 1982).
- *Cortical Quotient* (CQ): This is the only score besides the AQ that was mentioned

TABLE 3.5 Sections and subtests of the original *Western Aphasia Battery*.

AUDITORY-ORAL (AQ)				GRAPHEMIC	
I. Spontaneous Speech	*II. Auditory Verbal Comprehension*	*III. Repetition*	*IV. Naming*	*V. Reading*	*VI. Writing*
Interview	Yes/No questions	*Bed*	Object naming	Comprehend sentences	Name and address
Description of picnic scenario	Word recognition	*Snowball*	Word fluency	Commands	Write story about a picture
	Follow commands	*The telephone is ringing*	Sentence completion	Words	Write to dictation
		Pack my box with five dozen jugs of liquid veneer	Answer questions	Spelling recognition	

AQ			PQ
LQ			
CQ			
Auditory comprehension	Spoken expression	Reading & writing	Nonverbal skills

FIGURE 3.2   An overview of the summary scores for the *Western Aphasia Battery.*

in the original test manual. The CQ represents performance on all subtests, verbal and nonverbal.

Standardization and Interpretation

Typical scores were reported for 215 aphasic patients, 63 normals, and 53 nonaphasic brain-damaged patients (Kertesz, 1979). Normals had a mean AQ of 99.6. The tendency for anomic and conduction aphasias to be mild and moderate impairments is indicated in mean AQs of 83.3 and 60.5, respectively. Broca's and Wernicke's aphasias scored means of 31.7 and 39.0, respectively. Broca's aphasia had the widest standard deviation of all the aphasias. Persons with global aphasia had a mean AQ of 10.5.

Criterion-related validity was supported by comparisons to the NCCEA (Kertesz, 1982), PICA (Ross and Wertz, 1999; Sanders and Davis, 1978), and the *Lisbon Aphasia Examination Battery*'s quociente de afasia or "quotient of aphasia" (Ferro and Kertesz, 1987). The studies indicated that the WAB assesses aphasia like other batteries. To examine the specific goal of objective classification, Swindell, Holland, and Fromm (1984) compared WAB-derived syndromes to clinical impressions. Swindell found that the test agreed with clinical experience for 54 percent of the aphasic patients studied. Agreement was greater for nonfluent aphasias than fluent aphasias.

Shewan and Kertesz (1980) presented strong reliability, but Trupe (1984) found weak reliability in the content and fluency scales even after clarification and revision of scoring criteria. She concluded that it is difficult to use one fluency scale to characterize behavior consisting of multiple dimensions. She recommended that independent dimensions be rated separately as in the speech characteristics profile of the Boston Exam.

With respect to diagnosis, presence of a language disorder or "aphasia" is identified with an AQ cutoff score of 93.8 (Kertesz and Poole, 1974). In a study of prognostic indicators, aphasic people who surpassed the 93.8 score were considered to be "recovered" (Holland, Greenhouse, Fromm, and Swindell, 1989). Syndromes are identified according to patterns of performance with respect to the fluency scale and scores from auditory comprehension, repetition, and naming subtests (Table 3.6). Conduction aphasia, for example, is recognized by scores that are low in repetition relative to higher scores in spontaneous speech fluency and auditory comprehension. One perspective on diagnosis according to these criteria is illustrated in Figure 3.3.

Ross and Wertz (2003) suggested that "the use of cut-off scores for differentiating normal from aphasic performance is problematic" (p. 313). The problem is that the blind use of such scores for diagnosis can lead to identifying a mildly aphasic person as normal and vice versa. These investigators compared 18 aphasic and 18 normal adults matched for age and education. AQ and CQ scores overlapped between the two groups by 22 percent and 17 percent, respectively. For example, four of the aphasic participants had an AQ above the cut-off 93.8. So, it is possible to make a diagnostic error based on these summary scores alone. After a similar study focusing on mild aphasia, Ross and Wertz (2004) concluded that test scores may

TABLE 3.6   Criteria for classifying aphasias based on scores from the *Western Aphasia Battery.*

	FLUENCY	COMPREHENSION	REPETITION	NAMING
Global	0–4	0–3.9	0–4.9	0–6
Broca's	0–4	4–10	0–7.9	0–8
Isolation	0–4	0–3.9	5–10	0–6
Transcortical motor	0–4	4–10	8–10	0–8
Wernicke's	5–10	0–6.9	0–7.9	0–9
Transcortical sensory	5–10	0–6.9	8–10	0–9
Conduction	5–10	7–10	0–6.9	0–9
Anomic	5–10	7–10	7–10	0–9

Reprinted by permission from Kertesz, A., *Aphasia and Associated Disorders: Taxonomy, Localization, and Recovery.* New York: Grune & Stratton, 1979.

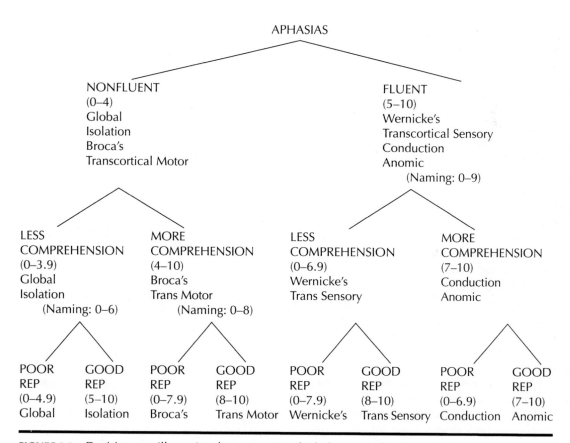

FIGURE 3.3   Decision tree illustrating the manner in which the WAB classifies aphasias according to scores for fluency, auditory comprehension, and repetition.

be helpful clinically for borderline patients with unclear symptoms.

A Short WAB

Crary and Rothi (1989) worked on a short WAB and discovered that four measures would be highly predictive of the standard AQ. These measures are the sequential commands and repetition subtests and the Information Content and Fluency ratings of spontaneous speech. However, considering that the AQ is normally computed based on a weighted formula for 10 scores, it was unclear how an AQ should be computed from these four specific scores. The new WAB-E comes with a short bedside version (Kertesz, 2006).

Comparing the WAB and the BDAE

Wertz (1983) had serious questions about the validity of the BDAE with respect to its classification of aphasias, and this concern later spread to the WAB. Wertz, Deal, and Robinson (1984) compared the two tests given to the same 45 aphasic patients with single left hemisphere occlusive lesions. There was only 27 percent agreement as to classification of these patients. In a follow-up study, Crary, Wertz, and Deal (1992) performed cluster analyses with each test. They found 38 percent agreement between BDAE diagnosis and cluster membership and 30 percent agreement with the WAB, leading to the conclusion that the tests classify aphasias differently.

In Ferro and Kertesz' (1987) comparison of the WAB to the similar Lisbon aphasia test, they found only a partial overlap of aphasia types derived from the tests. A major discrepancy was between global and Broca's classifications. The main issue was the amount of comprehension deficit that would turn a nonfluent patient into a global aphasic. Another problematic discrepancy was in diagnosing conduction aphasia.

These studies indicate that score-based diagnosis presents only an appearance of objectivity, because the score definitions are still based on a test author's criteria, and scoring is based on an examiner's judgment. Swindell suggested that clinical description be used to supplement scores for documenting diagnosis of a syndrome.

DIAGNOSING MODULAR IMPAIRMENT: PALPA

Some researchers in Europe have been critical of traditional aphasia batteries, saying they "were not designed primarily with the aim of elucidating the underlying nature of language disorder" (Byng, Kay, Edmundson, and Scott, 1990, p. 72). In 1992, they welcomed the "much-longed-for PALPA" (Marshall, 1996, p. 197), which they claimed "beautifully fills this gap" (Basso, 1996, p. 191). PALPA stands for *Psycholinguistic Assessments of Language Processing in Aphasia.* It was developed by Janice Kay, Ruth Lesser, and Max Coltheart in the United Kingdom and in the environment of the case study methodology of cognitive neuropsychology (Kay, Lesser, and Coltheart, 1992).

A few years later, the test manual's introduction was reproduced in the Clinical Forum of the journal *Aphasiology* (Kay, Lesser, and Coltheart, 1996a). In 2004, the test was examined in an entire issue of this journal, where the editor referred to an activity called "PALPAring" (Code, 2004, p. 75). However, PALPAring has been somewhat regional. In 217 citations of this test over 10 years, 139 were publications originating in the United Kingdom. The United States followed in second place with 34 (Kay and Terry, 2004). While lauding its goals, a few clinical aphasiologists have expressed some concerns about its many differences from the batteries discussed previously in this chapter. The PALPA has the following distinguishing features:

- emphasis on the word level
- flexible administration of subtests
- identification of impaired cognitive modules

Description

The PALPA consists of 60 subtests with an organization shown in Table 3.7. However, the authors

TABLE 3.7   A summary of most of the subtests for the *Psycholinguistic Assessments of Language Processing in Aphasia* (PALPA) (Kay, Lesser, and Coltheart, 1992).

SECTIONS	SUBTESTS	FUNCTIONS INCLUDED (SUBTESTS)
Auditory processing	1–17	Auditory lexical decision (5–6) Repetition (7–12) Rhyme judgments (14–15)
Reading and spelling	18–46	Letter discrimination (18–21) Visual lexical decision (24–27) Oral word reading (29–37) Spelling to dictation (39–46)
Picture and word semantics	47–54	Word–picture matching (46–47) Synonym judgments (49–50) Picture naming (53–54)
Sentence comprehension	55–60	Sentence–picture matching (55–56) Locative relations (58–59) Pointing span for noun–verb sequences (60)

recommend that the test not be given from subtest 1 to 60. Subtest selection should be flexible, and the test is "not designed to be given in its entirety to an individual" (Kay et al., 1996a, p. 160). Selecting a group of subtests may be based on a hypothesis of impairment, such as one that might focus on reading. Each subtest is introduced with instructions for administration. These introductions also contain "suggestions for where to go next," especially when a patient has difficulty with a subtest. Each subtest is scored for accuracy, and an examiner is also encouraged to pay attention to type of errors.

The auditory and reading sections through subtest 46 (three-fourths of the test) mainly deal with variables of word form, such as phonology and syllable length, or grammatical variables, such as morphology and grammatical class. They are considered to be tests of input processing. Only a few of these subtests deal with the relation of a word to another cognitive representation. That is, five subtests manipulate imageability as a variable (i.e., whether a word evokes a concrete visual image). Also, in subtest 38, a patient is asked to give a definition for a homophone (e.g.,

week, weak). The correct meaning must be related to a spelling rather than a sound. Similar subtests were inserted into the Boston Exam's third edition, including matching homophones (e.g., *mail, male*) and auditory-graphic grammatical morpheme matching.

The examination of reading input variables dominates the PALPA, especially with nine subtests involving oral word reading. The reading section responds to speech-language pathologists (SLPs) who have questions about subtle aspects of a patient's reading. Such questions may arise when a mildly aphasic outpatient makes an occasional error in reading aloud from a favorite novel. An important aspect of reading assessment is performance with nonwords (e.g., *bem*), which also infiltrated the third edition of the BDAE. Deficient pronunciation of nonwords is indicative of an impaired process for directly converting orthography to phonology.

Testing the meaningful use of words begins in earnest with subtest 47, which is the classical test of word comprehension by pointing to pictured choices. Much has been made of this subtest, especially because the authors recommended that this is "a good place to start an initial assessment of auditory processing . . . before going on to test auditory input processing skills" (Kay et al., 1996a, p. 177). Cole-Virtue and Nickels (2004) studied subtest 47 and concluded that the pictured choices have some confounds that might hamper interpretation, such as semantically similar distractors also being visually similar to the target word.

Standardization and Interpretation

The subtests were given to 25 individuals with aphasia and 32 individuals who were generally the partners of the aphasic participants. Performance by the aphasic patients is not reported in the manual. The norms consist of the mean and one standard deviation for the non-brain-damaged controls, data that appears at the beginning of most subtests. A diagnosis of deficit is judged to be two standard deviations below the controls' mean. The authors also recommend considering a score's relationship to chance when the response is a binary yes/no (i.e., 50 percent).

Interpretation of performance "is based on the assumption that the mind's language system is organized in separate modules of processing, and that these can be impaired selectively by brain damage" (Kay et al., 1996a, p. 160). The modules are illustrated in diagrams, or "models," showing the sequence of processing from one module to the next, a strategy that is explained more in Chapter 4. Any one of the models in the manual "forces one to think hard, and with precision, about the patient's performance . . ." (p. 173). The idea is to infer a specific cognitive impairment from a pattern of subtest scores. Relying on one subtest can be problematic. For example, giving a definition for a homophone (subtest 38) is confounded by verbal production, so that the comprehension process of interest can be masked by aphasic formulation problems. Once a decision on impairment is made, the isolated component becomes a target for treatment. Examples of how the PALPA is used for diagnosis appear in the journal *Cognitive Neuropsychology,* such as a case study of nonflu-

ent progressive aphasia (Tree, Kay, and Perfect, 2005).

The suggestions for where to go next are a useful guide to grouping subtests for the purpose of diagnosing impairments in particular components of the models. Marshall (1996) raised the possibility that "the PALPA expects too much of the practicing clinician . . . The PALPA calls for an alternative way of thinking about aphasia" (p. 198). However, some strategies are familiar to the most traditional clinical aphasiologists, such as comparing the same mode of output with different modalities of input to determine if a problem is output related (i.e., cannot produce the response in any condition) or input related (i.e., can produce the response to some input modalities but not others).

Limitations of the PALPA

The PALPA's allure is that its method systematically relates to a cognitive theory of language whereas other aphasia tests do not. Often the authors refer to their theoretical foundation in a broad sense or without qualification. However, some of the common features of aphasia batteries and psycholinguistic research are absent in construction and use of the PALPA. The test's authors acknowledged the following missing elements (Kay et al., 1996a):

- sentence production
- language use, such as inferencing (i.e., pragmatics)
- discourse-level functions

Stated reasons for these omissions include a desire to keep test administration simple and a preference for levels of language that are accessible with the modular theories of cognitive neuropsychology (see Chapter 4). Whereas the linguistic characteristics of sentence production have been important for diagnosis of syndrome, we shall see in subsequent chapters that diagnosis of syndrome is relatively unimportant in cognitive neuropsychology.

As indicated by comparisons of the WAB and BDAE, Robert Wertz has been concerned about all forms of assessment for aphasia. His main interest has been standardization (i.e., norms, validity, reliability). He was worried about some features of the PALPA, including its already recognized lack of breadth in assessing language functions (Wertz, 1996). The absence of norms for aphasia does not provide support for the judgment of deficit based on controls' standard deviations. Wertz also noted that the manual does not contain demonstrations of validity and measures of reliability. For validity, comparing this test to a similar test would have been difficult to do, because "a similar measure does not exist" (p. 185). The lack of evidence for reliability weakens the test as a measure of recovery, although administration of most tasks is fairly straightforward. Basso (1996) was less concerned: "For my part I do not think that a standardization would be of much help" (p. 191).

The PALPA's authors also recognized the absence of online testing, which is the case for all clinical batteries. However, online testing represents important components of language processing theory, such as lightening fast subconscious lexical processing and the automatic assignment of structure to sentences (see Chapter 5). Semantic memory imposes an organization on the activation of meaning, and this organization is missing from the modular theories that emphasize components of input and output (e.g., Ferguson and Armstrong, 1996). Context operates on these processes at sentence and discourse levels. What worries some aphasiologists is the limited language processing theory that supports the rationale for PALPAring. One response from the authors is that their "simple" model can be "a helpful way of *introducing* this way of assessing and thinking about language disorders, not because we believe it to be a particularly valid 'model' of language structure" (Kay et al., 1996b, pp. 203–204).

BRIEF TESTS AND BEDSIDE SCREENING

Regarding informal bedside screeening, Brookshire (1997) noted that "an unsystematic approach may lead the examiner to miss important signs and may invalidate comparisons of the patient's performance with that of other patients or with the same patient on subsequent tests" (p. 165). Standard screening protocols ensure that everyone in the clinic does the screening the same way. Large rehabilitation centers are likely to have their own standard protocol, and a few screening tests have been published.

In many rehabilitation settings, SLPs select subtests from a comprehensive battery. For a severe aphasia, we may select the easiest subtests in each modality to discover language abilities. For a mild aphasia, we may eliminate the easiest subtests or select a few of the most difficult ones to discover deficits. Impairment is more likely to appear with reading and writing tasks than with auditory-oral tasks. For focusing on basic auditory-oral communicative functions, we may postpone tests of reading and writing. Another approach is to employ a published screening test. In the shorter screening tests, each modality tends to be examined with items graded for difficulty rather than with whole subtests graded for difficulty.

The *Aphasia Diagnostic Profiles* (ADP) is intended to be more efficient than the BDAE and WAB for syndrome documentation (Helm-Estabrooks, 1992). Forty to 45 minutes of test time is divided into nine subtests. In addition to a classification profile, the ADP yields profiles for severity, alternative communication, and the communicative value of errors. The test was standardized on 290 adults with neurological impairments and 40 nonaphasic adults.

The *Aphasia Language Performance Scales* (ALPS) provides an informal standardized assessment in 20 to 30 minutes (Keenan and Brassell, 1975). The examiner can utilize objects in pockets and a patient's room for assessing comprehension and expression. Modalities are tested with four "scales," each containing a series of items increasing in difficulty.

Like the ALPS, the *Acute Aphasia Screening Protocol* (AASP) depends on objects reliably found in a patient's room such a pillow, window, and TV (Crary, Haak, and Malinsky, 1989). It should take around 10 minutes. The test begins with a quick check of attention and orientation and then assesses auditory comprehension and basic expressive abilities. The AASP includes a score for conversational style.

In its second edition, the ***Bedside Evaluation Screening Test*** (BEST-2) is a portable test that can be given in 20 minutes or less (Fitch West, Sands, and Ross-Swain, 1998). The use of magnetized objects from the first edition has been changed to the use of a picture book for all stimuli in the second edition. Assessment is speeded by the absence of a section for writing. Seven subtests are constructed for conversation, spoken production, auditory comprehension, and briefly for reading. The test was restandardized in 1996 on nearly 200 aphasic adults, and separate norms are provided depending on whether a patient is younger or older than 75 years. Confidence in the test was indicated by its use for measuring acute aphasia severity in an MRI study of early cerebral hypoperfusion (Fridriksson, Holland, Coull et al., 2002).

The following list exemplifies a growing selection of screening tests for aphasia:

- The ***Frenchay Aphasia Screening Test*** (FAST) was developed for use by nonspecialists, such as junior medical staff, nurses, and occupational therapists, to assist in identifying patients who have linguistic disturbances (Enderby, Wood, and Wade, 1997). Studies have shown positive correlation between the FAST and other tests (Al-Khawaja, Wade, and Collin, 1996; Enderby and Crow, 1996).
- For varied disorders, Tanner and Culbertson (1999) produced "quick assessments" including ***Quick Assessment for Aphasia,*** which can be given in under 20 minutes.
- Risa Nakase-Thompson, a neuropsychologist at Methodist Rehabilitation Center in Jackson, Mississippi, created the ***Mississippi Aphasia Screening Test*** (MAST). It can be given in 5 to 15 minutes. The clinician puts objects in front of a patient for pointing and naming. There are nine subtests, each with 1 to 10 items (Center for Outcome Measurement in Brain Injury, 2005).

SUPPLEMENTAL TESTS

Other tests are continually invented to help us deal with problems that the large batteries do not solve. One problem is posed by patients at each end of the severity continuum. We depend on retained abilities for a starting point in treatment, but a test battery may be so difficult for the most severe aphasic patient that it does not expose capabilities. Conversely for the most slightly impaired, a test may not be difficult enough to expose deficits that would point to goals of treatment.

The following are the main uses of supplemental tests:

- assess special aphasic populations such as the most mildly or severely impaired
- assess skills not represented in traditional batteries, such as functional communication
- more in-depth evaluation of a language skill, such as reading

For this chapter, only a few common tests of language functions are introduced. Other supplemental strategies of assessment will be presented in subsequent chapters, mainly because they illustrate how basic research and the health care system can have an impact on clinical practice.

Token Tests

The auditory language modality is usually the least impaired in aphasia (see Figure 1.1). Mild comprehension deficits are found in anomic, conduction, and Broca's aphasias. At the University of Milano in Italy in the 1950s, Ennio DeRenzi and Luigi Vignolo felt that it was difficult to detect mild deficits with the routine methods available at the time. Later the auditory sections of the PICA and BDAE were found to have low ceilings for aphasic patients, meaning that the challenging end of the tests does not have enough room for mildly impaired patients to show deficit (Morley, Lundgren, and Haxby, 1979).

DeRenzi and Vignolo (1962) created the Token Test to identify and measure subtle comprehension deficits. It was designed so that response would be based on processing language with minimal help from a situation, props, topic, or extraneous verbalization. The test is a series of instructions to identify and manipulate shapes of different shape, color, and size. With contextual factors cleared away, it focuses on the influence of linguistic length and complexity.

Boller and Vignolo (1966) published a complete list of commands, and so their version became the basis for most subsequent versions. The test has five parts. Parts I through IV contain 10 items each, and they differ according to information given about the tokens and length of command. Part V contains 22 commands of varying construction, and the commands are generally more complex than the items in previous sections. The complete test contains 62 items. The following illustrates each part of the 1966 version:

I. Touch the yellow rectangle.
II. Touch the large blue circle.
III. Touch the red circle and the yellow rectangle.
IV. Touch the small yellow circle and the large green rectangle.
V. (1) Put the red circle on the green rectangle.
  (11) Touch the white circle without using your right hand.
  (20) After picking up the green rectangle, touch the white circle.

Various scoring systems have been used. Originally, errors were counted for each element of each command, with total possible errors being 250. Most clinicians have followed Boller and Vignolo's (1966) recommendation of scoring each command as correct or incorrect and then having a best score of 62 (e.g., Swisher and Sarno, 1969; Gallaher, 1979).

Normative information must be pieced together from many studies (Table 3.8). Aphasic patients with mild comprehension deficit do poorly on Parts IV and V, indicating that initially undetected deficit can be exposed with the Token Test (Morley, Lundgren, and Haxby, 1979; Noll and Randolph, 1978). The test is very difficult for other aphasic persons, who perform much worse than RH-damaged patients and have lower scores than LH-damaged nonaphasic patients (e.g., Hartje, Kerschensteiner, Poeck, and Orgass, 1973). Problems with Part V in LHD nonaphasic patients led to a diagnosis of "latent aphasia" (Boller and Vignolo, 1966). Nonfluent and fluent aphasias score about equally, but specific syndromes differ. Wernicke's aphasia produces more errors than nonfluent aphasia (Mack and Boller, 1979; Poeck and Hartje, 1979).

The first abbreviated Token Test became the "Identification by Sentence" subtest of the *Neurosensory Center Comprehensive Examination of Aphasia* (Spreen and Benton, 1977). There are 39 items instead of 62. A 16-item version was equally capable of deficit identification (Spellacy and Spreen, 1969). Norms were also developed for a 36-item Token Test with a cut-off of 29 for identifying aphasic deficit (DeRenzi and Faglioni, 1978). DeRenzi eliminated the color blue because of problems that elderly adults have in discriminating between blue and green.

Revised Token Test (RTT)

McNeil and Prescott (1978) borrowed principles of the PICA to reduce inconsistencies in the family of Token Tests. The **Revised Token Test** (RTT) has structural balance with 10 sections and 10 commands in each section. A 15-point multidimensional scoring system is applied diligently to each element of each command, and a clinician ends up with a score for each subtest and an overall score. The RTT takes around 30 minutes

TABLE 3.8 Some sample scores on the Token Test by different groups (Noll and Randolf, 1978; Swisher and Sarno, 1969).

POPULATION	RANGE	MEAN
Neurologically intact adults	48–62	59.7
Mild aphasia	18–59	43.5
Wide range of aphasia severity	0–58	23

to administer. Several types of reliability are .90 or higher. The test has also been employed in research on auditory processing with aphasia (e.g., Hageman and Folkestad, 1986).

Testing time is cut about in half with the **Five-Item RTT.** It consists of the first five items of each subtest except for a complete subtest IX (i.e., 55 commands). Arvedson and her colleagues (1985) undertook a project to determine if the five-item version yields the same information as the full test. Results showed that the overall score predicted the overall score with the complete test. Arvedson suggested that the short version is substitutable for the overall score, but she was cautious about more specific analyses. Park, McNeil, and Tompkins (2000) found that test–retest, intra-rater, and inter-rater reliabilities are nearly as high as the full RTT.

Boston Assessment of Severe Aphasia (BASA)

Whereas the original Token Test was intended to assess aphasia at one end of the severity continuum, the *Boston Assessment of Severe Aphasia* (BASA) is directed at the other end (Helm-Estabrooks, Ramsberger, Morgan, and Nicholas, 1989). For severe language impairment, general batteries are often too difficult to expose communicative strengths that are reinforced in treatment. The authors distributed 61 items among sections for auditory comprehension, oral and limb apraxia, gesture recognition, oral and gestural expression, reading comprehension, and visuospatial functions. The clinician records a variety of responses, including gestural and affective responses. The BASA has detected significant improvements in communicative functions in severely impaired aphasic patients up to 18 months post onset (Nicholas, Helm-Estabrooks, Ward-Lonergan, and Morgan, 1993).

Reading Tests

For more thorough examination of a patient's reading capacities, clinical aphasiologists have created printed versions of auditory comprehension tests, borrowed reading batteries from the field of education, or created their own batteries of silent and oral reading tasks. The tests are considered when treatment objectives focus on a patient's reading needs, especially for mildly impaired patients wanting to return to jobs requiring reading skill.

Brookshire (1997) reviewed reading assessment extensively, having been particularly interested in paragraph-level tests. Nicholas and Brookshire (1987) used the *Nelson Reading Skills Test* (NRST) to examine inferencing in aphasic adults and also to evaluate the need to read pargraphs in order to answer test questions about them, called **passage dependency.** NRST paragraph tests were found to have better passage dependency than paragraph items in standard aphasia batteries (Nicholas, MacLennan, and Brookshire, 1986), indicating that the NRST is a more valid assessment of text comprehension. Some of the reading tests that Brookshire favors are summarized in Table 3.9.

The *Reading Comprehension Battery for Aphasia* (RCBA) is in its second edition (LaPointe and Horner, 1998). The main test contains ten subtests from word to paragraph levels. Unique sections include a subtest for functional tasks such as reading common signs, a checkbook, and a phone directory. A supplement (RCBA-S) was added for the second edition. It contains seven subtests exploring word-level reading in more detail. Subtests include letter discrimination and recognition, word–nonword discrimination, and oral word and sentence reading.

Aphasic patients are often meticulous readers. Van Demark, Lemmer, and Drake (1982) measured an average time of about 45 minutes to administer the main RCBA. They compared 19 nonfluent and 7 fluent patients. Both groups had PICA scores indicative of moderate impairment. With a maximum score of 100, the nonfluent group averaged 70.73, and the fluent group averaged 77.85. The mean and range for all patients were 71.34 and 31 to 97.

Boston Naming Test (BNT)

The BNT, first constructed to detect mild word-finding impairments, is now incorporated into

TABLE 3.9   Some reading tests from the field of education that have been suggested for use with aphasia.

TEST	READING LEVEL	DESCRIPTION	REFERENCE
Gates-MacGinitie Reading Tests	Grades 1–3	Word, sentence, and paragraph comprehension	Gates (1978)
Nelson Reading Skills Test	Grades 3–9	Word and paragraph materials at three reading levels	Hanna, Schell, and Schriener (1977)
Nelson-Denny Reading Test	High school through college	Word and paragraph materials	Brown, Bennett, and Hanna (1981)

the BDAE-3 (Kaplan, Goodglass, and Weintraub, 1983). The test contains 60 line drawings to elicit words of varied familiarity. It begins with simple words that are common in aphasia batteries such as *bed* and *tree,* and at the end it presents infrequent words such as *trellis, palette,* and *abacus.* Certain cues are provided when a patient is slow to respond, and testing stops after six consecutive failures. The score is derived from the total correct with the maximum being 60. Cued and uncued versions of the test proved to be reliable (Huff, Collins, Corkin, and Rosen, 1986).

Because of some of the vocabulary in the test (e.g., *protractor, tripod*), there have been several norming studies of the BNT (e.g., Henderson, Frank, Pigatt, Abramson, and Houston, 1998). Race has been an inconsistent factor, but education has been a regular factor. After a comprehensive review, Hawkins and Bender (2002) found that few norming studies have been representative of the general population. They recommended that norms be subdivided by level of education and that clinicians also consider premorbid vocabulary when using BNT scores to diagnose aphasia.

Nicholas and Brookshire were concerned that some of the pictures are ambiguous, capable of eliciting names other than the ones considered to be correct. They gave the test to 60 neurologically intact persons after changing some of the BNT's procedures. They wrote more explicit instructions, established a different cueing procedure, and de-

veloped a more elaborate response coding and scoring procedure. The patients averaged 54.5, which is close to the mean reported by Kaplan (Nicholas, Brookshire, MacLennan et al, 1989).

NOTES ON INTERPRETATION

The details of different aphasia batteries can distract us from our fundamental objectives. In the acute care setting, we are mainly involved in discharge planning. In the rehabilitation setting, we want to plan treatment so that it addresses a patient's communication problems *accurately.* Does the patient have a speech or language disorder? Is the language disorder aphasia? Does the patient have additional problems such as an agnosia, dysarthria, or a low level of arousal? Are clinical findings consistent with the medical diagnosis? Does the medical diagnosis present a favorable prognosis? No matter what test we use, our questions are the same.

"Too often examiners base their diagnoses on test results. They forget that tests do not diagnose problems; people do" (Fitch West et al., 1998, p. 20). We interpret our observations according to what we understand aphasia to be, namely, a disorder of language processing as opposed to hearing loss or a low level of consciousness. An inexperienced clinician may have a tendency to "overdiagnose" a patient who is not talking, especially in the first couple of weeks after onset.

The clinician may have the urge to say that someone has one or more of the main communicative disorders studied in graduate school, while forgetting that a patient may be silent for reasons that are unrelated to aphasia (see Chapter 2 on global aphasia). Sometimes it is more accurate to say that we cannot be sure of language abilities (or speech abilities) until the patient becomes more alert and has more energy.

As discussed previously, the possibility of diagnostic error exists with a dependence on test scores (e.g., Ross and Wertz, 2003). One source of error may be the potential for **cultural bias** in standardized tests for aphasia. The mistake would be to consider a low score as indicative of aphasia in individuals who may be at a cultural or linguistic disadvantage when taking a particular test. In one study, socioeconomically matched normal black Americans and white Americans submitted to administration of the oral expressive subtests of the *Boston Diagnostic Aphasia Examination* and the *Western Aphasia Battery* (Molrine and Pierce, 2002). There were no significant differences between groups with the subtests requiring convergence on a single response. Black Americans performed worse with word fluency subtests, in which participants had to rapidly produce a quantity of examples of a category in a minute or so (e.g., "Animal Naming" in the Boston Exam, second edition). However, black Americans also performed within normal limits. Molrine and Pierce concluded that "these common standardized aphasia assessment instruments were not unduly biased against Black test takers" (p. 147).

We want to determine the status of the four primary language modalities, no matter what test we use; and we want to determine the retained skills that can be useful communicatively. A test battery with 30 subtests does not mean that a patient could have 30 disorders. The 18 subtests of the PICA and the 46 subtests of the MTDDA do not mean that Porch and Schuell disagreed on the number of problems that could be diagnosed with aphasia. We know that aphasic people can have a few specific language disorders in word finding or sentence construction. In general, any test is harnessed to help us document our clinical observations of fundamental aphasic deficits and/or discover whether a patient has any of these disorders.

So, what do we do with the results, let us say, of 10 subtests and 10 items per subtest? We conduct three levels of comparison, summarized in Table 3.10. At the level of basic language functions, we compare listening, reading, speaking, and writing. We look for **common threads** such as problems with language in all modalities. Task comparison is essential because no single task is diagnostic of a disorder. For example, a low repetition score could be indicative of a hearing loss, short-term memory deficit, or motor speech disorder. In task comparison, we look for common threads such as difficulties only in tasks requiring lengthy verbal input or only in tasks requiring speech output. Within a single task, comparing items may direct us to specific problems for focusing treatment. A patient may make comprehension errors with particular sentence structures or may make particular types of errors in naming tasks (see Chapters 4 and 5).

As we identify specific language problems, we are starting to plan for language treatment. We **prioritize** with respect to a patient's communicative needs as well as the time we have. What will a patient be most motivated to work on? What is most likely to improve in the next month or so? What problems can the family help us with? For some patients, improving comprehension (e.g., yes/no response) goes a long way to improving communicative interaction. For some patients, reading or writing skills are relatively unimportant.

MARTIN EXETER'S INITIAL REPORT

Martin Exeter was transferred to the Rehabilitation Unit at Pocumtuck Medical Center five days after his stroke. His first day of rehabilitation included brief evaluations by a clinical neuropsychologist and physical therapist. A social worker

TABLE 3.10   Levels in analysis of aphasia batteries or supplemental tests.

COMPARISON	DEFINITION	DIAGNOSTIC ISSUES
Function	Comparing status of language modalities	Aphasia versus sensory loss, agnosias, or motor speech disorders
Task	Comparing task performances within a modality	Level of language impairment such as words, sentences, or discourse/text
		Impairment of a specific process such as word retrieval
Item	Comparing specific items within a task	Impairment of a specific linguistic feature such as verbs or passive sentences
		Impairment of a semantic category such as living things or vegetables

met with family members for a few minutes. Besides his wife Jackie, his daughter Julianna and son Peter were present. Martin and Jackie were married in their early thirties. Julianna was a sophomore in college and came home as soon as she heard the news. Peter was a junior in high school.

The SLP met the family to review her findings in initial assessment (Figure 3.4). The family wanted to know more about strokes and aphasia and the future. The clinician explained that they would have to wait and see how Martin was doing near the end of his inpatient stay, but his progress to date indicated that his aphasia should not keep him from taking care of himself at home. The clinician could not say at this time exactly how many inpatient sessions would be covered by their insurance, but she stressed the importance of their support. Each family member wanted to know what they could do to help, and the clinician assured them that their help would be very important in his language treatment. The clinician also wanted to observe the family's interac-

tion styles with Martin before making specific recommendations.

Julianna said she wanted to quit school to be with her father for a while. The SLP advised her that quitting school would not be necessary for her father's language rehabilitation, but that she would have to decide for herself. Jackie did not want Julie to quit school. The clinician asked Julie if she knew how quitting school would make her father feel, and Julie indicated that she would not tell him and hoped her mom and brother would keep it from him, too. The clinician thought that Julie's observations of her father in the hospital the next few days would help her make her decision.

Peter was quiet. The clinician asked him what sort of things he and his father did together. Peter started to answer but then left the room. Jackie said that Martin would take Peter to sporting events at the university. The basketball team was surprisingly good this year. They were looking forward to playing golf in the summer. Peter would want to know if his dad would be able to play golf again.

POCUMTUCK MEDICAL CENTER		
SPEECH-LANGUAGE PATHOLOGY		
Name: Martin Exeter	Location: Rehabilitation Unit	Date: 4-17-99

INITIAL EVALUATION SUMMARY

Dr. Exeter is a 55-year-old male who suffered an ischemic stroke on April 10, 1999. He is a professor at the university. After five days in acute care at this hospital, he was referred to the Rehabilitation Unit by Dr. Irving Waxman.

History

Medical diagnosis was a thrombotic stroke causing aphasia and moderate hemiparesis on the right side. There were no sensory deficits. A CT scan showed an area of infarction in the region of the left middle cerebral artery distribution, specifically in the inferior left frontal lobe sparing part of the 3rd frontal convolution but extending into the inferior parietal region and superior temporal region. After two days, Dr. Exeter became aware of his surroundings and was able to recognize hospital staff and family.

While in acute care, he was evaluated briefly by Patricia Burns, speech-language pathologist, who determined that Dr. Exeter has a severe aphasia, mild dysarthria, and no swallowing difficulties. He was able to answer a few simple questions, but was still in an acute confusional state at the time of evaluation. He was able to gesture most basic needs, and by the fourth day was able to produce a few words communicatively. It was recommended that he be transferred to the Rehabilitation Unit for further evaluation and determination of post-acute rehabilitation needs.

Subjective Observation

During initial interview, Dr. Exeter was attentive and cooperative. Normal conversation was overwhelming, but he understood simple instructions. He was still limited in verbal expression. He became somewhat agitated when he could not express himself.

Objective Language Evaluation

Dr. Exeter was given selected portions of the Boston Diagnostic Aphasia Examination to evaluate auditory-oral language abilities:

In auditory comprehension, he scored 64/72 for word comprehension, 10/15 for following commands, and 5/12 for answering questions about short paragraphs. Body part identification was not administered. In general, he had difficulty with the most complex material.

In verbal expression, he described the Cookie Theft picture producing six nouns, one verb, and one 2-word phrase that were appropriate. He scored 84/114 for picture naming and 20/30 for answering simple questions with one word. He was able to repeat short common words. He scored 4/16 in repetition of short phrases and sentences, a task that elicited more language than he could produce spontaneously.

Conclusions

Dr. Exeter has some functional comprehension and limited agrammatic verbal production. He can communicate most basic needs. His speech and test results conform to a pattern of severe but still evolving Broca's aphasia. Apraxia of speech is evident when repeating complex words and sentences. This diagnosis is consistent with site of lesion and accompanying hemiparesis. While individuals with this type of aphasia often make excellent progress, it is too soon to predict Dr. Exeter's outcome. However, his rapidly improving comprehension, relatively young age and good health, and motivation are all positive signs that he can progress a substantial degree.

Recommendations

(1) Dr. Exeter should receive language treatment to improve auditory comprehension, word-finding efficiency, and phrase length.

(2) Reading and writing abilities should be evaluated, especially because these skills are important to him with respect to his professional interests.

(3) The speech-language pathologist should meet with family members to answer questions and introduce them to the rehabilitation process.

FIGURE 3.4 Summary of Martin Exeter's initial speech and language evaluation in the Rehabilitation Unit.

SUMMARY AND CONCLUSIONS

Three comprehensive batteries reviewed in this chapter were introduced in a span of 15 years, between 1967 and 1982. Table 3.11 provides a historical perspective on most of the tests introduced here, especially in their relationship to other developments in clinical aphasiology. The motivation for developing new tests is likely to come from at least two sources, namely, changes in health care management and discoveries about the nature of aphasia that make a difference in rehabilitation.

Insurance companies do not tell SLPs to take 30 minutes for evaluation. Instead, time for evaluation is prioritized given a limit on the number of sessions that will be reimbursed. Clinicians have had to re-evaluate what is minimally needed to classify a patient for reimbursement and get therapy started. Fundamental diagnoses can be accomplished in an informal evaluation. Tests become important for documentation of deficit and setting baselines from which to measure progress. Time consuming reading and writing tests are not necessary to distinguish speech and language disorders and to identify language problems vital to everyday communication.

Beyond the initial evaluation, "diagnostic therapy" mines more useful discoveries about a patient as clinical interaction moves on. Refinements of diagnosis can be a problem-solving component of the treatment process.

TABLE 3.11   A chronology of assessments along with certain clinical developments.

DECADE	TESTS	CLINICAL THEORY AND RESEARCH
pre-1940s	Head's serial tests for aphasia IQ tests for neuropsychology	• Case studies to prove localization theories • Weisenberg and McBride's clinical studies
1940s	Schuell starts MTDDA	
1950s	Eisenson's test Research edition of MTDDA	• Wepman's central-transmission distinction
1960s	Token Test PICA	• Porch's test-based statistical prognosis
1970s	BDAE	• Lesion localization of syndromes • Wertz questions PICA-based prognosis
1980s	WAB Functional measures (Chapter 6)	• Wertz questions test-based classification • Model-based cognitive neuropsychology • Functional communication
1990s	PALPA BEST-2	• Managed care

MATCHING REVIEW_____

Match each familiar test abbreviation with one of its main features.

___ 1. MTDDA	a. bedside screening
___ 2. PICA	b. a test for auditory comprehension
___ 3. BDAE-3	c. reading for aphasia
___ 4. WAB	d. Schuell's long test
___ 5. PALPA	e. battery published with a Short Form
___ 6. ADP	f. the AQ
___ 7. BEST-2	g. first use of multidimensional scoring
___ 8. RTT	h. a syndrome diagnosis in 40 minutes
___ 9. RCBA	i. incorporated into a full battery
___ 10. BNT	j. looks for impaired cognitive modules

CHAPTER 4

INVESTIGATING APHASIA IN GENERAL

As a psychologist at the university, Martin Exeter's specialty was cognitive psychology. Long ago he learned that if he told people only that he was a psychologist, they would seek his help for emotional problems or make a joke about it. Experimental psychology is different. He enjoyed thinking scientifically and testing theories of the mind in the laboratory. His research dealt with language comprehension, and for most of his career he had not realized that psycholinguistic processes were a clinical concern. While preparing for his lecture in Europe, he was beginning to learn a little about aphasia.

The next few chapters deal with how discoveries are made about the underlying nature of acquired language disorders. The present chapter focuses on deficits that are common to most people with aphasia, especially problems of comprehension and word finding. Clinical implications are as follows:

- development of new supplemental assessments and measurement strategies
- new insights about language disorder that may focus treatment strategies

As part of the scientific foundation for clinical studies of word-level processing, we shall pay more attention to the automatic level of processing and the activation of stored information in lexical and semantic systems.

BASIC RESEARCH IN CLINICAL APHASIOLOGY

Clinicians support their beliefs about clinical practice (e.g., diagnosis) with personal experience, expert opinion, and experimental research.

Research can expand our viewpoint from personal experience but sometimes does not support expert opinion. Speech-language clinicians rely on a basic understanding of research to evaluate experimentally supported clinical claims. Three general topics in this section include styles of research, experimental design, and the influence of disciplines on the study of language disorder.

Data-Driven and Theory-Driven Research

There are two approaches to observing the effects of stimulus manipulations on responses, namely, data-driven and theory-driven approaches. To say that something "drives" a study is to state the primary motivation and background for designing an experiment.

Brookshire (1983) stated that the goal of research is "to demonstrate that manipulation of certain (independent) variables under controlled conditions affects other (dependent) variables in predictable ways" (p. 342). This turns out to be the goal of data-driven or empirical research. The following are examples of empirical questions:

- What is the effect of utterance complexity on pointing to pictures?
- What type of errors does a patient make in an object-naming task?

A theoretical interpretation is sometimes added after the presentation of an empirical study. This is called *post hoc analysis*. For example, an investigator may report finding more errors for more complex utterances when pointing to pictures and may speculate that the finding supports a theory of syntactic-processing impairment. This type of post hoc analysis is risky, because the method may not have been the best one for testing the proposed theory.

In a comment on data-driven studies of aphasic comprehension, Tyler (1988) suggested that "researchers have, on the whole, been primarily interested in whether a patient (or group of patients) has difficulty with particular types of linguistic information, but they rarely attempt to locate the source of the difficulty in a particular aspect of the comprehension process" (p. 376). In theory-driven research, a researcher uses a theory of mechanisms between a stimulus and response in order to arrange appropriate stimulus–response pairings and predict the effects.

Predictions establish a foundation for testing the validity of a theory. The author of a publication explains how a theory generated the experimental design and how results can be interpreted accordingly. Obtaining data becomes a means to an end, rather than an end itself. A theoretical account contributes to the **internal validity** of a study or whether we can establish a causal relationship between internal events and responses.

A rough example of a theory-driven study would be one intended to explain a patient's word-reading difficulty. Let us suppose that a researcher believes the impairment to exist in a grapheme–phoneme conversion process. This assumption motivates the researcher to look for sound-related errors in reading aloud (e.g., reading *ship* as "chip" instead of as "boat") and to present a task of reading aloud nonwords (e.g., *bemp*) that is dependent on grapheme–phoneme conversion. In this manner, the theory determines the method and guides interpretation of results.

Empirically speaking, we ask whether a response pattern can be related to characteristics of a stimulus. Theoretically speaking, we ask whether a response pattern can be attributed to an hypothesized hidden condition or process.

Clinical Research Designs

Any study consists of at least one comparison, such as comparing two patients with a particular procedure or comparing two procedures with one patient. This is similar to clinical diagnosis, in which we compare a patient's test score to a normal score. Also, we compare a patient's performances on numerous tasks to discern a common thread among the different scores.

In research, deficient or intact skills are identified with a between-group design when one group of participants is neurologically intact (Table 4.1). A comparison between brain-damaged and neurologically intact groups is less straightforward than a comparison between two neurologically intact groups. Two normal groups are expected

TABLE 4.1   Basic experimental designs and the empirical questions they answer.

DESIGN	COMPARISON	BASIC QUESTIONS	EXAMPLES
Between-group	Brain-damaged vs. neurologically intact	What deficits are caused by brain damage?	Trauma patients vs. normal participants
	Brain-damaged vs. brain-damaged	What behaviors can be linked to a specific neuropathology or site of lesion?	Anterior vs. posterior infarct
Within-group	Task A vs. task B	Is there a pattern of retained and impaired language abilities in an aphasic patient?	Comprehending words vs. naming objects
	Item A vs. item B	Can a patient have problems finding some words but not others?	Abstract vs. concrete words

to be alike in every respect except for the variable being studied. This assumption underlies use of the traditional t-test for comparing the average scores of two groups. However, this assumption does not usually apply when one group has brain damage (see Clark and Ryan, 1993; Duffy and Myers, 1991). Group description has improved over the years, increasing our confidence that two groups are homogeneous except for the variable being studied (Obler, Goral, and Albert, 1995).

A within-group design is employed for learning as much as we can about one group or a single case. An investigator may want to discover a unique pattern of performance among tasks or among items within a task. A single case is often examined when an investigator wants to use a large number of tasks to answer a very specific question. A group is preferred in order to increase the likelihood that results can be applied to a population. In either type of study, an informative participant description helps us determine the **external validity** or generalizability of findings to other patients (Brookshire, 1983).

Interdisciplinary Influences

Like other domains of communicative disorders, aphasiology draws upon basic sciences for frameworks about language functions and methods for studying them. Aphasiologists have varying experience with these sciences. A speech-language pathologist may have been mentored primarily in speech science, neurology, linguistics, or cognitive psychology.

Human language function is studied in two intimately related fields. **Linguistics** is the study of the structure of language (e.g., Akmajian, Demers, Farmer, and Harnish, 2001). Linguistic research is the logical examination of words and sentences. In the 1960s, linguists and experimental psychologists began to work together, forming the discipline of **psycholinguistics.** The data of psycholinguistics comes from people processing words and sentences in a laboratory (e.g., Gernsbacher, 1999). The initial question was whether linguistic theories have "psychological reality" for representing human knowledge.

Cognitive neuropsychology (CN) also has the goal of developing theories of normal language processing. CN is distinctive because it relies on brain-damaged participants, but it is divided between two approaches. In one, investigators study aphasia at word and sentence levels with psycholinguistic methods generally applied to groups of patients (e.g., Zurif, Gardner, and Brownell, 1989). Psycholinguists become interested in aphasia in order to extend the range of observations that bear on language systems (Dell, Schwartz, Martin et al., 1997). In the other approach to CN, investigators rely solely on single cases to test models of functions primarily at the single-word level (e.g., Rapp, 2001).

The literature contains numerous illuminating arguments among linguists, psychologists, and others over the best approach for answering questions about disordered language functions. Grodzinsky, Caplan, and Caramazza have debated procedural and statistical methodology for answering questions about deficits of sentence comprehension (e.g., Caplan, 2002; Caramazza, Capitani, Rey, and Berndt, 2001; Grodzinsky, Piñango, Zurif, and Drai, 1999). One argument has pitted advocates of participant groups against advocates of single case studies. Disagreement seems to be most contentious when the purpose of the research is to study relationships between function and brain location. Thinking of the case study approach, Harley (2004a) asked "Does cognitive neuropsychology have a future?" (p. 3). This question elicited some staunch defenses of CN (e.g., McCloskey, 2004). The aphasia laboratory is like a kitchen crowded with many chefs, each advocating a favorite approach to the study of behavior, the brain, and cognition (Table 4.2).

WORD PROCESSING

The clinical test of word comprehension is to present a word auditorily or visually and have a patient point to a picture. Nearly all aphasic patients have

TABLE 4.2   Disciplines that provide clinical investigators with experimental paradigms for the study of language impairments.

DISCIPLINE	ORIGIN	DOMAIN	PRINCIPAL METHOD
Linguistics		Form and structure of language	Logical analysis of sounds, words, and sentences
Behavioral psychology	Experimental psychology	Stimulus-response relationships	Learning experiments; empirical research
Cognitive psychology	Experimental psychology	Mental representations and processes in cognition	Group studies of task accuracy and response time
Psycholinguistics	Cognitive psychology	Mental representation and processes in language functions	Group studies of task accuracy and response time
Clinical neuropsychology	Clinical psychology	Cognitive dysfunctions caused by brain damage	Group studies of standardized test performance
Cognitive neuropsychology	Cognitive psychology	Mental representation and processes in cognition (including language)	Case studies of brain-damaged persons; many tasks presented

difficulty comprehending language at some level, but many do not have problems understanding single words. About 45 percent of aphasic subjects make no errors or are within normal range in a picture-pointing task (Schuell and Jenkins, 1961; Varney, 1984). A substantial deficit with individual words indicates severe receptive disorder.

If we are to understand comprehension disorder in cognitive terms, we should consider what happens mentally in a clinical word-comprehension task. Initially, the mind represents the stimulus, and the representation undergoes different levels of processing, shown in Table 4.3. The goal of accessing meaning can be impeded because of a problem early in the process. An elderly aphasic person could have hearing loss or a visual impairment that existed prior to stroke. To prevent these problems from interfering with assessing comprehension, we should make sure that such patients are wearing hearing aids or glasses.

Speech Perception

Perception results in the mental representation of a stimulus, called a **percept.** Investigators have

explored the possibility that aphasic people have a problem forming a percept of the speech signal, which might explain some comprehension deficits. Speech perception is assessed two ways:

- *discrimination* in which subjects make same–different judgments regarding CV-syllable pairs (e.g., /pa/, /ba/) or nonsense word pairs (e.g., *ursit, ursat*)
- *identification,* or "labeling," in which a patient points to a letter for the phoneme

Discrimination is easier for aphasic people, and labeling errors may be caused by a language deficit instead of a speech perception problem (Blumstein, Tartter, Nigro, and Statlender, 1984; Riedel and Studdert-Kennedy, 1985). Most aphasic patients are within normal range for discrimination. Most of those with a deficit improve to normal perception within four months after a stroke (Franklin, 1989; Varney, 1984). For others, deficits are stable over the first year (Gow and Caplan, 1996).

Is the speed of syllable production too fast for some aphasic listeners? In early studies, aphasic subjects perceived the order of two sounds only

TABLE 4.3   Functional levels of word processing beginning with sensation and concluding with comprehension.

FUNCTIONAL LEVELS	SUBJECTIVE EXPERIENCE	PROCESS	ASSESSMENT
Sensation	*I hear something.*	Initial detection of acoustic signal from the environment	Audiometric tests
Perception	*I hear the sound /metaphysics/.*	Mental representation of a lexical stimulus, called a percept	Discrimination; identification
Recognition	*It sounds like a word. I've heard that word before.*	Activation of word in lexical memory (match percept to lexical representation)	Word naming; lexical decision
Comprehension	*I know what that word means.*	Activation of concept in semantic memory (match lexical representation to concept)	Point to picture

when there was enough time between them. Normal intervals were too quick (Swisher and Hirsch, 1972; Van Allen, Benton, and Gordon, 1966). However, Riedel and Studdert-Kennedy (1985) found no support for the strong theory that the main deficit in aphasia is a problem with perceiving rapid auditory stimuli.

Sheila Blumstein at Brown University and Shari Baum at McGill University have been studying speech perception with aphasia for a couple of decades (e.g., Blumstein, Burton, Baum et al., 1994). They have compared nonfluent and fluent aphasias with respect to the influence of lexical knowledge on the perception of individual consonants. Is perception more accurate when a sound occurs in a word than in a nonword? Generally, aphasic patients have demonstrated a **lexical effect** in which perception was better with words than nonwords. This effect has been stronger or more consistent with nonfluent aphasia. A semantic bias in a sentence context also supported phoneme perception. Baum (2001) concluded that people with nonfluent aphasia rely on lexical and semantic information more than people with fluent aphasia, to compensate for any perceptual problems they might have.

Word Recognition

Hearing a word like *metaphysics* may induce a sense of recognition but not full comprehension. Recognizing something means that we have had some prior experience with an object or word and that a representation of this experience was stored somewhere. Recognition occurs when we match a percept to the stored representation. If we saw an object just a few seconds ago, then the stored representation may be active in working memory. However, usually we recognize people, places, and things with reference to a representation stored long ago in long-term memory. For recognizing common objects, we activate concepts stored in semantic memory. For recognizing words, we activate the lexicon stored in lexical memory.

Because word recognition requires contact with the mental lexicon, recognition tasks are employed to study lexical memory. As indicated in Chapter 1, our mental lexicon contains what we know about words. This includes what a word sounds like (phonology) and looks like (orthography). We may think about our knowledge of a word's form when we read a foreign word and realize we do not know its pronunciation or when we realize that there are words we use but do not know how to spell. Word form is represented as what is called a **lexeme.** Knowledge of words also includes their grammatical categories, such as knowing that *bank* can be a noun or a verb. Grammatical knowledge is called a **lemma** (Bock and Levelt, 1994).

The recognition tasks used to study access to the lexicon are "fast tasks." A **lexical decision task** (LDT) is usually used with aphasic patients. Most studies of normal adults employ visual word presentation. Usually a string of letters (e.g., BOOK or CHOT) is shown on a computer until a subject presses a YES or NO button indicating if the string is a word. The nonword is a structurally possible word, but researchers are mainly interested in response to the real word. It normally takes just over half a second (600 milliseconds) to respond to common words (Forster and Chambers, 1973). In one study, aphasic subjects were as fast as normal controls and, also like the controls, responded faster to common words than rare words (Gerratt and Jones, 1987). The results indicated that aphasic people are able to match the percept of a stimulus to a lexeme.

The instant of recognition is quicker than 600 milliseconds (msec). Psycholinguists want to locate the instant of matching a percept to a lexeme within this time frame. The goal is to determine what happens in the so-called *prelexical* period up to activating the stored lexeme. Afterward, response time is consumed by a *postlexical* phase involving at least the motor processes for pressing the button. Various experiments supported an estimate that lexical access normally occurs within 100 to 300 msec after stimulus presentation (Mc-Crae, Jared, and Seidenberg, 1990).

A **lexical priming task** focuses on the first 300 msec. In this paradigm, pairs of words are presented, one after the other. A **prime** (e.g., LOOK) is presented prior to the test word, now called the **target** (e.g., BOOK). Subjects listen to or look at the prime. They make the usual lexical decision response only to the target. Investigators are particularly interested in *subconscious response to the prime, which can be inferred from the prime's influence on the target.* A **priming ef-**

fect is indicated by a faster response for related prime–target pairs (e.g., LOOK-BOOK) than for unrelated pairs such as RAISE-BOOK. The prime is assumed to activate lexical neighbors in a network so a related target is "primed" for access. In studies of neurologically intact adults, an interval much less than 300 msec is placed between the prime and target so that fast prelexical automatic activation can be studied.

The word pair LOOK-BOOK is related phonologically or orthographically. An effect of this relationship is called **form priming.** Baum directed studies in which she presented such prime–target pairs auditorily. She manipulated the *interstimulus interval* (ISI), which is between the end, or offset, of the prime and the onset of the target. She found form priming in fluent and nonfluent aphasic subjects at a short interstimulus interval of 250 msec (Leonard and Baum, 1997). These results indicate that aphasic persons can activate related "lexical candidates" in less than 300 msec.

Word Comprehension

Word comprehension is viewed simply as attaching a meaning to a word. Meaning, in particular, is an important component of language processing, and it is considered to be stored as semantic memory. So, let us first come to an understanding of semantic memory, and then we will consider its role in word comprehension.

Semantic memory contains our information about the world. Its core is universal in the sense that most people have the same basic knowledge of living and nonliving things. Fringes of world knowledge vary according to locale, culture, and expertise. Psychologists are most interested in *natural* universal knowledge or, namely, how it is really stored in our heads (with "imperfections").

If our stored knowledge were to contain every object that we ever encountered, we might have difficulty recognizing new or unusual versions of common objects. Instead, semantic memory stores concepts. A **concept** is the simplest unit of world knowledge and may be defined as the mental representation of a class of objects or actions.

Concepts are stored separately from words. For this text, a concept will be represented in brackets. The concept [hat] may be a universal element of knowledge, but the word for it varies from language to language and is stored in lexical memory (e.g., *chapeau, cappello, hoed,* or *hat*).

Investigators agree that concepts are organized in some way. The prevailing view in psycholinguistics is that our knowledge store takes the form of a **semantic network.** In the spatial metaphor used to characterize this network, a concept is represented as a **node** connected to other nodes. A streamlined example is shown in Figure 4.1. A network permits a general category like [vehicle] or a general attribute like [red] to be recorded once. A network depicts the relatedness

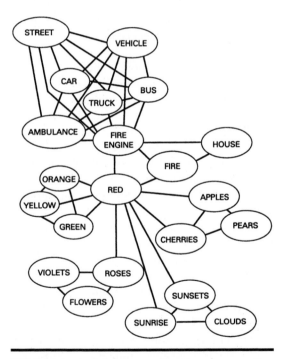

FIGURE 4.1 A simple semantic network suggestive of semantic relatedness or "distance" between concepts.

Reprinted by permission from Collins, A. M., & Loftus, E. F., A spreading-activation theory of semantic processing. *Psychological Bulletin, 82,* 1975, p. 412. American Psychology Association, publisher.

among concepts according to a distance metaphor. Related concepts are close together, like "neighbors" in the network, and less related concepts are more distant from each other. Relative distances between concepts lead to predictions of processing times from one node to another.

A clinical evaluation of conceptual knowledge is to have patients match or sort *objects* (not words) according to common categories. Some aphasic patients are normal when sorting objects into semantic categories (Milton, Wertz, Katz, and Prutting, 1981), but many others exhibit deficits and do worse than persons with right hemisphere damage (Gainotti, Carlomagno, Craca, and Silveri, 1986; Grossman and Wilson, 1987). Thus, there may be subtle changes in semantic memory for some persons with aphasia.

As mentioned earlier, the *clinical* examination of word comprehension has consisted of "slow tasks" in which a patient takes time pointing to an object in an array of pictures. With this task, researchers have tried to isolate the central disorder by using pictures for words that are phonologically or semantically related to the correct choice (Gainotti, Caltagirone, and Ibba, 1975). Aphasic people made more semantic errors than phonological errors. When foils were varied according to semantic relatedness, errors tended to be the picture most related to the correct one (Pizzamiglio and Appiciafuoco, 1971). These results indicate that aphasic word comprehension disorder lies in lexical-semantic relationships as opposed to phonological encoding.

In clinical studies, lexical-semantic structure is commonly studied with **word sorting** and other metalinguistic tasks. Patients group words on their own or according to categories stated by an examiner. When sorting words into requested categories, nonfluent and fluent groups have exhibited knowledge of categorical and functional organization (McCleary, 1988). In one study, a group of aphasic patients was able to match "high importance" attributes to a noun (e.g., *wings* to *bird*) but were deficient in matching "low importance" attributes (e.g., *sings* to *bird*) (Germani and Pierce, 1995). When deficits appear, they usually occur in posteriorly damaged fluent aphasias (e.g., McCleary and Hirst, 1986). Investigators started wondering if fluent aphasias are uniquely deficient in the lexical-semantic system.

To determine if a deficit in semantic or lexical-semantic knowledge contributes to a word comprehension deficit, studies include a comparison between a word comprehension task and a meta-linguistic semantic task with words or objects. In one study, 8 of 16 aphasic patients were identified as having deficient word comprehension (Chertkow, Bub, Deaudon, and Whitehead, 1997). Three of these 8 were "nonverbally preserved" according to a task involving objects, whereas five were diagnosed as being "nonverbally impaired." Thus, a clinically measured conceptual deficit may or may not accompany word comprehension problems.

Let us return to the picture choice task for a moment. Breese and Hillis (2004) compared this task with a rarely used word/picture verification task in which the patient decides whether a single picture is a match to the clinician's spoken word. About half of their 122 aphasic participants performed normally on both tasks. Of the others, nearly 80 percent performed worse with the verification task. Therefore, the verification task was significantly more likely to diagnose a word comprehension problem. This is one of many examples of task-dependent performance regarding a particular function and is suggestive of a clinical strategy in which a function should be assessed in different ways. The psycholinguistic function of comprehension ends in a person's head, and assessment tasks add other dimensions leading to a correct response. Verification could be more about making true/false decisions than about activating a meaning upon hearing a word.

When we hear or see a word like *bank,* we arrive at a meaning without cognitive effort. We have no mechanism for keeping comprehension from happening. Again, the process ends in our heads. The challenge for research is to establish a method that addresses this process with minimal interference from irrelevant processes. Arriving at such a method involves thinking about what word comprehension entails. To this end,

it is helpful to think of meaning as a conceptual structure in semantic memory. Researchers propose that word comprehension is an activation of a concept node in this network. Like the activation of a neuron, the activation of one node is likely to spread automatically to nearby semantically related nodes, a phenomenon known as **spreading activation.**

Automatic meaning activation is studied with a semantic priming task. In this task, a prime such as *bank* precedes a lexical decision target such as *money*. The decision is usually faster with a semantically related prime than with an unrelated prime (e.g., *baby*). This difference is called the **semantic priming effect.** The prime *bank* is presumed to activate nodes in its conceptual neighborhood, so that it is likely that the related target is active before it is presented. With an unrelated prime, it can be said that a subject's mind is somewhere else when the target is presented (e.g., in an area about babies).

Visual stimuli are more common than auditory stimuli in priming studies with neurologically intact adults. The interval between prime–target pairs is slightly different with visual stimuli and is called the *stimulus onset asynchrony* (SOA). The SOA is the time between onset of a visual prime (instead of offset) and the onset of a visual target. Semantic priming in normal adults can occur with as little as 16 msec SOA (Simpson and Burgess, 1985).

In aphasiology, early studies of semantic priming contained long intervals such as 500 msec (Blumstein, Milberg, and Shrier, 1982). Chenery, Ingram, and Murdoch (1990) compared groups of high- and low-comprehending subjects. Both groups showed semantic priming despite being impaired in a slow metalinguistic task of semantic judgments about word pairs. Baum (1997) found semantic priming to be consistent in nonfluent subjects but inconsistent in fluent subjects. Because of the long prime–target intervals, these studies could not determine if spreading activation in semantic memory is as rapid in aphasia as it is when the brain is neurologically intact. Nevertheless, the capacity for activation of concepts demonstrated that clinical tasks of word sorting tend to overestimate the extent to which a patient is impaired, probably because word sorting requires effortful decision making (Tyler and Moss, 1997).

A semantically ambiguous prime, such as *bank,* presents an opportunity to examine the possible activation of multiple concepts. If an isolated word automatically activates multiple meanings, then an ambiguous prime like *fan* should prime either *breeze* or *sport* as a target. In one study, patients with nonfluent aphasia had a priming effect for such ambiguous words with only a 100 msec interstimulus interval (ISI). Multiple-meaning activation occurred as quickly as it did in controls without neuropathology (Klepousniotou and Baum, 2005).

A more challenging method for examining ambiguous word comprehension is the use of word triplets, such as *coin-bank-money,* in which the middle position contains the ambiguity (Copland, Chenery, and Murdoch, 2002). In this task, researchers can examine the effect of a context on an ambiguous prime. The third word is still a target, which is preceded by two words occurring in sequence. To anticipate the processing of *coin-bank-money,* we should imagine the first word's activation of concepts (i.e., money related) and then the second word's activation (i.e., money related). The target should clearly be preactivated in this concordant condition. Now, let us consider a discordant condition in which the first word represents a meaning inconsistent with the target (e.g., *river-bank-money*). If multiple activation is automatic (i.e., in 100 msec), then *bank* should still activate helpful money-related concepts in addition to river-related concepts. If contextually irrelevant concepts are suppressed over time (i.e., given 1000 msec after the prime), then money-related concepts will no longer be active when *bank* is preceded by *river.*

Copland and his colleagues (2002) employed ISIs of 100 and 1250 msec with nine aphasic individuals. Like normal controls at the short interval, aphasic participants were primed when words like *bank* preceded targets like *money* no matter

what the first word was. This result indicates that aphasic individuals automatically activated multiple meanings when they heard an ambiguous word. When given more time between words, the normal controls were not primed in the discordant condition. That is, they had time to suppress irrelevant meanings of *bank.* The aphasic participants, however, continued to be primed in the discordant condition, indicating that they were slow or unable to use context to suppress alternative meanings of the ambiguous second prime. This failure to suppress alternatives has recently been hypothesized with respect to other locations of brain damage, as when a stroke occurs in the right hemisphere (see Chapter 11).

SENTENCE COMPREHENSION

When comprehension is tested with stimuli much longer than a single word, the impression is that all cases of aphasia have a comprehension deficit to some degree. Sentence comprehension is clinically assessed several ways. Patients choose a picture from a set, follow instructions with objects or tokens, answer yes/no questions, and verify the truth of a sentence relative to a picture. This section on sentence comprehension deals with this type of clinical evaluation and the manipulation of linguistic variables such as structural complexity, agent–object reversibility, and canonicity. Automatic sentence processing is discussed in the following chapter.

Structural Complexity

Clinical researchers are interested in general factors such as sentence length and complexity. Increasing the length of sentences can make them harder for aphasic people to comprehend. However, the effect of length is not straightforward. Longer sentences can also be easier. For example, *Which one is the knife?* is easier to understand when information is added: *Which one is the knife that cuts?* (Clark and Flowers, 1987; also, Gardner, Denes, and Weintraub, 1975; Pierce and

Beekman, 1985). Length sometimes adds facilitative informational redundancy.

For mildly impaired aphasic patients, comprehension difficulty may not show up until sentences are both long and complex. The Token Test reveals deficit in over 90 percent of aphasic patients (DeRenzi, 1979). In focusing on the role of syntax, researchers tested the hypothesis that aphasic persons comprehend sentences of the same length differently because of structural differences. In one study, Token Test commands were adjusted in order to examine syntactic complexity while controlling for length (i.e., 1b and 2b are each more complex than 1a and 2a):

(1a) Touch the red circle.
(1b) Touch each yellow circle.
(2a) Touch the small blue circle and the small red circle.
(2b) Before you touch the green square, touch the white circle.

Complexity reduced comprehension of short sentences. However, besides being more complex syntactically, 1b also requires more visual scanning of tokens. Similarly, structurally less complex 2a has a more complex response than 2b, indicating that mode of response in a task may obscure possible effects of linguistic variables (Curtiss, Jackson, Kempler et al., 1986).

The influence of early psycholinguistics can be seen when structural complexity was defined systematically according to linguistic theory. Shewan and Canter (1971) focused on passive and negative sentences. Three levels of syntactic complexity were identified according to number of transformations that were thought to modify basic subject-verb-object order (3a). The next structural level contained a single change that was either a passive or negative transformation (3b), and the third contained two transformations (3c).

(3a) The girl is reading a book.
(3b) The dogs are not chasing cats.
(3c) The milk was not drunk by her.

This comparison set the foundation for developing a clinical test called the **Auditory Com-**prehension Test for Sentences** or ACTS (Shewan, 1979). The ACTS contains 21 test sentences. Each sentence is read to a patient, who responds by pointing to one of four pictures. Three picture foils are based on systematic changes in the test sentence to facilitate error analysis. It takes about 15 minutes to determine effects of word familiarity, length, and syntax. A maximum score of 21 is based on number of correct responses, and error analysis identifies position of error in the sentence (i.e., first or second half) and grammatical category of error (i.e., primarily nouns or verbs).

Early studies addressed a very general question of whether aphasic patients have a quantitative or qualitative difference from normal comprehension. A quantitative deficit is indicated by more errors than a normal group. A qualitative deficit is suggested by an order of structural difficulty that differs from normal adults. The findings were that aphasic patients differ from normal in number of errors and response speed but do not differ according to order of difficulty (e.g., Shewan and Canter, 1971). This led to the conclusion that aphasic comprehension is an inefficient normal mechanism rather than a processing anomaly that does not occur in a normal language system.

Complexity is also increased by adding a subordinate clause to a main clause. Despite the fact that 4a is longer than 4b, 4a is structurally simpler than 4b, which has a center-embedded clause. The longer sentence is generally easier for aphasic people to understand (Goodglass, Blumstein, Gleason et al., 1979).

(4a) The man was greeted by his wife, and he was smoking his pipe.
(4b) The man greeted by his wife was smoking a pipe.

Butler-Hinz, Caplan, and Waters (1990) found a similar result. However, when verifying sentences with embedded clauses against a picture, four moderate to severe aphasic patientts demonstrated an ability to comprehend (Ni, Shankweiler, Harris, and Fulbright, 1997). These apparently conflicting results indicate that the demonstration of a comprehension deficit may be partly a function of the task and not the structure per se.

Word Order and Thematic Roles

When testing comprehension of single nouns, a patient does not have to detect a functional role for that noun. However, comprehending simple declarative statements entails figuring out who is doing what to whom. In a sentence, a noun becomes an agent or recipient of an action, an instrument, or a location. In linguistic terms, this means figuring out the thematic roles played by the nouns in sentences like 5a.

(5a) The nurse kissed the girl.
(5b) The girl drank the milk.

The order of nouns around a verb is one clue to their thematic roles. To assess the ability to capitalize on word order, clinical researchers employ **reversible sentences** in which the agent and recipient can be switched while preserving common sense. With respect to 5a, agent–recipient order is the only difference between related pictured options (e.g., *The girl kissed the nurse* or *The nurse kissed the girl*).

For aphasic patients, reversible sentences like 5a are more difficult to understand than nonreversible statements like 5b (Heeschen, 1980). In nonreversible statements, a semantic clue or constraint appears to be helpful. That is, the reversed option is implausible (i.e., milk cannot drink). Without such semantic aids, word location becomes paramount for understanding reversible sentences. The **reversibility effect** has become a central finding in studies of aphasic sentence comprehension, especially in the study of Broca's aphasia (see Chapter 5).

A patient may get a good score for nonreversible sentences merely by rejecting the absurdity of an implausible option instead of engaging in good syntactic processing. **Plausibility** may be a factor in reversible statements like 6b, in which the event is theoretically possible but unlikely, if not absurd.

(6a) The policeman arrests the thief.
(6b) The thief arrests the policeman.
(7) The woman greeting her husband was smoking a pipe.

Aphasic patients find comprehension easier when sentences correspond to their world (6a) than when sentences represent implausible events (6b) (Deloche and Seron, 1981; Heilman and Scholes, 1976; Heeschen, 1980; Kudo, 1984). In one study, plausibility did not matter when sentences like 4b became simply less probable, as in 7, according to Goodglass and others (1979). Many aphasic individuals seem able to use their knowledge of the world to facilitate sentence comprehension.

Similar to Breese and Hillis's (2004) study of word comprehension tasks, Mitchum, Haendiges, and Berndt (2004) showed that the task may or may not influence the ability to demonstrate sentence comprehension ability. Semantically reversible sentences were tested with two aphasic individuals using picture choice and sentence–picture verification tasks. One participant was better with picture choice, revealing a tendency to respond yes in the verification task, as if not paying attention to the stimuli or the task. The other participant had a tendency to treat the first noun as an agent for active and passive sentences in both tasks.

Canonicity

Early research determined that reversible passives like *The girl is kissed by the nurse* are harder for aphasic people to comprehend than reversible actives like 5a (e.g., Pierce and Wagner, 1985; Shewan and Canter, 1971). The problem with passives is often attributed to word order, because thematic roles are reversed from straight-shooting, active statements. The agent-action-recipient sequence in actives is known as the most typical or *canonical order* for thematic roles in English. Investigators wondered if difficulty with the passive exception is the tip of an iceberg, because there are other structural exceptions to canonical order.

Researchers have fiddled with sentences to determine whether aphasic difficulty can be attributed to the more general canonicity and not just to the passive exception. One trick is to create reversible clefted sentences such as 8a and 8b.

(8a) It was the woman that shot the man.
(8b) It was the farmer that the painter kicked.

In a study by Ansell and Flowers (1982), mildly aphasic participants had more difficulty with 8b than 8a, even though sentence structure is essentially the same. In fact, the canonical 8a was understood almost without error. Let us call this finding the **canonicity effect.** The key factor seems to be the deviation from canonical order in which, like passives, the recipient of the action is located before the verb and agent.

David Caplan (1987) argued that traditional forms of testing do not permit the study of important syntactic and semantic features. He preferred an **enactment procedure** in which patients manipulate toy animals in response to instructions. More types of errors are possible with this procedure, permitting more specific identification of difficulty. Caplan employed a *Thematic Role Battery* extensively to assess the ability to assign thematic roles to noun phrases in a variety of simple and complex reversible sentences. In one study, 14 structures generated a battery of 168 items (Waters, Caplan, and Hildebrandt, 1991).

Caplan found that patients can understand a variety of syntactic structures but comprehension gets worse as syntactic complexity increases. In particular, sentences preserving the canonical order of English (9a) were easier than deviations from canonical order (9b) (Caplan, Baker, and Dehaut, 1985).

(9a) The elephant hit the monkey that hugged the rabbit.
(9b) The elephant that the monkey hit hugged the rabbit.

In 9b, the recipient of *hit* (elephant) appears before the agent. Except for the most severely impaired, aphasic people use word order to comprehend but have difficulty when a sentence deviates from ca-

nonical order. Complexity effects were replicated with a two-picture choice task, indicating that Caplan's findings are robust across test procedures (Caplan, Waters, and Hildebrandt, 1997).

Caplan and Waters (2003) examined clefted sentences with an unusual procedure that detects increases in processing load within a sentence. Experimental participants heard sentences one segment at a time. When each segment was understood, participants pressed a button signaling presentation of the next segment and so on until the whole sentence was presented. The following shows a canonical subject cleft (10a) and a noncanonical object cleft (10b) with slashes indicating segment boundaries:

(10a) It was / the food / that nourished / the child.
(10b) It was / the woman / that the toy / amazed.

The investigators were interested in the time for reading each segment. The verb took longer than elsewhere in the sentence for object-cleft sentences (10b), but not for subject-cleft sentences (10a). This syntactic effect was consistent with Ansell and Flowers's (1982) finding that mildly aphasic individuals had more difficulty comprehending noncanonical object-cleft sentences. However, Caplan and Waters noted that one aspect of the results suggests an alternative explanation. The verb in (10b) occurs in a location that differs from the verb in (10a). All longer listening times occurred with the last word. This could have been an effect of *wrap-up* processing for final sentence interpretation, which is a phenomenon that may be independent of structure.

EXPLAINING SENTENCE COMPREHENSION DEFICIT

Let us recall Tyler's (1988) comment at the beginning of this chapter in which she wrote about extensive interest in discovering aphasic response to a variety of linguistic variables but little interest in locating the source of difficulty in the comprehension process. Complexity, reversibility, and canonicity effects describe results but do not explain them. That is, we should want to know what happens in the mind to cause these effects, because the disorder is in the patient's brain. Since 1988, interest has been shifting from empirical description to testing theoretical accounts of comprehension patterns.

A Language Disorder

It may seem obvious to suggest that impairment resides somewhere in the language comprehension system. Researchers have tried to uncover language processing problems by manipulating linguistic components of stimuli, such as syntactic or semantic features. Caplan (1987) suggested that "syntactic comprehension impairments are often independent primary disorders of sentence processing" (p. 323), rather than a result of some peripheral or general feature of cognition such as short-term memory. He also concluded that the syntactic processor is not impaired in an all-or-none fashion but rather is impaired partially (also, Caplan, 2002).

However, proposals of a disordered language processing mechanism have been pursued more vigorously in the study of syndromes. Especially in the study of Broca's aphasia (see Chapter 5), investigators have borrowed seriously from psycholinguistic paradigms for examining the obligatory processes of sentence comprehension. The rest of this section deals primarily with explanations of aphasia in general. With this perspective, investigators have turned to peripheral or general features of cognition.

Auditory Processing and Attention

As with words, explaining comprehension deficits begins with mental representation of the auditory stimulus. It was noted earlier that speech perception is not necessarily related to word comprehension deficit, but some still wondered if perception is related to sentence comprehension problems. In a comparison of perception to sentence comprehension, some patients with impaired perception passed a comprehension test, others with good perception had poor sentence comprehension

(Carpenter and Rutherford, 1973). Other researchers found minimal relationship between speech perception and comprehension (Baker, Blumstein, and Goodglass, 1981; Gandour and Dardarananda, 1982; Miceli, Gainotti, Caltagirone, and Masulo, 1980). Shewan (1982) concluded that explanations of language comprehension problems on the basis of perceptual disturbances "are no longer widely accepted" (p. 61).

One general question has been whether the auditory processing system in aphasia is fast enough to handle the normal rate of speech. Comprehension sometimes improves when rate is reduced or when pauses are inserted, indicating that aphasic auditory processing has slowed down (Blumstein, Katz, Goodglass et al., 1985; Poeck and Pietron, 1981). However, two- or five-second pauses did not matter for complex commands in other studies (Hageman and Lewis, 1983; Liles and Brookshire, 1975), and pauses did not help for a picture-pointing task (Blumstein et al., 1985). With the RTT, Brookshire and Nicholas (1984) found inconsistencies with reduced rate and four-second pauses and recommended that "previous reports of the effects of pauses and slow rate upon aphasic listeners' comprehension should be interpreted with caution" (p. 327).

Malcolm McNeil and his colleagues have argued that certain characteristics of aphasic behavior cannot be explained solely with respect to impaired language mechanisms (McNeil and Kimelman, 1986; McNeil, Odell, and Tseng, 1991). One of these characteristics is the variability or inconsistency of language behavior, such as naming an object one moment and not naming the same object a few moments later. McNeil suggested that a possible explanation lies in the influence of a multifaceted attention mechanism on the language system.

Two clinical research teams became interested in McNeil's ideas about aphasic variability. One team studied the effect of divided attention on sustained attention (Erickson, Goldinger, and LaPointe, 1996; LaPointe and Erickson, 1991). These investigators compared performance of an auditory vigilance task alone to performance of the same task in a dual-task condition. In one study, the vigilance task was verbal, involving listening to a series of words. In the other study, the vigilance task contained a series of tones. In both studies, aphasic participants could sustain auditory attention; but, unlike a control group, vigilance was reduced when participants had to sort cards at the same time. Another team also showed that aphasic individuals can differ from normals in attention to auditory stimuli (e.g., Peach, Rubin, and Newhoff, 1994). Thus, an aphasic patient may have some problems with verbal and nonverbal attention, especially under conditions of competing processing demands.

Short-Term Memory

In Chapter 1, short-term memory (STM) was identified as a temporary storage component of working memory. For a long time, it was thought that comprehension depends on a person's **immediate memory span.** Moreover, aphasic patients have had difficulty when asked to repeat a series of numbers or words of increasing length (Albert, 1976; Black and Strub, 1978; Cermak and Moreines, 1976; DeRenzi and Nichelli, 1975; Tanridag, Kirshner, and Casey, 1987). Although this deficit can occur for different reasons, the hypothesis is that a short memory span constricts comprehension for some patients.

Nadine Martin in Communication Sciences at Temple University has investigated the nature of STM measures in assessing aphasia. For example, Martin and Ayala (2004) tested 46 aphasic participants with five span measures: pointing spans for digits and words, repetition spans for digits and words, and pointing spans for blocks. One methodological issue was whether participants should be scored for serial order in addition to number of units recalled. Although Martin and Ayala thought that serial order would have been interesting, they preferred focusing on amount of information retained. Correlations were obtained between the span measures and several tests of word processing. In general, pointing spans for digits and words correlated with both phonologi-

cal and lexical-semantic tasks (i.e., word comprehension), and repetition spans for digits and words correlated only with phonological tests (e.g., phoneme discrimination). The nonverbal span test also correlated with phonological tests, indicating that these tests share general cognitive abilities. The main conclusion was that verbal STM tasks depend on lexical-semantic processing (Martin and Gupta, 2004).

Randi Martin in the Psychology Department at Rice University has been interested in the roles of phonological and semantic encoding in STM and their relationship to auditory sentence comprehension (Martin, 2001). After several studies of individual cases, she concluded that short-term retention of phonological information has little to do with complex sentence comprehension in aphasia. However, Martin and her colleagues "provided evidence that some types of span deficits do cause sentence comprehension difficulties for patients" (Martin and Miller, 2002, p. 305). The deficit pertains to retaining lexical-semantic information. The relationship to sentence comprehension is that aphasic individuals may have difficulty integrating word meanings into sentence-level meaning. One example was when several adjectives preceded a noun (e.g., *the rusty old red pail*). Some patients may not have retained *rusty* in order to connect it to *pail* (also, Martin and He, 2004).

Working Memory and Resource Allocation

The entire cognitive workload is managed in working memory (WM). STM span is one part of WM, namely, the brief retention of very recent input. Working memory includes cognitive work. For example, remembering digits in reverse order requires a mental manipulation beyond simple retention, namely, the reversal of presented digit order. This *digit span backward* test is closer to the spirit of evaluating working memory capacity (Wright and Shisler, 2005). Another way of thinking about workload management is to speak of the **allocation of resources** when performing a task.

Attention helps to manage the resources utilized for any task. **Focused attention** is studied by presenting two different stimuli or tasks and having subjects concentrate on one of them. **Divided attention** is studied with a dual-task paradigm. A participant is asked to perform two tasks at the same time, namely, the main skill being studied and a distractor task. The main task is often one that can be done well. If an aphasic person has a resource allocation deficiency, performance on the main task would be reduced in a dual-task condition when it would not be reduced normally.

There have been several proposals that aphasia includes a reduction of WM capacity. In one approach, investigators demonstrate that aphasic patients are deficient in managing simple concurrent tasks and then speculate that the deficit could be responsible for well-known comprehension problems observed elsewhere (LaPointe and Erickson, 1991; Peach, Rubin, and Newhoff, 1994; Tseng, McNeil, and Milenkovic, 1993).

The proposal also surfaces as an explanation of structural complexity effects across all cases of aphasia. One version is supported by experiments in which a general pattern of aphasic comprehension deficit was simulated with normal adults (Miyake, Carpenter, and Just, 1994). The investigators claimed to have shown how known comprehension deficits can be induced by a reduced WM capacity. A subsequent computer simulation of aphasia was also used to support this claim (Haarmann, Just, and Carpenter, 1997).

Another version of capacity theory came from Caplan and Hildebrandt (1988), who explained syntactic difficulties as a reduction of a resource system *specializing in syntactic processing*. Later, Caplan and Waters (1996) used a dual-task paradigm to test the hypothesis more directly. They selected aphasic patients who performed above average on a sentence–picture matching task and who had a clear complexity effect. Then, while responding to each item in the comprehension test, subjects repeated a sequence of digits within their digit spans. The effect of syntactic complexity was not increased in the dual-task condition, leading Caplan and Waters to conclude

that WM capacity may not be a factor for some patients.

A brief debate over the role of WM in comprehension and aphasia transpired between the Caplan–Waters team (1995; Waters and Caplan, 1996) and the Carpenter–Just group (Just, Carpenter, and Keller, 1996; Miyake, Carpenter, and Just, 1995). Caplan and Waters contended that WM operates with independent system resources including one for syntactic processing, whereas Carpenter and Just claimed that WM operates with a single resource pool. Caplan and Waters (1995) suggested that Carpenter and Just's simulations do not resemble aphasia in important respects. Each research team has stated that the other conducted invalid experiments and misinterpreted the opposition.

Shuster (2004) stimulated a lively debate in *Aphasiology*'s forum over resource allocation theory as it has been studied in aphasiology by McNeil and his colleagues (1991) and others (e.g., LaPointe and Erikson, 1991; Murray, Holland, and Beeson, 1997a). It is a small lesson in common research criticism, and Shuster's concerns were essentially as follows:

- Resource allocation theory is too broad and flexible to be falsifiable (i.e., it can explain any aphasic result).
- Other theories can explain the results used to support resource allocation.
- Methodology has been inappropriate (i.e., task switching instead of the more accepted continuous dual-task approach).
- Dual-task deficits have been found with other cognitive disorders (e.g., Alzheimer's dementia), so that we still need to know what causes the language problems of aphasia.

McNeil, Hula, Matthews, and Doyle (2004) were among the respondants. There was some agreement with the limitations of the dual-task methodology employed in the aphasia research. However, McNeil and his colleagues countered that the other theories cited by Shuster are no better than resource allocation theory. Shuster and Thompson (2004) were not convinced by McNeil's defense, so we should stay tuned for future forays into re-source allocation theory.

Why might aphasic individuals have problems with dividing attention? Murray, Holland, and Beeson (1997a) evaluated two possibilities. One is a reduced sense of effort or perception of task difficulty that might cause a person not to allocate resources in a difficult task. Another possibility is a reduced perception of accuracy (or lack of awareness of errors) that might cause someone to ignore the challenges of a task. Murray's aphasic patients were normal in monitoring their accuracy but had problems perceiving task difficulty after making lexical decisions under single task, selective attention, and divided attention conditions. Thus, aphasic people may not engage allocation strategies because of difficulty anticipating the effort required in certain linguistic processing conditions.

OBJECT NAMING

All aphasic people have some kind of difficulty with word finding, which is most often researched, assessed, and treated with an object-naming task (or "confrontation naming"). Geschwind (1967) wrote that "we are speaking of naming in the narrower sense and not of word-finding in the flow of speech" (p. 97). Object naming places word finding under a microscope in which we can examine mistakes with respect to a clear target. As indicated late in Chapter 3, naming errors may signify a disorder but do not necessarily signify aphasia. Geschwind wrote of aphasic misnaming and non-aphasic misnaming, implying that misnaming may be caused by an impaired language system or by another impairment.

Process Model of Naming

Causes of deficits can be hypothesized according to a process model for the naming task. Process models begin with processing the stimulus and end with the motor response for this task. One researcher proposed what happens in between: "the first step is the identification of the object as a member of a category whose stored representation provides a good match with the stimulus object. . . . Once a category representation has been activated, then the corresponding label is retrieved" (Brownell, Bihrle, and Michelow, 1986, p. 50). This thinking is consistent with the discipline of cognitive neuropsychology (CN).

The CN model of spoken naming in Figure 4.2 consists of independent processing components (in boxes) and the routes between them. This model operates serially, that is, with each process informing the next process, in order from

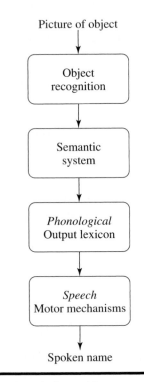

FIGURE 4.2 A typical cognitive neuropsychological (CN) model of object naming. Diagnosis entails determining the impaired component that is responsible for misnaming.

Reprinted by permission from Bruce, C. & Howard, D., Why don't Broca's aphasics cue themselves? An investigation of phoneme cueing and tip of the tongue information. *Neuropsychologia*, 26, 1988, p. 261. Pergamon Press, publisher.

the top down. **Object recognition** activates a concept in the **semantic system,** which then points to the **phonological output lexicon** guiding speech production. For writing, lexical representation is the *orthographic output lexicon.* Cognitive neuropsychologists tend to agree on the existence of a semantic and a lexical component, although terminology may vary slightly (e.g., "conceptual system," "speech output lexicon"). CN models may become a basis for the clinical diagnosis of disorders affecting naming. Such models are the basis for interpreting results of the PALPA (see Chapter 3).

Diagnosis is said to entail looking for location of the "functional lesion" responsible for misnaming. Is it in the semantic system or the phonological output lexicon? Before trying to answer these questions, we should realize that no single task leads to a diagnosis, because, like naming, each task utilizes multiple processes. Similarly, a single error can have different interpretations. Naming errors do not correspond precisely to syndrome diagnosis (LeDorze and Nespoulous, 1989; Mitchum, Ritgert, Sandson, and Berndt, 1990). The strategy in CN called **componential analysis** entails comparing performances on a few tasks (Table 4.4). Like analyzing a test battery, an investigator looks for common threads among deficient and intact performances. The assessment is truly theory driven, in that the investigator selects combinations of tasks that should logically help to determine the status of components in the model.

Semantic Impairment?

Aphasia has been quite broadly diagnosed as involving a lexical-semantic impairment. Now, the central question has become whether the impairment lies in either the semantic system or the lexical system (Nickels, 2001; Raymer, 2005). One challenge has been to tease apart effects of the semantic and lexical systems when designing experiments. Distinguishing a deficient semantic system from deficient lexical access is akin to distinguishing between misnaming due to unfamiliarity with an object and misnaming due to an inability to find the object's name.

A deficient semantic system is thought to send poor conceptual input to the output lexicon. From earlier in this chapter, we should be familiar with findings of intact semantic structure in some aphasic patients but not others. Investigators have found damaged semantic systems in a variety of neurological disorders including Alzheimer's dementia. A few experimental designs are used to see if a naming impairment can be attributed to a deficient semantic system.

One type of experiment is to compare naming errors to word comprehension. For example, Gainotti and his colleagues (1981) made this comparison with different types of aphasic patients.

TABLE 4.4 Differential diagnosis of naming difficulties based on a process model of object naming similar to Figure 4.2. Diagnosis of disorder is suggested with respect to component of principal deficiency.

PROCESS COMPONENT	DISORDER	RELATED TASKS
Object recognition	Visual agnosia	Match examples of an object; demonstrate use of object
Activation of semantic memory	Dementia or aphasia	Object classification; word–picture matching
Activation of lexical memory	Aphasia	Object naming; lexical decision task
Phonetic programming	Apraxia of speech	Complex word repetition
Motor execution	Dysarthrias	Oral mechanism examination

Comprehension was tested for error type, such as word form or semantic relationship. Although the number of semantic comprehension errors was related to word-finding difficulty in general, they found an inconsistent relationship between type of naming error and type of word comprehension problem. Thus, the problem was with function, not concepts.

Another exploration of the semantic system is to compare naming to metalinguistic tasks such as object sorting, which is similar to the strategy for studying word comprehension mentioned earlier in this chapter. Goodglass, Wingfield, and Ward (1997) studied rapid decisions about categorical relationships between objects as well as about semantic relationships between words and objects presented with a computer. Although aphasic patients were slower than normal on these tasks, performance did not predict naming performance.

We may suspect that conceptual deficits exist in severely aphasic individuals, especially those with significant impairment in word comprehension. Focusing on a group of eight such patients, Chertkow and his colleagues (1997) found that three were normal with a nonverbal task of associating related objects but five had deficits with this task. After comparing performances on a variety of tasks, these researchers concluded that the five aphasic individuals with additional deficit of object association had an impairment of "amodal" semantic processing. Thus, some severely aphasic people do not have a deeper semantic deficiency, but some severely aphasic people do.

One test of the semantic influence is Howard and Patterson's (1992) *Pyramids and Palm Trees*. Naming ability is evaluated in comparison to recognizing objects and comprehending words with a multiple-choice format. A clinician should be able to determine whether a patient has a central impairment of semantic knowledge or a problem accessing this knowledge with auditory or printed words.

A third type of evidence is the occurrence of category-specific naming deficits, especially when a patient has a comprehension problem in the same conceptual domain (e.g., musical instru-

ments). Category-specific deficits are seen mainly in a dissociation between inanimate and animate things. For example, Hillis and Caramazza (1991) described a double dissociation between two patients. Case PS named 39 percent of animals and 90 percent of inanimate objects. Case JJ had the reverse dissociation, naming 91 percent of animals but only 20 percent of inanimate objects. JJ also similarly favored animals for word comprehension and written naming.

The evidence for several hypotheses about the nature of category-specific deficits has been reviewed extensively, especially by Alfonso Caramazza and his colleagues at Harvard and in Italy (e.g., Chialant, Costa, and Caramazza, 2002; Shelton and Caramazza, 2001; also, Forde and Humphreys, 1999). One proposal, attributed to Warrington and Shallice (1984), has been called the *sensory functional hypothesis* (SFH). According to SFH, semantic memory is organized according to modality-specific subsystems, namely, visual-semantic properties and functional properties of objects. Living and nonliving things can be dissociated, because living things have a more visually based representation and nonliving things have a more functionally based representation.

Caramazza has considered the fundamental assumptions of the sensory-semantic theory to be mistaken and has presented cases that cannot be explained by this theory. He has preferred a *domain-specific theory* in which dissociations of semantic categories reflect an amodal conceptual organization of semantic memory (e.g., semantic networks and Figure 4.1). The nature of conceptual organization developed out of an evolutionary imperative for survival, such as "respecting distinctions between the animal and plant life categories" (Shelton and Caramazza, 2001, p. 439).

Capitani and others (2003) reviewed the vast literature on these deficits, most of which is based on the intensive study of individual cases. They found 79 case studies in which they considered the data to be sufficiently informative for identifying the categories for these deficits. The investigators catalogued the studies in various ways and even provided brief summaries of each case. In

61 cases, the deficit was clearly in the recognition and naming of biological categories consisting mainly of animals and fruits or vegetables. Forty-four percent of these were caused by herpes simplex encephalitis (HSE). Only three cases were caused by left hemisphere stroke. In the remaining 18 studies, the deficit was clearly in the recognition and naming of artifacts, and seven of these cases had left frontoparietal strokes. Therefore, the relevance of category-specific impairment for aphasia can be challenged.

This literature is focused on identifying deficits in single cases and debating commonalities among deficits that can contribute to the creation of CN theories of semantic knowledge. There is relatively little interest in explaining deficits with respect to etiology and less interest in putting the deficits in the context of clinical entities (e.g., aphasias). Therefore, it is difficult to present a picture for the practicing clinician. For example, we could suggest that clinicians examine comprehension and naming separately for animals, fruits and vegetables, and human-made objects (e.g., Boston Exam, third edition). Yet, it is difficult to say whether this is an efficient use of time when aphasia is probably more likely to consist of deficits across these categories.

Lexical Impairment?

Lexical variables pertain to characteristics of words per se, such as frequency of use and grammatical category. Common words are easier for an aphasic person to retrieve than rare words (e.g., Gardner, 1973). Grammatical category is usually studied by comparing nouns and verbs. For some patients, nouns are more difficult. Others display more difficulty with verbs, and others show no difference (Basso, Razzano, Faglioni, and Zanobio, 1990; Berndt, Mitchum, Haendiges, and Sandson, 1997). Berndt found that selective noun deficit is associated with severe word-finding disorder, and selective verb deficit can occur in fluent and nonfluent aphasias.

One indication of partial access to lexical form is the **tip-of-the tongue state** in which prop-

erties of a correct word are conveyed instead of the word itself. Barton (1971) instructed aphasic participants experiencing naming failure to point to the target word's first letter, number of syllables, and *big* or *small* to indicate the size of the target word. Patients guessed these properties accurately over 60 percent of the time in spite of being unable to say the word. It was as if an object activated the concept and parts of lexical form. In another study, some aphasic participants were less successful in reporting features of unspoken words, and a few others could not do it at all (Goodglass, Kaplan, Weintraub, and Ackerman, 1976).

Investigators also examined object familiarity by comparing the naming of common or "high-typical" examples of a category (e.g., *kitchen chair*) to uncommon or "low-typical" examples (e.g., *beach chair*) (Brownell et al., 1986). Normally, a basic name is elicited by highly typical examples (e.g., *chair*). Low-typical examples tend to elicit more subordinate labels than basic names (e.g., *beach chair*). Aphasic patients followed this pattern. They had difficulty producing subordinate names but conveyed the low-typical concepts with compensatory strategies. Instead of saying "race car," a nonfluent patient would say "car, goes fast." Fluent patients provided an attribute without the basic name. Because of this object recognition ability and communicative flexibility, Brownell concluded that the semantic system was intact. He located damage in the activation of particular lexical forms.

Psycholinguistic Study of Naming

CN models have been criticized for ignoring details about representation of information and how processes work in semantic and lexical systems. Psycholinguists put word finding within a spreading activation network and consider that lexemes are stored so they can slide quickly into sentences.

There are two fundamental positions on the naming process in psycholinguistics. One position is that semantic and lexical processes operate in a **serial** fashion. Activation spreads sequentially from semantic memory to lexical memory (Schriefers, Meyer, and Levelt, 1990). The other position is that the two systems are more **interactive,** meaning they operate simultaneously or "in parallel" (Dell and O'Seaghda, 1992).

Lyndsey Nickels at Birkbeck College in London conducted experiments comparing serial and interactive models in predicting relationships between certain variables and paraphasias (Nickels, 1995). The imageability rating of words was considered to be a semantic variable. Word length was a lexical variable. Word familiarity was thought to be related to both semantic and lexical modules. The interactive version predicts that all variables would affect both types of errors. A serial model is more selective, predicting imageability to be related to semantic errors and length to be related to phonological errors. Results supported the serial model.

Gary Dell proposed that word-form retrieval, called *lexical access,* requires two steps *after* semantic activation (Dell et al., 1997). In a spreading activation system, a concept cannot map to a word form directly as in Figure 4.2. Grammatical mediation is indicated by a high frequency of normal, phonologically unrelated word-finding errors within the same syntactic category (e.g., nouns for nouns, verbs for verbs). Therefore, the first step is lemma access or mapping a concept onto grammatical information such as syntactic category. The second step is lexical access or mapping the lemma onto phonological form. According to Dell, processing evolves as a series of "jolts" from semantics to sound. Originally he performed sophisticated statistical analyses of naming errors by normal and aphasic adults. He has also used computer simulations (i.e., computational modeling) of different versions of this theory to predict aphasic naming patterns (Dell, Lawler, Harris, and Gordon, 2004; Foygel and Dell, 2000).

The ***Philadelphia Naming Test*** (PNT) arose out of Dell and Schwartz's work (Roach, Schwartz, Martin et al., 1996). The unique contribution of this test is its error analysis and interpretation. The PNT consists of 175 nouns of different frequency and syllable lengths. Pictures are presented on a computer, and naming latencies are measured. The goal is to analyze errors according to "what they reveal about the mental processes underlying normal and pathological word retrieval" (pp. 129–130).

In another exercise of comparing theoretical predictions to cases, Caramazza has presented clinical data that fails to support interactive theories such as Dell's (Chialant et al., 2002; Ruml and Caramazza, 2005; Ruml, Caramazza, Shelton, and Chialant, 2000). The most striking counterevidence comes from cases who make only one type of naming error, namely, semantic paraphasias or phonemic paraphasias. Such cases indicate that levels or components of word finding were not interacting with each other.

Action Naming

Differences between nouns and verbs were mentioned earlier in the discussion of naming impairment at the lexical or lemma level. These dissociations have been classified as *grammatical category-specific deficits* in contrast to semantic category-specific deficits (e.g., Chialant et al., 2002; Laiacona and Caramazza, 2004). Consideration of grammatical category deficits begins with agrammatic patients who tend to omit closed-class words or grammatical morphemes while retrieving open-class words (nouns, verbs, adjectives). This problem is pursued in the next chapter. For now, we shall briefly examine differences of ability within the open-class category.

In the clinic, we may observe a dissociation between nouns and verbs in either direction. Some patients produce nouns much better than verbs (e.g., Jonkers and Bastiannse, 1998). Other patients produce verbs much better than nouns (e.g., Berndt, Haendiges, Mitchum, and Sandson, 1997). Investigators have reported that greater difficulty with nouns tends to occur in posteriorly lesioned individuals with fluent aphasias, whereas greater difficulty with verbs tends to occur in anteriorly lesioned individuals with agrammatic aphasia (Goldberg and Goldfarb, 2005). These tendencies have made it tempting to conclude that noun retrieval is located in a posterior cortical region and verb retrieval is located in the frontal lobe. However, exceptions have also been observed.

To be confident that the dissociation is truly between grammatical categories, researchers control for so-called nuisance variables, such as stimulus familiarity and visual complexity (Capitani et al., 2003). For example, a special problem in naming actions may be caused by the way that actions have to be pictured. Kemmerer and Tranel (2000a) investigated a number of variables in action naming with brain-damaged people who were either impaired or unimpaired in action naming. They found that stimulus variables of familiarity and complexity made little difference in the group data, but these variables did matter for a few participants. Researchers still institute the controls so results can be interpreted with minimal ambiguity.

Breedin, Saffran, and Schwartz (1998) explored the role of *semantic complexity* in the verb-retrieval deficits of eight aphasic patients. Some verbs are classified as "light" verbs (e.g., *go, have, do, get*), partly because they can be used as auxiliaries. The majority of verbs are "heavy" (e.g., *run, grab, sell*) partly because their meanings are more specific. Six of the eight aphasic participants in the study had more difficulty producing light verbs when telling a familiar story. Although verb difficulties were pronounced in some of these patients, others were only a little worse at naming actions (e.g., 83 percent) than naming objects (e.g., 88 percent).

Noun–verb dissociations were pulled into the semantic category debates by Bird, Howard, and Franklin (2000), who claimed that grammatical category dissociations can be explained with the same framework that has been used to account for the animate–inanimate dissociation for object naming. This framework follows the sensory functional hypothesis (SFH) cited earlier. They suggested that verbs are different because their meanings are heavily weighted with functional attributes, like inanimate objects. After Bird, Howard, and Franklin made their case, Shapiro and Caramazza (2001b) disagreed sharply with their theoretical assumptions and quality of evidence. The response prompted a further exchange of views (Bird et al., 2001; Shapiro and Caramazza, 2001a). In general, Caramazza and his colleagues have concluded that "grammatical effects cannot be reduced to a semantic deficit" and that the noun–verb dissociations arise at a level of lexical processing where grammatical information about words is represented (Chialant et al., 2002, p. 134).

PRODUCTIVE WORD FINDING

For clinicians to address a full range of word-finding conditions, Chapey, Rigrodsky, and Morrison (1977) argued that "divergent thinking" should be considered in addition to the "convergent thinking" in object-naming tasks. Confrontation naming converges on one idea and one response. In a divergent mode, we generate a quantity and variety of responses.

Word Fluency

The word fluency task involves producing a number of words to a single stimulus. Two types of word fluency tasks include producing words starting with a letter or words belonging to a conceptual category such as vegetables or countries. The task provides an opportunity for a different kind of qualitative analysis of word retrieval based on lexical-semantic connections. Letter-fluency tasks induce generation of words from a lexical base by having patients fish for commonalities of form. The categorical-fluency task induces generation of words from a semantic base. Productive strategies are identified as *clustering* (i.e., generation within semantic subcategories) and *switching* (shifting from one cluster to another) (Hough and Givens, 2004).

In a **categorical or semantic word fluency** task, a patient is asked to produce members of a semantic classification, often as many as possible in 60 seconds. The task has also been called "category generation" (Hough, 1989), "category naming" (Grossman, 1981), "word-naming" (Joanette,

Goulet, and Le Dorze, 1988), or a "controlled-association task" (Cappa, Papagno, and Vallar, 1990). In assessment, there is usually a limit of around 60 seconds for producing as many words as possible. Speed maximizes the number of words produced, but still the task can be highly strategic in the mind of the speaker.

Grossman (1981) used 10 categories such as sports, birds, furniture, tools, clothes, and weapons. Normal adults produced 14.66 words per category. Nonfluent aphasic patients produced 5.29 words, and fluent patients produced 6.71. These levels are fairly consistent. In another study, normal adults averaged 13.51 words per category and mildly impaired fluent aphasic persons produced 6.76 (Adams, Reich, and Flowers, 1989). The skill fluctuates as normal adults average 22.5 animal names in a minute but display a range of 9 to 41 words (Borod, Goodglass, and Kaplan, 1980; Goodglass and Kaplan, 1983). Persons with right hemisphere damage were also impaired, indicating that word fluency is sensitive to any brain damage.

The **letter word fluency** task was introduced by Borkowski, Benton, and Spreen (1967). They obtained data on production of "as many words as you can in 60 seconds" that begin with a particular letter. Six letters were difficult for normal adults; *J* elicited 4.83 associations. Moderate difficulty was observed with *N* (8.23). Easy letters for normal adults (*F, A,* and *S*) went into the aptly named and commonly used FAS test, with these three letters eliciting 10.22 to 11.50 words from persons without brain damage. Damage to the left or right hemisphere caused a large drop in production.

Persons with left hemisphere damage (LHD) did worse than those with right hemisphere damage (RHD) only for difficult letters. Persons with LHD, RHD, and bilateral damage were impaired in another study, and a discriminant analysis showed that only 48 percent of patients could be classified as to side of lesion using this method (Wertz, Dronkers, and Shubitowski, 1986). At around seven words per letter, the task did not clearly distinguish nonfluent and fluent groups studied by Collins, McNeil, Lentz, Shubitowski, and Rosenbek (1984).

In general, word fluency tasks present a challenge for any brain-damaged person, and we might be tempted to consider this test strategy for measuring progress in word finding. However, five administrations of the category test over a two-week period showed that word fluency can be quite variable with acute and chronic aphasia (Boyle, Coelho, and Kimbarow, 1991). A sample of individual ranges includes 1 to 8 words or 14 to 23 words for foods. For some patients, performance varied depending on the category used, such as 8 to 10 for animals and 9 to 17 for foods. This lack of consistency suggests that a single word fluency test is not a good diagnostic tool and that the value of word fluency is limited for measuring progress.

Words in Discourse

Words are produced naturally in an extended flow of interrelated words, often elicited by picture description. In a comparison with object naming, the two procedures were equally successful in eliciting nouns for nonfluent and fluent subjects (Basso et al., 1990). For action naming or verb finding, mildly impaired cases did better with description, leading to the conclusion that "performance on a single word confrontation-naming task may not be highly predictive of performance in connected speech" (Williams and Canter, 1987, p. 132).

Speaking rate differentiates nonfluent from fluent aphasias. Normal rate in words per minute (wpm) has been considered to be 100 to 175 wpm (Howes, 1964; Kerschensteiner, Poeck, and Brunner, 1972). Syllables per minute discriminated normal from aphasic groups (Yorkston and Beukelman, 1980). Normal elderly adults produced 193 syllables per minute. Mildly aphasic patients produced 121 syllables per minute. Kerschensteiner used the following categories to characterize variation among aphasic patients:

- *very slow:* 0 to 50 wpm
- *slow:* 51 to 90 wpm
- *normal:* above 90 wpm

Of 47 aphasic individuals, 17 were very slow, 13 were slow, and 17 were normal.

Quantification of elements is useful for measuring subtle progress in discourse production. Because counting number of units is biased by size variations among speech samples, most researchers utilize ratios (Table 4.5). A **type-token ratio** (TTR) is the number of different categories of items (i.e., types) relative to the total number of items produced (i.e., tokens). For measuring diversity of vocabulary, the TTR would be the number of different words relative to the total number of words. As variety of vocabulary increases, this TTR increases. The ratio is sensitive to sample size; "generally speaking the smaller the number of words spoken the larger the type-token ratio" (Fillenbaum, Jones, and Wepman, 1961).

READING WORDS

Word reading may be the fundamental problem for single-case cognitive neuropsychology. *Reading aloud* is the pivotal task. As with all task-related models, reading models are suggestive of hypotheses about the impaired component that could be responsible for a pattern of performance on a variety of tasks. When an impairment can be identified, the models indicate alternative routes

to successful reading. Reading problems are especially important to aphasic patients who want to use a computer at home and who are particularly fastidious about their spelling (Rapp, Folk, and Tainturier, 2001).

Figure 4.3 identifies common components of a CN model for reading aloud. CN models usually contain two routes from visual input to spoken response. In the primary or **lexical-semantic route,** a percept of the stimulus activates the lexicon (i.e., input-related form), which activates semantic storage, which then activates the lexicon again (i.e., output-related form) to guide speaking. A nonlexical or **conversion route** by-passes the semantic system, providing a capability for reading an unfamiliar word aloud (e.g., *Pocumtuck*). The ability to pronounce unfamilar words or nonwords depends on a rule-based spelling-to-sound conversion mechanism, called phonological reading.

Clinical investigators try to identify a component of the reading process that is responsible for symptom patterns in acquired dyslexias. In componental analysis, researchers manipulate stimulus variables and record spoken reading errors called **paralexias.** Stimulus variables and types of errors are shown in Table 4.6 (p. 89). Some variables relate strictly to word form, such as whether a string of letters is a real word, a nonword, or a

TABLE 4.5 A sample of ratios for measuring word production in spontaneous speech (Hier, Hagenlocker, and Shindler, 1985; Prins, Snow, and Wagenaar, 1978; Saffran, Berndt, and Schwartz, 1989).

MEASURE	RATIO	APPLICATION
Type-token ratio	Different words relative to total words	Patients with limited productive vocabulary
Anomia index	Pronouns relative to total nouns	Vagueness in anomic aphasia
Function word deletions	Omissions of closed-class words relative to total utterances	Grammatical deficits; free grammatical morphemes
Function word substitutions	Substitutions of closed-class words relative to total function words	Grammatical deficits; free grammatical morphemes
Inflected verbs	Verbs with inflectional endings relative to total verbs	Grammatical deficits; bound morphemes

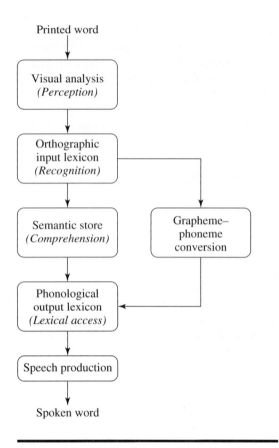

Printed word

Visual analysis
(Perception)

Orthographic
input lexicon
(Recognition)

Semantic store
(Comprehension)

Grapheme–
phoneme
conversion

Phonological
output lexicon
(Lexical access)

Speech production

Spoken word

FIGURE 4.3   Typical cognitive neuropsychological model of stages in reading words aloud. Functional equivalents are noted in parentheses.

pseudoword that comes close to being a real word. Other variables pertain to the semantic system, such as a word's concreteness or imageability. Assessment includes administering other tasks, such as word repetition to determine if a disorder is specific to one input modality.

One approach to diagnosis is to relate core performance patterns to classification of dyslexias (e.g., McCarthy and Warrington, 1990). Research often entails finding cases with basic symptoms of a category and then doing futher analysis to explain the symptom pattern according to the process model. Classification begins with a general distinction between *peripheral dyslexias* and

central dyslexias, roughly corresponding to the distinction between sensory and cognitive levels of function. Except for pure alexia, alexia without agraphia, these types of dyslexia are usually one part of a more pervasive disorder such as aphasia or attentional impairments.

The most common classification system is summarized in Table 4.7 (p. 90). In peripheral dyslexias, reading problems are caused by impairments outside the reading system. Central dyslexias are disorders of the reading process and can be a component of aphasia. The following are key characteristics of these impairments:

- In **phonological dyslexia,** there is a severe difficulty pronouncing nonwords, and familiarity is a strong factor. This disorder indicates that "the processes for pronouncing known words must be separable from those for pronouncing unknown words" (Ellis and Young, 1988, p. 211).
- In **surface dyslexia,** spelling-sound regularity is a strong factor. Nonwords and function words can be read aloud by the aforementioned phonological reading mechanism.
- **Deep dyslexia** is the reverse of surface dyslexia in the sense that nonwords and function words are harder to read than real content words. A patient makes a lot of semantic errors. Sometimes errors are visually mediated, such as reading *sympathy* as "orchestra." This error may have been accessed via the percept "symphony."

When a component process is impaired or a route is blocked, persons with acquired dyslexias appear to use compensatory strategies for reading aloud or for reading comprehension. A common strategy is called **letter-by-letter reading.** The key observation is an abnormally slow reading time, noted specifically by a large increase in reading latency as word length increases. It can take up to three or four seconds to read 3-letter words and a two-to-three second increase for each additional letter. A letter-by-letter reader is often identified as someone with pure alexia or vice versa. However,

TABLE 4.6   Symptoms observed in reading aloud as a function of word characteristics and paralexic error.

	SYMPTOM	DEFINITION	EXAMPLES
Stimulus factors	Word superiority effect	Real words more accurate than nonwords	*clean* better than *blean*
	Grammatical category effect	Difference between content words and function words	*tree* better than *the* *the* better than *tree*
	Concreteness or imageability effect	Concrete words more accurate than abstract words	*camera* better than *danger*
	Regularity effect	Regular words more accurate than irregular words	*mint* better than *pint* *cove* better than *love*
Paralexias	Visual	Looks like word	"plant" for *planet* "camping" for *campaign*
	Phonological	Sounds like word	"cambane" for *campaign*
	Regularization	Pronouncing an irregular word according to regular grapheme–phoneme conversion rules	"hayve" for *have* "sue" for *sew*
	Inflectional (morphological)	Changes structure, not grammatical category	"plant" for *plants* "running" for *run*
	Derivational (morphological)	Changes structure and grammatic category	"strange" for *stranger* "territorial" for *territory*
	Semantic	Similar meaning	"coast" for *seashore* "tear" for *crying*

reading one letter at a time is observed with various types of dyslexia. Other compensatory strategies include the following:

- *reading by sight* to compensate for the spelling–sound conversion problem in phonological dyslexia
- *reading by sound* to compensate for semantic route damage in surface dyslexia

Others take another route to diagnosis, bypassing classification of dyslexia and relating results of evaluation directly to components in a process model (e.g., Hillis and Caramazza, 1995a, 1995c). Hillis and Caramazza (1992) claimed that classification is abitrary and is "not informative with respect to the nature of damage that underlies the reading disorder" (p. 250). They argued that classification-based studies are "empirically inadequate" mainly because of incomplete testing biased to a classification. Also, classified cases can have different explanations (e.g., Berndt, Haendiges, Mitchum, and Wayland, 1996). Hillis and Caramazza advocated that "all theoretically relevant aspects of performance in language and other cognitive tasks should be considered in determining the level of impairment for every patient" (p. 251).

Investigators often avoid reporting diagnostic classification of aphasia syndrome and location of lesion. As a result, it can be difficult to relate the case to others in the clinic. Also, there does not seem to be a fixed relationship between dyslexia classification and diagnostic categories of aphasia.

TABLE 4.7   Types of dyslexia. Central dyslexias consist of phonological, surface, and deep types.

CLASSIFICATION	SYMPTOMS	DIAGNOSIS
Visual (peripheral)	Visual paralexias	Possibly "pure alexia"
	Reading one letter at a time	Usually left occipito-parietal lesion
Attentional (peripheral)	Visual errors with the left or right side of words	Attentional neglect of the left or right side of a word
	Cannot name parts of visual arrays but can name them in isolation	Right or left parietal lobe lesion
Phonological	Word superiority effect (real words much easier than nonwords)	Impaired conversion route
		Usually left posterior lesion
	Good nonword repetition (auditory input)	
Surface	Strong regularity effect	Damage to lexical or semantic stages of the primary route
	Regularization errors	Usually left posterior lesion
	No semantic errors	
	Nonwords and functors better than content words	
Deep	Mainly semantic errors	Impaired grapheme-phoneme conversion, or
	Visual and derivational errors	
	Strong word superiority effect	Damage to mapping input to semantics or semantics to output
	Content words better than functors	Left hemisphere lesion, including fronto-temporal lesions
	Concreteness effect	

Different types of aphasia can have the same reading impairment, and one type of aphasia, such as Broca's aphasia, can have different types of reading impairment. Thus, we cannot take a short-cut to diagnosing a reading impairment, such as diagnosing Broca's aphasia and then assuming that the patient has a particular reading disorder.

APHASIA IN BILINGUAL INDIVIDUALS

Michel Paradis (1998) of McGill University appeared to be a little uncomfortable contributing a chapter on aphasia in bilinguals for a book about "aphasia in atypical populations." He wrote that "there is nothing atypical about bilingual aphasics" (p. 35). Most of the world's population is bilingual. Paradis estimated that "there are over 150,000 bilingual aphasic patients in the United States today" (p. 37).

Grosjean (1989) defined bilinguals as "those people who use two or more languages in their everyday lives" (p. 4). He took a wholistic view of people who speak two languages. A bilingual person "cannot be decomposed into two separate parts . . . rather, he or she has a unique and specific linguistic configuration" (p. 6).

Does aphasia affect a bilingual person's languages equally or differently? In a review of cases reported over several decades, Albert and Obler (1978) found that each language seemed to be impaired. A patient's languages differed in severity of aphasia in 80 percent of the cases. In another retrospective study, Paradis (1977) found that 41 percent seemed to have aphasia equally between the two languages spoken, twice the proportion reported by Albert and Obler. Paradis noted other studies reporting as high as 90 percent having similar deficit across two languages. Small, controlled studies of aphasia in bilingual people, which began to appear in the 1980s, also revealed comparable deficits between languages (e.g., Vogel and Costello, 1986).

When there is a difference in aphasia between languages, is there a single basis for the difference? Long ago, Ribot and Pitres had different answers. The **rule of Ribot** ("primacy rule") stated that the native or first-learned language should be less impaired, which was supported in a study of some word-level tasks (Junque, Vendrell, Vendrell-Brucet, and Tobena, 1989). On the other hand, the **rule of Pitres** stated that the most frequently used language should be less impaired because of "habit strength." However, research has been unable to support that one rule or the other is dominant. **Alternating aphasia** is an unusual pattern in which expression with one language is impaired one day, and the other language is impaired the next day, and so on (Paradis, Goldblum, and Abidi, 1982). Any comparison between a patient's languages can be complicated by a dissociation between comprehension and expression. Good comprehension can be retained in two languages, while verbal expression is severely impaired in one language.

Impressions of bilingual aphasia were somewhat variable, because bilingualism is hard to study. Early case studies and the retrospective reviews were considered to be primitive (Solin, 1989; Zatorre, 1989). Albert and Obler (1978) were skeptical of their characterization of case studies, because patients with a discrepancy between languages were probably the more interesting to report. More importantly, bilingual individuals vary in a number of ways, including the following:

- proficiency in the second language
- age of learning the second language
- manner of learning the second language (e.g., naturally or formally)
- context of learning the second language (e.g., where it is predominant)
- affective factors such as cultural attitudes toward a language
- linguistic relationship between languages (some languages are more similar than others)

Also, the language behavior of a bilingual person varies according to the situation. When bilingual people converse with monolingual people, bilinguals enter a **monolingual mode** in which they deactivate the language not known by the monolinguals. When conversing bilinguals share the same two languages, the conversants enter a **bilingual mode** in which they activate both languages. An aphasic bilingual is likely to display different behaviors depending on the interactional mode necessitated by a clinician's linguistic status. Failure to consider the conditions in which multiple languages are evaluated has been one weakness in the study of aphasia's intrusion on the bilingual's linguistic skill.

A diagnostic dilemma is to distinguish aphasia from normal bilingual behavior, and one distinction has been suggested (Perecman, 1984). **Code switching** is normal and is defined as the alternating use of two or more languages in a conversation. It occurs when bilingual individuals are speaking to each other. Also, it is common in some bilingual environments but rare in others (e.g., Fabbro, 2001).

An aphasic person may exhibit **language mixing,** which is an inappropriate switching from one language to another such as in a conversation with a monolingual physician. It may also be considered to be part of the disorder when code switching is uncommon in the patient's community. Mixing may be indicative of a difficulty in accessing languages independently or a deficit in the ability to suppress a language that is not appropriate for the context. According to this distinction, code switching appears to be more intentional, whereas language mixing seems to be a more unintentional intrusion from another language. However, a distinction between switching and mixing is not always clear. They may be considered to be the same phenomenon, and the distinction is whether code switching (or mixing) is appropriate or inappropriate.

In one study, four Hispanic aphasic individuals conversed with neurologically intact Hispanic individuals in monolingual English, monolingual Spanish, and bilingual modes (Muñoz, Marquardt, and Copeland, 1999). Because normal participants exhibited code switching in the monolingual mode, this bilingual behavior was considered to be appropriate in the Hispanic community. The investigators concluded that decisions about the appropriateness of bilingual behavior should be made with respect to an aphasic person's bilingual community. The authors provided several examples of the code switching that occurred.

Paradis and Libben's (1997) *Bilingual Aphasia Test* (BAT) is available in several languages and includes the following three parts:

- *Part A:* patient's multilingual history
- *Part B:* comparative assessment of impairment in each language
- *Part C:* translation abilities and language interference detection

In any evaluation, we should first determine the following information about a patient prior to brain injury, perhaps, by interviewing a family member:

- relative ability in each language (linguistic level, style, reading, writing)

- situations and purposes for which each language was used (home, work, recreation)
- persons with whom each language was used (family, friends, colleagues)
- situations and people when in a monolingual mode
- situations and people when in a bilingual mode
- code-switching habits
- translation abilities

This information leads to assessment and treatment that are appropriate for a particular language. For example, we should not assess reading and writing in a language not used for these purposes. We should employ work-related content with the language used at work.

When evaluating each language, we obtain samples of language behavior in conversation and formal tests. Ideally, each language should be examined in each interactional mode, remembering that abilities in each language are not the same as the abilities of two monolingual persons. In the monolingual mode, conditions should lead to a deactivation of the language not being used, which is most likely to occur when the examiner truly does not know the other language. According to Grosjean (1989), pretending not to know the other language is rarely foolproof.

With a patient who speaks both English and Spanish, for example, a monolingual English-speaking person should do one evaluation and a monolingual Spanish-speaking person should do the other evaluation. A family member may be enlisted to translate and administer the aphasia test in the language not known by the clinician (e.g., Paradis and Goldblum, 1989). Vogel and Costello (1986) placed 30 minutes to two days between tests of object naming. The clinicians claimed that 15 to 20 minutes seemed too brief to minimize interference (or maximize deactivation of one language). Thirty minutes to one hour was sufficient for most participants. Paradis and Libben recommended assessing languages on separate days.

For obtaining behavior samples in the bilingual mode, the patient should feel comfortable code switching and borrowing. Translation abilities should be assessed by someone who knows both languages, and a bilingual family member or friend may be sought. Grosjean (1989) rec-ommended that we learn about how aphasia has affected the special skills used in the bilingual mode, such as whether the patient uses the "wrong" language, mixes languages to the same extent as before, or mixes in the same way as before. Has the ability to translate languages changed?

SUMMARY AND CONCLUSIONS

This chapter focused on what aphasic people have in common. Nearly everyone with aphasia has a problem with comprehension, although sometimes the problem is subtle and difficult to detect. A fundamental component of aphasia is some kind of difficulty retrieving words. The research supports two general objectives of treatment improving comprehension of spoken language and improving retrieval of words.

Also, we have the opportunity to work with culturally diverse communities and need to consider how aphasia affects a bilingual individual's use of each language.

Since 1960, basic research in clinical aphasiology has changed from a predominance of data-driven studies to the appearance of a steadily increasing number of theory-driven studies. Theory-driven research started out with tests of whether aphasia is a loss of knowledge or breakdown of process. Now, the research makes a distinction between automatic and controlled processing. Investigators figure out ways of doing studies that can address these distinctions in a valid manner.

In teaching cognitive paradigms to future specialists in cognitive-communicative disorders, two points stand out as being the most difficult:

- *Short-term memory (STM) is not the same as working memory (WM)*. STM is the temporary holding "buffer" in the processing system, and one approach to assessment is the memory span test. WM encompasses the entire processing "workspace," including a buffer to shelve some pertinent materials temporarily. One approach to assessing WM is the dual-task paradiagm in which a subject does two things at once.

- *Knowledge and process are interrelated but different aspects of a functional system.* Knowledge, such as the semantic network, is a "fixed" *structure* characterized by spatial metaphors. Spreading activation is a *process* occurring in a region of the network, and its duration can be measured. The "distance" between nodes in a network (i.e., their relatedness) is predictive of processing time, but distance (or relatedness) is an attribute of structure, not process.

What do we do when faced with multiple theories of the same thing? Is this a bad scientific situation? Focusing on one theory would certainly make learning aphasiology easier, and some researchers tend to advocate a single theory and then set out to prove it. However, when there are truly alternative explanations of something, other researchers set out to compare them in order to find the truth. For the sake of truth, it is better to know when an issue is not yet resolved and the nature of options left standing through the systematic evolution of research.

MATCHING REVIEW_____

Match the topics on the right with the names on the left. A topic may be used twice.

_____ 1. Alfonso Caramazza

_____ 2. David Caplan

_____ 3. Malcolm McNeil

_____ 4. Sheila Blumstein

_____ 5. Michel Paradis

_____ 6. Randi Martin

_____ 7. Lyndsey Nickels

_____ 8. Shari Baum

_____ 9. Cynthia Shewan

_____ 10. Nadine Martin

a. word-priming studies

b. *Auditory Comprehension Test for Sentences* (ACTS)

c. enactment procedure for sentence comprehension

d. attention and comprehension

e. STM and comprehension

f. category-specific semantic deficits

g. serial theory of paraphasias

h. bilingual aphasia

CHAPTER 5

INVESTIGATING SYMPTOMS AND SYNDROMES

Strokes cause aphasias. This chapter sharpens our focus on some symptoms and the syndromes introduced in Chapter 2. The syndromes characterize qualitative differences among aphasic patients. These differences make us wonder whether a single strategy for treating aphasia is appropriate and most efficient. The study of whether syndromes represent impairment of a distinctive psycholinguistic process has the following clinical implications:

- more specific diagnosis leading to more specialized treatments
- possibility of new methods for assessing automatic, obligatory processing

The identification of participants in research by syndromes enhances communication of research to all the readers, especially clinicians, who are familiar with this shorthand for patient identification.

We shall examine some features of language processing covered in the previous chapter and other features not covered. New features include syntactic processing and production of phonological form. Broca's aphasia has been the most scrutinized syndrome. Grodzinsky (1991) called it "the flagship of the neuropsychology of language." After an extensive presentation on Broca's aphasia, the chapter returns to stage theories of naming as a thematic current throughout the study of fluent aphasias.

AGRAMMATISM

So far, we have focused on production of words and have ignored the grammar of language production. Once researchers train their sights on

grammar, they think about Broca's aphasia. Agrammatism is the definitive feature of this syndrome. Many investigators prefer to say that these patients have "agrammatic aphasia."

Symptoms of Agrammatism

To look for problems with grammar, we must elicit sentences. Spontaneous speech is usually obtained through complex picture description or an interview. More restrictive procedures include the following:

- describe pictured actions or object locations
- complete a sentence or short story
- create a sentence given a noun or verb

Once sentences are elicited and transcribed, they are analyzed with respect to the presence or absence of standard features of grammar. A few guides have been developed to help us identify specific problems and to facilitate measurement of grammatical deficit (Table 5.1). These scales attend to lexicon, grammatical morphology, and syntactic structure. Some scales have a particular emphasis, such as grammatical morphology (Miceli, Silveri, Romani, and Caramazza, 1989) or phrase structure (Byng and Black, 1989). These orientations are indicative of the two broad features of grammar that are examined, namely, grammatical morphology or lexical characteristics (e.g., closed-class words) and syntax or structural characteristics (e.g., word order).

Historically, agrammatism (in English) has been thought to be "telegraphic" because of **omissions of grammatical morphemes.** These morphemes include *function words* (e.g., articles, conjunctions) and *inflectional endings* marking

TABLE 5.1 Analytical methods and measurements applied to the grammar of aphasic spontaneous speech production.

ANALYSIS	AUTHORS	SAMPLING	DESCRIPTION
Shewan Spontaneous Language Analysis (SSLA)	Shewan (1988)	Picture description	Profile of variables similar to Boston Exam; includes speaking rate and articulation rating
Grammatical morpheme measures	Miceli, Silveri et al. (1989)	Descriptions and narrations	Free and bound grammatical morpheme omission and substitution
Quantitative Production Analysis (QPA)	Berndt et al. (2000)	Fairy tale; first 150 words of narrative	Counts and ratio measures of lexicon, morphology, and sytactic structure
Predicate-argument analysis	Byng and Black (1989)	Fairy tale; unlimited amount	Counts of phrase and predicate-argument structures; related to production theory
Computer analysis	Thompson, Shapiro, Tait et al. (1995)	Cinderella story	More types of sentences, embedded clauses, verbs, and verb arguments

subject–verb agreement, verb tense, and case for nouns and conjugational forms in languages other than English. Closed- and open-class words are said to be free morphemes, because they stand alone. Inflections must be attached (i.e., bound morphemes).

For examples, let us look at a couple of descriptions of the Boston Exam's Cookie Theft picture:

- function word omission: "Mother washing dishes . . . water flows sink."
- inflection omission: "The mother is wash dish . . . the water flow from the sink."

Neat dissociations like this are rare, however. Usually agrammatism contains a mixture of function word and inflectional omissions.

Early scales by Saffran and her colleagues became the *Quantitative Production Analysis* (QPA) with a manual published for researchers (Berndt, Wayland, Rochon et al., 2000). One study was devoted to examining qualities of the QPA, such as demonstrating its reliability. Narrative productions

were obtained from 29 patients diagnosed as Broca's aphasic with the help of the Boston Exam. A cluster analysis highlighted variability of agrammatism, especially with respect to production of free and bound grammatical morphemes. That is, one subgroup produced more free-standing function words than bound morphemes, and another subgroup displayed the opposite pattern (Rochon, Saffran, Berndt, and Schwartz, 2000). These investigators also distinguished between *morphological agrammatism,* which emphasizes problems with grammatical morphemes, and *constructional agrammatism,* which emphasizes short and simple phrase structure (Linebarger, Schwartz, Romania et al., 2000).

Tesak and Niemi (1997) wondered if agrammatism is really like "telegraphese" or what Gardner (1974) called "telegramese." The importance of this question is derived from theories of agrammatism stating that patients with Broca's aphasia choose a "telegraphic register" as an adaptive strategy for dealing with their disorder. Tesak and Niemi compared agrammatism in four languages to telegrams written by a large group of normal subjects. One clear characteristic of normal telegraphese was an omission of function words ranging from 61 percent in Dutch to 77 percent in German. In agrammatism, there were 7 percent omissions in Swedish and 66 percent omissions in Dutch. Therefore, similarity between agrammatism and telegraphese depends on the language.

Instead of looking for linguistic forms in picture descriptions or fairy tales (Table 5.1), some investigators design tasks to elicit specific forms that have been observed to be problematic in spontaneous speech. Faroqi-Sah and Thompson (2004) focused on verb inflections, namely, V+*ing,* V+*ed,* and V+*s.* Eight agrammatic participants were instructed to describe a picture in a sentence starting with a cue word, such as the cue *yesterday* above a picture of a boy kissing a girl. There was considerable individual variability in patterns of inflection production, but 75 percent of responses contained inflected verbs. Yet, only 35 percent of the inflected verbs were accurate. Word frequency was a significant factor in determining the occurrence of errors.

It is important to note here that **grammatical morpheme substitution** occurs in other languages more than it does in English. Thus, omission can no longer be considered to be a definitive characteristic of agrammatism. After studying agrammatism in Italian, Miceli redefined the term as referring to "the omission of freestanding grammatical morphemes with or without the substitution of bound grammatical morphemes" (Miceli et al., 1989, p. 450).

Regarding structural or syntactic characteristics of agrammatism (or "constructional agrammatism"), two problems are considered most frequently. One is the **simplification** of sentence structure. In general, agrammatic patients do not use subordinate clauses as much as neurologically intact adults (Bastiaanse, Edwards, and Kiss, 1996). Instead of embedding a phrase with modifiers, an agrammatic patient sequences ideas as a series of simple structures. For example, instead of constructing a noun phrase such as *a large white house,* a patient may say "a large house, a

white house." A patient might say "girl tall and boy short" instead of "the girl is taller than the boy" (Gleason, Goodglass, Green, Ackerman, and Hyde, 1975).

In Chapter 4, we were introduced to the factors of structural complexity and reversibility for their influence on comprehension. Faroqi-Shah and Thompson (2003) used pictures to elicit active and passive sentences. Participants were instructed to describe the action in a picture by starting the sentence with the agent or object identified by an arrow. Patients with Broca's aphasia produced 60 to 80 percent of active sentences completely but produced only 10 to 30 percent of passive sentences completely. Difficulty was mainly in the omission of grammatical morphemes. Providing a printed inflected cue (e.g., *was hugged*) improved production of passives dramatically to about 80 percent. Reversible sentences tended to be more difficult to produce than nonreversible sentences.

In a linguistic study in the Netherlands, investigators compared agrammatic speakers to normal control speakers who were instructed to produce short utterances for describing drawings. The drawings were very specific, namely, circles and squares in different spatial arrangements. The aphasic participants were divided into a group with a mean length of utterance (MLU) below 3.0 and a group with an MLU above 3.0. Both control and aphasic participants reduced the complexity of their utterances. Aphasic speakers tended to use phrases like *square on* without completing the prepositional phrase. Aphasic speakers in general simplified structures like the controls who were instructed to use just two words. Also, patients and controls using shorter utterances produced more of them (de Roo, Kolk, and Hofstede, 2003).

The other possible structural or syntactic symptom of agrammatism is a **structural error** such as an illegal word order. For example, English does not allow structures like *man the* or *ing-walk,* but such errors do not appear to occur with aphasia (Bates, Friederici, Wulfeck, and Juarez, 1988). In one study, patients with Broca's aphasia reversed noun phrases 40 percent of the time when the phrases were alike in animacy (e.g., "The sink is in the pencil") (Saffran, Schwartz, and Marin, 1980). In Byng and Black's (1989) study, three-element utterances were nearly always in noun-verb-noun (NVN) order. Errors such as NNV were not observed, and the investigators concluded that reversal errors are rare.

The previous chapter cited studies indicating that people with nonfluent aphasia have more difficulty retrieving verbs than nouns. Saffran and others (1980) observed **verb-finding difficulty** in agrammatic patients. Then, a few studies found that action naming was more difficult than object naming in Broca's aphasia (e.g., Williams and Canter, 1987; Zingeser and Berndt, 1990).

In the past few years, several studies of verb retrieval in agrammatism have been directed by Roelien Bastiaanse at the University of Groningen in the Netherlands (with particular attention given to Dutch) and Cynthia Thompson at Northwestern University in Chicago (with particular attention given to English). Both investigators have found that people with Broca's aphasia have more difficulty retrieving verbs relative to nouns and that this difference is observed with production and not comprehension (e.g., Bastiaanse and Jonkers, 1998; Kim and Thompson, 2000). Moreover, Bastiaanse and Jonkers did not find a relationship between action naming and verb retrieval in spontaneous speech, prompting the conclusion that "a score on an action naming test is not a very good predictor for verb finding in daily life" (p. 966).

A special failure to activate verbs could have implications for sentence structure because of grammatical information carried by verbs. The grammatical information (or lemma-level representation) is known as *predicate-argument structure,* in which the verb is the predicate and attached noun phrases are its arguments. To simplify this linguistic construct considerably, let us think of the difference between transitive and intransitive verbs. Transitive verbs (e.g., *eat*) specify that they can take on themes (or direct objects). Intransitive verbs, such as *sleep,* cannot take on a direct object. Verb-argument structure specifies the "frames" that can accompany a verb. With Broca's aphasia,

producing transitive verbs is easier than intransitive verbs (Jonkers and Bastiaanse, 1997).

Another aspect of verb-argument structure is its complexity, presumed to reflect our knowledge of whether the verb can take one, two, or three arguments. Examples are as follows:

- one place: The dog is barking.
- two place: The boy is catching the ball.
- three place: The woman is giving the money to the girl.

Is this lemma knowledge related to an aphasic person's ability to name actions? For agrammatic participants with WAB AQs mostly in the 70s, Kim and Thompson (2000) found that action-naming accuracy was a function of verb complexity. One-place verbs were retrieved around 80 percent of the time, and three-place verbs were retrieved a little over 40 percent of the time. This relationship between verb complexity and naming agreed with earlier findings for putting verbs in sentences (Thompson, Lange, Schneider, and Shapiro, 1997).

Bastiaanse and Thompson (2003) got together to elicit declarative sentences and yes/no questions containing movement of part of a verb phrase from its usual position to the beginning of the sentence (e.g., *Is the convict kicking the sheriff?*). The researchers presented pictures consisting of a pair of reversed actions (e.g., convict kicking sheriff, sheriff kicking convict). They encouraged the use of a particular structure by priming, or modeling, a description for one picture, and participants were asked to describe the picture not modeled. All sentences were difficult for agrammatic participants to produce completely, but the yes/no questions were much more difficult. Bastiaanse and Thompson concluded that auxiliary movement is particularly challenging in formulating the agrammatic utterance.

Further study showed that not all agrammatic patients have problems producing main verbs, and the problem is not exclusive to nonfluent aphasias (Berndt et al., 1997; Miceli et al., 1989). Patients that have a special verb-finding problem tend to use common vague verbs in narration (e.g., *get, do, have*) and tend to simplify sentence structure more than patients with minimal verb retrieval problems (Berndt et al., 1997). Also, there is more variability. Some agrammatic patients produce more verbs in isolation than in sentences, and others produce more verbs in sentences than in isolation.

Because of exceptions to an old definition of agrammatism and because of more variation than is implied by the old definition, some aphasiologists have questioned whether agrammatism is a legitimate entity. Miceli and others (1989) were adamant, declaring that data "can no longer be ignored just for the obstinate protection of a fictional category of dubious theoretical value" (p. 475). Caplan (1991) suggested that variability of grammatical morpheme production in Broca's aphasia is indicative of the complexity of sentence formulation. In his opinion, agrammatism is an appropriate classification, and we just have to learn more about the intricacies of grammatical processes and be more flexible in defining agrammatism.

Explanations of Agrammatism

Initially, researchers attributed agrammatism to a vaguely specified dissociation of syntax from other components of language (Caramazza and Berndt, 1978). It was called the "no-syntax hypothesis" (Kolk and Van Grunsven, 1985). One problem with this hypothesis is that it is unclear as to whether it refers to syntactic knowledge ("competence") or syntactic processes ("performance"). This distinction is portrayed in various ways in the aphasiology literature. One approach to the dichotomy is to maintain the notion of competence as static knowledge but then to identify performance solely with working memory and resource limitations (e.g., Linebarger et al., 2000). However, this approach eliminates specific language formulation processes from consideration in the performance or process half of the dichotomy.

Is it possible that elements of language are missing because of a "loss of grammar" or erasure

of grammatical knowledge stored in long-term memory? A common strategy for evaluating the grammatical store is to compare performance on a number of different tasks. Schnitzer (1978) wrote that "a deficiency which affected all of the linguistic abilities would have to be either a remarkable coincidence or (more likely) a deficiency in the linguistic competence underlying all modalities" (p. 347). Caplan (1985) added that "disturbances found only in one language task have been considered to be disturbances in performance, sparing competence, while disturbances found in all language-related tasks reflect a disturbance of the central set of representations, that is, of competence" (p. 133). Success with any one language task indicates that knowledge is retained to some degree.

When studying a function such as verbal expression, the investigator might include a **metalinguistic task** to examine an area of knowledge. Such tasks require conscious judgments about language or about a language function, as in editing what someone has written. Common metalinguistic tasks include such things as arranging words or phrases into a sentence and deciding which of two sentences is correct. Metalinguistic tasks have been employed extensively, partly because they are thought to involve "shallow processing" (Linebarger, Schwartz, and Saffran, 1983) or may circumvent processes of comprehension and expression tasks (Baum, 1989).

The most common metalinguistic task for grammar is *grammaticality judgment*. The task is simply to detect errors or violations of linguistic rules. The ability of agrammatic subjects to detect morphological and syntactic violations of all sorts has been demonstrated repeatedly in many languages (Branchereau and Nespoulous, 1989; Devescovi, Bates, D'Amico et al., 1997; Linebarger, Schwartz, and Saffran, 1983; Shankweiler, Crain, Gorrell, and Tuller, 1989; Wulfeck, Bates, and Capasso, 1991). Kim and Thompson's (2000) agrammatic patients were able to recognize errors of predicate-argument structure. Exceptions may occur with complex sentences or demanding processing conditions (Haarmann and Kolk, 1994).

Grammaticality judgments support the view that people with Broca's aphasia retain the representation of phrase structure and grammatical morphology in long-term memory. Further evidence comes from the use of a "processing prosthesis" to ease the effort of resource allocation in working memory (Linebarger et al., 2000). Without being given any linguistic help, agrammatic patients improved grammatical structure when using a computer to substitute for short-term memory of formulated phrases (see Chapter 9). The computer made it easier to draw on intact stored knowledge.

Schwartz, Lingebarger, and Saffran (1985) noted that "it is one thing to describe agrammatism in syntactic terms and quite another to locate the responsible deficit in a mechanism that constructs syntactic representations" (p. 86). In order to explain sentence production behavior with a cognitive mechanism, we need some idea of what the mechanism is and how we go about evaluating it.

In search of a mechanism, investigators turned to Garrett's (1984) serial theory of sentence production for interpreting patterns of expressive disorder. Figure 5.1 summarizes processing subsystems and levels of mental representation computed by each process. Formulation begins with an idea and ends in two motor stages, namely, "regular processes" for speech programming and "coding processes" for execution of movement. Each process-generated representation informs the next process in sequence. The absence of a stimulus processing component indicates that this is a general theory rather than a task-specific model. It was mainly intended to account for normal errors or "slips of the tongue."

This model is more subtle than one that would have semantics, syntax, and the lexicon ordered in a row. For example, there is a syntactic component in two levels. Syntactic and lexical-semantic components are formulated interactively within each of these levels, making it possible for different language disorders to be caused by damage at one level. Also, the semantic and lexical components of naming theories discussed in Chapter 4 have been associated with the two linguistic levels

PROCESSES	REPRESENTATIONAL LEVELS	DESCRIPTION
Inferential	Message	idea to be conveyed (activation of semantic memory)
Logical & syntactic	Functional	conceptually specified slots for content words and specification of thematic roles (like deep structure)
Syntactic & phonological	Positional	syntactic frame (e.g., grammatical morphemes) and phonological form of words inserted into the frame (like surface structure)
Regular phonological	Phonetic	programming movement sequences
Motor coding	Articulatory	executing movement

FIGURE 5.1   Stages of sentence production according to Garrett (1984). In drawings of Garrett's model, the processes on the left are shown to generate the representational levels on the right.

of Garrett's theory (Brownell, Potter, Bihrle, and Gardner, 1986; LeDorze and Nespoulous, 1989).

Focusing on omission of function words, Garrett (1984) proposed that agrammatism is caused by a damaged positional-level mechanism because this is where function words are selected. Also, evidence of intact functional-level formulation is demonstrated by retention of basic canonical structure and logical location of agents and other thematic roles around a verb. Omission and substitution of grammatical morphemes as well as structural simplification have been interpreted as damage to the positional level (Caramazza and Berndt, 1985; Ostrin and Schwartz, 1986).

Garrett's theory was the basis for guiding and interpreting the analysis of Cinderella stories produced by 14 agrammatic individuals (Webster, Franklin, and Howard, 2001). The researchers segmented transcripts into utterances and analyzed each utterance with respect to grammatical features assumed to correspond to levels of the theory (i.e., thematic, phrasal, and morphological structure). The investigators did not appear to place the underlying disorder in either the functional or positional levels per se. Mainly they discussed how a deficiency in one feature may or may not be accompanied by successful production of another feature.

Linguistic theories are classified cognitively as **representational theories.** That is, they appear to capture the product of a formulation process. Two versions postulate a limitation on generation of a phrase structure or "syntactic tree." Caplan (1985) wrote of an "impoverished syntactic representation." People with agrammatism do not construct a hierarchical tree and, instead, activate a canonical linear subject-verb-object form through which any idea is conveyed. According to a slightly different view, agrammatic productions are the result of an "underspecified syntactic representation," in which a complete tree is formed but some terminal nodes are missing (Grodzinsky, Swinney, and Zurif, 1985).

Friedmann and Grodzinsky (1997; Friedmann, 2002) proposed the *Tree Pruning Hypothesis* (TPH) to account for agrammatic sentence production. According to TPH, the highest nodes in a structural representation are "impaired or inaccessible" or "do not exist." While the cognitive nature of this proposal is unclear, it does specify a subtle linguistic commonality among deficient productions with respect to agreement, tense, and types of questions. Other linguists have presented evidence that was not consistent with TPH (Burchert, Swoboda-Moll, and De Bleser, 2005; Wenzlaff and Clahsen, 2005). Therefore, this idea is in an early phase of development.

Kolk and Heeschen (1990) differentiated impairment symptoms attributable to a damaged processor (i.e., negative symptoms) from adaptation symptoms attributable to compensatory adjustments by the cognitive system (i.e., positive symptoms). They claimed that some symptoms of agrammatism are due to adaptation that is either *preventive* (before formulation is started) or *corrective* (after mistakes are made). Omissions are considered to be adaptive symptoms (e.g., telegraphic strategy) and substitutions are impairment symptoms. They were particularly interested in variability in a patient's agrammatic behavior with respect to the sentence production task. Task-dependent changes included reduction of grammatical morpheme omission in picture description relative to conversation, and increased substitution rates for picture description. This variability was considered to reflect some conscious use of strategy (Hofstede and Kolk, 1994).

Kolk and Heeschen's theory of impairment, called *synchrony reduction,* was that agrammatic patients are slow to activate structural representations. This slowness reduces the synchrony required to combine elements of a sentence and, thus, makes complex structures difficult to produce. Task effects pointed to consideration of reduced working memory capacity and the resulting reduction of resources available for complex formulation operations. That is, picture description supposedly requires fewer resources than conversation, thus, reducing the need to form a telegraphic strategy of omission. Strategic ellipsis (e.g., "more milk," "too late") was thought to be a preventive strategy intended to avoid computational overload that would occur if a complete sentence were attempted (Kolk and Heeschen, 1992).

ASYNTACTIC COMPREHENSION

Broca's aphasia is the clearest example of what used to be broadly termed "expressive aphasia." Auditory comprehension has been said to be "good" or "relatively preserved," at least relative to the overt agrammatism in language production. However, the *Boston Diagnostic Aphasia Examination* specifies a range from the 50th to 90th percentile for auditory comprehension (Goodglass and Kaplan, 1983). According to the *Western Aphasia Battery,* a patient can be between 4 and 10 points for this function (Kertesz, 1982). The manual for the *Auditory Comprehension Test for Sentences* (ACTS) shows where Broca's aphasia ranks relative to a maximum score of 21 and other syndromes (Shewan, 1979):

- anomic aphasia   14.8
- Broca's aphasia   12.5
- Wernicke's aphasia   9.7

Therefore, clinical measures indicate that substantial comprehension impairment can occur with Broca's aphasia, and it is in the middle of the pack relative to other syndromes. The next question became whether these patients have a particular kind of comprehension impairment, one that mirrors the agrammatic problems in verbal expression. The issues have two parts:

- Is the impairment isolated to one component of language?
- Is the impairment specific to one syndrome of aphasia?

Problem Identification

Early attempts to uncover a specific disorder focused on distinguishing between lexical and syntactic factors in comprehension. The most frequently cited study is Alfonso Caramazza and Edgar Zurif's (1976) comparison between re-

versible (1a) and nonreversible (1b) statements presented to patients with Broca's or conduction aphasia. Because comprehension was thought to be relatively good with these syndromes, structurally complex sentences were used to increase the likelihood that aphasic patients would make revealing errors.

(1a) The girl that the boy is chasing is tall.
(1b) The apple that the boy is eating is red.

Subjects chose interpretations from two pictures. Sometimes the foil differed according to a lexical element and, other times, according to a reversal of agent and recipient.

Two findings have had a tenacious influence. First, patients with Broca's aphasia had particular difficulty with reversible statements (1a). Second, they made more thematic role order errors than lexical errors. Caramazza and Zurif concluded that people with Broca's aphasia can use semantic or pragmatic constraints to comprehend thematic roles (e.g., apples do not eat) but are impaired when they must rely on the syntactic feature of word order. Suspicion of a special word order problem grew with studies showing particular difficulty with passive sentences (Schwartz, Saffran, and Marin, 1980) and mostly order errors when errors were made, even with reversible active sentences (Gallaher and Canter, 1982).

In Italy, Claudio Luzzatti and his colleagues (2001) tested agrammatic aphasias with simpler active and passive reversible sentences:

(2a) Mario cerca Flora. (Mario seeks Flora.)
(2b) Flora è cercata de Mario. (Flora is sought by Mario.)

Other sentences had agents and recipients that were the same gender. The twist in their four picture-choice method was to force a structurally based decision with sentences in which agent and recipient were different in gender. A reversal of agent and recipient of different gender generated two options. The same gender was in only one option. The results showed that participants comprehended sentences with high accuracy except for passive sentences with different gender. With this method Luzzatti exposed the structural problem with passive sentences and type of error by controlling for gender of agents and objects.

People with Broca's aphasia acquired a reputation for having difficulty with word order when it is the main cue to thematic roles. Some researchers started to identify Broca's aphasia according to an "inability to interpret other than simple active structures or semantically constrained sentences" (Rosenberg, Zurif, Brownell et al., 1985, p. 292; also, Shapiro and Levine, 1990). This "asyntactic comprehension" disorder has come to be diagnosed as the following:

- deficit with noncanonical reversible sentences (e.g., passives)
- significantly more order errors than lexical errors.

These criteria for identifying agrammatic comprehension can vary slightly, such as requiring only that a patient have a deficit with reversible sentences in general. Particular investigators may add a qualification that patients do well on word comprehension and grammaticality judgment tasks (Saffran, Schwartz, and Linebarger, 1998).

Next, we consider the methodologies and theories that have been aimed mostly at explaining the asyntactic pattern of comprehension. In this effort, procedures in the psycholinguistic study of sentence comprehension have been applied to the problem of figuring out what might be breaking down in the comprehension mechanism. When reviewing this literature, we discover some substantial disagreements. In particular, there has been disagreement over whether *the asyntactic pattern is confined to the Broca's syndrome* and whether *everyone with Broca's aphasia has this problem.*

Processes of Sentence Comprehension

The main task for the sentence comprehension system is thematic role assignment or, namely, figuring out who is doing what to whom. Like word comprehension, everyday sentence comprehension is the result of automatic obligatory

processes. According to Tyler (1987), core processes operate on a *principle of optimal efficiency* by assigning "an analysis to the speech input at the theoretically earliest point at which the type of analysis in question can be assigned" (p. 146). Core processes are supplemented with capacity-consuming controlled processes.

Sentence comprehension is assumed to rely on three subsystems: a lexical processor, a syntactic processor, and a semantic or interpretive processor (Figure 5.2). Some researchers focus on lexical access in sentences. Other researchers specialize in the assignment of syntactic structure to regions of sentences. Others are more interested in the ultimate interpretation of sentences, especially in a narrative context.

Some fundamental questions are entertained in most studies of normal adults. One is whether each processor, especially lexical access or syntactic parsing, operates as an autonomous subsystem. For example, does parsing occur without influence from lexical access or interpretations of nearby sentences? Figure 5.2a indicates that the parser is not left totally on its own. Another hypothesis is that all components are interdependent and operate in an interactive or parallel fashion (Figure 5.2b).

Two general strategies are used to study sentence comprehension. Most clinical assessments consist of **off-line** procedures in which patients respond after a sentence is presented. The procedures include the slow tasks of sentence–picture matching, sentence verification, and following directions. Response latency usually allows for a great deal of controlled processing to occur. The off-line approach measures the cumulative result of all processes or the *final interpretation* of a sentence, plus what goes into the task's response.

Online procedures, on the other hand, examine processing as it occurs "in real time." Patients respond to a point within a sentence, usually before its presentation is completed. Response time is indicative of relative processing load at that point. Inference about a process is based on the success of a theory predicting processing loads at key locations. The approach is said to detect

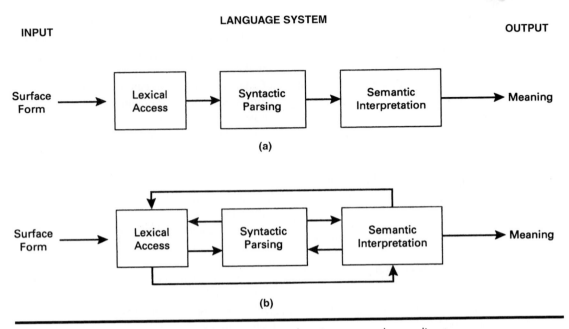

FIGURE 5.2   The major subsystems of sentence comprehension arranged according to (a) serial theory and (b) the preferred interactive-parallel theory.

intermediate interpretations within a sentence (Shapiro, Swinney, and Borsky, 1998). The variety of these methods is suggested by the listing in Table 5.2.

Lexical System

The primed lexical decision task introduced in Chapter 4 provides a look at the lexical processor in isolation. For now, let us consider the simple activation of meaning for Broca's aphasia.

Milberg and Blumstein (1981) had a surprising result with the semantic priming task. Patients with Broca's aphasia did not have a semantic priming effect. This result appeared to contradict the syntax–semantics dissociation proposed in the 1970s. These investigators decided to look more closely at the automaticity of semantic processing in Broca's and Wernicke's aphasia (Milberg, Blumstein, and Dworetzky, 1987). Patients with Broca's aphasia again had no semantic priming effects. The researchers concluded that agrammatic patients have a lexical-semantic impairment at the

automatic level of processing, which came to be known as the **automaticity hypothesis.**

Milberg and Blumstein's research design suffered some criticism (e.g., Baum, 1997; Hagoort, 1997; Ostrin and Tyler, 1993). One problem appeared to be the complexity of the task, because they used paired primes (e.g., *shore-bank*) before targets (e.g., *river*). Katz (1988) simplified the task by presenting semantically ambiguous one-word primes (e.g., *bank*) for targets such as *money* or *river*. This time, agrammatic subjects displayed semantic priming for both meanings of *bank*. This result was indicative of a basic finding in psycholinguistics, namely, that ambiguous nouns normally activate multiple meanings automatically (Simpson and Burgess, 1985).

Another problem with the early work was that Milberg and Blumstein relied on a long prime–target interval of 500 msec, which can allow for controlled processing to obscure capabilities at an automatic level. Later, shorter intervals were used. Tyler and others (1995) inserted 200 msec. Hagoort (1993, 1997) initially compared 100,

TABLE 5.2 Online (or on-line) methodology used to study lexical-semantic processes and syntactic parsing. Methods are distinguished based on whether the dependent measure is an intentional response by a participant.

	COMMON NAME	DESCRIPTION
Intentional response	Phoneme/word monitoring	Press button when hearing a specified sound or word in a sentence
	Cross-modal priming	Visual-lexical decision while listening to a sentence
	Self-paced reading time (SPRT)	Time to read a segment of a sentence, one by one, usually displayed left to right (also called *moving window task*)
	Self-paced listening time (SPLT)	Time to comprehend segments, one by one, presented over headphones (also, *auditory moving window*)
Unintentional response	Eye tracking (reading)	Measuring duration of eye fixations while reading a sentence
	Eye tracking (auditory stimuli)	Locating and measuring eye fixations on objects while listening to instructions
	Evoked potentials (EP)	Computed brain wave time-locked to a sentence location

500, and 1250 msec and, later, intervals of 300 and 1400 msec. Patients with Broca's aphasia displayed semantic priming at the short intervals. In cognitive terms, patients exhibited spreading activation to related concept nodes in a semantic network within 100 msec. The results led these investigators to reject Milberg and Blumstein's automaticity hypothesis for this syndrome. More recently, Blumstein found normal semantic priming with Broca's aphasia, but problems with subtle acoustic manipulations of the prime led her to maintain a notion that these patients have a "reduction in lexical activation" (Misiurski, Blumstein, Rissman, and Berman, 2005).

In a sentence, an ambiguous word activates multiple meanings instantaneously, even when prior context is suggestive of one interpretation (Seidenberg, Tanenhaus, Leiman, and Bienkowski, 1982; Swinney, 1979). This was evidence that lexical-semantic access operates as an autonomous or "encapsulated" system. Subtle features

of online research indicated that context selects interpretation a few syllables (or milliseconds) later. So, how do psycholinguists determine such things?

Swinney, Zurif, and Nicol (1989) borrowed a common online procedure to study multiple meaning activation in aphasia. In this case, an ambiguous word such as *plant* is presented as a prime in a spoken sentence such as 3.

(3) The gardener was responsible for watering every plant * on the enormous estate.

While listening to a sentence, aphasic patients made a visual recognition decision about letter strings (e.g., *tree* or *factory* or an unrelated word) shown immediately after the ambiguous prime (*). This auditory presentation of a sentence along with an online visual lexical decision is called **cross-modal priming.** Participants with Broca's aphasia were primed only for primary meanings (i.e., *tree*), unlike normal adults who are primed exhaustively for both dominant and secondary word meanings (i.e., *tree* and *factory*). Swinney concluded that patients with Broca's aphasia are slow in the autonomous access of meanings. That is, activation spreads to the closest nodes, but it is too slow to arrive at the more distant nodes in the time given in the experiment.

Baumgaertner and Tompkins (2002) examined the "slowed activation" theory with another cross-modal priming task, but they ran into problems. Biasing contexts were provided for the dominant and subordinate meanings of an ambiguous word (e.g., *ball*), as shown with the following truncated examples:

(4a) Dominant: The bowler focused on the pins and aimed the *ball* * until he was certain . . .
(4b) Subordinate: The debutantes waltzed with the young men at the *ball* * until all of them . . .

Lexical decision targets, called "visual probes," were displayed as the ambiguity (*) was heard. Surprisingly the age-matched controls did not prime for dominant meanings (e.g., *throw*) or subordinate meanings (e.g., *dance*) in either context, contrary to the automatic multiple activation that has commonly occurred before. This failure of the task "rendered results for the patient group uninterpretable" (p. 406). Maybe the sentences were too complex, or the targets appeared on screen too long. Sometimes experiments do not work out the way we hope, and it is admirable when this work is reported.

The proposal that exhaustive access of meanings is merely delayed should be tested with another lexical decision task (LDT) a few syllables later (Caramazza and Badecker, 1991). To check this out, Swinney's study was followed with a similar one that placed lexical decision five syllables after the ambiguous word (e.g., *plant*). Again, patients with Broca's aphasia were primed only for the primary word (Prather, Love, Finkel, and Zurif, 1994). It is still possible that these patients were slow to activate multiple meanings automatically. Using the evoked potential (EP) as an online procedure, others supported the possibility that people with Broca's aphasia use context to inhibit irrelevant meanings downstream from an ambiguous word (Swaab, Brown, and Hagoort, 1998).

In addition to word meaning, the lexical processor feeds grammatical information to the syntactic processor. This information is carried by free grammatical morphemes (i.e., function words), the morphological structure of words (i.e., inflections), and the argument structure of verbs. Researchers have wondered if patients with Broca's aphasia have as much trouble using grammatical morphemes in comprehension as they do for production. In the following paragraphs, this question is considered before addressing verbs.

A simple LDT was used for comparing access to open- and closed-class words (Bradley, Garrett, and Zurif, 1980). Diagnosis of deficit hinged on normal individuals, who had a frequency effect for open-class words but not for closed-class functors. People with Broca's aphasia did not exhibit this difference. The investigators proposed a **lexical hypothesis** stating that agrammatic comprehension is an impairment in accessing function words. However, several investigators could not replicate the frequency effect with normal adults, thereby, weakening the basis for claiming that aphasic patients are different (e.g., Petocz and Oliphant, 1988; Taft, 1990). Gordon and Caramazza (1983) could not replicate Bradley's findings for aphasic patients.

Studies had patients comprehend sentences in which functors matter for interpretation. Heilman and Scholes (1976) presented sentences like 5a and 5b in a picture-choice task with word-order and lexical foils.

(5a) She showed her baby the pictures.
(5b) She showed her the baby pictures.

In these sentences, position of *the* carries information about thematic roles of other words. Patients with Broca's and conduction aphasias had difficulty making word-order decisions. Elsewhere, those with Broca's aphasia uniquely failed to distinguish definite and indefinite articles (Goodenough, Zurif, Weintraub, and Von Stockert, 1977). Consequently, Broca's aphasia developed a reputation for being insensitive to free-standing grammatical morphemes. However, there was seemingly contradictory evidence because of appropriate response to sentences like *Bill walking the dog* and *Bill the walking dog* (Caplan, Matthei, and Gigley, 1981).

The online task of **word monitoring** was used to test the lexical hypothesis in real time. In this task, participants are instructed to press a response key when they hear a predetermined word as they are listening to a sentence. Like other online tasks, response time is considered to be indicative of processing load at the location of the target word. Agrammatic participants' response was slower to function words than content words, in contrast to normal controls (Friederici, 1983; Swinney, Zurif, and Cutler, 1980; Tyler and Cobb, 1987).

Accessing verbs may have a more direct influence on structural parsing because of the information that verbs carry about predicate-argument structure, discussed earlier in the chapter. Lew Shapiro was interested in the influence of verb complexity according to the number of nounphrase argument structures that can be attached to a verb. In particular, he looked for evidence of automatic activation of all possible argument structures, much like the multiple activation of lexical meanings illustrated by Swinney's research.

To test the multiple activation idea, Shapiro used Swinney's cross-modal priming procedure. Let us first look at the stimuli used for manipulating verb complexity.

(6a) The happy officer *put* * the new suit on * the shelf.
(6b) The sad girl *donated* * the new suit to * the charity.

The verb *put* is simpler than *donated,* because *put* takes on a single obligatory argument structure consisting of a theme (*new suit*) and location (*on the shelf*). On the other hand, *donated* allows two possible structures indicated partly by the optionality of location in 6b. Verbs like these were presented auditorily in similarly structured sentences (Shapiro and Levine, 1990).

Shapiro and Levine were interested in what happens at the site of the verb. Patients made visual lexical decisions at the verb in one condition and "downstream" in another condition. Patients with Broca's aphasia performed normally in that processing time varied with complexity at the point of contact with verbs, indicating that these patients activated multiple possibilities allowed by a verb. This effect dissipated downstream in a manner similar to what happens when mulitple meanings are activated. Fluent aphasic patients were not sensitive to argument structure. Another study also showed that patients with Broca's aphasia were sensitive to properties of verbs online, whereas patients with Wernicke's aphasia were impaired (Shapiro, Gordon, Hack, and Killackey, 1993).

In sum, different proposals have been put forth regarding the nature of lexical processing in Broca's aphasia. The notion of delayed lexical access was targeted at grammatical morphemes and, therefore, was related mainly to the characteristics of expressive deficits. Word monitoring provided some online indication that function words are problematic. In general, it is not clear how lexical deficits account for the asyntactic pattern. Lexical and/or semantic access for content words may not be as slow as once thought, but the possibility remains that word-meaning activation for sentences is a bit slow for some people with Broca's aphasia. Delays could throw off the assignment of syntactic structure, which is informed by word recognition.

Syntactic System

Syntactic parsing is the assignment of structure to a string of words. For now, let us get a better idea of what *syntax* or *structure* refers to, and then, we should have a perspective for evaluating clinical research on the processing of structure by aphasic individuals. The following *USA Today* headline, aided by its spacing, illustrates the assignment of structure for comprehension:

(7) Cruise ship dumping poisons
     seas, frustrates U.S. enforcers

If we stop at the end of the first line, it reads, "the ship is dumping poisons." When we continue to the next line, we have to correct the original structure so that the headline reads, "the dumping poisons the seas." The difference in meaning is slight, but this structural ambiguity (called a *garden-path sentence*) shows that structural relations determine the grammatical categories of the words. Of course, we cannot literally see the structure like we can see the words. Linguists provide us with "tree structures" to help us visualize these relations.

The next example comes from contrived headlines used in a study by Perfetti and others (1987):

(8)   Pentagon plans swell deficit

This is an example of a global ambiguity, because the sentence has two plausible interpretations derived from two possible assignments of structural relations among the words (i.e., the plans increase the deficit; the Pentagon plans a terrific deficit). In conversation, such ambiguities are resolved with prosody and additional words. Patients with Broca's aphasia had difficulties using stress and juncture to comprehend global ambiguities, such as *they fed her dog biscuits* (Baum, Daniloff, Daniloff et al., 1982).

Friederici (1988) proposed that parsing is impaired in Broca's aphasia based on evidence of intact knowledge and online tests of sensitivity to grammatical morphology. However, the early word-monitoring studies could have been indicative merely of recognition processes without implications for structural assignment. In a more recent use of word monitoring, the target word was placed immediately after inflected or uninflected words appearing in either a grammatical or ungrammatical context (Friederici, Wessels, Emmorey, and Bellugi, 1992). In general, people with Broca's aphasia displayed some deficient sensitivity to omitted inflection as a function of context, leading Friederici to conclude that syntactic information associated with inflection is not activated fast enough.

The theory of slow syntactic activation was supported by **syntactic priming** studies. Baum (1988) compared grammatical primes (e.g., *It's true that the boys*) and ungrammatical primes (e.g., *It's true that the boy*) presented prior to a target (e.g., *play*). Syntactic priming did not occur for subjects with Broca's aphasia as it did for normal controls with 500 msec between stimuli. Haarmann and Kolk (1991) varied stimulus onset asynchrony (SOA) and presented primes such as *We can* and targets such as *talk* or *nose*. Aphasic patients were facilitated at 1100 msec intervals but not at 300 or 700 msec. Additional evidence was provided by Blumstein, Milberg, Dworetzky, and colleagues (1991).

Tyler and her colleagues (1995) conducted a word-monitoring study leading to a different conclusion. Patients with Broca's aphasia listened to sentences with syntactic violations, such as 9.

(9)   They went into London chose to CARPETS and curtains.

The experimenters placed target words immediately after a violation or after the correct version in another sentence. The aphasic patients were sensitive to the violations, indicating that this study provides "no evidence supporting the claim that Broca patients are slow to access syntactic information in general or the more specific claim that they are slow to access members of the closed class" (p. 152).

Linguistic representational theories have been proposed to account for agrammatic comprehension. How such theories fit into a cognitive framework is unclear, but for this discussion it is assumed that they depict the result of a parsing operation. Caplan and Futter (1986) proposed a **linearity hypothesis** stating that agrammatic patients use a linear (or canonical) agent-action-recipient order to assign thematic roles for a sentence. This is why difficulty occurs with sentences structured differently.

Yosef Grodzinsky (1986, 1989) disagreed with Caplan by claiming that patients do generate hierarchical representations. Instead, impairment is an incomplete structural representation. For example, in linguistic theory of passives, a "trace" that designates thematic role is said to be left in the wake of movement of noun phrases (NPs) from their canonical position. Grodzinsky's **trace-deletion hypothesis** (TDH) states that agrammatic patients delete traces from structural representations and end up assigning thematic roles randomly. Grodzinsky believed that all of his patients diagnosed with Broca's aphasia had deficits only with sentences involving movement and traces. TDH may also be called "movement theory."

A foundation for argument was set by Berndt, Mitchum, and Haendiges (1996) who carried out a meta-analysis of reversible sentence comprehension in agrammatic aphasia. They concluded that the asyntactic pattern of deficit can occur with all types of aphasia, not just Broca's aphasia. Moreover, about one-third of those with Broca's aphasia were above-chance in comprehending reversible passives and, thus, did not conform to the asyntactic pattern. Grodzinsky and his colleagues (1999) did not care for how Berndt selected patients for analysis. A debate ensued regarding patient selection biases and statistical procedures (e.g., Caramazza et al., 2001). Caplan (2002) found Berndt's conclusions to be consistent with his research and considered them to be a problem for Grodzinsky's TDH. In general, the foundation for any theory of comprehension in Broca's aphasia was shaken, and research returned to taking one set of data at a time.

Several investigators decided to examine the basis for Grodzinsky's TDH. Support came from Friedmann and Shapiro (2003) who found a deficit (chance performance) in sentence–picture matching for Hebrew sentences involving noun-phrase (NP) movement. They suggested that aphasic people use an "avoid movement" comprehension strategy. Also, using the off-line procedures of picture choice or sentence–picture verification, researchers found results with other languages that were not consistent with a TDH explanation (e.g., Beretta, Piñango, Patterson, and Hartford, 1999; Burchert, de Bleser, and Sonntag, 2003; Caramazza, Capasso, Capitani, and Miceli, 2005; Luzzatti et al., 2001). One fairly consistent find-

ing continued to be the variability of people with Broca's aphasia.

The following Spanish active and passive sentences were used in a study of five monolingual agrammatic patients in Venezuela (Beretta et al., 1999):

(10a) El perro parece seguir al hombre.
(The dog seems to follow the man.)
(10b) El hombre parece ser seguido por el perro.
(The man seems to be followed by the dog.)

The active (9a) was understood above chance, and the passive (9b) was understood at chance. This result was consistent with the asyntactic pattern, but performance on other types of sentences in the study did not fit TDH expectations. This is important for Grodzinsky's theory, because his claim has been that asyntactic comprehension is a problem for any sentence containing constituent movement.

O'Grady and Lee (2005) proposed an alternative linguistic account of deficit in agrammatic comprehension, called the Isomorphic Mapping Hypothesis (IMH). In this case, patients have difficulty with sentences in which the order of NPs is not aligned with the temporal order of the depicted event.

(11a) She put the crayon on the pencil.
(11b) He tapped the crayon with the pencil.

In 11a, the agent acts on the crayon before the pencil, which is isomorphic with NP order in the sentence. In 10b, the agent picks up the pencil before tapping the crayon, which is inconsistent with NP order. In an enactment experiment with four participants who had Broca's aphasia, O'Grady and Lee found above-chance performance with isomorphic sentences and chance performance with nonisomorphic sentences. This is only a beginning from the IMH viewpoint.

Studies of processing address TDH with respect to traces. The cross-modal priming procedure provides an opportunity to test the psychological validity of any proposal that a patient has difficulty processing at the location of a trace or gap. Sometimes a gap involves movement, sometimes it does not. Zurif, Swinney, Prather and others (1993) presented the following types of sentences over headphones (gaps are designated by the symbol for a trace[t]):

(12a) The passenger smiled at *the baby* in the blue pajamas who [t] drank milk at the train station.
(12b) The passenger smiled at *the baby* that the woman in the pink jacket fed [t] at the train station.

In 12a, the gap is a pronoun. In 12b, there is a true empty space that is thought to function like the pronoun. That is, antecedents (e.g., *the baby*) are thought to be reactivated at the gaps; if this is so, then the gaps should prime related visual targets (e.g., *diaper*) for lexical decision.

Zurif and Swinney found that patients with Broca's aphasia failed to prime related targets at the gaps for both types of sentences, whereas normal controls evidenced antecedent reactivation. This research supports the notion that a trace has psychological reality. It also indicates that people with Broca's aphasia have a deficit in concept reactivation or priming at a gap. There is little help here for TDH, however, because only 12b contains constituent movement. Instead of movement, the common thread underlying deficient performance is the phenomenon of "gap filling" with an antecedent.

Blumstein and her colleagues (1998) discovered something different. They turned the cross-modal priming procedure into a unimodal priming procedure. Instead of presenting a visual-lexical decision at the gap, they presented an auditory target for lexical decision. The sentence was differentiated from the target by gender. The sentence was presented in a male voice, and the target in a female voice. We could call it a cross-gender priming task. Blumstein studied four types of sentences, and the semantically related lexical targets are shown beneath the trace location where they were presented. Sentences 13b and 13c were said to be noncanonical, containing movement of a recipient to an earlier position in the sentence.

(13a) Which *gun* did the trash collector find [t] in the alley?
       shoot
(13b) The *car* that the old lady was selling [t] needed many repairs.
       truck
(13c) The president visited the *city* that the big earthquake destroyed [t].
                town
(13d) The spy knew which *lock* the detective had opened [t].
       key

Seven participants with Broca's aphasia displayed priming effects, and so did a smaller group with Wernicke's aphasia. Thus, patients with either syndrome filled gaps in sentences involving movement, which is contrary to Grodzinsky's claim that such traces disappear and contrary to the findings of Zurif and Swinney. It is also possible that the antecedent concept simply maintained its original activation until the target was presented.

Especially when slowed processing is proposed, it may be useful to present targets later than the location of a gap in a cross-modal priming task. Burkhardt, Piñango, and Wong's (2003) patients with Broca's aphasia were not primed at the point of the trace, a finding similar to Zurif and Swinney's study. However, these participants were primed at a point later downstream and at a point where normal controls were not primed. Therefore, it appears that the participants with Broca's aphasia were delayed in reactivating antecedents.

In sum, linguistic studies identify structures that pose problems for people with aphasia, but they do not then specify the cognitive processing impairment. Difficulties with movement have been demonstrated in sentence–picture matching tasks, leading to the proposal that traces are deleted at some point in comprehension. With online tasks, deficits at a gap have been demonstrated with sentences not containing movement. In other online studies, people with agrammatism have shown a capacity for gap filling (or trace filling). Tasks that appear to detect automatic reactivation have had results that are somewhat different from the use of tasks that allow for strategic final interpretation and picture selection.

In conclusion, we should return to the beginning of this section on syntactic processing in which structure was illustrated with structural ambiguities. A large body of psycholinguistic literature is devoted to online demonstrations of automatic structural assignment (see van Gompel, Pickering et al., 2005, for a review of theories). In aphasiology, syntax has been studied mainly off-line or with respect to filling gaps. Caplan (2002) advised that "caution must be observed in taking the pattern of performance . . . in sentence–picture matching or enactment (off-line tasks) as definitive evidence for a deficit in the unconscious, obligatory construction of syntactic structures" (p. 333). He added that "few patients have been tested for online syntactic processing or for the ability to construct and interpret a large range of syntactic structures" (p. 335). In particular, there have been no reports of agrammatic patients being studied for the automatic assignment of structure at the location of structural ambiguities.

Semantic Interpretation

Semantic processing can be confused by bad information from damaged components of the system. For Broca's aphasia, the semantic constraint hypothesis states that intact semantic processes are a source of controlled or strategic adaptation to these limitations. Another possibility, suggested first by Schwartz and others (1980), stipulates that lexical and syntactic processes are intact and that asyntactic comprehension is actually based on an impairment in the final interpretive operation of assigning thematic roles. This is called the **mapping hypothesis,** and it has some clinical implications because of the promotion of "mapping therapy" (see Chapter 9).

The mapping hypothesis states that patients with clinical evidence of asyntactic comprehension fail to assign thematic roles to normally realized syntactic representations (Linebarger, 1990). With respect to the serial model of Figure 5.2a, the impairment can be said to be *between* the syntactic parser and semantic interpretation, where a mapping operation superimposes "who is doing what to whom" on a successful parse. Put more simply, the mechanism coordinates sentence meaning with sentence form. Empirical support for the mapping hypothesis is based on the claim that there is evidence of intact parsing despite the clinical evidence of sentence comprehension problems (i.e., difficulty with reversible sentences, role reversal errors dominating lexical errors).

Grammaticality judgments have been the main source of support for the mapping hypothesis (Linebarger, 1990; Linebarger, Schwartz, and Saffran, 1983). Success with grammaticality judgment in many studies suggested to Linebarger that the parser must be intact.

The main argument against the mapping hypothesis pertains to its reliance on off-line grammaticality and plausibility judgments as the basis for concluding that the syntactic parser is intact. Swinney and Zurif (1995) suggested that to diagnose the status of parsing, an experimenter should specify what a parser does and then design an experiment that addresses its characteristics. An experiment should also distinguish between a mapper and a parser in real time. At least, an investigator should consider that parsing has an automatic component and then test this characteristic accordingly.

Working Memory and Resource Theory

A reduction of working memory capacity is becoming a regular theme for explaining language deficits. As indicated in Chapter 4, the idea has been applied mainly to aphasia in general. One aspect of the theory is that a specific symptom, such as agrammatism, is not caused by a damaged component of a processing system. Instead the reduction of overall processing capacity may target one system more than others, such as the relatively demanding sentence processing systems.

This would give the appearance of a damaged component.

Several investigators have suggested that resource theory accounts at least partially for comprehension deficits in Broca's aphasia (e.g., Haarmann and Kolk, 1994; Swinney and Zurif, 1995). Using a sentence–picture matching task, Friederici and Frazier (1992) found an interaction between syntactic structure and processing demands of the task for agrammatic patients. The processing demands were manipulated by presenting pictures with a sentence or delaying the pictures after the sentence. The interaction was interpreted as the limitation of processing resources affecting syntactic processing more than lexical processing.

Friedmann and Gvion (2003) stretched short-term buffer demands for the comprehension of Hebrew sentences. Half the sentences were subject relatives (14) and half were object relatives (15), and the sentences varied in the amount of filler inserted into conveying similar actions (e.g., 14b, 15b). The following translations represent only some of the conditions in the experiment:

(14a) This is a guy with a beard that dresses the soldier.
(14b) This is the woman with the brown pants and the white shirt that hugs the woman.
(15a) This is the man that the boy catches.
(15b) This is the soldier that the doctor with the white robe draws.

A binary sentence–picture matching task included a single foil depicting a role reversal between agent and recipient. Individuals with agrammatic aphasia showed the familiar pattern of better comprehension of subject relatives than object relatives (see also Chapter 4). However, these participants were not affected by amount of filler (characterized by the authors as distances between an antecedent and a gap). Friedmann and Gvion concluded that these results do not support a working memory capacity reduction as the explanation for an agrammatic person's syntactic difficulties in comprehension.

Summary and Conclusions

Broca's aphasia is a swaggering flagship in a contentious sea. Theories of comprehension and production can be divided generally into linguistic theories and psycholinguistic theories. General agreement is found with respect to the status of linguistic knowledge or competence. People with Broca's aphasia have not lost their knowledge of lexical and syntactic features of the language they speak. Thus, investigators agree that impairments should be identified with processing. Researchers may differ regarding the characterization of processing, some limiting their scope of consideration to working memory and others also pondering specific processing components of sentence comprehension. The latter tend to reject notions of a totally demolished device in favor of some form of partial impairment, at least, for most patients of this type.

Agrammatism may be a problem either at Garrett's positional level or may be the result of reduced working memory capacity. The situation is more complex for comprehension (see Table 5.3). Some say the problem is slow lexical activation, and others say it is not slow. Some point to damaged parsing. Others claim that parsing is fine, and thematic mapping is impaired instead. While findings appear to be contradictory, such as response times at gaps, we should take a deep breath and realize that all sorts of methods are just being introduced. This is important for the clinical consumer of research to realize in case someone claims to have the answer.

ANOMIC APHASIA

Sometimes called amnesic aphasia, anomic aphasia is the mildest form of acquired language disorder. It gets relatively little attention in basic clinical research. Wernicke's aphasia seems to be studied much more frequently as a fluent contrast to Broca's aphasia.

Anomic aphasia is nearly the opposite of agrammatism. Comprehension seems unimpaired

TABLE 5.3 Summary of the theories of asyntactic comprehension. Only component-based theories are included. We should not forget the working memory hypotheses.

COMPONENT	THEORY	SHORT DEFINITION	METHOD
Lexical	Automaticity hypothesis	Slow activation of meaning in semantic memory	Semantic priming cross-modal priming
	Lexical hypothesis	Insensitivity to function words	Word monitoring
Syntactic	No-syntax hypothesis	General problem with structural knowledge or processing	Off-line comprehension tests
	Impaired parser	Slow assignment of structure	Syntactic priming
	Linearity and trace-deletion hypotheses	Simple or incomplete structural representation	Off-line comprehension tests
Semantic	Mapping hypothesis	Impaired assignment of thematic roles to intact parse	Off-line comprehension tests and grammaticality judgments

until we give the Token Test or assess reading. Function words are produced normally and content-bearing words are problematic. A patient fills word-finding gaps with generic terms and circumlocutions. Anomic aphasia is usually associated with a posterior lesion sparing Wernicke's area, but the same general characteristics can be observed after frontal lesions. A frontal anomic aphasia may be studied in comparison to posterior anomic aphasia (e.g., Kohn and Goodglass, 1985).

Divided Attention

Patients with frontal and posterior anomic aphasic can have attention problems while performing simple clinical tasks. Without a competing distraction, tasks of semantic categorization, grammaticality judgment, and sentence completion are done almost normally. However, patients drop below normal performance under focused and divided attention conditions. In a study of spontaneous picture description, a group with mild fluent aphasia (mostly anomic) had performance decrements in the dual-task condition that normal controls did not have (Murray, Holland, and Beeson, 1998).

The studies of attention and resource allocation indicate that mildly impaired patients should be assessed in optimal conditions to determine their peak capabilities. On the other hand, identifying the deficit may be important for functional communication, because some of these excellent communicators become distressed over language processing problems that arise when they are trying to get a ticket at an airport or participate in a gathering of friends.

Language Comprehension

Anomic aphasia has been examined rarely with lexical-semantic access paradigms. Chenery, Ingram, and Murdoch (1990) compared high- and low-comprehending aphasic subjects in a semantically primed lexical decision task. The high-comprehending group consisted of mostly anomic aphasia. This group was able to make controlled semantic judgments and displayed semantic priming with a 500 msec prime–target interval. Both performances indicated that semantic memory is largely intact and it can be activated normally when given plenty of time.

Regarding sentence comprehension, patients exhibited a normal sensitivity to function words in one study but had difficulty with inflections in a highly inflected language (Goodenough et al., 1977; Smith and Bates, 1987). Peach, Canter, and Gallaher (1988) compared patients with anomic and conduction aphasia in comprehending thematic information in active sentences. Both groups were accurate around 70 percent of the time and, like patients with Broca's aphasia, made significantly more subject–object order errors than lexical errors. Therefore, patients with anomic aphasia have a comprehension deficit. In clinical testing, it is most likely to be displayed with the Token Test and reading tests.

Word Retrieval

In general, naming accuracy with anomic aphasia is equivalent to Broca's aphasia, except when posterior and anterior anomic aphasias are separated (Table 5.4). The more frequently recognized posterior form has a more severe naming deficit than the anterior form. Groups do not differ in frequency of semantic paraphasias, so that this error by itself does not appear to differentiate type of aphasia. Anomic aphasia is distinctive in the use of circumlocutions when intended words are difficult to access (Kohn and Goodglass, 1985).

Good comprehension enables these patients to perform about equally when naming verbal descriptions and naming objects (Goodglass and Stuss, 1979).

Pashek and Tompkins (2002) studied 20 cases of mild aphasia with residual anomia. Word finding was better in narrative production than in picture-naming tasks. The basic conclusion was that confrontation naming is not predictive of word finding in narrative production for mild aphasia. This predictive weakness of the naming task has become a common finding (see Chapter 4).

People with anomic aphasia had been shown to be better at retrieving verbs than nouns, opposite the common finding with agrammatism (Miceli, Silveri, Villa, and Caramazza, 1984; Williams and Canter, 1987). A similar result in Pashek and Tompkins's study may have been confounded by word length and frequency. Bastiaanse and Jonkers (1998) did not find the double dissociation between nouns and verbs when comparing fluent and nonfluent aphasia. Anomic patients were like agrammatic patients in having more difficulty with action naming than object naming. These studies indicate that we should not necessarily expect a particular noun–verb difference in someone with anomic aphasia.

Those of us who are neurologically intact occasionally have a person's name on the tip of our tongue. We may say that it is a long name and

TABLE 5.4   Object-naming scores for the major syndromes.

	KOHN AND GOODGLASS (1985)	WILLIAMS AND CANTER (1982)	
		High-Frequency Words	*Low-Frequency Words*
Maximum score	85.0	20.0	20.0
Broca's	50.4	11.7	12.5
Anomic (posterior)	42.9	12.1	10.9
Anomic (anterior)	54.5		
Conduction	59.4	10.0	6.8
Wernicke's	39.1	7.8	6.1

begins with a certain sound. We may report the number of syllables. Do aphasic people enter a tip-of-the-tongue (TOT) state? If so, what does it tell us about the word retrieval system? Beeson and her colleagues in Arizona looked at these questions with respect to naming famous people. Before examining what happened, let us consider again the framework used for explaining naming or word-finding problems.

The framework continues to be two-stage theories of word finding that separate a lexical (or phonological) level from a semantic level (e.g., Figure 4.2). People with anomic aphasia exhibit two behaviors that are informative regarding the status of this system. One is the presence of word-finding gaps filled by generic terms such as *something* or *that thing over there.* The other is circumlocution, which is indicative of intact semantic activation (i.e., the concept to be conveyed) and a general capacity to retrieve lexical forms.

Ellis, Kay, and Franklin (1992) provided a guide for distinguishing between impairments at the semantic and lexical levels of word production. An impairment of the semantic system should result in word-finding problems because the semantic system informs the lexical system. As indicated in Chapter 4, pervasive semantic deficits in comprehension and object classification should be indicative of a problem in this system. Another clue would be word-finding deficits that are unique for particular semantic categories. We would suspect a disorder confined to the lexical system when object sorting and word comprehension are relatively intact. Case studies have demonstrated this approach to diagnosis (Franklin, Howard, and Patterson, 1995; Flude, Ellis, and Kay, 1989; Kay and Ellis, 1987).

Considering mostly scattered case studies, it appears that the word-finding difficulty in anomic aphasia can be attributed to a problem with accessing lexical form rather than a problem with semantics. Etiology may be important for understanding the occurrence of an exception. Patients with the diagnostic pattern of anomic aphasia were shown to have a semantic problem in one case and a lexi-

cal problem in the other case (Martin, Serrano, and Iglesias, 1999). The case with the semantic problem was caused by herpes encephalitis with extensive and deep temporal lobe damage.

What about the TOT state with anomic aphasia? When a patient could not name a famous person in Beeson's study, the patient was asked a series of questions about the person and the name (Beeson, Holland, and Murray, 1997). A group with anomic aphasia was compared to groups with Broca's and conduction aphasia. Performances with Broca's and conduction aphasia were similar with 64 to 70 percent ability to provide semantic information and 25 to 30 percent ability to identify the first letter of the first or last name. Patients with anomic aphasia were quite different. They were more accurate naming than the other groups (i.e., 60 percent accuracy). When they could not name, they produced semantic information 91 percent of the time but could identify the first letter only 7 percent of the time. These patients had a fairly intact semantic system but an occasional serious difficulty accessing an entire lexical form, or "access to phonology was more of an all-or-none phenomenon with the anomic group" (p. 333).

CONDUCTION APHASIA

The principal basis for diagnosing conduction aphasia is the severity of repetition impairment relative to a high level of auditory language comprehension and fluent spontaneous production. The main linguistic symptom is the occurrence of word production errors that sound like the intended word (i.e., phonemic paraphasias). In some patients, these errors are infrequent until the patient is asked to repeat, and errors increase as sentence length increases and familiarity decreases (Goodglass and Kaplan, 1983). Conduction aphasia is a relatively uncommon syndrome. It took Bartha and Benke (2003) five years to accumulate 20 cases for their research.

After reviewing the literature, Nadeau (2000) concluded that there are four variations of conduction aphasia based on the relative prominence of repetition deficit and/or phonemic paraphasias.

They are displayed in Table 5.5 because repetition and phonology comprise the main issues for conduction aphasia and because subtypes are likely to reappear in the future. Two subtypes are supported by only a few reported cases, one of which turns out to have been diagnosed as having transcortical motor aphasia (hence, good repetition). Bartha and Benke's (2003) definition for research selection is more familiar: "a profound deficit in repetition displaying phonemic paraphasias and self-corrections . . . in the absence of a severe language comprehension disorder" (p. 95). Nadeau's combination conduction aphasia seems to be closest to the classical clinical entity.

Language comprehension

Some standard tests of auditory and reading comprehension were given to 20 cases of conduction aphasia, resulting in a diagnosis of mild comprehension impairment (Bartha and Benke, 2003). As would be expected with mild comprehension impairment, 11 of these patients performed poorly with the Token Test.

There have been a few reports of asyntactic comprehension with conduction aphasia. Suspicion of syntactic comprehension deficit began with studies showing groups with conduction aphasia performing like those with Broca's aphasia (Caramazza and Zurif, 1976; Goodglass et al., 1979; Heilman and Scholes, 1976). In a study by Peach and colleagues (1988), subjects with conduction aphasia were very much like Broca's aphasia

in comprehending active sentences. Asyntactic comprehension was also reported in case studies (Caramazza, Basili, Koller, and Berndt, 1981; Friedrich, Martin, and Kemper, 1985). Such findings are problematic for the claim that this comprehension pattern is unique to Broca's aphasia.

Individuals with conduction aphasia were included in Friedmann and Gvion's (2003) study of short-term buffer demands on the comprehension of Hebrew sentences (see examples 14 and 15). Contrary to those with agrammatic aphasia, participants with conduction aphasia were well above chance in comprehending both subject and object relatives with the binary picture-choice task. This result is supportive of Grodzinsky's TDH in that the asyntactic pattern did not occur with a fluent syndrome.

Repetition and the STM Question

The unique deficit of repetition was purported initially to demonstrate the distinctiveness of memory stores through a selective impairment of short-term memory (Shallice and Warrington, 1977). STM is now identified as a **short-term buffer.** Input buffers retain stimulus representations briefly so that currently processed information can be related to previous input. Output buffers hold on to activated word forms while output processes act on them. Isolated memory span deficit signifies impaired phonological encoding and is considered to be evidence for "fractionation" of a phonological buffer from an articulatory buffer in working

TABLE 5.5   A proposal of variations in conduction aphasia (Nadeau, 2000).

SUBCATEGORY	CLINICAL PATTERN	
Repetition conduction aphasia	Severe repetition deficit and minimal or no phonemic paraphasias	Common
Reproduction conduction aphasia	Severe deficit in repetition of nonwords	One case
Phonological aphasia	Pervasive phonological paraphasias and minimal repetition deficit	Two cases
Combination conduction aphasia	Symptoms of both reproduction and phonological types	Common

memory (WM). Auditory verbal short-term memory was reduced in most of Bartha and Benke's (2003) 20 patients with conduction aphasia.

Impairment of a phonological buffer is illustrated by two cases. Each suffered a stroke with resulting symptoms of conduction aphasia. Case PV perceived speech normally in discrimination and rhyme judgment. She repeated single words but could not repeat digit and word sequences longer than three items. Retention time for subspan lists was reduced (Vallar and Baddeley, 1984). Case EA had an auditory digit span of 1.5 and displayed no recency effect for retaining items at the end of long lists. A deficit of phonological encoding was indicated when phonologically similar letters were harder to retain than phonologically dissimilar letters (Friedrich, Glenn, and Marin, 1984). Both cases had longer spans for visual stimuli, thereby, locating the problem in the auditory system.

EA continued to participate in case studies at least 15 years after her stroke (e.g., Martin, Shelton, and Yaffee, 1994).

When memory span was considered to be a gross indicator of processing capacity, researchers wondered about the impact of deficient STM on auditory language comprehension. As indicated previously, processing capacity is now examined with respect to working memory (WM) and resource allocation, and automatic processing is thought to take up little room in WM. With respect to the revised role of STM, the question is worded in terms of whether the phonological buffer is necessary for sentence comprehension.

To examine the role of the short-term buffer, let us look at the comprehension abilities of PV and EA. PV could comprehend long sentences of around 16 words. She displayed a variety of syntactic comprehension and judgment abilities except when anomalies occurred between widely separated elements in stories (Vallar and Baddeley, 1987). EA, on the other hand, was one of the cases with conduction aphasia shown to have asyntactic comprehension. Friedrich and others (1985) concluded that EA's phonological buffer impairment could not account for her pattern of sentence comprehension. Comprehension processes continued to

operate despite the STM disorder. One possibility was based on the assumption that "a phonological code . . . is the primary means by which important syntactic markers are represented" (p. 409). With her phonological buffer impairment, EA was not encoding grammatical morphemes.

Participants with conduction aphasia in Friedmann and Gvion's (2003) study were not affected by amount of filler. That is, these patients did not have a STM constraint when comprehending subject- and object-relative sentences. This result appears to contradict Bartha and Benke's (2003) finding of reduced STM, but comprehension may work differently from immediate recollection. In general, there is minimal or mixed evidence that a reduced STM accounts for repetition deficit or anything else in conduction aphasia.

Phonological Output Processes

Sound-related errors can be a distraction when listening to someone with conduction aphasia. A traditional approach to classification is to refer to all sound-related errors as phonemic paraphasias (Table 1.3). Recently investigators have been using a finer classification. Formal paraphasias are real words (e.g., *laser* for *razor*) and phonemic paraphasias are nonwords (e.g., *slazer*). The sound relatedness of errors suggests that word finding in conduction aphasia is different from the word-finding disorder in anomic aphasia. Conduction aphasia does not seem to involve the all-or-none retrieval found in anomic aphasia. Most sound-related errors are nonwords, but a few patients may produce a high rate of formal paraphasias (Gold and Kertesz, 2001). Current studies focus on nonword errors (e.g., Wilshire, 2002; Schwartz, Wilshire, Gagnon et al., 2004).

Studies of conduction aphasia tend to concentrate on the lexical stage of phonological output. Blumstein (1973) compared the conversational speech of patients with conduction, Broca's, and Wernicke's aphasia. She concluded that the groups were identical in the kind of phonemic errors produced. Perhaps influenced by this work, subsequent studies left the impression that any sound-level error was being called a phonemic paraphasia.

Because some of Blumstein's patients were fluent and others were nonfluent, researchers began to wonder if the widespread use of "phonemic paraphasia" was obscuring important differences in the speech of patients with different aphasias. This has been a particular concern regarding Broca's aphasia, which can be accompanied by motor system impairments of apraxia of speech (AOS) and/or mild dysarthria. There could be different levels of impairment associated with the distinction between phonemic and phonetic levels of speech production.

The ability to diagnose disorders at the phonemic and phonetic levels is partly a function of level of observation (Canter, Trost, and Burns, 1985). The usual clinical strategy is *perceptual analysis,* which involves classifying what we hear. *Acoustic analysis* records the speech signal with devices such as a spectrograph. Parameters of acoustic analysis include sound duration and voice onset time (VOT) for voiced sounds. Both of these approaches observe the external result of the production mechanism. *Internal analyses* depend on observing structures or events within the speech mechanism, such as evoked potentials in the brain stem, muscle contraction, or velar movement. As observation gets further from neurological events, the chance of misdiagnosis increases. Thus, the opportunity for error is greatest in perceptual analysis. Researchers thought that errors across syndromes in Blumstein's study sounded alike but were not necessarily the same disorder internally.

Many researchers set out to obtain relevant observations. Spectrographic measures showed longer sound duration in patients with Broca's aphasia than in the fluent aphasias (Williams and Seaver, 1986). Synergy in VOT was found with fluent aphasias but was lacking in Broca's aphasia or patients with diagnosis of AOS (Blumstein, Cooper, Goodglass et al., 1980; Itoh, Sasanuma, Tatsumi, Murakami, Fukusako, and Suzuki, 1982). Velar movement was asynchronous in nonfluent aphasia, whereas timing was normal in fluent aphasias (Itoh, Sasanuma, Hirose et al., 1983).

Seddoh and his colleagues (1996) found that patients with AOS had impairment of vowel and CV durational control and had more variability of duration than patients with conduction aphasia. Those with conduction aphasia were similar to normal controls. This sample indicates that nonfluent aphasia is accompanied by a disruption of the motor system, whereas motor function in fluent aphasias is normal.

Clinicians do not normally have such laboratory support. So, can we hear differences in the speech of nonfluent and fluent aphasias? Table 5.6 includes a summary of some differences uncovered in research. Two research teams studied naming and word repetition in Broca's, conduction, and Wernicke's aphasia (Canter, 1988; Canter et al., 1985; Manoi, Fukusako, Itoh, and Sasanuma, 1983). Conduction aphasia had more substitution errors taken from elsewhere in the same word, called transpositions. Buckingham (1989) called them "linear ordering derailments" that can be anticipatory (e.g., *papple*) or perseverative (e.g., *gingerged*). Speech with Broca's aphasia contained more transitional disruptions from one sound or syllable to the next. Errors increased as a function of motoric complexity in Broca's speech but not in fluent aphasias. All groups made one-feature errors, namely, an incorrect sound close to the target; three-feature errors were more likely in fluent aphasia.

Nickels and Howard (1995) have expressed an apparently different viewpoint regarding the distinction between apraxia of speech and fluent phonemic paraphasias. They stated that there is no reason to assume nonfluent and fluent phonological errors are different. The disorders are points on "a continuum of impairments to different aspects of the phonological encoding and motor programming process" (Nickels and Howard, 2004, p. 60). This argumentation was used to justify the inclusion of both disorders in one experimental group and has appeared in the participant description section of publications (e.g., Gordon, 2002).

On the other hand, different sites of lesion provides one reason to suspect that nonfluent and fluent phonological errors could be differ-

TABLE 5.6 Differential diagnosis of phonological disorders, including the terminology used to designate functional levels. Garrett's terminology (Figure 5.1) is represented in boldface.

DISORDER	CNS LOCATION	FUNCTIONAL LOCATION	SPEECH SYMPTOMS
Conduction aphasia	Posterior cortex	**Phonological process (positional level)** Premotor stage	Fluency More errors in final position Sequence errors Transpositions anticipatory perseverative No distortions
Apraxia of speech	Anterior, pre-motor cortex	**Regular phonological processes (phonetic)** Prearticulatory or motor programming	Laborious More errors in initial position Transition errors Distortions and substitutions
Dysarthria	Motor cortex and below	**Motor coding process (articulatory)** Execution	Varied distortion and substitution Respiratory and phonatory deficit Impairment at all functional levels

ent. Some could argue that research deeper than perceptual analysis also provides good reasons for making a distinction (as well as differences of treatment approach). Students of aphasiology should pay attention to slight shifts of wording, such as from a plural *phonological encoding and motor programming processes* to the singular *phonological encoding and motor programming process* used by Nickels and Howard.

Like theoretical options for other areas of language, phonological problems of conduction aphasia are investigated with respect to stage theory or interactive-activation theory. Caramazza and his colleagues (2000) studied a case in which semantic errors were absent and nearly all phonological errors in naming resulted in nonwords. They proposed an impairment that spared semantic processing and was specific to phonology. Wilshire and Fisher (2004) reported a case with exclusively phonemic and formal paraphasias and felt that explanation was served with an interactive-activation

account within the phonological component (i.e., pathologically rapid decay of phonological output representations). On the surface, these conclusions seem like a contradiction involving modular and interactive theories, but they are merely a paradox. One identifies impairment in phonology rather than semantics; the other is more precise about the phonological impairment.

Kohn and Smith (1990) worked on ideas about what happens to phonological output processing in fluent aphasias with many sound-related errors. In an extensive analysis of CM, they found that some errors were unlike normal errors. A few interactions occurred across several words in an utterance. In word interactions, a segment of one word is "copied" into another word. Kohn interpreted these behaviors as an "inability to clear a phonemic output buffer" (p. 133). That is, pieces of lexical items activated for previous production remain stuck in this temporary holding region of working memory.

Later, Kohn and Smith (1995) distinguished two types of phonological difficulty that are indicative of two stages in phonological output processing. The first stage is the activation of a stored "underspecified" *lexical-phonological representation*. Damage to this stage is indicated by greater difficulty in repeating and reading nonwords than real words. The lexical representation is sent to the second stage, which consists of sequential *phonemic planning* "from left to right." Damage to this stage, along with intact lexical activation, should cause errors that preserve or simplify the phonological structure of targets. Kohn and Smith concluded that fluent patients with lexical activation disorder made segmental errors with no position constraints, whereas fluent patients with phonemic planning disorder made errors that increased systematically from left to right.

In sum, phonemic errors in conduction aphasia are diagnosed as a disorder at a "prearticulatory" phonemic level in the language system, whereas AOS is a disorder in the articulatory or motor system. Like dysarthria or hemiplegia, AOS can accompany agrammatic aphasia because of site of lesion. AOS contributes to the nonfluency of these cases. Perhaps, we can say that the person with AOS produces an accurate lexical representation with difficulty, whereas conduction aphasia involves an inaccurate lexical representation produced smoothly. With respect to conduction aphasia, disorder underlying repetition deficit may converge on the disorder underlying phonological errors on the basis of phonological processing. That is, there may be a common disorder underlying impairment of a phonological input buffer and a phonological output buffer.

WERNICKE'S APHASIA

Wernicke's aphasia is the most severely impaired fluent syndrome, caused by a lesion in the posterior superior region of the temporal lobe. It is characterized by jargon and severe comprehension deficit. The term *jargonaphasia* is seen frequently in a presumed reference to patients with Wernicke's aphasia. According to Mitchum and others (1990), neologisms are so characteristic that Wernicke's aphasia is one of the few syndromes that can be identified by object-naming errors alone. Also, because of poor recognition of deficit, patients are not at all self-conscious about their neologisms and other paraphasias.

Despite the diagnostic signs of poor comprehension and jargon, we are likely to find studies including a group or a case purported to have Wernicke's aphasia but with test scores showing good comprehension and a surprisingly strong naming ability. One possibility is that the group consists of a well-recovered subgroup of this aphasia that had been found to have relatively small lesions (see Chapter 7). In a study by Faroqi-Shah and Thompson (2003), a group with Wernicke's aphasia had aphasia quotients (AQs) similar to a group with Broca's aphasia. Fluency scores were in the high range, but two Wernicke's participants had high comprehension scores. The authors explained that these patients had recovered from the low scores that are more definitive of this syndrome. A possibility in other research is that participants are misdiagnosed based on criteria that are too general, such as the existence of any comprehension deficit and/or simply fluency of verbal expression.

Word Comprehension

When syndromes are compared in tests of comprehension, this group usually makes the most errors along with global aphasia. Because of the severity of comprehension deficit, it is appropriate to focus on word comprehension in Wernicke's aphasia.

A patient may be with a group of people and act as if he does not even hear the conversations. Proximity of the lesion to the primary auditory area, as well as severity of deficit, led researchers to suspect that the processing of linguistic stimuli does not go beyond speech perception. The deficit appears to be like "pure word deafness" (Kirshner, Webb, and Duncan, 1981). Yet, speech perception deficits are not specific to this syndrome and are often not sufficient to reduce language comprehension substantially (Blumstein et al., 1977; Miceli et al., 1980). Nevertheless, variation of lesion size and location may create an "auditory-predominant" subgroup in which auditory processing is substantially below reading (Heilman, Rothi, Campanella, and Wolfson, 1979; Kirshner et al., 1989).

A loss or disorganization of semantic memory might reduce comprehension at the word level and produce paraphasias. In an object classification study, Wernicke patients were impaired in relating objects according to action, function, and physical attributes (Cohen et al., 1980). In another study, participants were shown three objects (e.g., apple, banana, pear) and, when ready, were then shown a series of test objects one at a time (e.g., peach, chair). They had to press a button indicating whether a test object belonged to the class of objects presented initially. Wernicke's aphasia did not exhibit a unique problem, indicating that semantic content and structure are preserved (Koemeda-Lutz, Cohen, and Meier, 1987).

Part of the surprising findings in Milberg and Blumstein's early work with semantic priming was that patients with Wernicke's aphasia had the priming effects that did not occur for Broca's aphasia (Milberg et al., 1987). Yet, Wernicke patients also had many more errors making lexical decisions, and they performed much worse than Broca patients in making judgments about the semantic relatedness of word pairs. In Hagoort's (1993) study with shorter SOAs (prime-target intervals), Wernicke's participants were primed like those with Broca's aphasia. Thus, the semantic system with Wernicke's aphasia may be intact structurally. Difficulties occur with slow tasks examining conceptualization at the controlled or strategic level.

Kiran and Thompson (2003) compared small groups with Wernicke's and Broca's aphasias on a category verification task. Word pairs were presented like a visual priming task, and only a 200 msec interval was placed between the words. The first word was a superordinate category (e.g., *vegetable*) and the second word was a typical exemplar (e.g., *tomato*), an atypical exemplar (e.g., *garlic*), or a nonmember (e.g., *rifle*). The participants were instructed to decide if the second word

belonged in the preceding category. The group with Wernicke's aphasia made more errors and were slower than the others; they also lacked a typicality effect that should have occurred with the short SOA and an assumption that spreading activation finds the most related nodes first. Although the Wernicke's group had the same *Western Aphasia Battery* (WAB) AQ as the Broca's group (like Faroqi-Shah and Thompson, 2003), the Wernicke's group displayed a unique difficulty making quick semantic decisions about words.

Sentence Comprehension

Wernicke's aphasia has been swept up with Broca's aphasia in efforts to determine if aphasias include a broad double dissociation of semantic and syntactic functions. The general hypothesis regarding Wernicke's aphasia has been that it might be a problem in the semantic domain while syntactic capacities remain intact.

Regarding activation of word meaning in sentences, four Wernicke participants were quite different from those with Broca's aphasia with the crossmodal semantic priming procedure (Swinney et al., 1989). The Wernicke patients seemed to be like normal adults, accessing multiple meanings automatically when the lexical decision task (LDT) was located right after the ambiguous prime. In the follow-up study in which the LDT was located five syllables after the ambiguous prime, the Wernicke patients continued to show activation of both meanings (Prather et al., 1994). This is unlike Broca's aphasia but is also unlike neurologically intact adults, indicative of a unique problem with Wernicke's aphasia. The problem appears to be a failure of context to bias or "penetrate" lexical access for the correct interpretation of the ambiguous word. It is as if the lexical-semantic system is stuck in a modular mode.

Caramazza and Zurif (1976) were perplexed about the performance pattern of five Wernicke patients in their pivotal study revealing asyntactic comprehension. These patients performed well on the task and had equal difficulty with syntactic and semantic factors. Caramazza and Zurif wrote frankly about the issue that introduced this section: "The good level of performance in the Wernicke's patients may have been due simply to a bias in the selection of patients; since patients had to have enough comprehension skills to be able to understand our instructions and perform the experimental task, we likely included only very mildly impaired, atypical Wernicke's aphasics" (p. 579).

Like other aphasias, processing canonical order appears to be preserved in Wernicke's aphasia (Bates et al., 1987a). Shapiro and others (1993) concluded that these patients, unlike Broca's aphasia, are impaired in activating verb-argument structures. The studies of gap filling leave us with findings that are as contradictory for Wernicke's aphasia as they are for Broca's aphasia. Zurif and others (1993) found that those with Wernicke's aphasia filled gaps, but those with Broca's aphasia did not. Blumstein and her colleagues (1998) obtained nearly the opposite result.

Nakano and Blumstein (2004) compared six Wernicke's to nine Broca's participants with a sentence-priming task in which the target was the last word. The target was syntactically viable but pragmatically either appropriate or unlikely (e.g., The kitten is drinking *milk/bourbon*). There were many subtle aspects to this experiment, and the two aphasic groups performed differently. The group with Wernicke's aphasia showed unique signs of deficiency in integrating semantic information.

The jury will be out for a long time regarding sentence comprehension in Wernicke's aphasia, because people with this syndrome should be difficult to test with sophisticated psycholinguistic procedures.

Word Retrieval

In clinical tests of object naming, patients with Wernicke's aphasia make more errors than those with other syndromes (Table 5.4). Patients also appear less likely to exhibit the tip-of-the-tongue (TOT) state (Goodglass et al., 1976). Unlike other syndromes, naming to description is more difficult than object naming, perhaps because of auditory comprehension deficit (Goodglass and Stuss, 1979). Kohn and Goodglass's (1985) naming study indicated that these patients do not differ from others in number of semantic and phonemic errors. Neologisms appear to set them apart (Mitchum et al., 1990).

Jargon consists of fluent verbalization containing lexical semantic and unrelated paraphasias and sublexical neologisms. We were introduced to this form of aphasia with Gardner's (1974) sample in the first chapter. It has complete sentences with lots of functors and inflections that seem to be in the right places. The sample is hard to interpret with one neologism (i.e., "repuceration") and words like *barbers* that have no apparent connection to context. Because of its minimal neologisms, we would refer to this sample as semantic jargon.

Unrelated and semantic errors indicate that people with Wernicke's aphasia can activate the lexicon. A semantic problem was indicated by the number of semantic paraphasias being correlated with number of semantic errors on a word-comprehension test (Gainotti, 1976). Rinnert and Whitaker (1973) inventoried relationships between semantic paraphasias and targets and compared them to normal word associations. Sixty percent of error targets corresponded to association norms for the error or the target. It was concluded that "semantic confusions are more like than unlike normal word associations" (p. 66). Thus, semantic errors may come from an intact semantic structure, which is consistent with semantic priming effects.

In his study of word fluency, Grossman (1981) examined the succession of words produced to a category such as "birds" (see Chapter 4). In contrast to nonfluent patients, those with Wernicke's aphasia were likely to produce words in the most distant bands of a category and words that did not belong in the category. Patients started producing examples of high typicality and progressed to examples of low typicality. They "often cross the borders around a referential field" (p. 327). Word fluency makes room for strategic processing, and patients with Wernicke's aphasia may be having difficulties using controlled word-finding strategies.

Neologisms tend to contain phonological sequences that are permissible in a patient's language. Exceptions are forms like *chpicters*. More examples come from samples of English provided by Buckingham and Kertesz (1976):

- "I appreciate that farshethe, because they have protocertive" (p. 66).
- "I would say that the mik daysis nosis or chpicters" (p. 70).

Investigators have distinguished two types. **Target-related neologisms** retain some phonological similarity to the target and could be roughly the same as sublexical phonemic paraphasias. **Abstruse neologisms** have little relationship to the target.

Patient LT was an elderly gentleman with a severe effortless jargon. He did not recognize his incomprehensible utterances and was surprised when he could tell that he was misunderstood. Robson and her colleagues (2003) examined his nonword responses in a naming task (e.g., neologisms). Many of these responses bore a phonological relationship to target words, and Robson found "no nonnative phonemes or violations of English phonotactic constraints" (p. 114). This indicated that the nonwords were generated by the lexical system rather than from some other source.

Hugh Buckingham (1981) asked "Where Do Neologisms Come From?" They could be an extreme manifestation of phonemic paraphasias, called the *conduction theory* (Kertesz and Benson, 1970; Robson et al., 2003). For the culprit to be a faulty phonological mechanism, a patient should produce a mix of phonemic paraphasias, neologisms, and ambiguous transformations. Also, the patient should not at the same time be producing other lexical paraphasias "or we could never, in principle, rule them out as possible inputs to the phonemic transformations" (Buckingham, 1981,

p. 50). This theory was ruled out at first, because patients exhibited no "middle ground" (Buckingham and Kertesz, 1976). Later, Buckingham (1987) would "not rule out the possibility that some bizarre lexical productions could stem from severe phonemic paraphasia" (p. 383).

Another proposal was that a patient has anomic aphasia but fills empty lexical slots with neologisms, called a *masking theory* (Buckingham, 1981). This would be an automatic or subconscious adjustment in the production system. When lexical activation fails, neologisms become "strings of well-formed phonemes or syllables that fill in the gaps and compensate for words not retrievable from the lexicon" (p. 198). Later, Buckingham (1987) suggested that a *random generator* of syllabic segments produces neologisms. In the context of masking theory, the random generator is assumed to fill gaps left by an underlying anomia. A lesion results in an abnormal process in addition to a damaged normal process.

Buckingham's ideas are similar to Kohn and Smith's stages of phonological output processing used to interpret sound-related errors in conduction aphasia. Abstruse neologisms could arise from damaged lexical activation. Target-related neologisms could arise from damaged phonemic planning (Kohn and Smith, 1995). If the latter is so, related errors should show the serial position effect from left to right found with conduction aphasia. In a study of neologistic naming errors, data did not conform to the discrete predictions of the theory. That is, related and remote neologisms did not differ with respect to serial position of phonemic errors (Gagnon and Schwartz, 1997).

Sentence Formulation

In a study of picture description, Wernicke patients generated as many words as normal individuals (Gleason, Goodglass, Obler et al., 1980). These aphasic participants produced many more verbs than nouns and used more indefinite "pointing" words (e.g., this, here) than normals and

Broca's participants. Schwartz (1987) suggested that the syntactic aspects of language formulation are relatively spared in jargonaphasia and, thus, are dissociated from lexical aspects.

There have been relatively few linguistic studies of syntax in jargon. It is a tough corpus, because it can be hard to tell a syntactic error from a semantic one. The inexquisite syntax spoken by neurologically intact persons also confounds interpretation. Picking over grammar in jargon leaves us wondering what can be called a deficit.

The classical idea is that jargonaphasia contains a symptom of commission called **paragrammatism.** This term is suggestive of a neat definitional opposite to agrammatism. According to definition, paragrammatism is the substitution of grammatical morphemes *in fluent utterance.* Having incorporated this notion in the Boston Exam, Goodglass and Kaplan (1983) stated that in paragrammatism "most inflections and small grammatical words fall smoothly into place, but with unsystematic substitutions or omissions of both grammatical morphemes and lexical words (i.e., nouns, verbs, adjectives), and tangled grammatical organization" (p. 7).

The logical notion of paragrammatism has run into a couple of problems. One is that some of the symptoms of commission suggested by this classification do not appear or are hard to find in fluent aphasias. In particular, the phrase-level order errors not found in Broca's aphasia were also not found in Wernicke's aphasia in a comparison of English, Italian, and German (Bates et al., 1988).

The other problem is that some people with Wernicke's aphasia exhibit some of the characteristics of agrammatism. In Gleason's study of discourse, these patients used fewer and simpler structures than normal controls. Phrases were sequenced instead of embedded. Because of the similarity of grammatical mistakes in Wernicke's and Broca's aphasias, investigators argued that there is no difference in syntactic disorder or that the traditional distinction needs "conceptual realignment" (Goodglass and Menn, 1985).

"We conclude that the contrast between agrammatism (attributed to Broca's aphasia) and paragrammatism (attributed to Wernicke's aphasia) has been greatly exaggerated" (Bates et al., 1991, p. 137).

In Faroqi-Shah and Thompson's (2003) study of cued sentence production, the group with mild Wernicke's aphasia did well producing active sentences (60 to 80 percent). Production of passive sentences was very impaired, with and without cues (10 to 30 percent). Production of passive sentences improved to 70 to 80 percent with a combined cue of the auxiliary and inflected verb. Reversible sentences tended to be more difficult for the group with Wernicke's aphasia. This group's errors differed from Broca's aphasia. The Wernicke's patients did not have grammatical morpheme omissions and seemed unable to access the passive structure.

UNIVERSAL APHASIA

The brain is, of course, a universal structure, and strokes are the same across cultures. However, aphasiology in the United States has been built on what Bates and Wulfeck (1989) called an *anglocentrism* in which aphasia has been studied mainly with respect to its appearance in English. Universal mechanisms of aphasia are more likely to be determined by comparing different languages. Most interest has been directed at grammatical features, with separate investigations of grammatical morphology and syntactic structure. One general basis for comparison is to determine whether the syndromes of aphasia have the same characteristics no matter which language is being used.

A few research teams have compared languages directly, called **cross-linguistic research** or comparative aphasiology. One team compared Broca's and Wernicke's aphasias in English, Italian, and German for comprehension and production (Bates and Wulfeck, 1989). A second team focused on production in a project called the

Cross-Language Agrammatism Study (CLAS I) involving 14 languages (Menn and Obler, 1990). Then, CLAS II published a comparison of Swedish, French, German, Polish, and English (Ahlsén, Nespoulous, Dordain et al., 1996). Also, smaller teams have formed, such as one comparing Dutch, German, Swedish, and Finnish (Tesak and Niemi, 1997) and another comparing English and Japanese (Menn, Reilly, Hayashi et al., 1998).

Language Comprehension

As we know from the study of sentence comprehension, universal thematic roles of agent and recipient are conveyed through linguistic cues such as word order and grammatical morphemes. English speakers rely a great deal on word order to signify agents and recipients of an action, whereas other Indo-European languages rely on a more intricate system of grammatical morphemes as well as word order for signaling thematic roles. For example, Italian signifies thematic role with inflectional case marking of nouns such as accusative (i.e., recipient role) and dative (i.e., indirect object or goal). French employs more determiners than English, such as distinguishing gender of nouns.

First, let us consider inflectional endings or case markings. Studies have shown that retention of grammatical knowledge is similar across languages (e.g., Wulfeck et al., 1991). In a comparison of Turkish and Hungarian, participants across three syndromes were impaired in using case markings to comprehend (MacWhinney, Osman-Sagi, and Slobin, 1991). As in studies with English, people with Wernicke's aphasia had more difficulty than those with Broca and anomic aphasia. The use of morphology to signal attachment (i.e., subject–verb agreement) was impaired in Broca's and Wernicke's aphasia in English, Italian, and German (Bates et al., 1987a). With other languages, patients with Broca's aphasia show difficulty with inflection but no problem in the use of semantic information (e.g., Smith and Bates, 1987; Smith and Mimica, 1984).

Aphasic patients retain a capacity for processing fundamental canonical order in many languages (Bates et al., 1987a; MacWhinney et al., 1991). We know that English speakers have difficulty understanding noncanonical expressions (e.g., passives). In English, the fundamental thematic sequence is subject-verb-object (SVO) as in *Mother bought bread*. In Japanese, canonical order is subject-object-verb (SOV) as in *Mother bread bought*. This difference gives an investigator an opportunity to test whether comprehension difficulty is related to a particular surface form or to the more universal attribute of canonicity no matter what the form is. Hagiwara and Caplan (1990) found that sentences with the Japanese canonical SOV order were understood with less difficulty than deviations from this order. This suggests that canonicity is a more important factor than surface structure.

Researchers have compared word order and inflections for sentence comprehension. In an order-dependent language like English, word-order errors were easier to identify than inflection errors, whereas in an inflection-dependent language like Italian, inflection errors were easier to identify (Wulfeck et al., 1991). Regarding Italian, asyntactic comprehension appears to affect inflection more. In a pattern opposite of that found in English, German and Italian patients relied on word-order cues in an apparent compensation for morphological deficit (Bates et al., 1987a). In Turkish and Hungarian, switches of order did not pose a problem when case markings were available (MacWhinney et al., 1991).

Language Production

Cross-linguistic researchers suspected that agrammatism would be manifested differently depending on the importance of grammatical morphemes in a language. Perhaps the most striking discovery was the variability of agrammatism among languages and among patients within languages. This was surprising to English-speaking aphasiologists who had become comfortable with thinking of agrammatism as a symptom of omission. Patients with Broca's aphasia substitute grammatical morphemes more often in other languages. Substitution errors for inflections and function words occur in German (Bates, Friederici, and Wulfeck, 1987b), Hungarian (MacWhinney and Osman-Sagi, 1991) Italian (Miceli et al., 1989), French (Nespoulous, Dordain, Perron et al., 1988), and Hebrew (Grodzinsky, 1984). Omissions do occur more often in English than in other languages.

Tesak and Niemi (1997) found that the ratio of omission to substitution is quite variable among languages with 66 to 1 percent in Dutch and 7 to 4 percent in Swedish. The range is from nearly complete absence of substitution to equal rates of substitution and omission. Table 5.7 summarizes other findings.

The occurrence of morphological substitutions in Broca's aphasia has implications for the traditional dichotomy between agrammatism and paragrammatism (i.e., ommission vs. substitu-

TABLE 5.7   A sample of small-scale crosslinguistic comparisons to English, published in a two-year period.

LANGUAGE COMPARED TO ENGLISH	SUBJECTS	KEY FINDING	REFERENCE
French	Nonfluent aphasia	Sensitivity to morphological grammatical markings in comprehension similar in the two languages	Nicol, Jakubowicz, and Goldblum (1996)
Chinese	Broca's aphasia Fluent aphasia	Morphological and syntactic limitations comparable in English and the Cantonese dialect of Chinese	Yiu and Worrall (1996)
Japanese	Varied aphasias	In narration, pragmatic positioning of protagonist at beginning of sentences, called empathy, is preserved in both languages	Menn, Reilly, Hayashi et al. (1998)
Dutch, French	Broca's aphasia	Negative sentences more difficult than positives for French and English, not for Dutch; linguistic form of negation differs from Dutch, indicating the linguistic form is the problem instead of negation per se	Rispens, Bastiaanse et al. (1997)
Dutch, Hungarian	Fluent aphasia	Some structural simplification of verbal expression in all languages, especially in using subordinate clauses	Bastiaanse, Edwards, and Kiss (1996)

tion). Substitution errors, which are difficult to detect in English, occurred with similar frequency in Broca's and Wernicke's aphasia in German (Bates et al., 1987b). In studies of German and Dutch aphasias, Heeschen and Kolk (1988) detected differences in spontaneous speech in which Broca's aphasia has a higher proportion of omissions to substitutions, whereas Wernicke's aphasia has a mixture or a predominance of substitutions.

Regarding structural characteristics of sentence production, cross-linguistic studies addressed the status of word order in picture descriptions (Bates et al., 1988). Phrase-level morphological sequence errors, defined early in Chapter 5, did not occur in English, Italian, and German for either Broca's or Wernicke's aphasia. To study preservation of canonical order, three-element productions were examined. Canonical SVO order was used 81 percent of the time across syndromes and the three languages. Order around a preposition was correct across syndromes and languages about 70 percent of the time. These results were well above chance, and aphasic patients did not differ from normals. The canonical order of SOV also appeared to be preserved in Turkish speakers (Bates and Wulfeck, 1989). Resiliance of canonical order appears to be a universal feature of aphasia. Sometimes, canonical order is overused as a "safe-harbor," especially for speakers of Italian and German.

Sign Language

American Sign Language (ASL) is expressed in a visuospatial mode and possesses grammatical features akin to spoken languages. "Despite the important differences in form, signed and spoken languages clearly share underlying structural principles. Like spoken language, sign language exhibits formal structuring at the lexical and grammatical levels, similar kind and degree of morphological patterning, and a complex, highly rule-governed grammatical and syntactic patterning" (Poizner, Klima, and Bellugi, 1987, p. 21).

Researchers at the Salk Institute for Bilingual Studies in California have studied deaf persons who suffered single strokes in the left or right cerebral hemisphere. Those with left-hemisphere damage (LHD) had disorders similar to the aphasias observed in spoken languages (e.g., lexical and grammatical deficits). Those with right-hemisphere damage (RHD) did not exhibit language problems. More recently, 11 deaf individuals with LHD performed worse than 8 with right hemisphere damage on three tasks of comprehending ASL from single signs to complex commands. Deficits increased with damage to the left temporal lobe. Thus, ASL comprehension is lateralized to the left hemisphere and depends on the temporal lobe, much like language for the hearing population (Hickok, Love-Geffen, and Klima, 2002).

Corina (1999) conducted a critical analysis of the Salk group's work with ASL with regard to what the research might say about the specialization of the left hemisphere for a signal or modality independent language processor. He distinguished between "domain-specific" language capacities (i.e., either signed or spoken language) and "domain-general" capacities (i.e., across signed and spoken languages). He was unhappy with the general level of previous research and advocated a more rigorous specification of general and specific processes and more appropriate methods for testing hypotheses about them.

For something a little different, let us consider "Maureen," a deaf woman who was bilingual in spoken English and British Sign Language (BSL). She had acquired some speech before contracting meningitis at 18 months, learned lip reading, and began to learn BSL when she entered school at age 5 (Marshall, Atkinson, Woll, and Thacker, 2005). When she was 70, she had a left hemisphere stroke. The stroke rendered her unable to sign, but she could understand gestures and could produce spoken words occasionally. She could be cued to say nouns when presented a sign. Maureen's dissociation between signs and gestures reinforced the linguistic and left-hemispheric nature of sign language.

MARTIN EXETER'S APHASIA

In the acute period, Martin Exeter appeared to have severe aphasia. His early confusion included problems with understanding what people were saying to him. He could not answer their questions. When questions required a simple nod for *yes* or a frown for *no,* he would often indicate yes for no and no for yes. His CT scan indicated to the doctors that the global condition would probably be temporary. Then, even in his first week in the rehabilitation unit, his language comprehension started improving and he was saying more words. His aphasia was taking on the appearance of Broca's aphasia. A brief aphasia test indicated that he was able to understand simple sentences. His aphasia would change more in the next few months.

During the two weeks or so after his stroke, Martin's "comprehension" was splitting between an improving recognition of what was going on around him and a persistent difficulty with understanding language. It was not until Martin started language treatment that the speech-language pathologist began analyzing his comprehension more than the initial assessment was able to do. Passive sentences were difficult for him. He made mostly thematic role order errors. He was able to name more than half the pictures shown to him. He could produce only one or two words with a great deal of effort when answering a question. He used nouns, adjectives, and sometimes a verb.

Occasionally, instead of making the effort to answer, he would say "I can't talk any more" surprisingly easily. When he got especially frustrated, he would blurt out "I don't want to do that anymore." A graduate student getting experience by working at the hospital asked if this meant that Martin had fluent aphasia. The SLP explained that these were only automatic phrases that he said a lot. The student was asked to notice the general nature of his propositional speech, rather than focus on a single utterance. His usual conversation consisted only of a painstaking word here or there.

SUMMARY AND CONCLUSIONS

One approach to reducing health care costs is for a rehabilitation team to develop more specific therapies for disabilities (Dobkin, 1995). The opportunity for more specific language therapies is suggested, in principle, by an increase of precision in the observation of behavior and in the diagnosis of a patient's disorder. In the clinic, we may need to look more closely, for example, at the phonological configuration of sound-related naming errors. By addressing the main aphasic disorders, Chapter 5 focused on characteristic symptoms of these disorders. These symptoms drew our attention to linguistic components of comprehension and expression (Table 5.8).

Collecting a substantial experimental group of participants with a specific syndrome presents a challenge for the study of aphasia. Unlike the study of captive college students, aphasic participants have to be discovered and tested one at a time. For research conducted in one location, it may take a few years to develop a statistically viable group representing an uncommon syndrome. Moreover, new developments in research may make it tempting to change theory and procedures along the way. Collaborative research with multiple locations may produce a group more quickly, but it heightens the demand for demonstrating reliability among experimenters.

In this chapter, a prominently displayed development is the online examination of sentence comprehension. When this paradigm gives us a better idea of what is going wrong in a patient's

TABLE 5.8 Summary of topics covered in Chapter 5.

LINGUISTIC COMPONENT	SYNDROME	SYMPTOM
Phonology	Conduction aphasia	Phonemic paraphasias
Morphology	Broca's aphasia	Agrammatism
Syntax	Broca's aphasia	
Lexical-semantics	Anomic aphasia Wernicke's aphasia	Circumlocution Neologisms, jargon

language system, then assessment procedure may be supplemented accordingly. Clinical professionals will be especially responsive if psycholinguistic paradigms identify impairments reliably and the diagnosis makes a difference in treatment accuracy and efficiency. A psycholinguistic device would address the automatic subconscious processing that goes into everyday language comprehension and formulation. It would treat cognitive processing as the time-based phenomenon that it is.

However, much is undecided. Asyntactic comprehension is one example of a clinical pattern with multiple explanations. The asyntactic pattern of a canonicity effect and order errors could be caused by an impaired language processor or reduced working capacity. No single theory has overwhelming support, especially in the absence of comparisons to alternatives. As Blumstein stated, we do not yet know what causes asyntactic comprehension. This lack of definite answers excites scientists and annoys clinicians. It is a wide open area of research, and it makes for interesting conferences.

One way to approach theories is to read articles (and listen to speakers) with a fair-minded skepticism. Some seemingly competing theories may be more paradoxical than contradictory, because they were based on different experimental methods. A

lexical theory of sentence comprehension deficit may make sense, because the experiment was lexical. A syntactic theory may make sense, because the experiment tapped into structure. Working memory may seem to explain comprehension deficit, because the experiment challenged working memory. Few experiments combine an examination of lexical, structural, and memory factors for a single problem. In other instances, only the wording of a theory may be special, and we should not let different wording for an established idea pass as a different or new theory.

One promising development in aphasiology was illustrated in a study at the University of Maryland School of Medicine by Berndt, Mitchum, and Wayland (1997). They compared predictions from three different theories of asyntactic comprehension, and then let the chips fall where they may. The three theories were the trace-deletion hypothesis, a grammatical morpheme filter hypothesis, and the increasingly visible capacity constraint hypothesis. Although the capacity constraint hypothesis was most consistent with the results, the conclusions are not really all that important at this point. What is important is that the investigators did not appear to be invested in proving one theory, and we are waiting to see if they started a trend.

MATCHING REVIEW_____

Match the topics on the right with the names on the left. One topic may be used twice.

_____ 1. Myrna Schwartz   a. verb-finding problems

_____ 2. Hugh Buckingham   b. problem of asyntactic comprehension

_____ 3. Cynthia Thompson   c. trace-deletion hypothesis (TDH)

_____ 4. Bartha and Benke   d. cross-modal priming

_____ 5. Elizabeth Bates   e. mapping hypothesis

_____ 6. Swinney and Shapiro   f. conduction aphasia

_____ 7. Yosef Grodzinsky   g. neologisms in Wernicke's aphasia

_____ 8. Roelien Bastiaanse   h. cross-linguistic research

_____ 9. Caramazza and Zurif   i. American Sign Language

_____ 10. Bellugi, Klima, and Hickok

CHAPTER 6

DISCOURSE AND FUNCTIONAL COMMUNICATION

Audrey Holland (1975) pointed out that aphasic people communicate better than they talk, and her encouragement got us thinking about functional rehabilitation in the United States. The examination of aphasia in functional terms has been influenced from several directions, including the following:

- theoretical and experimental influences, guided by linguistic pragmatics (and sociolinguistics) frequently applied to other cognitive impairments
- influences outside the United States, where many clinicians have taken a functional approach to assessment and treatment
- influences within the United States, where changes in the health care system forced clinicians to "do more with less"

A recent development can be said to be an integration of these concerns, such as applying methods of conversation analysis to functional assessment. As Holland implied, the implications of language difficulties for a person's quality of life can be anticipated with some homespun common sense.

The World Health Organization's former classifications of activity limitation and participation limitation coincide with the functional or pragmatic aspects of aphasia. These classifications have become a ubiquitous foundation for the discussion of functional rehabilitation. The progression of WHO terminology is worth remembering, simply because the previously recommended terms appear in relatively current literature. As indicated in Chapter 1, we continue to rely on these concepts for identifying levels of dysfunction and rehabilitation: In this spirit, this chapter emphasizes activity limitation or "disablement" but con-

cludes with a brief introduction to assessment for participation limitation.

Aphasia threatened Martin Exeter's career as a professor. He had to cancel his lecture in Europe. However, it did not take long for his vocational prospects to be put aside, because daily living demanded his total concentration for the first few months after his stroke. Daily living included the ability to communicate his wishes and ideas. It included connecting with his wife, children, and friends. In addition, if he could communicate better, then perhaps he could salvage at least parts of his career.

PRAGMATIC LANGUAGE

The traditional clinical concern with relating words to objects is not the whole story regarding the language system. Taking a communication perspective, we must consider the language system as it operates in natural context. For example, we might consider how a process model of naming operates when people are talking to each other or how a model of reading works when thumbing through a phone book. The study of natural language use is called **pragmatics.** Relevant observations consist of language behavior in relation to context. Tirassa (1999) argued that we should still be concerned with cognitive processes and drew attention to *cognitive pragmatics,* defined as an interest in the mental processes responsible for the functional or natural use of language. Examples include comprehending a speaker's intent and repairing a defective utterance in conversation.

The language system's contexts have been said to be **external** to a speaker, such as a communicative situation, and **internal,** which consists of world knowledge and emotional states. Functional tasks rely on these contexts in different ways. Conversation is more *situation dependent,* because many referents exist in the participants' surroundings. Reading is more *knowledge dependent,* because interpretation depends heavily on the reader's knowledge (and imagination). "Rarely can we look around the room to make sense of what we have just read in a book" (Smith, 1982, p. 82). The plausibility effect (Chapter 4) is one indication of how world knowledge facilitates language comprehension.

Let us focus on the messages expressed or understood in real-world language use. There is "a gap between the semantic representations of sentences and the thoughts actually communicated by utterances" (Sperber and Wilson, 1986, p. 9). A **speaker's meaning** can differ from the literal or acontextual semantic representation of a sentence called **sentence meaning** (Gibbs, Jr., 1999). In a notorious murder case in England, a teenager's life hinged on his intent when he said "Let him have it, Chris" to a friend pointing a gun at a policeman. In this case, meaning lies in the speaker's intent and a listener's interpretation. Ambiguity is created by the situational context. Did the speaker mean "give him the gun" or "shoot him"?

How do we study or evaluate the exchange of hidden intentions? A solution to this problem includes finding some clear differences between sentence meanings and speaker meanings that can be presented in experiments. One approach to distinguishing these meanings was Searle's (1969) contention that the basic unit of communication is the *speech act.* Speech acts include asserting, greeting, warning, and requesting. When we politely ask "Can you open the door?" we are making a request rather than literally asking about someone's ability to open the door. The act of requesting is part of speaker meaning, and patients can produce speech acts mainly because it does not take much verbalization to greet, warn, request, and so on (Ulatowska, Allard, Reyes et al., 1992).

Indirect speech acts have been investigated with aphasic patients in the form of indirect requests. In one study, video vignettes contained a situation followed by a request (e.g., "Can you open the door?"). Another actor made either an appropriate response to speaker meaning or a pragmatically inappropriate literal response (i.e., "Yes"). A mixed group of aphasic participants usually responded to speaker meaning, indicating their ability to relate the situation to the utterance (Wilcox, Davis, and Leonard, 1978). This ability was unrelated to clinical measures of literal comprehension. Other investigators have supported the conclusion that aphasia does not impair the capacity to make nonliteral interpretations (e.g., Foldi, 1987).

Inference is the general psycholinguistic mechanism for making nonliteral interpretations. A relatively simple type of inference is to add information not explicitly stated in a sentence, called an elaborative inference. An example is to hear "The woman stirred the coffee" and think of [spoon]. Inferencing in comprehension is often referred to as mental *inference generation,* not to be confused with verbal production. Inference is also considered to be a mechanism used in the comprehension of metaphor, a topic that we visit with respect to the study of right hemisphere dysfunction in Chapter 11.

Do aphasic individuals generate inferences without being asked to do so explicitly? A cross-modal priming task is suited to answer this question. In one study, pairs of sentences were presented such that the first sentence should leave one impression, but the second sentence should change that impression, called *inference revision* (Wright and Newhoff, 2004). An example follows:

(1a) Bill bumped the car in front of him while going around the curve.   *accident*
(1b) At the end of the ride, Bill got out of the bumper car.   *fair* or *accident*

The first sentence, 1a, is likely to activate the concept of a traffic accident, but 1b shifts the scenario to a ride at a fair. In the task, a spoken sentence (prime) preceded a visual word target such as those following the example sentences. After hearing each sentence, aphasic participants made lexical decisions about word and nonword targets. Priming of *fair* would be indicative of inference revision. If *accident* continued to be primed after the second sentence, then participants would be presumed to have failed to revise their inference about the depicted scenario. So, how did the aphasic participants do?

Nonfluent and fluent aphasic groups had fairly moderate-to-mild impairments determined with the *Western Aphasia Battery* (WAB). Neurologically intact participants and participants with nonfluent aphasia activated the intended meanings for each sentence in a pair. Although most of the fluent group had WAB aphasia quotients (AQs) well into the 80s, this group included several participants who generated the first inferences (e.g., accident) but not the revisions (e.g., fair). Therefore, with mild fluent aphasia, a person can have a subtle deficit inhibiting an inference that is no longer appropriate and, thus, has trouble arriving at a full interpretation of a speaker's intended meaning.

DISCOURSE AND TEXT

Discourse has been used to refer to numerous things, but here the term refers broadly to units of language larger than a sentence (e.g., Carroll, 1999). Monologue and dialogue are examples of discourse and share features of processing simply because each entails dealing with strings of sentences. Dialogue is the same as *conversational discourse.* For reading and writing, this level of language use is known as *text.* We can continue to think about pragmatics, because language is normally used at the level of discourse, and the discourse itself provides a linguistic context in which single words and sentences are usually understood and produced.

The special qualities of discourse come from interrelationships among statements known broadly as **coherence.** A conversation of alternating single sentences makes sense because the statements are about a single topic holding them together. Coherence is studied at two closely related levels. The local or *microstructural level* pertains to the overlap of meaning between sentences. This local level overlap is known as **cohesion.** It is the minimum level of discourse and needs only pairs of statements to be studied. The global or *macrostructural level* pertains to broad themes and structural schemes. It is necessarily invoked with a length of three or more statements.

One type of cohesive device in microstructure is **anaphora,** which is a lexical unit that refers to information presented previously. One type of anaphora is the pronoun, which can serve the function of *coreference.* That is, a pronoun and antecedent can refer to the same referent. Lexical coreference occurs when a noun, such as a superordinate term, refers back to a specific or subordinate term. In 2, the determiner or definite article *the* signals that a particular *vehicle* should already be known to a reader or listener.

(2)   A bus came roaring around the corner. The vehicle hit a pedestrian.
(3)   We checked the picnic supplies. The beer was warm.

In 3, the noun phrase *The beer* seems to refer back to something in the previous sentence, but there is no explicit antecedent for it. A reader or listener makes what is called an instantiation inference in which beer is assumed to be among the picnic supplies. When coreference and inference come together, it is called a **bridging inference.** In comprehending discourse, a bridge is often needed when a distant antecedent has vanished from the short-term buffer (Fletcher and Bloom, 1988).

Macrostructure is the "upper limit of structural organization" where an entire discourse or text is held together (Stubbs, 1983). The topic or **theme** of a discourse contributes to coherence at this level, as every statement is expected to be related to the overall theme in some way. For example, a text may be about nuclear disarmament or a conversation may be about Uncle Fred. Also, types of discourse possess an overall **structure** leading to expectations for what comes next. The following are some discourse types:

- **narrative,** or a story which is commonly said to have a beginning, middle, and end
- **exposition,** such as a lecture, which may include research presentation with methods, results, and so on
- **procedures** or **routines,** telling how to perform the steps of a task, such as making a sandwich
- **description,** or a characterization of an event or scene

Communicative competence includes knowledge of these forms. Besides clinical studies of picture description, narration or storytelling is the most frequently studied form of discourse, perhaps, because its structure is more apparent and familiar than the other forms.

Story grammars are theories of our knowledge of narrative structure. These grammars specify storytelling functions and how they are organized. Thorndyke's (1977) hierarchy branches into functions of *setting, theme, plot,* and *resolution.* Then, *plot* branches into multiple *episodes,* and an episode contains a *subgoal, attempt,* and *outcome.* Stein and Glenn's (1979) grammar has a plot starter called the *initiating event.* We may recognize a setting such as "Once there was a wily fox who lived in a forest." A plot is initiated when "one day the fox left the forest to explore a henhouse in a nearby village." Studies of reading time and recall support the notion that a story grammar has psychological reality (Mandler, 1987).

Like a theory of any cognitive function, a minimal account of discourse comprehension contains a knowledge structure and a processing system. Semantic memory has to contain more than object concepts, and so the network is broadened to account for knowledge of complex situations generally known as **schemas.** For example, we have a schema for weddings. Our schema for narrative structure (i.e., story grammar) lets us know when someone is telling us a story about a wedding. Processing is con-

strained by what is called the **bottleneck problem.** That is, only small chunks of a discourse can squeeze into working memory as we listen or read. Theories of comprehension propose different levels of representation for holding previous input temporarily and for accumulating a representation of the entire discourse (Kintsch, 1994, 1998).

DISCOURSE COMPREHENSION WITH APHASIA

Tests of discourse-level comprehension have been used mainly for identifying subtle comprehension deficits. The usual clinical method is to read a paragraph to a patient or ask a patient to read a paragraph. Then we ask questions about what was just heard or read, thereby testing recall as well as comprehension. In aphasia batteries, many questions can be answered without having heard or read the paragraphs (Nicholas et al., 1986). This off-line approach differs from online comparisons of information load at specific points in a text. For example, in a "moving window" paradigm, portions of a text are shown one at a time. A patient presses a button causing one portion to disappear and the next one to appear (e.g., Haberlandt and Graesser, 1990).

Few studies of aphasia have targeted microstructural comprehension of cohesive devices. Chapman and Ulatowska (1989) presented short vignettes in which two characters were introduced in the first sentence and a subsequent sentence referred back to one of the characters, as in 4.

(4)   The customer shouted angrily at the waitress that the meal was awful.
The waitress was new at the job and did not know how to respond.
or
She was new at the job and did not know how to respond.

Participants were given response cards showing the two characters and were asked questions such as "Who was new at the job and did not know how to respond?" Aphasic patients responded less accurately with the pronominal anaphor than the lexical anaphor (see also Kahn, Joanette, Ska, and Goulet, 1990).

The *Discourse Comprehension Test* (Brookshire and Nicholas, 1993) contains 10 stories played to patients on a tape recorder, and each story is followed by eight yes/no test questions. Some test questions address **main ideas** considered to be central to the theme of the story, and other questions address **details** peripheral to the story line. Inferencing is assumed to be assessed by presenting questions about information that is implied in a story.

Aphasic patients made more errors than neurologically intact individuals on the *Discourse Comprehension Test*. Yet, normal and aphasic groups displayed the same pattern with respect to type of question. Both groups did better with main ideas than details and did better with explicit information than with implied information (Nicholas and Brookshire, 1995a). In another study, patients with Broca's and conduction aphasias performed poorly in recalling main ideas (Christiansen, 1995b).

Nicholas and Brookshire (1995a) found both quantitative and qualitative similarities among aphasia, RHD, and traumatic brain injury. They noted that "this does not necessarily mean that the underlying reasons for their performance deficits are the same" (p. 78). They acknowledged that "evaluation of the underlying reasons . . . would appear to be a productive area for future research" (p. 78).

APHASIC DISCOURSE PRODUCTION

Aphasic discourse production is evaluated for somewhat different reasons. One is to determine the nature of impaired word finding and syntax in a natural productive circumstance (i.e., spontaneous speech). The other reason is to determine a patient's abilities with respect to discourse-specific functions. When evaluating discourse, we should consider the method for *elicitation* and the method for *analysis* somewhat independently. For example, we can elicit a narrative (i.e., discourse level) but analyze only word finding (i.e., word level).

Elicitation Method

Stimuli and instructions determine whether a patient's discourse is a narrative, procedure, or description (Table 6.1). The types of discourse in the table are produced as **monologue,** that is, with the patient talking and the clinician listening. Description, narration, or exposition can also arise in **dialogue** such as an interview (e.g., *I'd like to ask some questions about your job*) or a conversation (e.g., *What do you think about the President's problems*?). In some studies, an interview is said to be the means for studying conversation.

The early clinical discourse research could be somewhat confusing. The main problem was that varied types of discourse were called "narrative." Ehrlich (1988) asked patients to tell "everything you see happening . . ." in a complex picture and called the result "narrative discourse." On

TABLE 6.1 Methods for eliciting different kinds of monologue. Description has been the most commonly elicited form in clinical evaluation.

	VISUAL STIMULUS	INSTRUCTION
Description	Complex picture	Tell me everything you see in this picture.
Procedure	None	Tell me how you make a sandwich.
Narration	Complex picture	Tell me a story about this picture.
	Picture sequence	Tell me the story being told in these pictures.
	None	Tell me the story of Cinderella.

the other hand, others instructed patients to tell a story about a picture when the goal was to elicit a story (Liles, Coelho, Duffy, and Zalagens, 1989). Mentis and Prutting (1987) asked for procedures but called the result narrative.

Clinical researchers have been interested in whether the condition for eliciting discourse makes a difference in observations of language production. The concern is whether standardized test conditions are valid with respect to the way an aphasic person talks in natural circumstances. In one study, a test of describing object functions was compared to conversation (Roberts and Wertz, 1989). Utterances and clauses were longer and word finding was more accurate in conversation, but syntactic structures were formed better in the object-function test. Another study showed that some discourse conditions such as describing pictures of the Kennedy assassination elicit more words than describing the Cookie Theft picture (Bottenberg, Lemme, and Hedberg, 1987). Thus, a full picture of sentence-level capacities may require observation in formal and natural conditions and with different topics.

Doyle and others modified a story-retelling procedure so that it could be presented with a computer (Doyle, McNeil, Park et al., 2000). They selected 12 stories from Brookshire and Nicholas's *Discourse Comprehension Test* and created six-frame drawings representing each story. The audio version was synchronized with the pictures for computer presentation. Aphasic individuals' story retelling was analyzed according to several variables. The investigators were particularly interested in whether four subsets of three stories each would produce comparable results. It turns out that there was no significant difference among the four subsets for any of the language measures, indicating that 3 stories should be as informative diagnostically as 12.

Discourse Analysis

First, the transcript of a patient's discourse is parsed into units for various purposes. One purpose is to have a frame of reference for comput-

ing density of different forms, such as number of words per sentence or number of sentences per episode in a story. Also, investigators like to have a basis for examining meaningful relationships among elements of a discourse. The most common units include the following:

- **sentence,** a syntactic unit containing a subject and predicate
- **T-unit,** a syntactic unit containing a main clause and attached subordinate clauses
- **p-unit (proposition),** an informational unit defined as a predicate and its arguments

A sentence may be the most ambiguous of the three. Mentis and Prutting (1987) divided spoken narratives into sentences according to pauses and intonation, which may not correspond to punctuation in text or a transcript of spoken narration. Several others have utilized T-units (e.g., Liles et al., 1989; Ulatowska, Freedman-Stern, Doyel et al., 1983). An example might be the following: *The heroic policeman who apprehended the thief turned over his weapon before the investigation began.* The ambiguity of syntactic units is that this could be a sentence or a T-unit containing the equivalent of two or three sentences and three propositions (e.g, *the policeman apprehended the thief; the investigation began*).

Choice of units can be related to the level of analysis. For example, p-units may be recorded with little regard for grammatical precision because of an interest in examining the ability to tell a story. Levels are designated broadly as "within-sentence" **microlinguistic analysis** of lexical and grammatical forms (see Table 5.1) and "between-sentence" **macrolinguistic analysis** of the unique properties of discourse at microstructural and macrostructural levels. These levels of analysis are summarized in Table 6.2.

In a cohesion analysis, the first thing to look for is the presence of cohesive elements such as pronouns and nouns preceded by *the*. Investigators may stop there (e.g., Bloom, Borod, Obler et al., 1995). However, other researchers look for a **cohesive tie** between an element and an antecedent. Incomplete ties are noted when an antecedent

TABLE 6.2   Basic types of discourse analysis.

LEVEL	ANALYSIS	MEASUREMENT APPROACH	REFERENCE
Microlinguistic	Informativeness	Counting main concepts	Nicholas and Brookshire (1993)
		Counting propositions	Joanette et al. (1986)
	Grammar	Counting omissions and substitutions of grammatical morphemes	Haravon, Obler, and Sarno (1994)
Microstructural	Cohesion	Counting cohesive elements (e.g., pronouns) and clear connections to antecedents (i.e., cohesive ties)	Lemme et al. (1984)
Macrostructural	Story grammar	Rating scale of narrative organization	Bottenberg et al. (1987)

cannot be found. In a study of interviews with fluent aphasic patients, they produced a normal number of cohesive elements but also produced more incomplete cohesive ties than controls, indicating that pronouns and definite articles were difficult to interpret (Glosser and Deser, 1991).

Narration has been employed to study global themes and structure. With a story-recall task, Gleason and others (1980) found aphasic patients were deficient in number of thematic statements. They tended to reiterate major themes and omit details. In another study, patients displayed intact narrative form and did not differ from controls in the number of actions expressed. They were deficient in producing certain components such as setting, resolution, and evaluation (Ulatowska et al., 1983). Bloom and others (1995) rated stories according to accuracy, completeness, logic, and whether they had a beginning, middle, and end. They found overall story structure to be preserved but coherence reduced in other respects.

We might imagine that fluency distinguishes syndromes of aphasia with respect to microlinguistic features. Early research distinguished narrative styles in Broca's and Wernicke's according to word finding and grammatical characteristics (Gleason et al., 1980). More recently, Christiansen (1995b) compared Broca's, conduction, and

Wernicke's aphasias. She evaluated production by rating the relevance of propositions in stories told from cartoons. Fueled by their press for speech, patients with Wernicke's aphasia were distinctive in producing more irrelevant statements than the other patients. Those with Broca's and conduction aphasia were more coherent.

Then, Christiansen (1995a) focused on mildly fluent aphasias. She compared syndromes according to the occurrence of so-called coherence violations, namely, information gaps, repetitive propositions, and irrelevant propositions. The patient groups displayed different kinds of problems. Those with mainly word-finding deficits of anomic aphasia produced mostly information gaps and fewer propositions than the other groups. Patients with conduction aphasia produced more repetitions than other violations, which was considered to be a compensation for grammatical difficulties. Those with mild Wernicke's aphasia produced more irrelevant propositions than other violations and seemed to produce more description than narration.

Aphasic sentence-level language deficiencies can mask capacities at the discourse level, but aphasia also seems to attack local-level discourse functions directly such as coreferential cohesion. Yet, we do not know if poor cohesion is secondary to word-finding deficit or an impairment of a process unique to establishing cohesive ties. People with aphasia produce recognizable narrative structure. That is, someone with anomic or Broca's aphasia can tell a good story with circumlocutory or agrammatic statements. Generally, aphasia seems to impair microlinguistic parameters while preserving macrolinguistic parameters.

Informativeness

Some aphasiologists are interested in measuring the informativeness of discourse. They look for the presence of predefined content units without regard to their relationships to each other. Measurements address the density and rate of content production in narration and other types of discourse. The main objective is to have a reliable measure that discriminates aphasia from normal performance.

Initially, Yorkston and Beukelman (1980) divided Cookie Theft descriptions into content units the size of a word or short phrase. A **content** unit was considered to be "a grouping of information that was always expressed as a unit by normal speakers" (p. 30), such as *cookies, from the jar, mother,* and *in the kitchen.* A mildly aphasic group did not differ from normal elderly subjects in amount of information, but these patients were much less efficient with 18.7 units per minute compared to the control group's 33.7 units per minute. Other investigators supplied profiles for severely impaired patients according to this method (Craig, Hinckley, Winkelseth et al., 1993).

At the Veterans Administration Medical Center in Minneapolis, Linda Nicholas and Robert Brookshire worked on improving content analysis. In particular, they wanted a system that is not tied to a particular picture and can be used with any stimulus. They started by counting the most informative words in a narrative, which they called **correct information units** (CIU) (Nicholas and Brookshire, 1993). The basic measures were the percent of words that are CIUs and the number of CIUs per minute. These measures separated aphasic patients from normal controls. Later, the

investigators determined that obtaining 300–400 words from four or five stimuli lead to the most reliable informativeness score (Brookshire and Nicholas, 1994).

Nicholas and Brookshire turned their attention to a more elaborate system for identifying **main concepts,** still being especially concerned with establishing a reliable measure that is sensitive to deficit (Nicholas and Brookshire, 1995b). Main concepts are statements that form a "skeletal outline" of the essential information in pictured stories. One study showed that aphasic patients produce fewer complete and accurate concepts and more incomplete and inaccurate concepts than neurologically intact individuals. Other researchers counted units of particular kinds of information in a narration (Bloom, Borod, Obler, and Gerstman, 1992).

Can the CIU method be applied reliably to aphasic persons' natural conversation? Oelschlaeger and Thorne (1999) investigated this question with a 50-year-old individual diagnosed as having conduction aphasia. Clinicians counted words reliability, but interrater reliability for CIUs was low. Nearly three-fourths of disagreements were attributed to insufficient scoring rules for the original measure, and one-fourth of the disagreements were due to scorer error.

McNeil and Doyle and their colleagues (2001) created their own information unit (IU) analysis for the procedure cited earlier, now called the Story Retell Procedure (SRP). An IU was a "word, phrase, or acceptable alternative from the story stimulus that is intelligible and informative and that conveys accurate and relevant information about the story" (p. 994). The investigators found the procedure to be reliable and later discovered that calculating *rate* (i.e., percentage of IUs per minute) distinguished aphasic patients from normal controls better than the percentage of IUs per se (McNeil, Doyle, Park et al., 2002).

Do Nicholas and Brookshire's measures correspond to impressions of informativeness? Doyle and others (1996) asked volunteers to rate the informativeness of several narratives produced by aphasic patients. The investigation indicated that the CIU and main concept measures are strongly related to the subjective judgments and, thus, are valid measures of perceived informativeness.

CONVERSATION

The dynamic interaction of conversation differs from formal clinical interactions. For example, tests and treatments tend to have a patient either comprehending repeatedly or producing utterances repeatedly; whereas participants take turns talking in the give-and-take of conversation. This section covers two distinctive aspects of conversation:

- exchange of new information
- management of turn taking

The study of conversation has slightly different orientations. Besides our interest in how aphasia appears in a natural activity, we want to know whether patients have any difficulty with the unique features of conversation.

New Information

Conversation is conducted as if there were a tacit agreement or "social contract" between participants. Grice (1975) called it the **principle of cooperation.** According to Grice's "maxims," a speaker tries to be informative, truthful, relevant, and concise, and a listener assumes that this is what the speaker is trying to do. Let us focus on the informativeness maxim as we turn our attention to **shared responsiblities** of participants in a conversation. More specifically, we shall pay more attention to a clinician or others engaged in conversation with an aphasic person.

The informativeness maxim gives us another way of examining speaker meaning. It states that a speaker tries to convey **new information** in addition to rehashing information a listener already knows. Comprehension is said to be a process of relating new information to information already known, called given or old information. A speaker uses linguistic devices to help a listener identify what is new and what is old. For example, a pronoun signals that we are referring to information

that a listener should already know from a previous utterance, the situation, or knowledge of the world. When a speaker estimates what a listener already knows, a speaker is said to be assuming the point of view of the listener or what is now being called "theory of mind" (see Chapter 11).

Conditions can be devised to observe a patient conveying new information. A blunt procedure is to put a barrier between a patient and a listener so the listener does not see the patient's stimuli. Another method is to provide both participants with their own set of pictures of slightly differing events. Aphasic patients can be quite good at verbalizing distinctive enough information about a particular picture so listeners can choose the same picture (Busch, Brookshire, and Nicholas, 1988). Another approach is to switch listeners, so that a patient may talk to one who is already familiar with a message or another who is unfamiliar with the message. Thus, we try to minimize or control a **listener's prior knowledge** of a patient's topic or meaning. Also, we may record the *listener's* comprehension accuracy in addition to recording the patient's expressive behavior.

At the University of Illinois, Julie Hengst (2003) employed a barrier activity to study **referencing** by young adult aphasic patients and family members. The linguistic notion of a word referring to a concept now becomes a collaborative communicative act in which partners work together to convey reference to an object in mind or in the situational context, also known as *referential communication.* In one *referencing task,* a partner directs the other to place a picture in a location on a board, but the partners are unable to see each others' workspace. Hengst found that all participants were successful in exchanging information, with the aphasic individuals communicating occasionally with partial words, spellings, and paraphasias. The method and participant behaviors are reminiscent of a treatment procedure known as PACE, which is presented in Chapter 10.

Another dimension of listener knowledge is captured in the **familiarity of a listener** to a speaker. Clinicians, spouses, and strangers contribute differently with respect to world knowledge and communicative strategies. Stimley and Noll (1994) had familiar and unfamiliar examiners administer the four verbal subtests of the PICA to aphasic patients. The patients scored significantly better on the most difficult subtests with the unfamiliar examiner. One explanation was that a patient may reduce effort assuming that the familiar clinician already knows some things about the patient's communicative style.

Familiarity of a listener may not affect a patient's storytelling behavior (Bottenberg and Lemme, 1991; Brenneise-Sarshad, Nicholas, and Brookshire, 1991). In a study of conversations with patients who had Broca's aphasia, Doyle and others (1994) manipulated familiarity of the communicative partner, conversational method (i.e., open topic and constrained topic), location (i.e., at home or a simulated home environment), and number of participants (i.e., dyad or triad). Only conversational method affected the use of statements, requests, answers, and ambiguities.

In general, investigation of shared information has suffered from the absence of clear connection between the experimental manipulations and the measure of patients' behavior. The measure is often one that has already been developed for general purposes. Explanation can be facilitated with a study derived from a theoretical framework that links the measure to variables. That is, a framework would indicate why chosen independent variables *should* affect the chosen dependent variables.

Conversational Management

Now, we consider interactive characteristics of conversation. Clinical investigators have borrowed methods from sociolinguistics and anthropology or have invented their own approaches. Generally, attention is given to the local management system of turn taking or the global structure of any conversation whether it be face-to-face or over the telephone. Like trying to tame a wild horse, clinicians are working on reliable methods of observation directed by frameworks specifying structural features of conversation.

Mildly to moderately impaired aphasic people tend to conform to conversational rules. In the typical conversation, speaker turns rarely overlap (i.e., simultaneous talking), and gaps between speakers often span less than a second. This precision stems from an inherent predictability of a speaker turn, which enables a partner to anticipate when a switch from speaking to listening will occur. We may be concerned about the comprehension deficit and press for speech of Wernicke's aphasia. However, these patients also appear to be sensitive to turn-taking conventions (Schienberg and Holland, 1980).

There are different types of turn sequences. One is the **adjacency pair,** in which a speaker turn (first part) is followed by a predictable response from the other speaker (second part). For example, a greeting is followed by a greeting; an answer follows a question. Other types of turn sequences may encompass three or four turns. One of these is the **repair sequence,** in which a speaker's turn is modified because it failed to convey a message. We might anticipate that repairs are frequent in conversation with an aphasic person, because either the patient or another speaker does not get a point across.

Lubinski, Duchan, and Weitzner-Lin (1980) referred to repairs as "hint-and-guess" sequences in conversation with aphasic patients. A patient's speaking turn consists of a hint, and a listener guesses the patient's intent. The patient may attempt a repair in the third turn of the sequence. A repair may be self-initiated (without prompting) or other-initiated (with prompting). It may be a self-repair by the patient or an other-repair by another participant. Neurologically intact adults prefer self-initiation and self-repairs. Other-repairs are rare, and when they occur, they are usually modulated with prefaces such as "You mean . . . ?" or addendums such as " . . . , I think."

Ferguson (1994) studied precursors of repairs in conversations between aphasic patients and either familiar individuals living with the patients or less familiar individuals who were visiting the patients. In particular, she looked for *trouble-indicating behavior* by either participant, such as commenting about a word-finding problem or failing to continue in the conversation. Then she examined types of repair, called *repair trajectories*. Of course, normal participants indicated more trouble and used more repairs when interacting with aphasic partners compared to interacting with other normal partners. Visiting participants made more other-repairs than subjects living with the aphasic participants, indicating that unfamiliar partners are more likely to seek a "speedy remedy" for trouble.

Ethnography and Conversation Analysis

The topic of ethnographic research (also known as "qualitative research") is an extension of the previous section on conversational management. The ethnographic approach originated in anthropology and sociology with the main goal of studying human behavior in its natural state (Mey, 2001; Schiffrin, 1994). In clinical aphasiology, a great deal of this research has been cultivated in two regions. Louisiana has been the home of collaboration between Nina Simmons-Mackie at Southeastern Louisiana University and Jack Damico at the University of Louisiana at Lafayette. Qualitative research also has been pursued in the United Kingdom at the University of Newcastle upon Tyne by Ruth Lesser, Lisa Perkins, and Anne Whitworth, as well as at University College London by Ray Wilkinson.

Ethnographic research consists of special methods for observing behavior and for analysis of that behavior. Unlike structured discourse research, behavior is not elicited with a contrived stimulus or task. Researchers aspire to obtain data that is "authentic." Ethnographic aphasiology also relies on detailed case studies. Like cognitive neuropsychology, it consists of many observations of a single case, but, unlike cognitive neuropsychology, the research is mainly empirical with questions such as "Is repetition a naturally occurring behaviour in the conversation of a person with aphasia?" (Oelschlaeger and Damico, 1998, p. 972). "Naturalistic observation" in the form of taking field notes has been used to gather infor-

mation about the activities of older people with aphasia compared to healthy older people (Davidson, Worrall, and Hickson, 2003). Often it is said that analysis is guided by the data. For example, Madden and others (2002) classified instances of an aphasic individual's laughter and observed that it was frequently associated with trouble spots in a conversation.

For obtaining authentic conversations, researchers leave recording equipment in the home and train participants in its use so that naturalness is not compromised by the presence of an investigator. In one study, researchers arranged a particular time of day for recording (e.g., Perkins, Crisp, and Walshaw, 1999). In another study, a couple received no instructions on the conditions or frequency of recording (e.g., Oelschlaeger and Thorne, 1999). This method generates multiparty conversations as well as several dyadic interactions with routine communication partners.

A formalized analysis of natural conversation is quite naturally called **conversation analysis** (CA). For the study of brain-damaged patients, guidelines began with Perkins, Whitworth, and Lesser's (1997) *Conversation Analysis Profile for People with Cognitive Impairment* (CAPPCI) (also, Lesser and Perkins, 1999). From this foundation they developed the similar *Conversation Analsyis Profile for People with Aphasia* (CAPPA) (Booth and Perkins, 1999; Booth and Swabey, 1999). An investigator may focus on a feature of conversational management and present a transcript of dyadic turns that exemplifies a participant's realization of that feature. In one study, researchers observed that "speaking for" behavior by a nonaphasic spouse occurred often in semistructured interviews with six couples (Croteau, Vychytil, Larfeuil et al., 2004).

The researcher describes the behavior and compares it to what is known about normal conversation. CA "is informed by two domains of data: prior aphasiological knowledge and the experience and expertise of conversation analysts with talk and conduct in interaction among language-unimpaired speakers" (Heeschen and Schegloff, 1999, p. 365). Interpretation consists of "explaining the essence of the social phenomenon and its meaning in the participants' lives" (Damico and Simmons-Mackie, 2003, p. 133), including detection of motivation (Oelschlaeger and Damico, 1998).

CA was used to identify strategies that distinguished nonaphasic conversational partners who had been judged as "good" from partners judged as "poor" (Simmons-Mackie and Kagan, 1999). For example, during repair sequences, the good partners tended to use strategies that were "face saving" for their aphasic partner. These partners would adopt communicative behaviors used by the person with aphasia such as gestures. The poor partners relied only on talking, such as asking the person with aphasia to talk instead of gesturing; and the poor partners tended to focus on getting information, rather than fostering a positive relationship.

Hengst and her colleagues (2005) concentrated on *reported speech*, which is the restating of what someone said at another place and time. It may be produced as a direct quote or indirect paraphrase. Cognitively speaking, reported speech would be a sign of good episodic memory. Hengst videotaped conversations between seven mildly to moderately aphasic individuals and their routine partners at home and other settings such as restaurants, stores, and a high school football game. In this instance, a researcher was present but functioned primarily as an observer. Both partners produced reported speech, the neurologically intact partners producing it more often.

Ethnographic research is certainly different from standardized assessment and cued elicitation of specific sentences. Naturalistic data gathering is usually accompanied by analysis of conversational behavior. So far, there appears to be little integration of formal linguistic interests with naturalistic ones. For example, agrammatism could be examined in transcripts of conversation with the experimenter absent to determine if the findings from picture naming or elicitation are consistent with real life. However, ethnographers do not appear to be studying auxiliary movement. We may think of clinical ethnography as being at an early

stage, roughly equivalent to the time-consuming earliest studies of child language acquisition. The latter contributed to focusing research on important behaviors, which led to the development of efficient clinical assessments. Ethnographic research is said to consist of "rigorous qualitative methodologies" (Hengst, 2003), and it may stimulate more controlled studies that tap into the cognitive pragmatics of conversational behaviors.

NONVERBAL MODALITIES

One option for maximizing functional communication is to supplement or replace impaired language functions with another means of communicating, especially for the acute period following stroke or for chronically severe or global aphasia. This section identifies capacities for nonverbal communication, or what Hengst (2003) called "nonverbal resources." For now, we shall focus on behaviors elicited in formal conditions that determine a patient's capacity. Later, we shall examine more natural communicative conditions in which gesturing accompanies speech.

Assessing Limb Movement

Limb apraxia is a disorder of skilled movement (or **praxis**) that cannot be attributed to paralysis. A movement, such as brushing teeth, can be performed in natural circumstances but not when a patient is asked to perform the action. Thus, the disorder may not be experienced until it is diagnosed in the clinic (DeRenzi, Motti, and Nichelli, 1980). Limb apraxia occurs mainly when there is damage to the left parieto-temporal lobe boundary (DeRenzi and Lucchelli, 1988). Because of this posterior location, patients with this disorder often do not have hemiplegia.

Evaluation is usually done in conditions of imitation, movement on command, and natural or spontaneous movement. Movements are classified according to *transivity,* such as transitive actions on objects (e.g., dialing a phone) or intransitive actions without objects (e.g., an OK sign), and according to *complexity* such as a single movement (e.g., drinking) or a sequence of movements (e.g., making coffee). Clinical researchers often study transitive movements as **pantomime** or pretended movement without the object in hand (i.e., "mime").

To facilitate diagnosis, researchers have categorized movement errors, especially for mimed transitive gestures such as combing, hammering, erasing, or smoking. Rothi and others (1988) looked for content errors (e.g, wrong pantomime), temporal errors (e.g., wrong sequence of movements), and spatial errors (e.g., unusual amplification of movement). In a comparison of aphasic people to normal controls, several error types were never or rarely produced by any patient. These included unrelated, sequencing, amplitude, and unrecognizable errors.

One observed spatial error is the use of **body-part-as-object** (BPO), such as puffing on a finger when asked to mime smoking a cigarette. The BPO error differs from what Raymer and others (1997) called **body-part-as-tool** (BPT) errors in which someone actually uses a body part as the tool. Examples of the latter include using a straightened finger as a toothbrush or pencil when miming the appropriate action, as opposed to pretending to hold the toothbrush or pencil. In comparisons among brain-damaged groups and normal controls, researchers have reached opposite conclusions regarding whether BPT responses are symptoms of deficit (e.g., Duffy and Duffy, 1989; Haaland and Flaherty, 1984; McDonald, Tate, and Rigby, 1994). That is, normal adults do these things, too. Subsequent research demonstrated that a truly pathological BPT error occurs only after a patient is reinstructed to pretend to hold the tool (Raymer et al., 1997).

Duffy and Duffy's (1989) *Limb Apraxia Test* (LAT) is one device for assessing praxis. The LAT relies on the imitation task to specify response parameters precisely, minimize verbal instruction, and minimize the influence of cognitive problems that may appear when making movements on command. The test also avoids conventional intransitive gestures. Eight subtests are constructed according to the following factors:

- movement with and without objects
- simple (i.e., one to three components) and complex (i.e., four to six components)
- sequenced (i.e., complete movement) and segmented (i.e., one component at a time)

Scoring is based on the PICA's model of a multidimensional system. A control group showed that there is no difference between left and right hand performance of the tasks. Sixty-eight percent of LHDs performed beneath the range for normal controls.

The *Test of Oral and Limb Apraxia* (TOLA) by Helm-Estabrooks (1991) evaluates movement a little differently from the LAT. The section on oral apraxia instructs a patient to perform nonrespiratory actions with the mouth such as "lick a lollipop" and respiratory actions such as "cough" and "blow out a candle." Oral and limb movements are observed first on command and then by imitation. Transitive and intransitive gestures are compared. An early version of this test was correlated with a rating of spontaneous gesture, indicating that TOLA may be predictive of natural gestural use (Borod, Fitzpatrick, Helm-Estabrooks, and Goodglass, 1989).

The Question of Asymbolia

Two origins of miming deficit have been considered when it occurs with aphasia (Wang and Goodglass, 1992). One possibility is that pantomime deficit is a manifestation of limb apraxia. The other possibility is that language and pantomime deficits are part of a broad disorder that could be called "asymbolia." In 1870, Finkelnburg described the case of a pious Catholic woman who could not initiate the sign of the cross and another case of a violinist who was able to play by ear but could not read musical notation (cited in Duffy and Liles, 1979).

Some gestures are more symbolic than others. Comparable to verbal language, a symbolic gesture has a somewhat arbitrary relationship to its referent. For example, a salute does not share physical characteristics with a referent, and yet its meaning is known by a community. On the other hand, gestures can be a natural expression of emotion, such as a clenched fist or a frown. The physical similarity between a gesture and its referent is known as the gesture's *iconicity*. Iconic gestures, such as pantomime, are replicas of their referents. *Intentionality* is another variable, and aphasic patients retain unintentional or subpropositional emotional expression or reaction (Buck and Duffy, 1980; Gardner, Ling, Flamm, and Silverman, 1975). The question is whether aphasia necessarily includes deficit with intentionally or propositionally symbolic behavior such as appropriate use of the OK sign.

Investigators tried to separate cognitive and motor factors in gesture production. Duffy and Duffy (1981) found that miming the use of objects was correlated with severity of aphasia and that apraxia contributed little to pantomime performance. In another study, aphasic patients without limb apraxia were impaired for imitating American Indian Sign Language (Amer-Ind) and American Sign Language (ASL) (Daniloff, Fritelli, Buckingham et al., 1986). ASL contains many arbitrary symbols, but Amer-Ind is loaded with pantomimic representations of referents.

Because of the possibility of a motor confound, many investigators decided to study **pantomime recognition.** It also provided an opportunity to determine whether a central disorder can be inferred from coexisting receptive and expressive deficit. To assess recognition, a researcher produces a pantomime, and a participant identifies the referent in a set of pictures. Evidence of asymbolia with aphasia came from a group mean deficit (Duffy, Duffy, and Pearson, 1975), correlation with a measure of overall language ability (Duffy and Duffy, 1981), and correlation with receptive language ability (Ferro, Santos, Castro-Caldas, and Mariano, 1980). Aphasic patients also had more difficulty recognizing pantomime than facial emotion (Walker-Batson, Barton, Wendt, and Reynolds, 1987), and posteriorly damaged subjects had particular difficulty verifying a mimed action that was physically similar to an action on an incorrect object (Lambier and Bradley, 1991).

The studies mentioned so far relied on the average performance of an aphasic group. When the number of aphasic individuals below a cut-off score was computed, the proportion of individuals with recognition deficits varied from 41 to 74 percent (Gainotti and Lemmo, 1976; Seron, Van Der Kaa, Remitz, and Van Der Linden, 1979; Varney, 1982). Range of aphasic individuals in Duffy and Duffy's study overlapped considerably with the normal range. Some studies showed no relationship between pantomime recognition deficit and severity of aphasia (Daniloff, Noll, Fristoe, and Lloyd, 1982; Feyereisen and Seron, 1982). Therefore, many aphasic persons do not have pantomime recognition deficit, indicating that this problem is not a necessary component of aphasia.

Meanwhile, other researchers claimed that pantomime deficit in aphasic patients is a movement disorder or a manifestation of limb apraxia (e.g., Kertesz, Ferro, and Shewan, 1984). Like Duffy and Duffy (1981), Wang and Goodglass (1992) found pantomime recognition and production to be correlated with each other and with auditory comprehension, but, unlike the Duffy findings, pantomime abilities were not correlated with severity of aphasia. Wang and Goodglass were concerned about use of the PICA in the Duffy study as a measure of aphasia, because this battery contains subtests of gesturing with objects. Wang and Goodglass also found a strong correlation between miming and a measure of motor praxis. Using a sophisticated analysis of their own data, Duffy, Watt, and Duffy (1994) concluded that pantomime impairment has both a symbolic and motoric basis.

Most investigations of the asymbolia question have relied on pantomime as an example of symbols. Because pantomime may not be truly symbolic because of its iconicity (Peterson and Kirshner, 1981), the issue of whether aphasia is a sweeping asymbolia may not be clearly resolved by this research. Moreover, a clinician is concerned about the communicative avenues available to aphasic persons. The research shows either that pantomime can be one option with little training for some patients or that pantomime has to be trained for other patients.

To determine whether miming is available, a test of pantomime was developed. The ***Assessment of Nonverbal Communication*** (Duffy and Duffy, 1984) contains two tests of recognition and two tests of production. For recognition, a videotaped demonstration can be obtained for maximizing consistency of presentation. Response is made with a choice of four pictured objects. One expression test models the naming task in that the examiner shows a picture of an object, and the patient demonstrates its use. Finally, in a "referential abilities" test, the patient's gesture is evaluated by a third person who must decide what was conveyed by choosing one of four pictures. One foil is an object that would be used in the same location in space as the correct object, thereby requiring a precise gesture.

Drawing

Although many of us would say we are not artistic, most of us can draw to some degree. Because the right hemisphere is thought to be responsible for visuospatial skills, we might expect aphasic patients to have retained whatever drawing skill they had. However, right hemiplegia can restrict the usually preferred side for writing and drawing. This may be one reason why 30 to 40 percent of patients with left or right hemisphere strokes have some degree of drawing deficit as tested by copying tasks (e.g., Arena and Gainotti, 1978; Carlesimo, Fadda, and Caltagirone, 1993).

Chapter 11 has a discussion of drawing from the perspective of constructional skills in right hemisphere dysfunction. One point in that chapter is that drawing difficulties with LHD are different from those with RHD. Patients with LHD generally include accurate details and preserve the overall structure of an object, but they draw slowly and very simply (e.g., Gainotti, and Tiacci, 1970; Swindell, Holland, Fromm, and Greenhouse, 1988). What is important for the present discussion is whether drawing with aphasia is recognizable or can convey meaning to an observer.

In one study, clinicians examined copying and sketching ability of three severely aphasic individuals with right hemiparesis and little drawing experience. The patients were right-handed and drew with the left hand. All three produced intelligible copies and sketches of objects. The wives of two of the patients were surprised with their husbands' newly discovered artistic skills. The study demonstrated that drawing can be a communicative option (Kashiwagi, Kashiwagi, Kunimori et al., 1994).

Conversational Gesturing

Gesturing serves at least two functions during conversation. As discussed early in this chapter, one function is communicative with either the automatic gestures that show emotion or the volitional gestures that express ideas. Gestures are also used for signaling conversational moves, thereby regulating an interaction. Clinical researchers are especially interested in severely nonfluent or global aphasias for whom gesturing may be considered to be a compensatory behavior (Simmons-Mackie and Damico, 1997).

Simmons-Mackie and Damico (1996) employed their ethnographic approach to identify **discourse markers** that nonfluent aphasic people employ in managing conversational interaction. They observed the following markers in two patients:

- initiation or alerting (e.g., raised finger indicating desire to begin or maintain a speaking turn)
- termination or reorientation (e.g., hand clasp to end a failed communicative attempt)
- participant role request (e.g., eye gaze and body movements to relinquish speaking turn)
- affiliation or politeness (e.g., "Is good" as a response to an offer)
- truth level (e.g., "I don't know" amidst trying to convey something)

Other research has shown that severely nonfluent patients indicate when they are not comprehending, and they signal for help from a clinician (Herrmann, Koch, Johannsen-Horbach, and Wallesch, 1989).

Researchers have also studied whether communicative gestures arise naturally in communicative situations. Severely aphasic patients displayed better gestural ability in a new information condition than in a formal test of limb apraxia (Feyereisen, Barter, Goossens, and Clarebaut, 1988). Yet, communicative use of gesture decreased when a barrier was placed between patients and partners, indicating that patients are sensitive to the viability of gesture as a communicative option (Glosser, Wiener, and Kaplan, 1986). Gesturing style in Broca's and Wernicke's aphasia corresponded to the nature of their verbal expression (Duffy, Duffy, and Mercaitis, 1984). In Hengst's (2003) study with a barrier task, participants tapped into several nonverbal resources including displaying cards over the barrier, hand and facial gestures, full body postures, and drawing in the air.

In developing the ***Boston Nonvocal Communication Scale,*** Borod and others (1989) measured spontaneous use of gestures during informal activities especially when interacting with others. Seven types of behavior were rated on a four-point scale for frequency of occurrence. Behavioral categories included greetings, pointing, indicating yes or no, and using pantomime or drawing to communicate. Spontaneous gestures were used less often by a globally aphasic group than by other groups.

More recently, aphasic patients were videotaped while describing a complex picture to someone who had not seen it. Then they were asked questions to create a more interactive condition (Hadar, Wenkert-Olenik, Krauss, and Soroker, 1998). The researchers tracked gestures that supplemented meaning conveyed with language. Also, aphasic patients were divided into some unusual categories (i.e., conceptual, semantic, and phonologic groups). The findings indicate that patients with conceptual deficits beyond aphasia gestured differently from normal controls. Pantomimes were sometimes unrelated to associated words. Patients with deficits restricted to word finding gestured most like controls.

OVERALL FUNCTIONAL STATUS

At rehabilitation centers, a patient's functional independence is commonly rated soon after admission and at discharge. Professionals generally use rating scales to assess *activities of daily living* (ADL), and these scales encompass the domains of several rehabilitation services. Subscale ratings are usually obtained for each activity or function. A full-scale score addresses overall dysfunction. One of the original rating scales is the **Barthel Index** for ten activities of daily living including ambulation, feeding, bathing, and dressing (Fortinski, Granger, and Seltzer, 1981; Mahoney and Barthel, 1965). Current scales are used to track progress, measure functional outcomes, and assist in determining costs of rehabilitation.

A national task force developed the **Functional Independence Measure** (FIM) (State University of New York, 1990). It is a widely used multidisciplinary scale intended to measure overall severity of disability or "burden of care." It consists of 18 items classified into the following six subscales:

- self-care (eating, grooming, bathing, dressing, toileting)
- sphincter control (bladder and bowel management)
- mobility (bed, chair, toilet)
- locomotion (walking or wheelchair, stairs)
- communication (comprehension, expression)
- social cognition (interaction, problem solving, memory)

These subscales are grouped into *motor* and *cognitive* domains with communication and social cognition included in the latter. Each member of the rehabilitation team uses a fairly reliable seven-point scale for rating abilities in his or her domain (Hamilton, Laughlin, Granger, and Kayton, 1991). The speech-language pathologist (SLP) rates functional comprehension and expression, reserving lowest ratings for complete dependence on a helper and highest ratings for independence requiring no helper.

The FIM is now a trademark of the Uniform Data System for Medical Rehabilitation, a division of UB Foundation Activities, Inc. It has been used to document a patient's status on a minimum set of skills at hospital admission and discharge and has been incorporated into Medicare and Medicaid's system for reimbursement (Chapter 8).

The **Functional Assessment Measure** (FAM) was incorporated into the FIM resulting in an outcome assessment called the FIM+FAM (Hall, Hamilton, and Keith, 1993; Hawley, Taylor, Hellawell and Pentland, 1999). The FAM adds 12 items to the FIM's 18, producing the 30-item FIM+FAM. The developers had traumatic brain injury in mind, so the FAM added more items for assessing communication and cognition. For example, there are additional items for reading and writing. This measure has a rating scale for each item, rather than a single general scale, and these scales can be viewed at the website for the Center for Outcome Measurement in Brain Injury (www. tbims.org/combi).

ASSESSING OF FUNCTIONAL COMMUNICATION

Although functional assessment has been mandated by legislation and payment providers, some devices have been around since before the mandates. The main idea is to ensure that services are helping a patient progress in activities that are essential for daily living and, thus, maximize independence from the health care system. Newer methods are influenced by the currently reduced time for assessment.

Communication Profiles and Scales

The **Functional Communication Profile** (FCP) is a rating scale for mostly language functions of "everyday urban life" (Sarno, 1969). A clinician estimates (or predicts) abilities in five categories: movement, speaking (e.g., saying nouns, noun–verb combinations), understanding (e.g., for conversation, television, movies), reading, and other (e.g., writing, calculation). Functional performance is defined as the use of language "without assistance, cues, or artificial conditions." The

estimates are obtained from informal interviews and formal test performances. While the interview is freshly in mind, each item is rated on a nine-point scale. The FCP has been used to study recovery not detected by a traditional aphasia test (Sarno and Levita, 1979). Wertz and others (1981) modified the FCP so family or friends would rate a patient's communication, and the researchers called this modification the *Rating of Functional Performance* (RFP).

Prutting and Kirchner (1987) devised a **pragmatic protocol** that addresses 30 features of conversation. It has sections for rating verbal aspects (e.g., topic selection and initiation, turn-taking behaviors), paralinguistic aspects (e.g., intelligibility, prosody), and nonverbal aspects (e.g., proximity, posture, gesture). Each behavior is rated as appropriate, inappropriate, or not observed. Profiles were reported for 11 LHDs and 10 RHDs in 15 minutes of conversation with a familiar partner.

Designed for patients in acute care, the **Inpatient Functional Communication Interview** (IFCI) was developed in Australia and described in a book chapter by McCooey, Toffolo, and Code (2000). The clinician investigates a list of twenty-three communication situations, mainly through a bedside interview. The situations are classified by (A) basic need, (B) present health care need, and (C) social need. The following are some of the items listed according to classifications assigned by the authors:

- responding to his or her name (A)
- telling about any pain or discomfort (B)
- giving information regarding progress (B)
- telling if he or she is hungry or thirsty (A)
- calling for a nurse (B)
- asking for something to read (C)

This short list is indicative of what a clinician considers when visiting a patient in the hospital. Each item is scored for whether communication is successful using any means. Implementation of this idea was illustrated with a brief case study in McCooey's chapter.

Patrick Doyle and his colleagues translated the logical concept of "burden of stroke" into an assessment tool called the **Burden of Stroke Scale** or BOSS (Doyle, McNeil, Hula et al., 2003). An interviewer assists a patient in reporting activity limitations in areas that include mobility, self-care, sleep, cognition, and social relations. Doyle was interested in obtaining a measure of the psychological distress associated with each of these areas. In particular, the BOSS contains a *Communication Difficulty* (CD) scale and a *Communication Associated with Psychological Distress* (CAPD) scale. The researchers administered these scales to 281 stroke survivors in the Pittsburgh area. They found that the CD and CAPD distinguished communicatively impaired survivors from those who were not communicatively impaired, substantiating validity of the scales (see also Doyle, Hula, McNeil et al., 2005).

Communication Activities of Daily Living (CADL-2)

Holland and her colleagues reduced the original CADL in number of items and administration time, resulting in CADL-2 (Holland, Frattali, and Fromm, 1999). It is still an assessment of interpersonal interaction and of solving common communication problems. The following seven areas are evaluated:

- reading, writing, and using numbers
- social interaction
- divergent communication
- contextual communication
- nonverbal communication
- sequential relationships
- humor/metaphor/absurdity

To make presentation easier, the authors eliminated features of the first edition such as role playing and some props. Access to a working phone is still required. The number of items was decreased from 68 to 50, causing test time to decrease from 40 to 30 minutes. In addition to the examiner's record booklet, the CADL-2 provides a booklet for a patient to mark a birthday party on a calendar, fill out an address form, and make a short shopping list while looking at a color photograph of the fruits and vegetables section of a supermarket. Scoring is done with a three-point scale applied to each item, with the best score per item being a 2. Maximum score is 100.

Ross and Wertz (2002) included the CADL-2 in a study of relationships among several tests of aphasia and a general estimate of quality of life. Eighteen chronically aphasic patients averaged 74.9 on the CADL-2. There were no significant correlations between quality of life and Holland's test as well as the WAB. Therefore, a measure of activity limitation (or disablement) does not necessarily correspond to a patient's feeling of life satisfaction.

Mahendra (2004) translated the CADL-2 into Hindi and modified it for an illiterate population in India, providing an example of how a test needs to be modified to be used in a different culture. The CADL's restaurant menu was changed to reflect Indian cuisine and included photographs of selections, which is common in India and helpful for illiterate individuals. Bus schedules are uncommon in India, and people in rural areas do not relate to the car speedometer problem. Some could not state their complete home addresses, not because of aphasia, but because they tend to identify their houses by structural features and landmarks. In all, the investigator deleted 14 items to create a culturally appropriate CADL-2 of 36 items with a maximum score of 72.

Functional Assessment of Communication Skills (ASHA-FACS)

In 1992, the American Speech-Language-Hearing Association sponsored the development of a universal measure of functional communication. ASHA sought advice from an international panel. The developers especially wanted to assess the use of language and other communicative skills in activities of daily life. The result is the *ASHA Functional Assessment of Communication Skills* (ASHA-FACS), which covers four domains summarized in Table 6.3. A field test version with 44 items was described for initial publication (Frattali, Thompson, Holland et al., 1995).

To obtain observations, the clinician becomes familiar with a patient's communicative behavior and solicits judgments of family members and other caregivers. Each of the items is rated according to two scales. One is a seven-point scale of Communicative Independence. The other is a five-point scale of Qualitative Dimensions of Communication, which is intended to assess the nature of functional deficit. As reported in 1995, a second pilot test produced data on 32 patients with aphasia due to stroke and 26 patients with traumatic brain injury. One study found that the ASHA-FACS and the WAB are strongly correlated (McIntosh, Ramsberger, and Prescott, 1996).

Other Assessments

The *Amsterdam-Nijmegen Everyday Language Test* (ANELT) has been revised a couple of times during the course of its development (Blomert, Kean, Koster, and Schokker, 1994; Blomert, Koster, Van Mier, and Kean, 1987). It is a measure of verbal communicative abilities exhibited in verbally presented, functional scenerios like the following:

- The kids on the street are playing football in your yard. You have asked them before not to do that. You go outside and speak to the boys. What do you say?
- You have an appointment with the doctor. Something else has come up. You call up and what do you say?

Verbal responses are evaluated according to an A scale for understandability of the message independent of linguistic form and a B scale for intelligibility of an utterance independent of content or meaning. Two equivalent versions of the test (i.e., ANELT I and ANELT II) permit measuring progress without the bias of a learning effect.

The **Communicative Effectiveness Index** (CETI) attempts to reach into a patient's daily life (Lomas, Pickard, Bester et al., 1989). A family member or friend is asked to rate communicative ability for 16 situations that were determined to be most important to family members. Situations include getting someone's attention, having coffee-time visits and conversations, conveying physical problems such as aches and pains, starting a conversation with people not close to the family, and conversing with strangers. Ratings are based on a scale with respect to "not at all able" at one end and "as able as before stroke" at the other end.

TABLE 6.3   Domains assessed with the ASHA-FACS. Only some of the 44 items are listed under the domains (Frattali et al., 1995).

SOCIAL COMMUNICATION	COMMUNICATION OF BASIC NEEDS	DAILY PLANNING	READING/WRITING/ NUMBER CONCEPTS
Uses names of familiar people	Recognizes familiar faces or voices	Tells time	Understands signs
Explains how to do something	Expresses feelings	Dials the telephone	Follows written directions
Participates in telephone conversation	Requests help	Keeps appointments	Writes or types name
Understands nonliteral meaning and intent	Responds in an emergency	Follows a map	Completes forms
			Makes money transactions

Another approach to measuring pragmatic skills, similar to parts of the CADL, comes from observing real-life interactions that some have decided to call *service encounters*. In such encounters, information, goods, or services are exchanged in face-to-face interaction or over the telephone. Togher, Hand, and Code (1997) evaluated patients making two types of telephone calls. One task was to call a bus service for information that would be helpful for organizing a group outing. Another task was to call the police to find out how a brain-injured person gets a driver's licence reinstated. As we might gather from the tasks, the patients in these cases had a relatively high level of language ability after traumatic brain injury.

Transcripts of the service encounters were assessed with a Generic Structure Potential (GSP) analysis. This analysis begins with dividing the conversations into speaking turns (or "moves"). The turns are classified as to the presence of obligatory elements in the encounter, such as a greeting, service request, service enquiry, closing, and goodbye. Other elements may be predictable deviations from the type of patient being evaluated. Togher looked for incomplete, unrelated, or inappropriate reponses. The investigators found that their patients differed from controls who engaged in the same encounters.

ASSESSING LIFE PARTICIPATION

The problems of life participation pertain to the extent of an aphasic individual's involvement in his or her social environment. Increasing this involvement has become the primary objective of *social and life-participation approaches* to treatment (Elman, 2005; Simmons-Mackie, 2001). Digging deeper into the implications of aphasia, clinical specialists have become interested in the notion of **quality of life** (QoL) for representing outcome of rehabilitation. This "intuitively appealing" phrase has been formalized "not only as an aggregate of broad domains but as the product of personally weighted life domains filtered through the individual's own perspective" (Hirsch and Holland, 2000, p. 37). That is, QoL means

many things depending on the individual, and perhaps the most potent indicator of a patient's progress is whether he or she perceives that life is getting better after the acute turmoil of stroke.

The study of QoL with aphasia, as a general concept, has a long history. This history may not be recognized by some contemporary scholars, because the issues were not identified as QoL or with the goal of developing outcome measures. Instead, the issues were discussed with respect to "emotional and psychosocial adjustment," "role changes," and so on (e.g., Davis, 1983). In today's terms, health care professionals are interested in the impact of medical conditions, known as *health-related quality of life* (HRQoL, HRQOL, HR-QOL). Psychologists and physicians have produced several precedents for monitoring a patient's satisfaction with life and, therefore, documenting outcomes of their therapies (see Bowling, 2004).

The World Health Organization developed one example of a general health-related QoL measure. The brief *WHO Quality of Life* questionnaire (WHOQOL-BREF) poses 26 questions with each to be rated on a five-point scale (WHOQOL Group, 1998). Some of the questions are listed as follows:

- How would you rate your quality of life?
- To what extent do you feel your life to be meaningful?
- How safe do you feel in your daily life?
- Are you able to accept your bodily appearance?
- How satisfied are you with the support you get from your friends?
- How satisfied are you with your transport?

This questionnaire is being translated and standardized in countries around the world. The WHOQOL-BREF was more sensitive in identifying aphasia than the Psychosocial Well-Being Index (PWI) scale for aphasia noted in Table 6.4. The items distinguishing aphasia from neurologically intact adults had to do with independence, social relationships, and the environment (Ross and Wertz, 2003). Also, with narrow exceptions, these QoL measures did not correlate with traditional language and communication tests, indicating that perception of QoL is unrelated to severity of aphasia (Ross and Wertz, 2002).

Since the mid-1990s, Carol Frattali at the National Institutes of Health in the United States and Linda Worrall of the University of Queensland, Australia, accumulated and disseminated information for speech-language pathologists (SLPs) related to the functional consequences of aphasia, including its impact on quality of life. They were especially concerned about the documentation of functional outcomes of aphasia rehabilitation. The

individualized perspective on what goes into a QoL has probably been the greatest challenge for developing a measure and documenting outcome of treatment. For example, returning to work may be seen by one person as enhancing QoL or by another person as diminishing QoL.

Variation on method includes the source of information. For **self-report** from an aphasic patient, original questions or statements may be simplified (Hoen, Thelander, and Worsley, 1997). The *Dartmouth COOP Charts* (for a primary care "cooperative") are a general health-related measure and may be good for aphasic patients, because

TABLE 6.4   A sampling of quality of life measures. There are many others (see Bowling, 2004).

	ASSESSMENT	DESCRIPTION	REFERENCE
General	*Ryff Scales of Psychological Well-Being*	Measures agreement on 24 statements in 6 areas	Ryff (1989)
Health-related	*Sickness Impact Profile* (SIP)	136 items in 12 categories of daily life	Bergner et al. (1981)
	Dartmouth COOP Charts	Illustrations for 9 questions about well-being	Nelson et al. (1987)
	WHOQOL-BREF	Short version, 26 items in 4 domains	WHOQOL Group (1998)
Stroke-related	*Stroke-Specific Quality of Life Scale* (SS-QOL)	49 items in 12 domains	Williams et al. (1999)
	Stroke Impact Scale 2.0 (SIS)	64-item self-administered questionnaire; 8 domains	Duncan et al. (1999)
	Stroke and Aphasia Quality of Life Scale-39 (SAQOL-39)	39 questions in 4 domains	Hilari et al. (2003)
Aphasia-related	*Code-Müller Protocols* (CMP)	Rating anticipation of change in 10 areas	Code and Müller (1992); Hemsley and Code (1996)
	Psychosocial Well-Being Index (PWI)	11 questions about participation and life satisfaction	Lyon et al. (1997)
	Aachen Quality of Life Inventory (ALQI)	Pictorial version of a pared-down SIP	Engell et al. (2003)
	Quality of Communication Life Scale (ASHA QCL)	15 minute administration	Paul et al. (2004)

each question and response options are illustrated with drawings. The scales address nine areas including daily activities, physical fitness, and quality of life, and they take about three minutes to administer (Nelson, Wasson, Kirk et al., 1987). In Germany, an adaptation of the *Aachen Quality of Life Inventory* (ALQI) consists of transforming items (e.g., *often alone*) into pictorial form (e.g., a person sitting alone). Ratings are depicted with a thumbs up or thumbs down and a neutral, frowning, or weeping face (Engell, Hütter, Willmes, and Huber, 2003).

The American Speech-Language-Hearing Association has published the *Quality of Communication Life Scale* (ASHA QCL) for neurologically impaired populations. It takes around 15 minutes to administer and is recommended as a complement to the ASHA-FACS for documenting outcomes (Paul, Frattali, Holland et al., 2004).

Cruice, Worrall, Hickson, and Murison (2003) gave a few QoL measures to moderately or mildly aphasic patients. These measures included the *Dartmouth COOP Charts* and an adapted form of the Ryff scale (Hoen, Thelander, and Worsely, 1997). Impairment measured with the WAB and disability measured with the CADL were correlated to scores on QoL measures, which supplied evidence that language, communication, and life satisfaction are interrelated. Later, these investigators compared QoL responses from aphasic patients with **proxy reports** using the same measures (Cruice, Worrall, Hickson, and Murison, 2005). The proxies were mainly spouses and children, and they were significantly more negative in their rating of quality of life, physical functioning, overall health, and vitality. They agreed with the aphasic patients for rating physical fitness, feelings, and daily activities. Cruice and her colleagues concluded that proxies do not reliably reflect the life satisfaction of aphasic patients. The apparent overlap of items indicates that ratings may depend on the scale being used. Qualitatively oriented clinicians advocate that outcome documentation be person centered or patient generated, apparently meaning that information should come from the patient rather than others (Worrall and Cruice, 2005).

In conclusion, there are many scales for measuring satisfaction with life. Health-related scales have been devised with stroke, traumatic brain injury, heart disease, and other medical conditions in mind. These scales tend to be standardized for validity and reliability. However, the aphasia-related measures provided through the 1990s tended to be nonstandardized (Hirsch and Holland, 2000). There are also scales for caregiver burden, which are cited in Chapter 10. Ross and Wertz (2003) concluded that "no comprehensive, conceptually coherent, psychometrically sound assessment of QOL with aphasia exists" (p. 362; also, Ross and Wertz, 2005). Others have argued that there are plenty of excellent assessments (Worrall and Cruice, 2005). Formal measurement of QoL with aphasia is relatively new, and the recently published ASHA QCL may be part of the evolution. Also, it is not clear how third-party payers value such measures relative to a patient's simply returning to work. Meanwhile, concerned clinicians recommend that patients or proxies should have the opportunity to supplement whatever scale is used with information that is most relevant for them.

MARTIN EXETER'S FUNCTIONAL SKILLS

Jackie Exeter quickly discovered that Martin could communicate better than he could talk, even during his acute hospitalization. It made sense to try writing at first, but this effort showed that aphasia affects both modalities. Many residual communicative sensitivities were drawn from an intact right hemisphere and intact structures involved in new learning and memory of his life before his stroke. For example, just a few days after the stroke, it was evident that he knew where he was and recognized his family and friends. Doctors and nurses became familiar quickly. A few words referred to Europe and his job.

Communicative intent was apparent when considering words, left-handed gestures, and slightly asymmetrical facial expressions. He gave a thumbs up to his worried son, Peter. When Julianna showed up in his room for a second visit,

Martin frowned a little and muttered something that sounded like "school" and a question. When she said she would go back to school as soon as she knew he was OK, Martin smiled. As the days became weeks, he could get across basic needs, but his language impairment was keeping him from conveying details. Jackie had to ask many questions. Sometimes listeners were not sure if he was talking about the present, past, or future unless the topic became apparent. Martin made a great deal of progress over the months after the stroke.

SUMMARY AND CONCLUSIONS

This chapter concludes a series of three chapters about the basic study of the language and communication problems of aphasia. It is essential background for understanding the nature of aphasia and for asserting an expertise in aphasiology. Clinical practitioners may identify with these objectives as well as be somewhat tolerant of the well-worn axiom that research begets clinical method. Research foretold clinical practice, for example, when studies by Harold Goodglass went into creating the Boston Exam. Furthermore, some aphasiologists have deftly applied the expertise of independent sciences, and this attention to the expertise of others will continue (see Table 6.5).

Meanwhile, Chapter 6 put the impaired language system into the contexts of its use. It began with pragmatics (e.g., inference, discourse) and proceeded to activity limitation (e.g., conversation, compensatory communication) and finally to participation limitation (e.g., quality of life).

TABLE 6.5 A chronology of outside influences on clinical aphasiology.

DECADE	DISCIPLINE	EARLY REFERENCES
pre-1900	• Medicine/neurology (localization)	• Broca in 1861; Wernicke in 1874
pre-1940	• Educational psychology (testing)	• Weisenburg and McBride (1935)
1940s	• Clinical neurology	• Goldstein (1942); Luria (1966)
1950s	• Clinical/counseling psychology • Experimental design and statistics	• Eisenson (1949); Wepman (1951) • Schuell and Jenkins (1959, 1961)
1960s	• Structural linguistics • Behavioral psychology • Neoclassical neurology	• Goodglass and Mayer (1958) • Brookshire (1967); Holland (1970) • Geschwind (1965)
1970s	• Speech and hearing sciences • Clinical psychology (test theory) • Transformational linguistics • Cognitive neuropsychology	• Shankweiler and Harris (1966); Swisher and Hirsch (1972) • Porch (1967) • Shewan and Canter (1971) • Shallice and Warrington (1970)
1980s	• Psycholinguistics (automaticity) • Psycholinguistics (online) • Neurolinguistics	• Milberg and Blumstein (1981) • Swinney, Zurif and Cutler (1980) • Caplan (1987); Grodzinsky (1986)
1990s	• Crosslinguistics	• Bates and Wulfeck (1989); Menn and Obler (1990)
2000s	• Ethnography	• Simmons-Mackie and Damico (1997)

Along this journey, we visited tests and scales that may be used to document an aphasic patient's functional outcome. Measurements may emerge out of an area of investigation that is relatively new for clinical aphasiology, namely, qualitative research or ethnography. Nurtured by laboratory science, some of us are not sure of what to make of this new kid in town. Finally, quality of life is a longstanding concern in new clothing with fresh energy for developing documentation.

We shall revisit most of these topics later in the book. We now have a foundation for chart-ing goals and imagining procedures in pragmatic treatment. Functional rehabilitation addresses compensatory communication, conversation, and participation in life (Chapter 10). We also have a foundation for learning about the pragmatic language difficulties that are unique to right hemisphere stroke (Chapter 11) and traumatic brain injury (Chapter 12). Of course, all of this matters for people with Alzheimer's disease and other dementias (Chapter 13).

MATCHING REVIEW

Match the test or measure on the left with the problem area on the right.
One problem area may be used more than once.

_____ 1. Discourse Comprehension Test

_____ 2. correct information units (CIUs)

_____ 3. Conversation Analysis (CA)

_____ 4. Limb Apraxia Test (LAT)

_____ 5. FIM

_____ 6. FCP

_____ 7. Burden of Stroke Scale (BOSS)

_____ 8. CADL-2

_____ 9. ASHA-FACS

_____ 10. WHO Quality of Life questionnaire

a. discourse analysis

b. main ideas and details

c. life participation measure

d. gesturing

e. scales of functional communication

f. includes communicative disress

g. test of solving communication problems

h. a patient's overall functional status

i. ethnographic method

CHAPTER 7

RECOVERY AND PROGNOSIS

"Marty talks for a living," Jackie Exeter thought during those first few days in the hospital when she realized Martin was safe but unable to muster more than a few words. They would have to cancel his speech in Brussels. A more important concern was that Martin talked for fun. Talking was a major part of who he was and who they were together and what they did with their friends. "Would he talk again?" "How long would it be before they would have a normal conversation?"

Besides the Exeters, payment providers have a stake in what can be expected from recovery from stroke. In this chapter, we will explore the facts obtained from behavioral measurement in clinical research. A great deal of the information pertains to the factors that enable clinicians to make general predictions about amount of recovery and its eventual outcome. What happens in a patient's head, neurologically or cognitively, is explored at the end of the chapter.

STROKE AND FUNCTIONAL OUTCOMES

Chapter 2 explained why structurally intact regions far from the site of infarction are dysfunctional during the acute period. Rapid early improvements are the result of a subsiding diaschisis. Lifting the cloud of global confusion reveals the *sparing* of regions of the brain rather than recovery from infarction per se.

It is characteristic of stroke that most patients improve regardless of whether they enter rehabilitation. This is called **spontaneous recovery.** A general impression of recovery was obtained in a longitudinal study of 92 patients with ischemic

stroke (Skilbeck, Wade, Hewer, and Wood, 1983). The investigators followed functions of daily living with the Barthel Index for two to three years postonset. They measured statistically significant progress during the first three months postonset. Between three and six months, improvement occurred but was not significant, and no change was measured after six months.

Health care professionals and payment providers want to know the **functional outcome** of services provided in the hospital. *Outcome* is a term that is currently used to refer broadly to the benefits of medical and clinical treatments. Desired results are specified according to objectives, and preserving life is the desired outcome of emergency diagnosis and treatment of stroke. For long-term rehabilitation, outcome measurement has become the means of documenting whether functional therapeutic objectives are being attained (see Chapters 6 and 10).

One outcome indicator is a patient's discharge destination. Physicians would like to predict whether a stroke patient will eventually be discharged to home (a good outcome) or long-term institutionalized care (a poor outcome). In one study, 172 patients were examined initially during the first two weeks after onset (Henley, Pettit, Todd-Pokropek, and Tupper, 1985). Researchers recorded information about medical history and obtained CT scans, measures of sensory and motor functions, a rating of activities of daily living, and a couple of measures of cognitive functions. CT scan data were not predictive of discharge outcome. Predictors of independent living included attentiveness, cooperation during testing, and high scores on motor-sensory and cognitive evaluations.

The *Functional Independence Measure* (FIM) has become a common measure of functional outcome in trauma-related rehabilitation programs as well as stroke-related programs (Cook, Smith, and Truman, 1994). The FIM has also been evaluated for its predictive value. When administered six days after admission to an acute care hospital, the FIM is helpful in predicting discharge to home, a rehabilitation center, or a nursing home (Mauthe, Haaf, Hayn, and Krall, 1996). When the scales are given during admission to a rehabilitation center, around two months after stroke, the severity level of the full-scale is suggestive of outcome after 60 days of therapy (Oczkowski and Barreca, 1993). The FIM is also predictive of "burden of care" at home, measured according to the minutes of assistance per day provided by a caregiver (Granger, Cotter, Hamilton, and Fiedler, 1993).

MEASURING RECOVERY OF LANGUAGE

Recovery of language has been documented in a variety of circumstances, including studies in which untreated patients were compared to treated patients. We find information about spontaneous recovery in this research. In one study, "patients were prevented from attending therapy by extraneous factors, such as family or transportation problems, but were willing to come back once again to the unit after six months or more in order to take the second examination" (Basso, Capitani, and Vignolo, 1979, p. 191). Elsewhere, "inclusion of a no speech therapy group was considered ethically acceptable because there was considered to be reasonable doubt whether the speech therapy service available to these patients was effective" (Lendrem and Lincoln, 1985, p. 744).

We may measure either **clinical improvement** in tasks used for clinical assessment or **functional improvement** in solving communicative problems of daily living. It has been suggested that "improvement which is not reflected in the patient's daily life is not improvement in fact" (Sarno, Sarno, and Levita, 1971, p. 74). Most investigators have measured clinical language behavior with the *Porch Index of Commu-*

nicative Ability (PICA) or the *Western Aphasia Battery* (WAB).

Robert Wertz, first with the Veterans Administration and then at Vanderbilt University, has directed studies of recovery and treatment efficacy. He has been particularly interested in the performance of various clinical tests, and this interest has been on display here in Chapters 3 and 6. His work included comparison of impairment-related tests and functional tests and scales (e.g., Ross and Wertz, 1999). From a large study covering intervals up to one year after stroke, he compared the PICA and two functional measures introduced in Chapter 6, namely, his RFP and the pragmatic protocol. These measures were not correlated with respect to measuring change at any point in the first year, indicating that impairment and functional (or pragmatic) tests measure different aspects of recovery (Irwin, Wertz, and Avent, 2002). For the purpose of documenting a patient's progress, this research indicates that one type of testing cannot substitute for the other.

It would be good to remind ourselves of the scores associated with these tests (see Chapter 3). The following sections introduce the fundamental components of recovery. Most data is from clinical measures taken from patients in rehabilitation programs, but studies of spontaneous recovery are given special mention. The reader will discover that *variability* is a central theme. Moreover, research has shown that predictions differ depending on the component of recovery, especially when considering amount, outcome, and rate of recovery (Connor, Obler, Tocco et al., 2001; de Riesthal and Wertz, 2004).

Proportion of Patients that Improve

What is the likelihood that language ability improves at all after stroke? In early studies, only about 50 percent of patients made recognizable improvement according to general rating scales or vaguely reported testing methods (Basso et al., 1979; Godfrey and Douglass, 1959; Marks, Taylor, and Rusk, 1957). Then, according to the more sensitive PICA measurement, 90 percent of untreated patients were found to improve over the first 10 weeks postonset (Lendrem and Lincoln, 1985). The proportion dropped to 79 percent between 10 and 22 weeks. Thus, standardized and reliable measurement has painted a more hopeful picture than cautious clinical judgments.

Amount

Reliable measurement enables us to quantify progress without relying solely on subjective judgment. Amount of improvement is determined by subtracting an earlier test score (i.e., pretest) from a later score (i.e., posttest). The result is a "difference score" or "change score." Change scores have been reported for a variety of intervals between the first and second test.

In studies of recovery, *initial scores* have been obtained at different times postonset. Sarno and Levita (1971) obtained functional ratings on 28 patients at bedside within two days postonset, when some had "a total lack of responsiveness and, quite probably, total absence of consciousness" (p. 177). Researchers often prefer to wait until the medical condition stabilizes and pattern of language deficit is apparent before giving the first comprehensive test. Therefore, the first score may be obtained around one month after onset (e.g., Deal and Deal, 1978; Wertz, Collins, Weiss et al., 1981), sometimes depending on the time of admission to a rehabilitation center (Pickersgill and Lincoln, 1983).

In studies of spontaneous recovery, the *final score* may not always be obtained at the point of maximum recovery. Investigators tend to give the final test at three or four months postonset, thus, possibly not detecting all the progress that might have been made. Lendrem and Lincoln (1985) retested at 6-week intervals beginning at 10 weeks postonset and concluding at around 8 months.

In studies of patients in rehabilitation, the final test has been often given around one year postonset (e.g., Wertz et al., 1981). Also, change scores were based on final scores at termination of treatment (Deal and Deal, 1978) or *peak scores* achieved before treatment was terminated (Bamber, 1980; Hanson and Cicciarelli, 1978). Thus, investigators have reported end points tied to slightly different clinical circumstances, such as a decision to end treatment as opposed to the continuation of treatment.

The most consistent fact arising out of this inconsistent research is that aphasic patients are widely variable in amount of recovery. This is a central clinical problem, making prediction seem to be impossible. In one study of mostly untreated subjects, the WAB's Aphasia Quotient (AQ) progressed an average of 16.64 percentage points (Kertesz and McCabe, 1977). Yet, one subgroup improved 5.16 points; and another, 36.80 points. The PICA has yielded ranges of spontaneous progress of 0.34 to 2.72 (Deal and Deal, 1978) and −0.49 to 5.18 overall response level points (Lendrem and Lincoln, 1985). Therefore, a group mean is not indicative of individual progress.

Treated aphasic patients display similar variability. Three small-sample studies had remarkable agreement in average amount of change measured with the PICA over the first year postonset (Table 7.1). Just looking at change scores,

TABLE 7.1   Amount and variability of change in PICA overall scores in three studies of mixed aphasic groups.

	N	INITIAL	FINAL	CHANGE	RANGE
Hanson and Cicciarelli (1978)	13	9.48	12.72	3.24	0.98–4.29
Deal and Deal (1978)	17	9.14	12.52	3.38	0.51–7.16
Bamber (1980)	13	8.40	11.65	3.25	0.10–6.18

we may be tempted to inform the Exeters that Martin is likely to improve around 3.30 points in the first year. Unfortunately, we cannot promise this improvement for anyone. A treated aphasic client may improve between 0.10 to 7.16 response level points.

A final comment has to do with how we interpret a change score. Researchers speak of "significant progress" with respect to an objective statistical analysis. In Lendrem and Lincoln's (1985) repeated administrations of the PICA, spontaneous progress did not become statistically significant until five months postonset. Some clinical researchers distinguish between *statistical significance* and *clinical significance* of recovery data. With a large experimental group, a small change score may be statistically significant; but it may not represent a meaningful change in a patient's life. For an individual patient, a small change may be clinically significant depending on what it represents functionally (e.g., progress in answering yes/no questions amidst a battery of tests).

Final Outcome

What will an aphasic person be like at the end of recovery? The aforementioned final or peak scores are a numerical indication of level of language ability that can be attained around a year after stroke. In research, the end of recovery is usually demonstrated with a series of measures showing a **plateau** of slightly variable scores. These scores indicate that the final linguistic outcome usually falls short of normal function.

In their study of spontaneous recovery over four months postonset, Kertesz and McCabe (1977) reported that one-fifth of 93 subjects attained levels above the cut-off AQ of 93.8 on the WAB. Twenty percent of this group had hemorrhages and traumatic injuries. Later, Kertesz (1985) categorized outcomes of mostly untreated patients with AQs taken at an average of two years postonset. He placed 27 percent in the excellent category (75–100 AQ); 24 percent were good (50–75); 24 percent were fair (25–50); and 25 percent ended up in the poor category (0–25).

The final scores in Table 7.1 are indicative of average PICA overall outcomes for thromboembolic patients in treatment until a year postonset. However, outcomes ranged from 8.69 to 14.88 across the three studies. Thus, many were far from a neurologically intact group that scored between 13.40 and 14.99 overall (Duffy et al., 1976). About one-third of the aphasic patients represented by the table reached into this "normal" range. The highest levels after a year were auditory comprehension and word repetition, which were around or above 14.50. Verbal subtests averaged 12.52, whereas describing the function of objects lagged behind at 10.87 (Hanson and Cicciarelli, 1978).

Aphasic patients do not return to normal function, because the loss of brain cells is permanent. These cells do not grow back. This difficult reality restrains recovery. To the extent that *recovery* implies a cure, there is an uneasiness over the use of this term. Some clinicians prefer to speak of "progress" or "improvement," instead of recovery. In this chapter, all three terms are used somewhat interchangeably because *recovery* has a common usage with a mutual understanding of the constraints on it.

Saying that a patient might end up with a 12.00 on the PICA does not say much about the *quality of life* that can be achieved. Schuell and her colleagues (1964) documented the number of patients that returned to school, entered vocational training, or re-entered employment. In her youngest group with "simple aphasia," 14 percent entered school or vocational training, and 19 percent resumed employment. In a group with a diagnosis similar to Broca's aphasia, 33 percent entered vocational training, and 27 percent found employment. Schuell explained that the less impaired aphasic clients had more difficulty accepting employment that was less demanding than their previous jobs. The more successful group seemed more determined to improve and to adjust realistically to deficit. Among the most impaired groups, no one entered vocational training or became employed.

Rate

Although final outcome varies, we may still wonder how long it takes to get there. Payment providers are particularly interested in the length of time that progress can be expected. It is one thing to say that a patient may improve 3.30 points, and it is another thing to say that it will take four months or four years. Our information comes from research that has regularly employed certain time frames, namely, from onset to 3 months, 3 to 6 months, 6 to 12 months, and beyond 12 months. Most data comes from the first 12 months.

One of the most consistent findings is that progress is more rapid in the first two or three months postonset than in any period thereafter. This recovery curve is illustrated in Figure 7.1. Lendrem and Lincoln (1985) found statistically significant progress between 4 and 22 weeks (1 to 5.5 months). A comparison of 10 weeks to 34 weeks yielded change that was not significant. The shape of this curve applies to both spontaneous recovery and progress during rehabilitation. For one group of aphasic patients receiving language treatment until 11 months postonset, 65 percent of their progress occurred within the first four months (Wertz et al., 1981).

Duration of spontaneous recovery has been an important consideration with respect to determining the efficacy of treatment. For patients in a rehabilitation program, clinicians are tempted to conclude that progress can be attributed to a treatment when the improvement is observed after spontaneous recovery is assumed to have run its course. Since a study by Butfield and Zangwill (1946), the belief has been that spontaneous recovery lasts around six months, so that it is safe to say that any progress afterward is caused by therapeutic intervention. However, this belief has been difficult to substantiate because of the reluctance to withhold treatment for more than three or four months postonset.

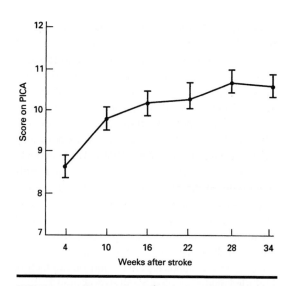

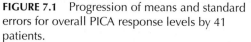

FIGURE 7.1 Progression of means and standard errors for overall PICA response levels by 41 patients.

Reprinted by permission from Lendrem, W., & Lincoln, N. B., Spontaneous recovery of language in patients with aphasia between 4 and 34 weeks after stroke. *Journal of Neurology, Neurosurgery, and Psychiatry,* 48, 1985, p. 747. British Medical Association, publisher.

Kertesz and McCabe (1977) discovered spontaneous progress after 6 months. Wernicke's aphasia showed substantial gains between 6 and 12 months. Also, recovery in terms of overall function may mask progress that continues for specific functions (e.g., Hagen, 1973). With statistical analysis of change scores, the magnitude of difference is a function of the interval between measures. An amount of progress achieved in 3 months may be achieved again over the next 18 months.

Rate of recovery is also highly variable among individual patients. In studies of treated patients, one took over 7 months to improve 4.01 points overall on the PICA, whereas another took about 8 months to improve only 0.98 points (Bamber, 1980; Hanson and Cicciarelli, 1978). Also, duration of recovery may be quite different between patients improving the same amount. Two patients improved almost 3.00 points but took about 4 and 19 months to do so. Two others, who improved

4.84 and 5.22 points, took 7.7 and 30.4 months, respectively.

Substantial progress has been found in some cases receiving treatment well beyond the first year (e.g., Broida, 1977; Sands, Sarno, and Shankweiler, 1969). A group of 35 patients with infarcts, hemorrhages, and one trauma were given the PICA at 3, 6, 12, 24, 36, and 55 months postonset (Hanson, Metter, and Riege, 1989). These patients were receiving varied amounts of individual treatment until 24 months and mostly group treatment after 24 months. Many patients showed steady and substantial improvement in the overall score until 24 months. After this point, patients either held steady or declined. Those that declined tended to have the mildest aphasias, and contributing factors included declining health and depression.

Pattern

An overall measure is less informative than attending to specific communicative functions. An overall measure may also be misleading. A patient may progress substantially in one function while regressing in another, but this result would balance out in an overall score. Just as a patient-group mean may not reflect individual scores, a patient's overall change score may not be indicative of individual test or skill changes. Most comparisons in the research have been between auditory comprehension and oral expression.

Spontaneous recovery for the four months postonset was differentiated according to eight subtests of the WAB (Lomas and Kertesz, 1978). The observations included two auditory comprehension tasks, one repetition test, and five expressive tasks mainly requiring word retrieval. The investigators concluded that comprehension fares better than verbal expression in early spontaneous recovery. Auditory comprehension has had a better outlook for treated patients, as well (Basso et al., 1979; Kenin and Swisher, 1972; Prins, Snow, and Wagenaar, 1978).

Following recovery to its peak with the PICA, Hanson and Cicciarelli (1978) found a different pattern. Verbal functions improved more than auditory functions. However, auditory functions reached their peaks sooner than expressive functions (i.e., around 5.5 months vs. over 8 months). Amount of progress in auditory functions may be smaller, because this initially less impaired function reaches a test's ceiling. Standard tests may keep us from observing further progress. Also, when a patient is followed long enough, verbal expression may overtake auditory functions in amount of progress.

Another approach to following the changing pattern of aphasia is through the WAB's filter of syndrome diagnosis. Kertesz and McCabe (1977) recorded "transformation from one clinically distinct group to another as defined by the subscores on subsequent examinations" (p. 15). Thirty-three percent ended up with a syndrome that differed from the initial diagnosis. "Broca's, conduction, and Wernicke's aphasics usually become anomic aphasics when recovery reaches a plateau" (Kertesz, 1979, p. 99).

In Pashek and Holland's (1988) study, evolution of aphasia took two paths. One was a rapid day-to-day fluctuation, sometimes back and forth between syndromes during acute hospitalization. The other path was gradual over weeks or months. Fluent aphasias rarely evolved to nonfluent aphasias.

In a retrospective study, researchers found records of patients who had at least two WABs within the first two months poststroke (McDermott, Horner, and DeLong, 1996). Those who changed syndromes progressed a significantly greater amount than those who did not change syndromes, indicating that good recovery pushes a patient through different patterns of impairment.

APPROACHES TO PROGNOSIS

The documentation of amount, rate, and final outcome of recovery demonstrated that it is nearly impossible to predict the long-range future based on an early and general diagnosis of aphasia. We must identify more specific factors that are related in some way to whether a patient does or does not get much better.

Porch, Collins, Wertz, and Friden (1980) identified three strategies of prediction:

- **behavioral profile approach** which involves "evaluating the aphasic patient with a variety of listening, reading, speaking, and writing tasks; constructing a profile of his performance; and comparing this profile with the change made by previous patients with a similar profile" (p. 313)
- **statistical prediction** or the use of early test scores to predict subsequent test scores, perhaps, with a mathematical formula
- **prognostic variable approach** in which we compare "a patient's biographical, medical, and behavioral characteristics against how these variables are believed to influence change in aphasia" (p. 312)

The behavioral profile approach, employed by Schuell and others (1964), is not used often except for the extent to which initial syndrome diagnosis is known to imply a pattern of recovery. The goal of statistical prediction is implied in any attempt to relate an initial test score to later scores. This goal was thought to have been achieved with the PICA for aphasic patients (e.g., Porch, 1981; Wertz, Deal, and Deal, 1980). The most common clinical strategy, however, is the prognostic variable approach.

Rational use of prognostic variables depends on a body of investigations into factors that are thought to be predictive of recovery. A "real factor," such as size of lesion, is one that has a direct influence on the recovery process. Other factors, such as the timing of initial test, may be useful predictors but do not influence recovery per se.

Prognostic indicators fall into two other broad categories (Table 7.2). *Endogenous factors* are attributes that a patient brings to rehabilitation. The clinician can do nothing about many of these factors (e.g., size of lesion, age). *Exogenous factors* are external to patients and are often a function of clinical decisions or circumstances. Timing of initial evaluation is a predictor that depends on when treatment is initiated or when a referral is made.

TABLE 7.2 Many of the factors studied as to whether they have a relationship to recovery from stroke.

ENDOGENOUS		EXOGENOUS
Neurological	*Functional*	
Size of lesion	Severity of deficit	Timing of initial test
		Language treatment
Site of lesion	Syndrome	
	Age	
	Gender	
	Race	
	Handedness	

Speech-language pathologists (SLPs) try as soon as possible to predict whether a patient's prospects are at least favorable or unfavorable. First, we gather pertinent information regarding medical history, neurological diagnosis, and initial test results. The collective impact of the factors is estimated, and prediction is framed in general terms. Perhaps the most striking development in the past 20 years has been the investigation of brain imaging for providing concrete clues to a patient's future. What we know about the main factors is presented in the following sections.

TYPE OF STROKE

The gradual recovery described so far is mainly characteristic of thromboembolic cases. Hemorrhage is likely to have different outcomes because the hematoma "displaces the fibre bundles without completely destroying them" (Basso, 1992, p. 340). Hemorrhage appears to produce alternating periods of progress and plateau; and recovery may not begin for months following a small intracerebral hemorrhage (Rubens, 1977a). In Kertesz and McCabe's (1977) study of spontaneous recovery, some patients with hemorrhage had large and rapid recovery, whereas others had little or no recovery.

Two other studies showed better recovery with hemorrhage than ischemic stroke. Holland and others (1989) gave the WAB at discharge and at one and two months postdischarge. Type of stroke had a moderate influence on progress during this period, with hemorrhage being more favorable than infarction. Basso (1992) reported on a comparison of 46 patients with intracerebral hemorrhage and 101 patients with infarctions. These patients were examined less than six months postonset and then six months later. More patients with hemorrhage had substantial recovery. The most significant progress occurred in reading and writing.

Nagata and others (1986) studied neurological factors in recovery, especially by measuring cerebral blood flow during a period beginning at two to four weeks postonset and concluding at least three months after onset. In a group with infarction, blood flow gradually improved and was correlated with recovery. Among patients with hemorrhage, blood flow was highly variable and was not related to recovery. Their explanation pointed to the instability of compression by a hematoma on adjacent brain tissue.

SEVERITY OF IMPAIRMENT

For infarction, **severity of brain damage** need no longer be estimated from behavioral examination. Neuroimaging permits a physician to look at the damage relatively soon after a stroke. The hope has been that characteristics of the lesion would provide a concrete aid in predicting a patient's linguistic outcome. In general, larger lesions are related to less recovery, which is most evident when comparing very large and very small lesions (Goldenberg and Spatt, 1994; Kertesz, Harlock, and Coates, 1979; Knopman, Selnes, Niccum, and Rubens, 1984; Mazzoni, Vista, Pardossi et al., 1992).

Naeser and her colleagues (1998) examined 12 aphasic patients one year and then 5 to 12 years poststroke. They found that lesion borders had expanded over this period of time. The reason for this slight but statistically significant increase in lesion size is not understood. The possibilities include degeneration of adjacent cells, a hypoperfusion creating the appearance of degeneration, or problems in other small arteries (although no patient had been diagnosed with a second stroke). Curiously, Naeser also found significant progress in naming and phrase length in patients with nonfluent speech. Evidently the gradual expansion of lesion borders had no negative effect on the patients' language behavior.

A modern EEG technique was administered to 23 aphasic patients at two weeks after stroke and then at what was characterized as "outcome" but was actually was at only two months postonset (Szelies, Mielke, Kessler et al., 2002). The scalp recordings of electrical activity were taken while the patient was at rest and while taking the Aachen Aphasia Test. The investigators focused on the Token Test component of the battery for their measure of language dysfunction. Activity in regions of infarction was related to Token Test performance at two months, but it appears that more research needs to be done for EEGs to be used in individual prognosis.

Speech-language pathologists suspect that **severity of dysfunction** can be predictive of recovery. The general belief has been that "there is a negative correlation between severity of aphasia in the early recovery period and the amount of improvement which occurs during the recovery process whether or not speech therapy is given" (Sands et al., 1969, p. 204). That is, the more severe the impairment before one month postonset, the smaller the change score. However, there are some exceptions around the edges of this generalization.

In a few studies, initial severity of overall language impairment around one month after onset was unexpectedly correlated in a negative direction with amount of recovery by patients with thromboembolic stroke (Bamber, 1980; Hanson and Cicciarelli, 1978). That is, patients with the most severe disorders tended to change the most. However, the lowest initial PICA overall scores were 5.85 and 6.63. Later, de Riesthal and Wertz (2004) pored over data from a large treatment study conducted in the 1970s (see Chapter 8). They found that initial PICA scores correlated positively with outcome but, like the previous studies, correlated negatively with size of change score in the first year poststroke. In general, initially more severe aphasia was predictive of a larger amount of progress but was also predictive of a poor outcome. This still may not contradict findings that the most severe aphasias do not result in much change, if these studies did not include the most severe aphasias. In addition, correlations are disrupted by the problem of ceiling effect when including initially mild aphasias with little room to improve with common aphasia tests.

The value of severity of deficit as a predictor may depend on when the first test is administered. Wallesch, Bak, and Schulte-Mönting (1992) found the first two weeks to be an unstable platform from which to predict recovery. Severely impaired patients were unpredictable, which was one reason for delaying a prognosis for Martin Exeter until the end of the acute period. On the other hand, Mazzoni and others (1992) found that distinguishing severe from moderate impairment at 15 days postonset was related to spontaneous recovery over the subsequent six-month period. It is possible that the platform begins to become more stable at the end of the first two weeks.

Lomas and Kertesz (1978) studied spontaneous recovery with 31 aphasic subjects divided into four groups based on initial levels of comprehension and verbal fluency. These groups were tested within one month postonset and were retested two and one-half to four months later. Relative amounts of progress are shown in Figure 7.2. The low-fluency/high-comprehending group made the most progress. The low-fluency/low-comprehending (i.e., "global aphasia") made the least progress. The two high-fluency groups (i.e., "posterior aphasias") made moderate amounts of progress. Pattern of improvement varied among these groups. Patients with low comprehension improved mainly in receptive functions, whereas those with high comprehension improved receptively and expressively. No group improved in word fluency in the early months postonset.

Initial severity of auditory comprehension deficit appears to be a factor. In a study by Gaddie

and others (1989), high-comprehending patients made much more recovery of *expressive* language than low-comprehending patients. However, initial severity of comprehension deficit may not be predictive of recovery of *comprehension* with severe aphasia. Also, good initial word comprehension is predictive of good recovery in naming (Knopman et al., 1984). Like the PICA and other

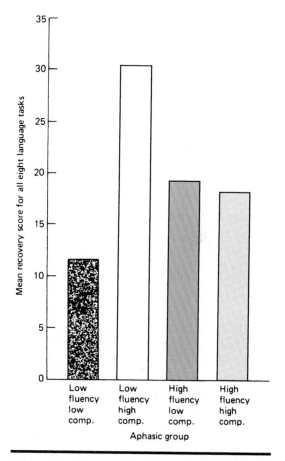

FIGURE 7.2 The overall amount of spontaneous language recovery differs among groups defined according to level of comprehension and fluency. These amounts are from the first four months after onset.

Adapted by permission from Lomas, J., and Kertesz, A., Patterns of spontaneous recovery in aphasic groups: A study of adult stroke patients. *Brain and Language, 5,* 388–401, 1978.

early language tests, initial Token Test score was positively correlated with outcome but negatively correlated with amount of change (de Riesthal and Wertz, 2004).

TYPE OF IMPAIRMENT

Site of lesion and type of aphasia are interrelated factors. Syndrome has been studied according to the general distinction between nonfluent and fluent disorders or according to specific syndromes. Investigators have found that size and location of lesion may be prognostic indicators with respect to particular syndromes.

Site of Lesion

Site of lesion in the left hemisphere has a pronounced effect depending on whether it is in the primary language zone around the Sylvian fissure or in the borderline areas encircling the primary language zone. The latter tends to cause transcortical aphasias. Recovery occurred more often in patients with penetrating trauma in marginal zones than in those with perisylvian damage, and several with marginal damage made rapid and complete recovery (Luria, 1970b). Rapid and near-total recovery of transcortical aphasias has been observed by Rubens (1977a) and Kertesz and McCabe (1977).

Deficits caused by **subcortical lesion** recover differently from those caused by cortical stroke. Using SPECT to measure hypoperfusion to other regions of the brain, Vallar and others (1988) found that improvement of blood flow is related to the best recovery. In distinguishing between thalamic and nonthalamic sites of damage (see Chapter 2), we should again be cautious in thinking about aphasic-like symptoms because of the possibility that some of the language deficits are not genuine aphasias.

With thalamic hemorrhage, aphasic symptoms disappeared completely by the end of the second month (Rubens, 1977a). Patients in Kirk and Kertesz's (1994) study were retested with the WAB at 3, 6, and 12 months. Several patients with predominantly thalamic infarcts recovered completely or dramatically by 3 months postonset. One patient with symptoms of Wernicke's aphasia did not improve much, and one with early diagnosis of global aphasia was much improved in comprehension and repetition by the 6-month measure.

Kennedy and Murdoch (1991) assessed four cases with nonthalamic or capsulostriatal hemorrhage at 3, 6, and 12 months postonset. Each case had some aphasic symptoms at 3 months, but two of these cases had AQs above the 93.8 cut-off for language deficit in most of their assessments over time. Regarding cases in Kirk and Kertesz's study, those diagnosed with anomic aphasia either recovered completely by 3 months or were still mildly anomic. Symptoms of global aphasia occurred with lesions extending into white matter posterior to the capsulostriatal region, and symptoms persisted for several months. The investigators concluded that subcortical language deficits generally resolve dramatically over time.

Broad Classification of Dysfunction

Dividing aphasic patients according to dichotomies has produced inconsistent results. Patients with expressive or nonfluent aphasia have been found to make more progress than receptive or fluent aphasias (e.g., Butfield and Zangwill, 1946; Godfrey and Douglass, 1959). In other studies, nonfluent and fluent aphasias did not differ (McDermott et al., 1996; Prins et al., 1978; Sarno and Levita, 1979). In the study by Mazzoni and others (1992), however, nonfluent aphasias had less progress in verbal expression and in reading and writing than fluent aphasias. The dichotomy may be too broad for meaningful study of recovery, especially when researchers are so varied in selecting patients in each of these categories.

Research focuses increasingly on the major syndromes. In Kertesz and McCabe's (1977) study of spontaneous recovery, data within each group represented varying time intervals after onset, and some individuals were followed much longer than others. Starting at a mean AQ of 85.5, anomic aphasia was similar to global aphasia in having the smallest amounts and slowest rates of progress. Lendrem and Lincoln (1985) compared four syndromes with the PICA overall score. Pashek and Holland (1988) followed short conversations throughout acute hospitalization; and then, starting at one month poststroke, the WAB was administered regularly until 7–12 months poststroke.

Global or Severe Aphasia

We are especially concerned about prospects for patients with chronically global or severe aphasia. Holland, Swindell, and Forbes (1985) followed patients who presented with global aphasia when admitted to the hospital. Short conversations were recorded daily during acute care, and the WAB was given at regular intervals until a year poststroke. Some cases evolved to other forms of aphasia by the time of acute hospital discharge, whereas others remained globally aphasic for months. A sign of whether a patient might remain globally aphasic was whether verbal expression changed rapidly in the conversations. Those with chronic global aphasia exhibited minimal or no change during hospitalization.

In Kertesz and McCabe's study of patients who were not receiving language treatment, global aphasias changed by an average AQ of 5.16 in contrast to a nearly 37-point improvement by nonfluents with Broca's aphasia. When 13 patients with global aphasia were diagnosed within the first 30 days, 4 remained global and 7 evolved to Broca's aphasia within the next two or three months (McDermott et al., 1996).

Pockets of progress in specific functions can occur. During early spontaneous recovery, low-comprehending patients improved in comprehension but not expression (Lomas and Kertesz, 1978). Within one year postonset, seven severely impaired patients receiving treatment made significant gains in auditory language comprehension and gesturing; and most of this progress occurred between 6 and 12 months postonset (Sarno and Levita, 1981).

Size and site of lesion can vary. Using CT scans, Ferro (1992) found five types of lesion that caused global aphasia in the first month poststroke:

- *Type 1:* large middle cerebral artery infarction encompassing anterior and posterior regions
- *Type 2:* anterior infarction with variable damage to underlying deep nuclei and white fiber tracts
- *Type 3:* subcortical infarction
- *Type 4:* parietal infarction involving supramarginal and angular gyri
- *Type 5:* simultaneous infarctions in frontal and temporoparietal regions

Based on a comprehensive aphasia battery, the subcortical group (Type 3) had the best prognosis. Some cases with circumscribed anterior (Type 2) or subcortical lesions (Type 3) "recovered completely" after six months (see also Kirk and Kertesz, 1994). Good progress could be characterized as improving to a Broca's or transcortical aphasia, which is consistent with Kertesz and McCabe's observation of global aphasia. Prognosis was very poor, however, for patients with large Type 1 infarctions.

Naeser (1994) reported on her team's retrospective study of global aphasia in which the first clinical test was given between one and four months poststroke, and a second test was given over a year later. She separated cases into two groups. In one group, cases had a cortical and subcortical lesion across frontal, parietal, and temporal lobes. The other group was the same except for an absence of damage to Wernicke's area. This group had a significantly greater recovery of word comprehension, but there were no differences between the groups in measures of language production.

Brookshire's (1997) review of early studies of global aphasia led him to conclude that "the presence of global aphasia at 1 month post onset is an ominous prognostic sign" (p. 247). However, preliminary research indicates that progress is possible in some cases. The problem lies in identifying the cases that are most likely to improve. Positive indicators are lesions that are mainly subcortical, the absence of damage to Wernicke's area in the temporal lobe, and probably a corresponding early improvement in auditory comprehension.

Wernicke's Aphasia

Wernicke's aphasia is also a severe impairment, but with fluent verbal production. These patients displayed a bimodal distribution of recovery in Kertsz and McCabe's study. Some improved little. Others improved by at least 20 AQ points. Four of 13 ended up in the anomic category according to WAB profiling. Patients with higher initial test scores and less jargon did better than others. Lendrem and Lincoln found that Wernicke patients had poorer outcomes at eight months than the other syndromes. Frequently flat lines of recovery are displayed in Figure 7.3.

Kertesz and others (1993) wanted to determine if lesion size and location would be predictive of recovery in 22 cases of Wernicke's aphasia diagnosed between 14 and 45 days poststroke. Patients were grouped according to whether they had good, moderate, or poor recovery after one year. Poor recovery was related to damage extending beyond Wernicke's area to the supramarginal and angular gyri bordering the parietal lobe. Good recovery to high AQ scores was associated with small lesions sparing much of the superior and middle temporal gyri.

Naeser (1994) reported results of a similar strategy in which patients with Wernicke's aphasia were classified at six months as having good or poor recovery. Differing from Kertesz, Naeser could not find a relationship between recovery and damage to the parietal lobe. However, there was a distinct relationship to the amount of damage to Wernicke's area. All patients with good recovery had damage in half or less than half of Wernicke's area, whereas all poorly recovered cases had larger lesions.

Cases of Wernicke's aphasia have also appeared in neuroimaging studies of ways the brain may reorganize for recovery. This research is presented near the end of this chapter.

Broca's Aphasia

In Kertesz and McCabe's study, four patients with Broca's aphasia had spontaneous improvement averaging 36.8 AQ points. Compared to the

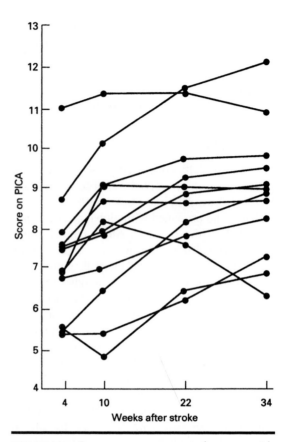

FIGURE 7.3 Spontaneous recovery of persons with Wernicke's aphasia. Note that starting as high as 11 is unusual for this diagnosis.

Reprinted by permission from Lendrem, W., & Lincoln, N. B., Spontaneous recovery of language in patients with aphasia between 4 and 34 weeks after stroke. *Journal of Neurology, Neurosurgery, and Psychiatry,* 48, 1985, p. 746. British Medical Association, publisher.

others, this syndrome had the greatest amount of recovery and had varied outcomes of fair, good, and excellent. Figure 7.4 shows the variability of PICA overall scores over eight months postonset. With respect to early evolution, patients with Broca's aphasia either remain in the same category or progress to a milder, more fluent form (McDermott et al., 1996).

Naeser (1994) reported on a comparison between a small group with Broca's aphasia and others with more severe expressive deficit of either

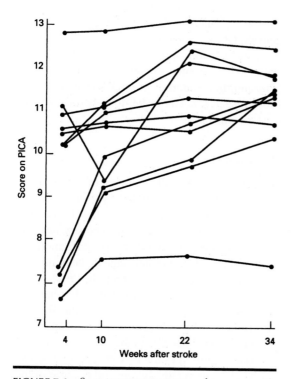

FIGURE 7.4 Spontaneous recovery of persons with Broca's aphasia.

Reprinted by permission from Lendrem, W., & Lincoln, N. B., Spontaneous recovery of language in patients with aphasia between 4 and 34 weeks after stroke. *Journal of Neurology, Neurosurgery, and Psychiatry*, 48, 1985, p. 745. British Medical Association, publisher.

no speech or mainly stereotyped words or phrases. No single lesion site could discriminate between these groups. However, cases with Broca's aphasia had less damage in two subcortical areas.

Conduction Aphasia

Conduction aphasia has been judged to be between Broca's and anomic aphasias in overall severity of language impairment. Patients seem to remain in a milder form of conduction aphasia or follow the fluent route to anomic aphasia, sometimes within the first three months (McDermott et al., 1996; Pashek and Holland, 1988). In Kertesz and McCabe's (1977) study, conduction

aphasia had an amount of recovery comparable to Broca's aphasia and reached nearly maximum AQs in some cases. Most anomic, conduction, and transcortical aphasias had excellent outcomes; and many rose above 93.8 for the AQ.

One case was followed by Gandour and others (1991) for six months after onset. BH developed conduction aphasia after a second stroke. He could follow simple commands and produced fluent utterances with occasional paraphasias. However, when asked to repeat "No ifs, ands, or buts," he said "sucklent incadiblems." BH evolved from a "reproduction" form of conduction aphasia (i.e., reading aloud as impaired as repetition) to a "repetition" form (i.e., reading aloud resolved). Chronic short-term memory impairment was indicated by improvement in Part V of the Token Test but not in Parts III and IV. Phonemic paraphasias were rare one month poststroke and were nonexistent five months later.

OTHER FACTORS

Several other factors have been studied extensively or have been suspected to be prognostic based on common sense or theories of functional organization of the brain.

Age at Onset

Chronological age may be more of a predictor than a real factor. Kimmel (1974) wrote that "when we find age changes or age differences, it is important to keep in mind that these findings only point to changes that occur with age but do not indicate the possible causes of these changes" (p. 33; see Tompkins, Jackson, and Schulz, 1990). Growing older is accompanied by changes in biological function, susceptibility to disease, and cognitive and social changes.

The experimental support for a patient's age as predictor has been mixed. Correlations between age and recovery were not significant in several studies (e.g., Basso et al., 1979; de Riesthal and Wertz, 2004; Keenan and Brassell, 1974; Kertesz and McCabe, 1977). Yet, Sands and others (1969) called age the most "potent" variable that influenced recovery, because five patients making the most change averaged 47 years of age and five making the least change averaged 61 years. Holland and others (1989) found age to be a strong predictor over two or three months postonset. McDermott and others (1996) found patients younger than 65 making more progress than patients above 65. A similar result occurred with respect to age 70 (Pashek and Holland, 1988).

In sum, Pashek and Holland warned that age by itself is a precarious predictor, and older patients may differ according to whether they have dementia and other pathologies. Basso (1992) concluded that age is not a very important factor in recovery. We may contemplate age as a favorable or unfavorable indicator with respect to extremes, especially when youthful middle age or older adulthood is accompanied by medical or motivational conditions that create a positive or negative climate for therapeutic success.

Gender

Gender is considered a factor because of the possibility that men and women differ in distribution of cognitive functions between the hemispheres (e.g., Moir and Jessel, 1991). The suspicion has been that verbal and nonverbal capacities are more evenly distributed in women, whereas men have the more familiar asymmetric division of labor. However, a great deal of data supporting this idea is indirect, based on comparisons between verbal and nonverbal tasks thought to be related to one hemisphere or the other. If the difference is true, women should have a more favorable prognosis because the RH already has more linguistic capability. This issue has been difficult to address because of the amount of research done in male-dominated veterans' hospitals.

Gender was found not to be a factor in several studies (e.g., Kertesz and McCabe, 1977; Lendrem and Lincoln, 1985; Sarno and Levita, 1971). However, it was a factor in the predicted direction in a few other studies. In a study of nearly 400 patients, females did improve more than males in spoken language but not in auditory comprehension (Basso, Capitani, and Moraschini, 1982). In cases of severe aphasia, women had more improvement than men in auditory comprehension (Pizzamiglio, Mammucari, and Razzano, 1985). More research needs to be done before we can trust this factor.

Handedness

Handedness or overall *laterality* of motor functions are commonly assessed by clinical neuropsychologists. For reasons similar to gender, handedness could be a clue to recovery because of evidence that left-handed people have more bilateral representation of language in the brain than right-handers (Springer and Deutsch, 1998). However, these differences apply to half of left-handers at the most. This factor is of particular interest with respect to right- and left-handed people who get aphasia after damage to the left hemisphere.

Data on this question is scarce, partly because left-handers are relatively rare and because of the tendency to study only right-handers. In a study of traumatic injuries, Luria (1970b) found an effect of familial left-handedness in right-handers. That is, pure right-handers without family history of left-handedness did not recover as quickly. Basso and her colleagues (1990) found that non-right-handed patients with stroke-related aphasias did not differ from right-handed patients. Borod, Carper, and Naeser (1990) followed the progress of left-handed patients and found patterns of change that were similar to right-handers.

Race

Race was considered in Holland and others' (1989) multivariate analysis of spontaneous recovery up to three months postonset, and they found that it did not matter. Wertz, Auther, and Ross (1997) compared African Americans and Caucasians across the course of a 44-week treatment study that began a month poststroke. Progress was measured with the PICA, Token Test, and a word fluency task. The two clinical groups did not differ in initial severity and in amount and rate of improvement of auditory and oral language skills over 10 months.

Time of Initial Test

The recovery curve (see Figure 7.1) tells us that amount of recovery depends on when we initially test a patient after stroke. We can expect a smaller amount of improvement the later a patient is referred. Pickersgill and Lincoln (1983) measured overall progress of 1.01 points with the PICA over an eight-week period, much less than the change scores in Table 7.1. However, patients were tested initially at an average of five months postonset at the time of admission to a rehabilitation program.

Yet, the timing of first test within the first two months is probably unrelated to change measured over a year, as indicated in Bamber's (1980) study and in an analysis of data reported by Hanson and Cicciarelli (1978). Thus, starting treatment anytime within two months is not likely to be predictive of subsequent progress, but a program started much later is likely to be accompanied by less improvement.

Additional Considerations

There are other factors that make sense but have not been studied much. In one study, *history of previous stroke* did not matter with respect to progress over the first three months (Holland et al., 1989). *Length of hospital stay* was a moderate predictor, as 20 days or less was more favorable than 21 or more days. Like age, this is one of those indicators tied to more direct or "real" influences such as the reasons for a short stay (e.g., smaller infarct, less severe deficit, good medical condition).

Other contemplated factors are *education* and *estimated premorbid intelligence,* and de Riesthal and Wertz (2004) found that neither correlated with language outcome one year after stroke. A retrospective review of hospital records indicated that neither education nor *occupation* relates to rate of recovery, although these indicators of

"socioeconomic status" were related to early severity of aphasia and severity years later (Conner et al., 2001).

A more exotic possibility is that *morphological asymmetry* or a person's brain size can affect recovery. Burke and his colleagues (1993) reviewed some previous work indicating that globally aphasic patients with a *right* hemisphere larger than the left recovered better than patients without this asymmetry of brain structure. Others found no relationship between structural asymmetries and recovery. Burke's team decided to do their own study and reviewed medical charts at the Albuquerque VA Medical Center from 1976 to 1986. They came up with a different result.

Burke's team compared the relative size of each hemisphere on CT scans to PICA overall scores recorded initially at one month poststroke and at one-month intervals until a year poststroke. Posterior width asymmetry favoring the left was associated with a faster rate of recovery and higher outcome at one year than right posterior asymmetry or equal hemisphere size. This so-called occipital asymmetry included portions of Wernicke's area and the temporoparietal boundary. Their conclusion was that a larger posterior *left* hemisphere is a more efficient language processor and provides more intact brain for facilitating recovery. More research probably needs to be done before neurologists routinely measure brain size as a clue to prognosis.

MAKING THE TARGETED PROGNOSIS

The variability in Figures 7.3 and 7.4 indicates that predicting recovery is a challenging problem. What do we say to a patient and family regarding the patient's prospects? Similarly, what do we say in a discharge staffing? As indicated before, we generally follow the so-called *prognostic variable approach* for any of these scenerios, and much depends on the time postonset of the decision and the period of recovery being considered. That is, acute phase prognosis is likely to be expressed differently than postacute phase prognosis; and predicting the next two weeks (short-term goals) is a little easier than predicting the next year and beyond (long-term goals).

A clinician's overarching desire is to be as positive as possible, especially for encouraging a patient and family members to do the work of rehabilitation. The data tell us that people with a stroke do not return to the way they were before. The data also tell us that we can be more positive when predicting some progress than when predicting recovery.

During the acute phase, shortly after the stroke, the doctor is likely to ask the family to be patient and wait and see. Because of diaschisis (or remote effects), it is difficult to know the pattern of dysfunction and how serious the permanent impairments will be. The doctor can be vaguely positive if the lesion is small, the patient is middle-aged and otherwise healthy, and the family is supportive. If the lesion is large and the patient is elderly and weak, it is still best to wait a few days to see if the patient shows signs of gaining physical strength and psychological vigor.

Speech-language pathologists may be more comfortable making a general prognosis during the subacute (or postacute) phase, soon after admission to a rehabilitation unit. At this time, we can obtain a better picture of the fundamental impairment. A patient's outlook is related to (a) severity of aphasic impairment, especially amount of residual language comprehension, and (b) amount of progress made since the stroke and in the first few days of rehabilitation. Then, prognosis becomes defined by realistic objectives. What are a patient's desires?

- substantial improvement in spoken language?
- reading the newspaper again?
- writing letters to the editor?
- making communication better than it is right now?
- maintaining personal relationships?
- returning to work?

Returning to work is an example of a general goal that may need to be modulated by realism, and this is likely to be a process that takes place over several months. Paul Berger had to adjust his sights, as he attempted to return to his position in Washington, D.C.'s real estate development department and had some difficulties (Berger and Mensh, 2002). How realistically positive we can be depends on the severity of impairment in skills required for each activity. Predicting a return to work may require evaluation by a state department of vocational rehabilition. The main point is that prognoses can be targeted toward realistic possibilities, and all of the factors should be considered at a staffing and with the patient and family.

BILINGUAL RECOVERY

Does a bilingual person recover languages differently? Exceptions to the equivalent recovery of two languages have long been associated with the rules of Ribot and Pitres (see Chapter 6). The rules indicated that any difference would have something to do with which language is the native tongue and/or which is the most familiar language.

- *rule of Ribot* ("primacy rule"): the first learned or native language recovers first
- *rule of Pitres:* the most frequently used language recovers first

Obler and Albert's (1977) review of the literature indicated that Pitres's rule describes recovery more often than Ribot's rule. That is, the most recently used language recovers faster more often than the other languages. The reliability of this characterization is confounded by definition of most frequent/familiar language, partly because functional bilinguals use two languages depending on the situation.

Paradis (1977) got a different impression from his review of 138 cases of bilingual aphasia reported in the literature. He found many possibilities (Table 7.3). Contrary to the previous emphasis on differential recovery, nearly half the cases improved according to a **synergistic** pattern in which progress in one language is accompanied by comparable progress in the other language. Subsequently, Paradis and others (1982) described another category. In *alternate antago-nism* (or "seesaw recovery"), "for given periods of time, the patients could speak only one language, and the available language would alternate for consecutive periods" (p. 56). A critical suspicion regarding reports over the past century is that cli-nicians may be more inclined to report differences between languages or that journals may be more inclined to publish them.

On a smaller scale, Fabbro (2001) reported on the severity and recovery of aphasia by Friulian-Italian bilinguals who live in the Friuli, the province of Udine in northeast Italy border-ing Slovenia. Code switching rarely occurs. Of the 20 individuals studied, 65 percent exhibited the synergistic parallel pattern of recovery in which Friulian and Italian were impaired equally and recovered at the same rate. This percent-age is more in line with Paradis and Table 7.3. The other patients had a version of the syner-gistic differential pattern, depending on which language was more severely impaired at the beginning.

EXPLAINING RECOVERY

One of Julianna Exeter's friends told her, "I heard that the right side of the brain takes over or that you can teach the right side to talk."

Now, we consider changes in the brain that may occur after a stroke and that may allow re-covery to occur. Two general types of changes are considered. One is the structural repair of dam-aged regions, and the other is a compensatory contribution from structurally intact regions such as the right hemisphere.

Early in this chapter, it was stated that cor-tical cells do not grow back. However, neuro-scientists have not given up on exploring the possibility that there can be some **repair** of the damage or a restoration of the damaged region. *Spontaneous regeneration* of damaged nerves was demonstrated in animals in the 1930s and 40s by Weiss and Sperry. Sperry cut the optic nerve of salamanders. The nerve regenerated, and sight was restored. The optic nerve in mammals, however, does not regenerate. After damage to the motor cortex on one side in adult rats, den-dritic arborization or "sprouting" occurred nearby and in the opposite hemisphere (Keefe, 1995; Rose, 1989). Findings with mice are suggesting to researchers that the injured brain "remodels itself."

Other theories of recovery are based on the global notion of the brain's **plasticity** or flexibil-ity. A child's brain is maximally flexible as it is continually learning new things. However, does the adult brain make adjustments subsequent to

TABLE 7.3   Patterns of recovery between languages in bilinguals (Paradis, 1977).

PATTERN	DEFINITION	PERCENTAGE
Synergistic (parallel)	Two languages progress at the same rate and were similarly impaired at the beginning; nearly identical recovery curves	41
Synergistic (differential)	Two languages improve at the same rate but were impaired to different degrees at the start; curves separate but parallel	8
Selective	One language improves but the other does not improve	27
Successive	One language recovers after another; one seems dormant while another is progressing, and the dormant language starts improving weeks or months later	6
Antagonistic	One language progresses but the other regresses	4
Mixed	Two systematically intermingled languages	?

stroke? According to **functional substitution,** a structurally intact area assists in or takes over an impaired function. Like the comforting thought from Julianna Exeter's friend, the right hemisphere (RH) may take over language functions to such a degree that it becomes a substitute for the damaged left hemisphere (LH). This used to be called the "spare tire" theory.

Another dimension of substitution pertains to whether the RH (or any intact region) had a capacity for the impaired language function before the stroke. *Spontaneous substitution* would indicate that language skills already existed in the substituting region. A demonstration of this in normal adults would contribute to this theory of recovery. *Therapeutic substitution,* on the other hand, would be indicated if the RH became more involved because of language therapy. This would suggest that the RH did not have an important role in the rehabilitated function before the stroke. For a long time, these were handy logical possibilities. Then researchers started to look for a basis for believing, at least, that the role of the RH changes after stroke.

One group of studies relied on indirect "observation" of brain function with techniques for studying functional asymmetry (Moore, 1989). Presenting stimuli simultaneously to each ear, called dichotic listening, is one of these techniques. Normally there is a right-ear advantage (REA) in response to verbal stimuli, which is considered to be indicative of the expected LH role in verbal processing. Curiously, various studies have shown a left-ear advantage (LEA) in aphasic people. This LEA has been interpreted as the RH taking a greater role in language function. However, the basis for this possibility rests with a comparison to what is typical or to a normal control group, not a comparison of poststroke and prestroke laterality.

Other indirect evidence for a shift of language function has come from presentation of words to the visual fields. Ansaldo, Arguin, and Lecours (2002) published a study of patient HJ who had a severe aphasia and who was asked to make lateralized lexical decisions at 2 months, 6 months, and 10 months poststroke. He responded faster with words in the left field (RH) than with words in the right field (LH) at 2 and 6 months postonset. An early pattern was that the RH was faster with high-imagery words than low-imagery words, a common finding with neurologically intact individuals. At 10 months, however, responses of the hemispheres were equivalent. This sign of an improving LH coincided with "some recovery" of verbal expression. The authors speculated that the hemispheres changed and that each hemisphere contributed to HJ's progress in different ways at different times.

Now, scientists can observe brain function more directly after stroke with neuroimaging techniques. These methods have usually consisted of measuring cerebral metabolism with PET scans or blood oxygen levels with fMRI while a patient performs a simple language task. Some studies entailed simply comparing a patient to normal controls, whereas other studies consisted of repeating tests after a stroke so a participant served as his own control. Repeated testing is considered to be stronger evidence for changes in a person's brain (Thompson, 2005); these studies are cited in Table 7.4. In general, the data so far indicate that changes in the LH near the infarct may be more impressive than changes in the RH's role in language function.

In the few studies that have compared aphasic patients to controls, the aphasic individuals had recovered to some degree. Three of these studies similarly found greater activation in the RH during simple lexical tasks (Cao, Vikingstad, George et al., 1999; Gold and Kertesz, 2000b; Weiller, Isensee, Rijntjes et al., 1995). A third study was less clear for fMRIs conducted during a covert word-finding task (Perani, Cappa, Tettamanti et al., 2003). Again, without repeated measurement, we do not know if these findings represent change.

In Italy, Cappa and his colleagues (1997) obtained PET scans from eight aphasic patients two weeks after stroke. In the acute stage, there was diminished metabolism in both hemispheres, indicative of diaschisis. Then, metabolism in-

TABLE 7.4   Some studies of changes in the cerebral hemispheres with measures
repeated beyond the acute phase.

BRAIN IMAGER	REFERENCE	LANGUAGE TEST	FINDING SUMMARY
SPECT	Mlcoch et al. (1994)	Speech fluency	Nonfluent aphasia; poor recovery associated with hypoperfusion
	Mimura et al. (1998)		20 patients; first year, changes in LH function; RH changes after first year
PET	Cappa et al. (1997)	Token Test, naming	At 6 months, metabolism increased in LH and RH
	Karbe et al. (1998)	Token Test, word repetition	At 12–18 months, recovery related to increased metabolism near infarct (LH)
	Warburton et al. (1999)	Verb retrieval	Little evidence of RH activity
fMRI	Thulborn et al. (1999)	Sentence reading	Increased RH activation of Wernicke's area homologue
qEEG	Szelies et al. (2002)	Aphasia battery	After 2 months, changes in LH including language areas

creased significantly in both sides of the brain for all subjects six months later. Moreover, changes in Token Test comprehension and spoken naming were correlated more with specific changes in the right hemisphere than in the left.

In Germany, Hans Karbe and his colleagues (1998) believe that they found physiological evidence of left brain reorganization associated mainly with improvement in Token Test scores. PET scans were obtained three to four weeks after stroke and then over a year later for seven severely aphasic patients. Metabolism was measured while patients did a word repetition task. As a presumed compensatory response one month after stroke, areas of both hemispheres were activated that are not normally active for the repetition task. The best language recovery over the following year was related to restored metabolism in the left superior temporal lobe, not increased metabolism in the RH. The investigators concluded that "left hemispheric structural reorganization is significantly more effective than the right hemispheric compensation" (p. 227).

Only one study of repeated fMRIs is reported in this text. Thurlborn, Carpenter, and Just (1999) followed a case of Wernicke's aphasia for whom an fMRI had been done fortuitously prior to his stroke. Along with a sentence-reading task, it was repeated at three and nine months after the stroke. The investigators found increased activation in the homologue RH Wernicke's area over time.

MARTIN EXETER'S RECOVERY

Martin Exeter was progressing more rapidly than many persons with aphasia (Table 7.5). His improvement in comprehension accuracy in the first two months was important for conversation. He could answer questions about what he was trying to convey, and he could detect when he was misunderstood. In the first few months, he was having a hard time managing his frustration. Just naming a picture never felt particularly "good." He would humor the therapist with a smile, but it was not what he was used to thinking of as an accomplishment.

TABLE 7.5   Some progress notes concerning Martin Exeter's functional progress.

TIME POSTONSET	LANGUAGE	FUNCTIONAL SKILLS	LISTENER'S BURDEN

2 months	Sporadic comprehension
	Pretends to read newspaper
	Word-finding delays
	Agrammatic phrases
		Gets basic ideas across
		Supplements with gesture
		Depressed and reclusive
			Lots of yes/no questions
			Anxiety over
			    impatience
			Jackie speaks for
			    Martin sometimes

6 months	Mildly agrammatic sentences More fluent but still slow Reads headlines and first paragraphs Writes short phrases	Gets most ideas across Sense of humor returning Avoids work-related topics Invites friends to house	Fewer questions Jackie more patient Close friends adjusting

12 months	Slow but nearly complete sentences
	Reads newspaper articles slowly
		Practices with computer
		Pursues social situations
		Cannot follow
		    conversations
			Minimal burden for
			    dinner conversation

18 months	Aphasia not apparent to strangers
	Martin senses word-finding
	    problems
	Reads professional articles slowly
	Writes with computer very slowly
		Friendly debates too fast to
		    get the fine points
		Thinks about returning
		    to work
			Patient with his
			    misinterpretations
			Balancing
			    encouragement
			    with reality

Over time, word finding quickened and grammatical morphemes filled gaps. His verbal production became generally more fluent. His therapist would report that he seemed more like someone with anomic aphasia than Broca's aphasia. By 18 months after his stroke, Martin was nearly his former self in everyday conversations with family and friends.

In two years, it was difficult for a stranger to tell that Martin had a language disorder. However, he could tell that his processing system was im-perfect. He remained quiet in social gatherings, because his friends talked too fast and took turns too quickly. His confidence was still shaken. He was slow finding words about obscure or complex topics. Even with these difficulties, he was beginning to contemplate a return to teaching. The stroke did not destroy his memory of the issues he had wanted to debate with students and colleagues. Yet, reading journals was laborious, and writing a couple of sentences would sometimes take an hour.

SUMMARY AND CONCLUSIONS

Important decisions about services are based on notions of recovery. Recovery is greatest and swiftest during the first two or three months post-onset and slows down until six months after onset. Some believe that language does not improve after six months or a year. However, recovery has been demonstrated in some patients up to one year and, in a relatively few patients, beyond one year. The problem with these observations is their variability. We need to have a way of managing a case-load based on an ability to predict who is likely to progress the most in the least amount of time.

The referring physician is interested in a speech-language pathologist's (SLP) opinion about prospects for recovering language, especially if the patient is provided language treatment. We want to be sure that the physician and family are also thinking about recovery of communication, which involves more than language per se. We also make a point of documenting recovery of language comprehension as well as verbal expression, considering that physicians often focus only on speech.

Like the physician, SLPs shy away from prediction during the first week after onset. We are more willing to make a general prediction later in the first month. Our prognosis pertains to the likelihood that a patient can benefit substantially from treatment. This is close to a binary decision, namely, either a patient can benefit from treatment or treatment is not likely to help. Of course, the physician's opinion regarding type, size, and site of lesion is important. Our job is to document initial severity of deficit and follow a patient's early spontaneous progress. A focal infarction preserving the comprehension area along with some early spontaneous progress are all fairly positive signs.

Although this chapter presented recovery by patients in rehabilitation programs, it avoided discussing treatment as an exogenous factor. Evidence for the effects of treatment remains to be considered in the following chapters.

CHAPTER 8

PRINCIPLES OF LANGUAGE RESTORATION

A speech-language pathologist came to Martin Exeter's bedside in the Stroke Unit and quickly evaluated his language abilities and oral motor function (including swallowing). She recommended some communicative strategies for him and his family, and offered encouragement to everyone. This was fine, but Jackie was particularly impressed that the therapist had started by explaining who she was and what Martin could expect when he started rehabilitation. "I know. You know what you want to say, but cannot think of the words right now." This person understood the problem.

Martin's rehabilitation went through four phases. He was transferred from the Stroke Unit to the Rehabilitation Unit of Pocumtuck Medical Center where he received subacute inpatient therapy for about a month, following the recommendations in his initial clinical report (see Figure 3.4). Then, he began the chronic phase by returning to the Rehabilitation Unit as an outpatient for about three months. He took a "vacation" from therapy for a couple of months, until he heard about a university-based program in another state. After three months at the university, he returned home and began his own regimen of daily language exercises. Thinking about returning to work, he sought help at the speech-language clinic in his own university. The variety of rehabilitation settings is summarized in Table 8.1.

Poststroke care has become the responsibility of a **rehabilitation team.** Besides a speech-language pathologist (SLP), the team minimally includes a physical therapist, occupational therapist, and social worker.

- *Physical therapy:* to improve strength and range of motion of large muscle groups. The therapist's concerns include ambulation and transfers between bed and wheelchair.
- *Occupational therapy:* self-care, work, and play activities. The therapist is particularly concerned with manipulation of utensils for grooming, eating, and other self-care tasks.
- *Social services:* for psychological, residential, and vocational needs; and discharge planning.

Reasons for more integrated teamwork in recent years include the sharing of reimbursement resources. In many rehabilitation centers, team members meet regularly so that, for example, language treatment can be coordinated with occupational therapy.

This chapter begins a set of three devoted to the SLP's multiple approaches to treatment for aphasia. This first chapter introduces a variety of considerations focusing on the language impairment. The general principles should establish the fundamental thought underlying this endeavor regardless of rehabilitation setting and constraints. This thought also goes into proposals and procedures for cognitive impairments surveyed in Chapters 11 and 12. We start with principles of cognitive stimulation, including an occasional comparison to behavioral methods that are common throughout speech-language pathology.

COGNITIVE STIMULATION

The fundamental strategy of stimulation facilitation originated in the clinical work of Hildred Schuell. Her contemporaries followed her lead (e.g., Darley, 1982; Eisenson, 1984), and she con-

TABLE 8.1 Rehabilitation settings in the United States, including common estimates of length of stay as inpatient or length of therapy.

SETTING	TYPE OF CARE	NOTES	LENGTH OF THERAPY
Acute care hospital	Inpatient Acute	Ensure survival Discharge when medically stable	Less than 7 days
Rehabilitation hospital	Inpatient Postacute or Subacute	Often in acute care facility Therapy as soon as possible Short-term treatment	Less than 4 weeks
Rehabilitation center	Outpatient Chronic	Independent facility Long-term rehabilitation	Weeks or months
Home health care	Residential Chronic	Patient's home Home Health Agency (HHA)	Weeks or months
Nursing home	Residential Chronic	Skilled nursing facility (SNF) Private practice contracts	Weeks or months
University clinic	Outpatient Chronic	Supervised student practicum Experimental treatments	Months to years

tinued to influence prominent clinicians such as Brookshire (1997), Duffy and Coelho (2001), and Shewan and Bandur (1986). The term *cognitive* is added to the notion of stimulation in order to indicate the approach's reliance on understanding the nature of aphasia. Clinicians think about treatment of comprehension and formulation processes.

Targets of Treatment

Schuell stated that "what you do about aphasia depends on what you think aphasia is" (Sies, 1974, p. 138). Brookshire (1997) has elaborated: "Most clinicians and investigators agree that aphasia is not a loss of language (either vocabulary or rules) but is the result of impairments in processes necessary for comprehending, formulating, and producing spoken and written language" (p. 249).

Brookshire advocated a *treat underlying processes approach* which steers clinicians away from replicating tests and toward cognitive processes assumed to be responsible for impaired performances. Treating a process should lead us away from targeting specific stimuli and responses and toward targeting general processes or abilities

that may underlie a patient's response pattern. In principle, "treating a general process may affect several specific communicative abilities that depend on the process" (Brookshire, 1997, p. 249). For example, when targeting the process of word finding, a clinician may employ word-production tasks not used in assessment, increasing the likelihood of improving divergent abilities and sentence production. The idea of treating underlying processes, originating with Schuell, is currently refined by various assumptions about the nature of language processes (see Chapter 9).

Current clinical practice tends to target general processing systems such as comprehension. When therapy is said to target comprehension, a clinician is speaking of a mental process, not a behavior. A behavior consists of pointing to pictures in response to spoken sentences, and one of Brookshire's points was that the comprehension system is built to deal with a variety of stimulus–response relationships.

In behavior modification, the target of a treatment is a particular behavior without consideration of underlying processes. A target may be pointing to a picture, giving yes/no responses to questions, producing the auxiliary *is,* or saying certain social phrases such as *I am fine.*

The Task

The activities of language treatment are similar to research and assessment. In research and assessment, tasks are designed for observing failures and successes. In treatment, some of the same tasks are carefully chosen for eliciting a patient's best performances. Brookshire, Nicholas, and others (1978) studied 40 videotaped treatment sessions conducted in various regions of the United States. The clinicians did basically the same thing when administering treatment. That is, all therapy tasks contained the following components:

- clinician's stimulus
- patient's response
- clinician's feedback

Any treatment task consists of the clinician's stimulus and the expected response. When working on comprehension, the stimulus is a word or sentence. The response tends to be nonverbal so production difficulties do not distract from comprehending (e.g., pointing to a picture). When working on production, the minimal stimulus may be a picture of an object, and the patient is asked to make a verbal response. Table 8.2 shows some basic tasks for some general objectives.

SLPs are interested in improving rather than just observing a patient's response. We help the patient by modifying or supplementing a stimulus or by providing informative feedback. For example, in a comprehension task, we may simplify a linguistic stimulus to improve the response. For a naming task, we may supplement a picture with hints about an object's name.

Among the types of behavior modification technique, **operant conditioning** has been preferred for modifying volitional behavior. A patient responds to a stimulus and is rewarded after an adequate response. Operant treatment for aphasia was common in the 1960s (e.g., Brookshire, 1967; Holland and Harris, 1968). It then faded from clinical aphasiology for a while and reappeared in the early 1980s in conjunction with efficacy research.

Because behavioral treatments are geared to specific responses, there may be a tendency to *treat to the test.* In this approach, "the clinician identifies tests in which a patient's performance is deficient and constructs treatment tasks that mimic the content and structure of those tests" (Brookshire, 1997, p. 248). For example, a naming task in treatment is likely to be quite similar to the naming task in assessment. Holland and Sonderman (1974) devised a task similar to the Token Test for treating auditory comprehension.

One key feature of a therapy task is the **number of items,** for example, whether a patient hears 10 different words or 50 different words. Shewan and Bandur (1986) put stimulation techniques together in a package called Language Oriented Treatment (LOT). "In LOT the same stimuli are not used over and over again . . . different stimuli at a comparable level of difficulty are presented to elicit responses" (p. 13). A patient could say "car" in response to "You buy a ___," "You wreck a ___," and "You fix a ___." Conversely, more than one response may be acceptable for one stimulus (e.g., You drive a *car, Ford, bus* and so on).

TABLE 8.2   Some basic tasks in treatment of aphasia.

AREA TO IMPROVE	CLINICIAN'S STIMULUS	PATIENT'S RESPONSE
Auditory comprehension	Says a sentence while showing three pictures	Points to one of the pictures
Reading comprehension	Shows a sentence while showing three pictures	Points to one of the pictures
Spoken word finding	Shows a picture of a common object	Says name of the object
Written word finding	Shows a picture of a common object	Writes name of the object

The key is that the particular words or sentences presented or produced do not matter as long as the targeted process is being exercised. In fact, it may be advantageous to vary item content, because progress may be more likely to generalize to untreated stimulus-response content that depends on the same process (Thompson, 1989). In the jargon of behavioral modification, this principle is known as "training sufficient exemplars."

Behavioral methods have entailed the training of specific sets of responses to a small set of stimuli. Thompson and Kearns (1981) trained the production of 10 names to 10 pictures until a patient reached a criterion of success. That is, the same items were elicited repeatedly. Kearns and Salmon (1984) trained the auxiliary *is* in 10 specific sentences. A small number of specific items is especially common when working with a severe impairment.

Adequate Stimulation and Good Response

SLPs start therapy with what a patient can already do, which is demonstrated directly or indirectly in initial testing. That is, we rely on tasks that produce a high frequency of accurate responses without training. This is known as the **success principle.** Brookshire (1997) wrote that "a good general rule is to keep patient performance at 60% to 80% immediate correct responses during the beginning of a given task" (p. 225). Starting at 80 percent accuracy or higher is possible when including slow responses.

Following the success principle ensures that a patient is practicing normal processing. Repeated failure, in effect, is the practice of an ineffective or aberrant cognitive process. Also, errors beget errors. Brookshire (1972) discovered that erroneous naming on one trial increased the likelihood of error on the next trial. Brookshire and Nicholas (1978) found that three or four consecutive errors reduced the chance of subsequent correct response to almost nil. When a patient starts making 30 percent or more errors, we adjust the task to make it easier, or we switch to a different task in which normal processing is resumed. As noted

in later chapters, this principle is known as "errorless learning" in some circles.

Schuell said that "I do not teach aphasic patients words. I stimulate language processes and they begin to function. Words come out that I never used" (Sies, 1974, p. 138). In the stimulation approach, the antecedent event is the driving force behind improving responses, as opposed to the consequent event in behavioral therapy. Darley (1982) suggested maximizing the "arousal power" of a stimulus, and Duffy and Coelho (2001) recommended that stimulation be strong enough to elicit a response without forcing it. Rosenbek and his colleagues (1989) wrote that "our feeling that good clinicians can—by their stimulus selection, ordering, and presentation—elicit responses from all but the most severe or sullen patients, causes us to emphasize antecedent over consequent events" (p. 137).

Schuell added that "I am going to depend largely on auditory stimulation, because I think language is most dependent on this perceptual system" (Sies, 1974, p. 139). Another reason for relying on the auditory modality is that it is the least impaired of the language modalities. Schuell believed in bombarding a patient with stimulation and requiring many successful responses, making therapy quite different from the other hours in a patient's day.

From a baseline of auditory stimulation, the power of input is often increased with **multimodality stimulation** (Duffy and Coelho, 2001). This usually entails supplementing an auditory stimulus with a printed word or sentence. However, if we restrict our thinking to modalities, we risk forgetting that the main target is a process. For example, when the goal is to improve word finding and the task is picture naming (a visual stimulus), a combined auditory and printed stimulus may provide the word to be retrieved. When this happens, it is no longer a word-finding task. The task becomes reading aloud (or repeating). For example, combined auditory and visual stimulation is *process consistent* if each is a contribution to comprehension, such as an auditory and printed version of a single statement, or a drawing that helps someone comprehend a question. For the naming task, multimodality stimulation might be the first sound and first letter of a target word.

Feedback for Errors

In operant training, "consequences of the behavior serve to control the frequency of its occurrence" (Mowrer, 1982, p. 204). Reinforcement should increase the frequency of a desired behavior, and negative feedback (or "punishment") should decrease the frequency of errors or undesirable behavior. Clinicians usually employ verbal praise such as "good" or "nice job," called **incentive feedback** (Brookshire, 1997). Kearns and Salmon (1984) presented redeemable coupons and tokens after correct responses.

In operant conditioning, errors may be "consequated" by verbal punishment. Tonkovich and Loverso (1982) administered a "verbal reproof" such as *No, that wasn't right*. Thompson and Byrne (1984) simply said *No, not quite*. A computer may be programmed to emit a "cheerful sound" after a correct response and a "negative tune" after an error (Scott and Byng, 1989).

Restimulation is the alternative to verbal reproof after a patient makes an error. Brookshire (1997) noted that "many clinicians tend to avoid negative feedback, perhaps because they do not wish to discourage their patients" (p. 230). Schuell and others (1964) stated that "the objective is to get the language processes working, not to teach the patient that whatever he says is wrong" (p. 342). According to this philosophy, the stimulus was probably not adequate if a patient fails to respond, and we *stimulate the patient again* instead of correcting errors.

There should be little need for restimulation, when stimulation is planned to be powerful enough to elicit a good response most of the time. When the occasional inadequate response does occur, we first say "Let's try it again," and then repeat the initial stimulus. If simple repetition does not work, we repeat the stimulus, supplemented with cues, such as the first sound in a naming task. However, if a patient exhibits frustration and starts

making errors at a frequency of more than 30 percent, then we modify the task so the stimulus is more powerful. That is, the restimulation becomes the antecedent event for the modified task.

Brookshire (1997) suggested that "incentive feedback does not play an important part of treatment of most brain-damaged adults" (p. 229). Most patients are self-motivated. Many know their target and are aware of the difference between their response and their target. For most aphasic patients, Brookshire preferred **general encouragement** that is not necessarily contingent on adequacy of response (e.g., "You're doing fine," "You're doing much better today").

Another option is **information feedback.** That is, we point out the degree to which a response approximated the instructed expectation (e.g., "It's not a complete sentence" or "Close, but you should have put *was* in front of the verb"). Brookshire recommended information feedback for self-motivated clients who are unaware of the target or the relationship between the target and an inadequate response. Simple positive feedback after correct responses may be considered to be informative.

In sum, clinicians have taken different approaches to the treatment of aphasia. These differences are illustrated in behavioral and stimulation methods. The main contrasts are summarized in Table 8.3.

PROGRAMMED STIMULATION

How does treatment progress over time? Principles of programmed learning keep stimulation treatment on a track defined by a goal. Treatment changes across sessions because a patient changes. Stable treatment is a sign of a stable patient. LaPointe (1985) referred to the overall approach as programmed stimulation (see Table 8.4). A treatment may be plotted broadly as starting with maximum dependence on the clinician for response (e.g., imitation) and proceeding gradually in the direction of the patient's becoming independent of the clinician. This principle may define a procedure within one task in a session or define increases in task difficulty over days or weeks.

TABLE 8.3   Comparison of cognitive stimulation and operant conditioning in carrying out a treatment task.

COMPARISON	COGNITIVE STIMULATION	OPERANT CONDITIONING
Theoretical assumptions	Belief that aphasia involves impaired cognitive processes and preserved linguistic knowledge	No assumptions about the nature of aphasia
Targets of treatment	Treatment of cognitive or psycholinguistic processes	Treatment of particular behaviors in relation to environmental events
Obtaining an accurate response	Behaviors naturally elicited by a stimulus most of the time	Modeling when responses are not forthcoming naturally
Therapeutic mechanism	Power of a stimulus to elicit a response repeatedly	Behavior changed through consequences or the clinician's feedback
Number of items in a task	Large number of different stimulus items that may vary from session to session	Restricted number of stimulus items repeated across sessions
Feedback on error	Restimulation	Punishment

Historically, long-term treatment of aphasia has been a series of little victories. Principles of programmed learning state that moving from an initial behavior to a terminal behavior requires small steps. The idea is that if the next step is similar to the current step, then capacities shown in the current step should transfer readily to the next step. The same processes are being used in each step, and the next step should present an easily surmountable new obstacle.

In principle, a small step is created by changing only one variable in the current task. These variables exist mainly in the clinician's stimulus and client's response. We may make a stimulus sentence slightly more complex, or we may increase the length of verbal response that we instruct a patient to produce. One approach to stimulus adjustment is called **fading,** in which we gradually remove supportive cues so the stimulus becomes more like what would occur in real life.

TABLE 8.4   Programming terminology applied to stimulation treatment.

TERM	DEFINITION	EXAMPLE
Initial behavior	Starting point of a treatment plan	Names actor in picture of simple event
Terminal behavior	End point of a treatment plan	Complete statement of simple event
Program	Steps from initial behavior to terminal behavior	(1) Names actor (2) Names action (3) Produces actor and action (4) Produces the complete statement
Response criterion	Basis for going from one step to the next	Each step is 90% accurate before changing response instruction

Formal programs usually include a somewhat flexible response criterion as the basis for moving to the next step. In Shewan and Bandur's (1986) LOT, a 70 percent criterion is frequently recommended. A patient has to achieve this level of accuracy on consecutive blocks of 10 trials before processing is considered sufficient for handling the next level of difficulty. Brookshire (1997) suggested a 90 to 95 percent criterion, especially because a task should start at a 70 to 80 percent level.

In the United States, however, program-driven treatment for aphasia has become more of an ideal than a reality. With managed care, the traditional principles of programming might be modified in at least two ways. The terminal behavior is more likely to be functional, such as requesting an item at a grocery rather than just producing a particular linguistic form. Second, a step of progression is more likely to represent changes in multiple variables rather than just one at a time. Many patients skip steps successfully, anyway; small steps may be quite inefficient for cases that show bursts of improved processing. For example, once a patient starts producing verbs regularly, other elements of a sentence may naturally follow without specific treatment. It may be more useful, in this case, to shift stimulus conditions to real-life communicative problems or settings.

MEASUREMENT AND GENERALIZATION

The health care system demands that clinicians document whether a patient is getting better. We can take three approaches to measuring progress during a period of treatment:

- charting performance of treatment tasks
- repeating a standardized test (e.g., "pre–post test")
- regular probing with specific goal-related tasks that are independent of treatment

Probably the least time-consuming approach is to measure performance in the task(s) used as treatment. The practice of setting criteria for changing tasks indicates that clinicians measure performance in treatment activities (e.g.,

LaPointe, 1985). A change of 70 to 95 percent accuracy would indicate that a patient is improving (as well as becoming successful with increasingly difficult tasks). Graduate students are often required to measure treatment as part of their clinical training.

Measuring the treatment, however, presents conflicts between some principles of treatment and the need for reliability of a progress measure. One conflict is between starting treatment at a high rate of accuracy (e.g., 80%) and starting measurement at a low baseline for showing clear change (e.g., 20%). Another conflict is between a flexible responsiveness to patients in therapy and the consistency required for reliable measurement.

The conflict between flexibility and consistency can be resolved by employing separate tasks for conducting treatment and measuring progress. Treatment can be flexible and at a high rate of success, and measurement can be consistent and can begin at a relatively low level. One implication of this separation is that the task used for measurement is likely to differ from the task used as treatment.

This fortuitous difference provides an opportunity to measure generalization (Kearns, 1989). Clinical researchers commonly distinguish acquisition and generalization. **Acquisition** refers to a new behavior appearing consistently during a training activity. In terms of learning theory, a patient is said to have acquired the behavior. Yet, our goal is that a patient use a new behavior beyond the therapeutic task. **Generalization** refers to progress in "something else," either in other conditions or with untrained responses. Studies of treatment often contain measures of both acquisition and generalization.

The types of generalization consist of stimulus and response generalization, and maintenance (Table 8.5). The importance of stimulus generalization has been known for a long time. For example, the last step of Taylor and Marks' (1959) classic naming program was the use of their core vocabulary in "everyday life without the help of a picture, a word card, or a therapist" (p. 16). In addition, response generalization should occur with

TABLE 8.5 The three types of generalization.

TYPE	DEFINITION	TREATMENT	TRANSFER
Stimulus	Trained response to stimuli that differ from treatment	yes/no to a list of questions	yes/no to other questions at home
Response	Untrained response to the stimuli used in treatment	Says "car" to picture of a Toyota	Says "Toyota" to same picture
Maintenance	Trained stimulus-response pairs after completion of treatment	Says 10 food names in 60 seconds	Same outcome six months later

improvement in a general process such as word finding. As Schuell stated, words start coming out that she never used in therapy.

Stimulus and/or response generalization can be observed with what researchers call a **generalization probe.** A probe takes a few minutes to administer and is usually given at the end of a session. Thus, it is sometimes called a post-session probe. Postsession probes are given daily, on alternate days, or once per week. Reliability is maximized by using at least 10 items and, of course, by administering the task the same way each time.

A systematic approach to probing is illustrated with *matrix training.* One example comes from a study of gesture training (Tonkovich and Loverso, 1982). The basic idea was to train a few signed agent-object messages with the hope of improved gesture production in 25 additional combinations not trained (Figure 8.1). Edges of the matrix defined training items (T). Other items (I) were for assessing transfer a short distance from training

	MILK	COKE	TEA	COFFEE	JUICE	WATER	BEER	WINE
SPILL	SPILL MILK **T**	SPILL COKE **T**	SPILL TEA **T**	SPILL COFFEE **T**	SPILL JUICE **E**	SPILL WATER **E**	SPILL BEER **E**	SPILL WINE **E**
DRINK	DRINK MILK **T**	DRINK COKE **I**	DRINK TEA **I**	DRINK COFFEE **I**	DRINK JUICE **E**	DRINK WATER **E**	DRINK BEER **E**	DRINK WINE **E**
BUY	BUY MILK **T**	BUY COKE **I**	BUY TEA **I**	BUY COFFEE **I**	BUY JUICE **E**	BUY WATER **E**	BUY BEER **E**	BUY WINE **E**
POUR	POUR MILK **T**	POUR COKE **I**	POUR TEA **I**	POUR COFFEE **I**	POUR JUICE **E**	POUR WATER **E**	POUR BEER **E**	POUR WINE **E**

T = Training Items (7)
I = Intramatrix Generalization Items (9)
E = Extramatrix Generalization (16)

FIGURE 8.1 A matrix of verb + object pairs for training gesture and sign combinations. T = items trained, I = generalization items within the training matrix, and E = generalization items outside the training matrix.

Reprinted by permission from Tonkovich, J. & Loverso, F., A training matrix approach for gestural acquisition by the agrammatic patient. In R. H. Brookshire (Ed.), *Clinical aphasia conference proceedings.* Minneapolis: BRK, 1982, p. 284.

(i.e., untrained combinations of trained verbs and nouns). Pairs outside the matrix (E) were for assessing transfer a greater distance from training (i.e., both elements not trained). All subjects improved with untreated gestures. Three of four patients reached the level of 100 percent accuracy achieved in acquisition of the seven treated pairs.

A treatment activity and a generalization probe are linked by a goal. The treatment is the means to achieving the goal. The generalization probe tells us whether we are meeting the goal. Because a treatment is a means to an end, goals and measures pertain to behaviors that differ from the treatment. For example, a treatment may consist of imitation tasks, but our goal is *not* to make a patient a better imitator. Instead, our goal may be to improve spontaneous verbalization. We can document progress toward meeting this goal by measuring spontaneous verbalization, not by measuring the imitation used as the therapy. Another example is shown in Table 8.6.

As indicated earlier, the notions of improving a process and achieving generalization are the theoretical and empirical sides of a coin. Generalization is the observation of improvement in something other than the treatment. Improving a process is a likely explanation of the generalization. That is, generalization occurred because a process was improved. Examples of this relationship will be introduced in the next section on word finding and repeatedly in the next chapter.

Another theme that appears more later is that there are two fundamental approaches to maximizing generalization, namely:

- improving treatment of impaired processes (e.g., more accurate diagnostically)
- making therapeutics more functional or more authentic

It is hoped that examining the probing methods in research gets the idea of generalization across, but measuring generalization in clinical practice may be somewhat different. For example, the concept of distance between the treatment and generalization probe may come into play. A clinician may be more interested in naturalistic changes (i.e., more distant) than improvement with untreated words or sentences with the same clinical task (i.e., less distant).

WORD FINDING

One of the main goals in Martin Exeter's early language treatment was to improve word-finding efficiency. This was not unusual, because every patient has some kind of word-finding problem. Technique usually revolves around the object-naming task. A week after his stroke, Martin named common objects promptly and without help around 50 percent of the time. The therapist found that a hint or cue would raise his word finding to about 80 percent. Therefore, this is where treatment began. The goal was for him to be naming at 80 percent without hints in a couple of weeks.

Cue Responsiveness

If an aphasic cannot bring forth an intended response himself, it is sometimes possible to lead him to do so by eliciting a response first in a more automatic way and then in more and more voluntary ways by gradually withdrawing the facilitations incorporated in the stimuli. This passage from more automatic to more voluntary constitutes the core of rehabilitation. (Basso et al., 1979, p. 192)

We use cues to elicit words automatically or without training. Several studies have been done to

TABLE 8.6   The relationship of a treatment and a measure to a goal.

BEHAVIORAL GOAL	TREATMENT PROCEDURE	GENERALIZATION PROBE
Improve naming from baseline of 40% to 80%	Sentence completion at 90% accuracy	Simple naming using words not practiced in treatment

determine the arousal power of cues for aphasic patients. Naming cues fit into two broad categories (Table 8.7). Semantic cues provide information about the target word's meaning, and the most frequently studied version is a carrier phrase conveying superordinate, functional, or locational information (e.g., "It's a sport"). A purely semantic cue provides no intentional information about the target word's form. Cognitively speaking, semantic cues may be said to activate an area in semantic memory. A lexical or phonological cue provides information about a word. It is usually the first sound or syllable (e.g., "It starts with /b/"). It gives no additional information about meaning. Cognitively speaking, lexical cues point to a form in the mental lexicon. Either type of cue is more effective in eliciting names than a picture alone (Stimley and Noll, 1991).

In the research, cues have been presented either prior to showing an object, called *prestimulation* (Pease and Goodglass, 1978; Stimley and Noll, 1991), or they have been presented as restimulation after naming difficulty or naming error (Li and Williams, 1990; Kohn and Goodglass, 1985; Love and Webb, 1977). Generally, cues are more effective as the severity of naming deficit decreases. A phonological cue is more effective than semantic cues and other lexical cues such as a printed or rhyming word. In one study,

phonemic cues elicited names about 50 percent of the time, and semantic cues were effective around 30 percent of the time (Li and Williams, 1989).

Some exceptions have been observed. The greater power of phonemic cues applied to nouns but not to verbs. For an action-naming task, phonemic and semantic cues were equally effective around 40 percent of the time (Li and Williams, 1990). Semantic cues were more effective for verbs than for nouns.

Phonemic cue superiority was slightly more pronounced for Broca's aphasia relative to aphasia in general. Some investigators left the impression that phonemic cues are especially useful for cases of Broca's aphasia that have the most difficulty in naming (Bruce and Howard, 1988; Love and Webb, 1977). Regarding the fluent aphasias, cues were more effective for conduction aphasia than the other fluent syndromes. Cues have been least productive for Wernicke's aphasia.

Self-Cueing

If an aphasic person can identify the first letter of a word in a tip-of-the-tongue (TOT) state and retrieves words when a clinician provides the first sound, then maybe the patient can generate his or her own cues to facilitate retrieval. This would make the patient more independent of the

TABLE 8.7 Common cues used to facilitate spoken object naming. Carrier phrases create syntactic probabilities that may be helpful.

SEMANTIC CUES	EXAMPLE	LEXICAL CUES	EXAMPLE
Definition	"It uses ink and you write with it."	Phoneme (first sound/syllable)	"puh"
Function	"You use it for writing."	Rhyming word	"It's not ten; it's a ___."
Semantic associates	"Pencil," "ink," "It's like a pencil."	Spelling	"p-e-n"
		Printed word	PEN
Sentence completion	"A ball-point ___." "You write with it. It's a ___."	Modeling	"pen"
Location	"You find it on a desk."		

clinician. It sounds like a good idea. It was reported first by Berman and Peele (1967). They described training a patient to write the first letter, sound it out, and generate his own carrier phrase; but they did not submit the program to experimental scrutiny.

Bruce and Howard (1988) studied possiblities with 20 persons who had Broca's aphasia, only half having been helped by clinician-generated phonemic cues. These researchers figured that the patients should be able to point to the first letter of a word that cannot be retrieved, sound out (or recode) the letter, and use the sound as a cue. Yet, only six patients could identify first letters when failing to name objects. None retrieved words when identifying the first letter. Only two could sound out letters, and none displayed all three abilities. Attempts to train the recoding skill were laborious.

Theory-Driven Naming Therapy

A great deal of literature since around 1990 has been devoted to theory-motivated treatment of naming or word finding. Fortunately, Lyndsey Nickels of Sydney, Australia, has contributed several essays and an ambitious review with comparison charts (Nickels, 2002). A few groups of clinical researchers have produced several case studies. The United Kingdom has been a hub for cognitive neuropsychological studies, beginning with the work of David Howard and continuing currently with his colleagues, Julie Hickin, Wendy Best, and Ruth Herbert. Anastasia Raymer has pursued a similar theoretical approach in the United States.

Of course, a theory-motivated approach does not necessarily require that the theory be the serial-stage naming model of cognitive neuropsychology. Mary Boyle, Carl Coelho, and others have worked with a different theoretical take on the problem, namely, an interactive-activation theory that is common in psycholinguistics.

The model of object naming (see Figure 4.2) is a frame of reference for establishing objectives and explaining results of a therapy procedure. The arousal power of cues is considered to be evidence that aphasic impairment lies in lexical retrieval instead of being a loss of lexical storage (Howard, Patterson, Franklin et al., 1985a). Phonological cues are superior to semantic cues possibly because the stimulus object already activates semantic memory through the object recognition capacity of most aphasic persons. Thus, semantic cues may be redundant; the aphasic person, who knows what he or she wants to say, still needs help for accessing or retrieving the word. One thought has been that a stroke raises the thresholds for lexical activation and that form-related cues lower the threshold or raise the activation level.

Treatments have been designed to repair the semantic system (Nickels and Best, 1996), the phonological output lexicon (Bastiaanse, Bosje, and Franssen, 1996; Miceli, Amitrano, Capasso, and Caramazza, 1996), or the route between semantic and lexical systems (Marshall, Pound, White-Thomson, and Pring, 1990). The therapies are classified as two general types, namely, phonological (or lexical) treatment and semantic treatment. Neither of these therapies represents a consistent set of tasks. To speak of a semantic treatment, for example, is to speak of a variety of treatments. Also, the idea behind many of the studies is to match a treatment with a presumed semantic or phonological impairment.

Semantic treatments steer a patient toward activating concepts associated with words. A unique feature is that patients are not required to produce a word during the therapy, as if the semantic system is to be exercised in isolation of word finding. That is, activation of the semantic system precedes the lexical access in Figure 4.2. One version of semantic treatment centers around word comprehension (Byng et al., 1990). This *picture–word matching* technique may be supplemented with a semantic judgment task. Progress in naming, especially regarding untreated items, has been mixed (Nickels and Best, 1996b) if not somewhat disappointing (Pring, Hamilton, Harwood, and Macbride, 1993).

Another version of semantic therapy is called *semantic feature analysis* (SFA), in which the object in a naming task is accompanied by various cues. An object is placed in the center of a feature analysis chart containing cues to various types of conceptual associations (e.g., "is used for ___," "has ___," "reminds me of ___"). A patient is asked to complete the phrases and write answers in boxes surrounding the object. Boyle and Coelho (1995) tried this procedure with a patient diagnosed with Broca's aphasia. Naming treated and untreated items improved, but spontaneous speech did not get better. Lowell, Beeson, and Holland (1995) tried SFA for three cases with fluent aphasias, and two of the patients improved in naming. Subsequent studies again showed generalization to untreated items with fluent and nonfluent aphasias (Boyle, 2004; Coelho, McHugh, and Boyle, 2000). Investigations of SFA do not seem to have been aimed at a specific semantic impairment but, instead, use theory to specify the nature of the therapy.

Phonological treatments rely on the type of cueing called "lexical." Phonological treatment focuses on sound structure, whereas orthographic treatment focuses on written structure or spelling. Because both are directed at word form, both can be identified under the more general classification of lexical or "word" treatments (e.g., Carlomagno, Pandolfi, Labruna et al., 2001). The empirical precedent of phonemic cue superiority would predict continued effectiveness as a treatment procedure for individuals.

Howard and his colleagues (1985a) administered a phonological treatment to determine the therapeutic value of lexical cues. Eight patients were given a package of word repetition, rhyme judgment, and rhyming cues. Phonemic cueing was superior to no cueing for one session; but, after a 30-minute interval "filled with general chat and a cup of coffee," trained names were retrieved no better than before treatment and no better than names that were not cued. Later, a similar treatment without rhyming cues was given to 12 patients for four days across one week or eight days

across two weeks (Howard, Patterson, Franklin et al., 1985b). Six weeks later, the superiority of treated items faded. Howard's studies raised a question as to whether only a few sessions of lexical cueing is sufficient to restore the retrieval process for lasting use.

Raymer and others (1993) administered a phonological treatment to patients with Broca's aphasia. Detailed analysis indicated that one patient's disorder was squarely in the phonological output lexicon, whereas the other three had a "lexical-semantic impairment." Each patient received the same naming procedure consisting of three levels of restimulation. Upon a patient's failure to name an object, the clinician tried a rhyming cue, then the initial phoneme, and then the word itself for repetition. The therapy was given for 15 to 20 sessions. Some cases improved in the naming of untreated items and in word production on tasks not used in therapy (i.e., reading aloud and written naming). There was no clear relationship between treatment effects and diagnosis.

Phonological and orthographic cues were presented one session per week for eight weeks to aphasic patients more than one year after stroke in a study by Hickin, Best, Herbert, and colleagues (2002). Twenty words for treatment were chosen by the patient. If a patient did not respond to the first sound or letter, more of the word was presented until imitation achieved success. Pre- and posttreatment testing with 200 words showed improvement.

Phonological and semantic treatments have been compared. One comparison showed the two procedures to be equally effective but with limited generalization (Howard et al., 1985b). Le Dorze and others (1994) alternated two versions of semantic therapy, one involving word forms and the other without word forms, with a single patient. Naming improved for items drawn from the procedure involving words but not for items drawn from the other procedure, indicating that including words in a semantic task is important. There was no difference between phonological and semantic cueing for action-naming treatment (Wambaugh,

Cameron, Kalinyak-Fliszar et al., 2004). One research method is to provide one approach as a base treatment (e.g., semantic treatment) and compare the base with and without the other treatment (e.g., phonological or orthographic). Drew and Thompson (1999) were more impressed with the results of a combined treatment than with semantic treatment alone.

Those who have been studying theory-driven naming treatments have been well aware of their limitations. From her review of the literature, Hillis (2001) noted most of the following characteristics of the results from case studies:

- Patients with the same diagnosis do not respond well to the same treatment.
- Patients with the same diagnosis respond well to different treatments.
- Patients with different diagnoses respond well to the same treatment.
- Too often, the treatments fail to generalize to other items and other tasks.
- The diagnostic methods are time-consuming.

Nickels (2002) summarized the situation succinctly: "We still cannot predict which therapy will work with which impairment" (p. 959). Moreover, the variety and quality of experimental designs used to examine the same basic questions need to be critically examined. Yet, some clinical aphasiologists believe that we have the capability of targeting naming treatments to underlying phonological and semantic impairments (e.g., Fink, Brecher, Sobel, and Schwartz, 2005).

Can we generalize these studies to real clinical circumstances? Experimental treatments are often provided months and years after stroke, and they may be relatively infrequent and spread out over time. Thus, the experiments may not be representative of the timing and intensity of treatment in rehabilitation centers. Basso (2005) reviewed pertinent studies and concluded that increased frequency and longer duration of direct language treatment results in better communicative improvement. More functional therapies, however, may not need to be drawn out for a long time (see Chapter 10). Certainly the effectiveness of theory-

driven naming procedures is not known for the subacute phase of recovery.

In addition, advocates of more functional or social approaches to treatment may question the communicative value of the gains in picture naming and other simple tasks that have been demonstrated with these methods, especially for the time allotted to treatment in most rehabilitation settings in the United States. How we view these treatments depends partly on the distance of generalization that is achieved.

Other Naming Treatments

The main variant of phonological or semantic treatments is to combine elements of each, which is probably the most common form of cueing treatment in a rehabilitation center. Robson and others (2004) applied a mixed semantic-lexical procedure to the treatment of proper and common nouns. In a preceding study, 20 aphasic patients named family members better than common objects. Famous people and places were the hardest to name. The semantic treatment had a comprehension component and a lexically cued naming component. After five weekly sessions, 10 patients, mostly many months poststroke, improved equally with treated common and proper names, but they did not improve much with untreated items. One participant was evaluated for word finding beyond the naming task and was found to have improved. Despite this limited demonstration of generalization, the authors were enthusiastic about the gains in naming.

In Philadelphia and Finland, Nadine Martin, Ruth Fink, and Mattie Laine tried a slight variant of naming therapy called *contextual priming*. Naming was preceded by repetition, which was intended to facilitate naming. The treatment occurred in the following sequence:

- spoken word–picture matching
- repetition of the name
- independent naming ("delayed repetition")

Semantic context conditions focused on words from a category such as animals or professions, whereas phonological context conditions focused on a particular sound. Of the two cases studied, one displayed more improvement than the other, and generalization was inconsistent (Martin, Fink, and Laine, 2004). Various aspects of the treatment manipulations were studied further with 11 patients (Martin, Fink, Laine, and Ayala, 2004).

Kiran and Thompson (2003b) tried a different approach for obtaining generalization of naming therapy for two fluent aphasic patients. Whereas we would usually do naming therapy with easy or familiar objects, the investigators started therapy for a category (e.g., birds) with semantically difficult or atypical items (e.g., *penguin*). This treatment generalized to untreated, easier, or typical items in the same semantic category (e.g., *robin*). However, treatment with easy items did not generalize to difficult items in the same category. It was thought that the treatment with more difficult items challenged word retrieval to a point that the process functioned better when it came time to try easy items. We shall return to the notion of training more difficult items in the next chapter.

COMPUTER-ASSISTED TREATMENT

"Teaching machines" were part of the wave of programmed instruction in the 1960s. These devices provided automated presentation of stimulus "frames" and feedback upon response (e.g., Holland, 1970; Sarno, Silverman, and Sands, 1970). The machines were quickly reviled by Wepman (1968) as being a "devil's box" coming between a therapist and a patient. Now, computers are a ubiquitous fixture in clinics as well as patients' homes.

We have become familiar with the essential role of computers in studying the automatic processes of language comprehension and production. For about 20 years, Richard Katz (2001) has been showing us how computers can supplement standard treatment. Companies such as Parrot Software have developed sophisticated programs for work on reading comprehension, semantic categorization, visual attention, short-term memory, and reasoning. The software is capable of providing hints to correct response and data on performance over time, including how often the patient requested hints.

Let us consider a commercial naming program in which a photo of an object appears, and the patient is to type the name. If the patient needs help, the clinician or patient can use the mouse to click on one of three types of cues (i.e., first letter, brief description, carrier phrase). However, here is where we might become concerned about the computer. A gorgeous banana split appears on the screen. A patient types out "fudge." The computer says this is incorrect. The patient might just as well have typed "mars." Because of such glitches, the clinician usually runs through a program before leaving a patient to run it alone. Fortunately, many aphasic patients will chuckle over the computer's aphasia and just move on to the next stimulus.

Computer-assisted treatment is evolving rapidly. Some of the recent developments include:

- a program in Philadelphia called *MossTalk Words* (www.MossTalk.com), which provides auditory and written cues for naming and is clinician assisted or self-guided (Fink et al., 2002)
- *Multicue,* a program in the Netherlands for naming therapy in which the patient selects his or her best cueing hierarchy (Doesborgh, van de Sandt-Koenderman, Dippel et al., 2004)
- in the United Kingdom, remote delivery of word-retrieval therapy without a therapist present (Mortley, Wade, and Enderby, 2004)

Studies of computer-assisted language treatment have been analyzed recently, and several authors suggest that better designed studies are needed (Fink et al., 2005; Wallesch and Johannsen-Horbach, 2004; Wertz and Katz, 2004). We shall return to computers later with regard to supplementing or replacing severely impaired verbal functions and helping aphasic people participate in an electronic society.

GROUP TREATMENT

A great deal of treatment during and after World War II was conducted with patients in groups

(Huber, 1946; Sheehan, 1946; Wepman, 1951). The large number of patients in military hospitals made groups necessary, but it also came to be viewed as a valuable supplement with dynamics that do not occur in individual treatment. Most clinicians do not utilize groups as a substitute for individual treatment.

Because groups can be constituted for different purposes, there is no single entity for which the label "group therapy" suffices. When someone reports that group therapy was conducted, we can assume only that it involved two or more clients. Generally, groups are formed for the following purposes:

- *treatment* of cognitive and psycholinguistic impairments
- *maintenance* of communicative gains achieved in prior treatment programs
- *transition* from a treatment program to real life (i.e., community reintegration)
- *support* for patients and/or families while the patient is undergoing other treatment programs

Multiple purposes can be operative for a single group, such as the support that patients provide each other as they work on cognitive or communicative treatment goals. Groups for any purpose may include family members or volunteers used in ways reported in Chapter 10 on functional rehabilitation.

EFFICACY OF STANDARD APHASIA TREATMENT

A speech-language pathologist (SLP) is required minimally to document whether a patient is progressing during the period of treatment. Because managed care also encourages that treatment be attempted as soon as possible, it is often provided during the period of maximum spontaneous recovery in the context of a rehabilitation team. In these circumstances, we cannot determine whether language therapy is the cause of progress. This section presents some studies that have addressed whether language treatment makes a difference in a patient's recovery. For those wanting to do proper clinical investigations, several sources are available (e.g., Kazdin, 1998; Morgan, Gliner, and Harmon, 2006).

The Meaning of Efficacy

Bloom and Fischer (1982) wrote of the "three *eff*'s" of accountability in clinical practice. *Effort* is documented as the number of patient visits and the length of a visit. *Efficiency* is a measure of effort with respect to time (e.g., visits per day). However, working hard and efficiently does not guarantee the third *eff, efficacy,* which is the effect of a treatment on recovery of language skills.

Some clinicians have brought the notion of functional improvement to bear on an additional distinction between efficacy and *effectiveness,* the latter referring to whether treatment causes a change in functional abilities or in daily life (e.g., Brookshire, 1994). This fine-tuning of our wording appears to have some inconsistency, as Robey and Dalebout (1998) distinguished between the benefit of "treatment delivered under ideal conditions" as efficacy and "treatment delivered under routine conditions" as effectiveness (p. 1227; also, Wertz and Katz, 2004).

A generalization probe per se does not provide evidence for efficacy or effectiveness of treatment, because other factors could account for progress any time postonset (e.g., neurological changes, medications, living environment, other activities). Demonstration of a cause–effect relationship has obligatory and optional components. The obligatory component is to control for other factors that could be present while treatment is being administered. The optional component lies in the type of progress measurement chosen, namely, the extent to which treatment causes generalization beyond the treatment.

Large Group Studies

Because of the difficulties in conducting large-scale comparisons of treated and untreated groups, only a few such studies have been reported. For an ideal examination of efficacy, the only difference between the groups should be that one is receiving a treatment and the other is not receiving a treatment.

The largest efficacy study in terms of number of participants was carried out in Italy (Basso, Capitani, and Vignolo, 1979). Most subjects had aphasia caused by stroke. The researchers used the size of treated and untreated groups to maximize their similarity. Participants entered the no-treatment group, because they "were prevented from attending therapy for extraneous factors, such as family or transportation problems" (p. 191). It took 30 years to complete the study, but the comparability of groups was still weakened by the nonrandom selection. Not being able to attend therapy may have made the untreated subjects differ from treated subjects in other respects, such as communicative environment or motivation to get better. Yet, the groups were similar in educational and socioeconomic levels, and in distribution of types of aphasia, etiology, and gender.

The treated and untreated groups were subdivided according to the time postonset that treatment was initiated. Some subjects received treatment less than two months after onset. Others began treatment between two and six months postonset, and other patients did not start treatment until after six months. The dependent variable was the percentage of patients making a substantial improvement of at least two points relative to

a five-point scale. Main results are summarized in Table 8.8. At each period, the proportion of subjects making such progress was higher in the treated group. Percentages were lower but the differences between groups were still pronounced after six months. The study showed that treated patients are more likely to make substantial improvement than untreated patients, but the study did not indicate relative amounts of progress with respect to measures that were developed long after this major undertaking had begun.

In Canada, Shewan and Kertesz (1984) compared three treated groups with an untreated group "who did not wish or who were unable to receive treatment" (p. 277). The groups ranged from 23 to 28 subjects with ischemic or hemorrhagic strokes. The therapies consisted of language-oriented treatment (LOT), stimulation-facilitation therapy, and an unstructured support therapy provided mainly by nurses. LOT was the decision-making process for treatment developed by Shewan (Shewan and Bandur, 1986), and stimulation therapy was associated with Schuell's methods (Duffy and Coelho, 2001). Few details about differences between procedures were reported. Treated patients received three hours of treatment per week for a year.

Progress was measured with the *Western Aphasia Battery*'s Language Quotient (LQ) and Cortical Quotient (CQ) and with the *Auditory Comprehension Test for Sentences* (ACTS) at

TABLE 8.8   Percentage of substantially improved patients in each of six groups (Basso et al., 1979). Groups were defined as treated or untreated and whether treatment was initiated within 2 months, 2–6 months, or after 6 months postonset.

	TIME POST ONSET		
	< 2 months	*2–6 months*	*> 6 months*
Auditory Comprehension			
Treated (N = 107)	88	65	50
Untreated (N = 86)	50	48	16
Oral Expression			
Treated (N = 162)	59	39	29
Untreated (N = 119)	33	9	4

regular intervals beginning within the first month and then at 3, 6, and 12 months postonset. With an analysis of covariance for the last LQ, treatments together produced a better outcome than choosing not to have treatment. Both treatments by SLPs had a better outcome than no-treatment, whereas the unstructured group did not differ significantly from no-treatment. There was no difference between LOT and stimulation therapy. The treatment effect occurred mainly in the 6-to-12-month period postonset.

Poeck, Huber, and Willmes (1989) followed the progress of 68 treated aphasic patients with the *Aachen Aphasia Test* in Germany. The treated subjects were compared with the spontaneous recovery of 92 patients in 17 departments of neurology where aphasia treatment was not available at the time. Treatment was said to be similar to Shewan's LOT, but it was three times the amount. It was given in five 60-minute individual sessions and four 60-minute group sessions per week. Treatment periods lasted six to eight weeks. The treated group was divided into an early group receiving treatment between one and four months postonset and a late group treated between four and 12 months postonset. For some in the late group, treatment occurred beyond the final measurement of spontaneous recovery. A "chronic" group started after 12 months.

The progress of each treated patient was computed by correcting for spontaneous recovery. That is, treatment effects were determined by "subtracting" the control group's spontaneous recovery from the progress that occurred. With these corrections, significant treatment effects occurred for 78 percent of the early group and 46 percent of the late group. Poeck and his colleagues thought that these estimates were low because of the strictness of the correction. No correction was made for the chronic group, but 68 percent showed significant improvement, which should be of interest to those who believe that progress cannot occur after the first year.

Small Group Comparisons

Several studies with smaller groups and/or less experimental control have been reported. Wep-

man (1951) found that 68 aphasic patients, whose treatment had begun at least six months postonset, improved in grade level from 3.8 to 9.1. Fourteen cases reported by Broida (1977), where treatment was started at least 12 months postonset, improved an average of 10 overall percentile points on the PICA. Three patients improved as much as 19 and 22 points. Hagen (1973) compared treated and untreated groups in a study that "commenced when all subjects were discharged from the physical rehabilitation program six months post-onset" (p. 456). The treated group had substantial progress in language functions for which the untreated group had no improvement. Other investigators have found impressive progress in patients whose treatment was not started until four to seven months after onset (Butfield and Zangwill, 1946; Deal and Deal, 1978).

Holland (1980b) bumped into some data pertaining to treatment efficacy during standardization of the CADL. Twenty-eight patients were retested at intervals varying from 8 to 15 months, and the first test was given no sooner than 4 months postonset. Many patients improved in their test scores. Thirteen receiving treatment had significantly more improvement than the 15 who did not receive treatment. The groups turned out to be comparable in several prognostic factors. This "post hoc" study had its weaknesses; but if Holland had not known the basic principles of designing efficacy research, then she would not have recognized her accidental study.

Treatment Comparisons

In the United States, a massive project was undertaken to compare individual treatment with group treatment (Wertz et al., 1981). Several VA Medical Centers participated in a fastidious effort to match treatment groups according to several criteria and assign patients randomly to each group. For over three years over one thousand patients were screeened, and 67 met the criteria. Eight hours of treatment per week was started at one month postonset. Each group received treatment for 11 weeks or until about four months postonset. Due to attrition, a total of 34 patients were followed for 44 weeks or until about a year postonset.

The only difference between treatments was that individual treatment had greater progress in the PICA overall score than group treatment. Otherwise, both methods were similar in being accompanied by significant progress. The only suggestion of treatment efficacy per se was a common one. That is, significant improvement occurred after six months, the point at which spontaneous recovery is believed to have ceased.

The next report from the cooperative study addressed a comparison between two other categories of treatment (Wertz, Weiss, Aten et al., 1986). One type was treatment in the clinic by an SLP. The other was a home-based treatment by a volunteer who had received six to ten hours of training. The treatments began about seven weeks after onset. Eight to ten hours per week were devoted to the treatments for 12 weeks. Comparisons to periods of no-treatment were introduced partly by using these groups as their own controls. That is, treatment was followed by 12 weeks without treatment. Yet, because the spontaneous recovery curve biases this design to favor the period of treatment, a deferred-treatment group was added. This group, beginning about eight weeks postonset, had 12 weeks without treatment followed by 12 weeks of clinic treatment.

The progress made by the clinic-treatment group was significantly greater than that made by the deferred-treatment group over the first 12-week period. The home-treatment group was between these groups, not differing significantly from either one. The three groups did not differ from each other at the end of the 24-week study period or about eight months postonset, indicating that delaying treatment for a while does not matter ultimately.

A summary of the major group studies is shown in Table 8.9.

Intensity of Treatment

Basso (2005) scrutinized the efficacy literature to examine the question of how intensive and prolonged treatment should be to produce the best results. Treatment was not effective when it was provided an average of two hours per week for an average of 23 weeks or a little over five months. Treatment *was* effective when it was provided about nine hours per week for 11 weeks. Thus, more intensive treatment for a shorter duration had the better outcomes.

Pulvermüller and others in Germany have been developing *constriant-induced* (CI) therapy, which

TABLE 8.9   Characteristics of the large studies of treatment efficacy.

INVESTIGATORS	LOCATION	GROUP COMPARISON	INITIATION (POSTONSET)	INTENSITY AND DURATION
Vignolo and Basso	Italy	Stimulation treatment No treatment	Within 2 months 2–6 months After 6 months	
Shewan and Kertesz	Canada	Language-oriented stimulation Unstructured support No treatment	1 month	3 hours/week 52 weeks
Poeck, Huber, and Willmes	Germany	Language-oriented No treatment	1 month 4 months	9 hours/week 6–8 weeks
Wertz and many others	USA	Individual treatment Group treatment	1 month	8 hours/week 44 weeks
Wertz and many others	USA	Professional treatment Volunteer treatment	7 weeks	8–10 hours/week 12 weeks

consists of intensively scheduled or "high doses" of language activities at least three hours per day for a few consecutive days. A group of 10 patients received 30 to 35 hours of CI, and this massed practice appeared to produce better results than more conventionally scheduled therapy (Pulvermüller, Neininger, Elbert et al., 2001). At the time of this publication, the Department of Veterans Affairs in the United States was recruiting participants for a clinical trial to be conducted in Houston, comparing constraint induced language therapy (CILT) to a traditional multimodal communicative treatment (U.S. National Institutes of Health, n.d.).

Studies Showing No Effect

Two group studies indicated that treatment has little effect. A study by Sarno, Silverman, and Sands (1970) has been trotted out in support of opinions that aphasia therapy is of little value. Their comparison of treated and untreated groups consisted of patients who were severely impaired at 27 to 41 months postonset. Therefore, the study was restricted to a particular group with a poor prognosis and to a period after stroke when treatment is not usually provided.

Another study stirred some controversy. Lincoln and her colleagues (1984) tried to randomly assign patients to treated and untreated groups. The treated group was to receive two hours of therapy per week for 24 weeks for a total of 48 hours of treatment. There was no difference between groups at the end of the study period, over eight months postonset.

Several SLPs published a letter in *Asha* magazine expressing serious reservations about Lincoln's study (Wertz, Deal, Holland et al., 1986). For example, there were no criteria to ensure that patients had aphasia. There was no evidence that subject assignment produced matched groups, a possibility weakened by 134 dropouts over four weeks before the study began. After the study began, about 74 percent of the treated subjects dropped out at some point. The two hours of therapy per week were considered to be "minimal" for most clinics, and only a few patients actually received the full 48 hours of therapy. The letter from the SLPs sug-

gested Lincoln's study proved that "when one does not treat patients who may or may not be aphasic, those patients do not improve" (p. 31).

Robey's Meta-Analysis

At the University of Virginia, Randall Robey (1998) has analyzed studies of efficacy with a technique called meta-analysis. It is "a mathematical means for synthesizing independent research findings scattered throughout a body of literature" (p. 173). In a tutorial, Robey and Dalebout (1998) advised that "science requires converging evidence from all independent experiments as the basis for a compelling conclusion" (p. 1227). They suggested that "thoughtful reviews of salient literature" are insufficient for this purpose. A meta-analysis of independent experiments determines the *weight of scientific evidence* bearing on a research hypothesis.

Robey's first report dealt with 21 studies and addressed general questions about efficacy. The study showed that recovery of treated patients was nearly twice the recovery of untreated patients when treatment was begun during the acute period. There was a smaller effect favoring treated patients when treatment was started after the acute period. The requirements of meta-analysis dictated that more studies had to be found to address more specific questions about amount and type of treatment.

A later analysis included 55 studies, and Robey (1998) replicated the results of the smaller study. Focusing on amount of treatment, the strongest effects occurred for moderate amounts started in the acute or postacute periods (i.e., 2–3 hours/week) in comparison to low (i.e., less than 1.5 hours/week) and high amounts (i.e., more than 5 hours/week). In an attempt to compare types of treatment, Robey noted that the most frequently reported type was "not specified," and most specified types were not studied often enough to meet statistical requirements for comparison. Regarding severity of aphasia, it was especially telling that no study examined mild aphasia explicitly. Severe and moderate aphasia had strong treatment effects in the acute stage.

Limitations of Group Efficacy Research

Robey (1998) concluded that the group investigations substantiate the value of standard treatments for aphasic people in general. Few studies have been replicated and, "as a result, many outcomes are singular observations and practically independent of all others" (p. 183). For more specific information, the research has shown mainly that intensive individual treatment does not differ greatly from intensive group treatment (Wertz et al., 1981) and that two similar language treatments administered by an SLP are equally effective with respect to clinical tests of language ability (Shewan and Kertesz, 1984).

Group studies have high hurdles to overcome. The main challenge lies in establishing a no-treatment control group that is comparable to a treated group. Self-selected groups (i.e., according to patient choice, not random assignment) run the risk that "the characteristics causing a subject to be assigned to a no-treatment group may also affect how they perform on the measures used to assess the effects of treatment" (Brookshire, 1994, p. 7). In addition, the treatments studied may not be typical of current clinical practice. Robey (1998) was concerned about the failure to report information. For example, "an ambiguous or absent description of a treatment protocol under test is a troubling matter" (p. 183).

Robey concluded that the basic issue regarding treatment efficacy has been settled and that resources should now be directed toward answering more specific questions. He suggested that future studies establish a criterion for meaningful or beneficial change. Clinicians have turned to single-case experimental designs as one means of answering the more specific questions (see Chapter 9), and a meta-analysis indicated that treatment effects were large in the studies reviewed (Robey, Schultz, Crawford, and Sinner, 1999).

Evidence-Based Practice

The efficacy research contributes to our ability to realize an evidence-based practice (Cornett, 2001), a concept borrowed from the relatively new move-

ment toward establishing evidence-based medicine (EBM). An evidence-based clinical practice is one that applies research data to clinical decision making, whether it is diagnosis or treatment. For example, Ross and Wertz (2004) invoked this concept as a rationale for using tests to differentiate mild aphasia from the normal effects of aging. The additional goal is to choose treatments for which there is good scientific evidence of their effectiveness. Some of this evidence comes from specific treatment studies, such as those reported earlier for naming therapies or others reported in Chapter 9. Chapter 10 cites efforts by the American Speech-Language-Hearing Association to assist SLPs in this regard.

MEDICAL TREATMENTS

A caregiver may say to an SLP, "I heard that there are drugs that can cure aphasia." SLPs have been interested in the possibility that **pharmacotherapy** can directly affect the brain's language functions (e.g., Helm-Estabrooks and Albert, 2004). There have been some useful analyses and reviews of the literature (e.g., Shisler, Baylis, and Frank, 2000).

Steven Small (1994, 2002, 2004) of the University of Chicago has made some valuable contributions toward our understanding of medications and their potential impact on aphasia recovery. One area of investigation is the use of medicines for enhancing the production neurotransmitters. These drugs include *bromocriptine* (a dopamine agonist) and *piracetam* (cholinergic facilitation). Favorable results with respect to language improvement appear to have been mainly with those who had nonfluent aphasia (e.g., Gold, VanDam, and Silliman, 2000). Also, the intravenous administration of *phenylephrine,* which elevates blood pressure, led to improvement of language functions (Hillis, Kane, Tuffiash et al., 2001). This improvement was associated with reperfusion of intact cortical regions.

Small has identified drugs to avoid in aphasia rehabilitation (also, Goldstein, 1998). These drugs include *diazepam,* which can cause anxiety, *haloperidol,* which can cause psychosis, and *phenobarbital* which can cause seizures. He warned that it is important "to insure the appropriate neuro-biological substrate for this [behavioral] treatment (or, more concretely, to insure that this substrate is not pharmacologically inhibited from responding to the therapy)" (Small, 2002, p. 407).

Some publicity has been given to repetitive *transcranial magnetic stimulation* (rTMS) as a treatment for depression and other psychiatric problems. A handheld coil (or wand) generates magnetic field impulses, which stimulate nerve cells in targeted cortex. It is thought to have potential for reorganizing brain functions. Based on functional imaging of increased or high activation levels in the right hemispheres of patients with nonfluent aphasia, Naeser and her colleagues (2005) explored the potential of rTMS for four cases with nonfluent aphasia ranging 5 to 11 years poststroke. After 10 days of application over the right homologue of Broca's area, these patients improved in picture naming. Naeser recommended further investigation.

HEALTH CARE TOPICS

The health care system in the United States is driven by the desire to provide maximum benefit at minimal cost. Health care professions have provided input to this system with information about the amount and type of services needed to achieve maximum benefits.

Reimbursement

Managed care has transformed reimbursement for medical and rehabilitative services in the United States. We have become familiar with the **health maintenance organization** (HMO), which is a private insurance plan that contracts with a medical group or groups to provide a full range of health care services to enrollees who pay a fixed monthly fee. A medical group tends to be a **preferred provider organization** (PPO), which is a network of health professionals approved by an HMO to provide services to plan members at a discount. One early development was the use of *diagnosis-related groups* (DRGs) as a basis for reimbursement. DRGs are a classification of hospital inpatients with implications for likely utilization of resources. Table 8.10 presents some basic terminology regarding reimbursement.

Medicare is an insurance program provided by the United States government for persons over age 65. The program consists of two parts.

- **Part A** provides necessary inpatient medical services within the first 90 days in a hospital and the first 100 days in a skilled nursing facility (SNF). Now a hospital receives a single payment per patient.
- **Part B** pays for subsequent physician-prescribed services in a hospital, clinic, or at home. A clinician submits a short certification form to the physician, noting planned visits per week and an anticipated maximum duration of treatment. Certification also requires a brief statement of short-term goals that are within a patient's immediate grasp and long-term goals for the duration requested.

The Balanced Budget Act of 1997 changed Medicare reimbursement dramatically. For Part B, the significant change was the introduction of an annual $1,500 cap on services per patient. One

TABLE 8.10 Terminology for reimbursement in managed care.

TERM	DEFINITION
Co-payment	Additional fee for a service paid by insurance plan members
Prospective payment system (PPS)	Payment determined before provision of services, rather than the former *retrospective payment* following services
Fee-for-service	Payment for each service provided (discouraged in managed care)
Capitation (CAP)	Payment per person; fixed monthly payment for all medical care of an individual (encouraged in managed care)

cap is to be shared by speech-language pathology and physical therapy, while occupational therapy has its own cap. The cap applies to inpatient rehabilitation, rehabilitation centers, and home health agencies. It does not apply to outpatient clinics in hospitals. The cap does increase with inflation, and the latest figure was $1,740. Pressure from rehabilitation interests led Congress to suspend the cap for a period of time. However, it was reinstated in January 2006, accompanied by automatic and manual categories of exceptions to the cap. Exceptions are automatic for certain conditions, including swallowing evaluations. Manual exceptions require a formal request supported by documentation. Staying abreast of legislative developments can be done by checking the website for the American Speech-Language-Hearing Association (www.asha.org).

Medicare has instituted an **Inpatient Rehabilitation Facility Prospective Payment System** (IRF PPS), which can be found at the website of the Centers for Medicare & Medicaid Services (www.cms.hhs.gov/providers/irfpps). The IRF PPS utilizes information from a patient assessment instrument (IRF PAI), which relies mainly on the FIM (see Chapter 6).

Frymark and Mullen (2005) studied the influence of the IRF PPS on speech-language pathology services. They obtained outcomes data reflecting a period before and after implementation of the payment system at several rehabilitation units and hospitals. There was a decline in speech- and language-related lengths of stay, and SLPs attempted to compensate by increasing their services. Despite these efforts, fewer patients achieved multiple levels of functional progress than they did before the payment system was implemented. Furthermore, the FIM demonstrated less progress than a national outcome system developed by ASHA. Frymark and Mullen concluded that the PPS presents a challenge for SLPs in providing quality care.

At a community hospital in Madison, Wisconsin with an inpatient rehabilitation program, sources of reimbursement were Medicare (58 percent), Medicaid (4 percent), HMO/PPO (23 percent), and fee for service (15 percent) (Odell, Wollack, and Flynn, 2005).

Medical Records

In 1996 the U.S. Congress enacted the **Health Insurance Portability and Accountability Act** (HIPAA; pronounced "hippa") to standardize the electronic exchange of all health care data. In April of 2003, the Secretary of Health and Human Services authorized the "Privacy Rules" aimed at safeguarding the confidentiality of an individual's health information. These rules are intended to prevent someone from using or disclosing personally identifiable health information without the patient's consent. The rules also protect participants in research, and Horner and Wheeler (2005) published an article in *The ASHA Leader* explaining how the rules apply to research practices.

Quality of Care

The health care system has several mechanisms for providing **quality improvement.** Quality is evaluated with respect to standards developed by each health care profession. One standard is the **care path** or **critical pathway,** which is a hierarchy of steps or protocols for rehabilitation of each disorder (Cornett, 2001). Care paths guide decisions about diagnostic and treatment services for each patient, and each decision is documented in a patient's records. This documentation is one basis on which a *utilization review* can evaluate the appropriateness of services at a health care facility (see Table 8.11).

A hospital has a critical path for stroke with hemiplegia. Speech-language evaluation should be on this path. When it is not on the critical path, SLPs would advocate for its inclusion. The following care path, without a decision hierachy, outlines basic stages in speech-language services for someone with aphasia:

- receive referral or consultation from a physician
- review medical chart
- evaluate patient at bedside

TABLE 8.11 Accreditation agencies.

LEVEL	AGENCY	MISSION	WEBSITE
Hospitals and other facilities	Joint Commission on Accreditation of Healthcare Organizations ("Jayco")	Improves safety and quality of health care through accreditation and related services; founded 1951	www.jcaho.org
Rehabilitation facility	Commission on Accreditation of Rehabilitation Facilities (CARF)	Provides accreditation for a variety of human services; founded 1966	www.carf.org
Speech-language pathology	American Speech-Language-Hearing Association (ASHA)	Quality indicators program (replaced Professional Services Board); since 1959	www.asha.org
Neurogenic disorders	Academy of Neurologic Communication Disorders & Sciences (ANCDS)	Promotes quality service by developing guidelines for training practitioners and standards for clinical practice; founded 1983	www.ancds.org

- report results of evaluation to physician (in medical chart)
- administer standardized language evaluation in clinic
- report results of evaluation and recommendation for treatment
- document treatment goals and plan
- administer treatment
- document progress relative to goals

Ethical Practice

The Code of Ethics of the American Speech-Language-Hearing Association addresses the following:

- providing services with the appropriate clinical certifications
- maintaining adequate records of professional services
- engaging in any form of dishonest practice or misrepresentation of services or outcomes

Minimal documentation includes the basis for diagnosis and ongoing records of treatment objectives, procedures, and measures of progress. Possible misrepresentation includes diagnosis of a nonaphasic cognitive impairment as aphasia, prediction of recovery for a patient with progres-sive disease, and documentation of progress when there has been no progress.

Beauchamp and Childress (1994) help us iden-tify fundamental ethical issues, based on a construct developed in the 1970s by a national commission for the protection of human subjects (also, Strand, 1995). Conflicts can arise between three legitimate considerations identified in Table 8.12. Regarding patients' autonomy, patients have "a common law right to choose what care they will or will not ac-cept" (Mariner, 1994, p. 43). A corollary to the clini-cian's beneficence or desire to "do good" is the need to prevent harm, called *nonmaleficence*. Third, there is society's need for justice or fairness in distribution of services given limited resources. Conflicts can be minimized by conducting a clinical practice with in-tegrity and by following ASLHA's code of ethics.

NOTES FROM THE CLINIC

Clinical objectives and decisions change as a func-tion of time poststroke. Acute therapy differs from therapy in the chronic phase. Fundamentally, we should think of treatment as evolving across the phases of recovery, which coincide with changes in setting, physical health, and attitude. Of course, the primary determiner of the treatment itself is the patient's impairments, needs, and wishes.

TABLE 8.12 Framework for discussing ethical issues and conflicts.

COMPONENT	DEFINITION	POTENTIAL CONFLICT
Patient's autonomy	Or "respect for persons"; the right of an individual for self-determination	*Patient vs. clinician:* a patient does not want therapy that a clinician thinks is needed
Professional's beneficence	The desire to contribute to another person's welfare and protect another from harm	*Clinician vs. patient:* a clinician prescribes a communication board that a family member refuses to acknowledge
Social justice	Fairness in distribution of services given limited resources (third-party considerations)	*Clinician vs. third party:* a speech-language pathologist prescribes care that a third party is unwilling to pay for
		Third party vs. clinician: a third party pays for services that are inappropriate or unnecessary

Acute Stage

As stated in Chapter 2, acute care is aimed at survival, ensuring that a patient can leave the hospital. For an ischemic stroke, the hospital stay averages around four days. In this time the SLP can do little more than evaluate the patient for swallowing and reassure the patient and family that rehabilitation for speech and language difficulties is available. The patient is usually changing rapidly in the first few days for the reasons cited in Chapter 2. If the patient is still in the Stroke Unit after four or five days, the SLP may conduct a bedside evaluation and counsel the patient and family regarding communicative strategies.

Martin had several factors going for him. He had suffered a focal infarction with some immediate spontaneous recovery. He was relatively young at age 55 and in good health besides his stroke. He was oriented to his surroundings and quite aware of his deficits. He was highly motivated and had a supportive family willing to participate in treatment.

Subacute Stage

Once a patient is admitted to a subacute rehabilitation unit or hospital, an SLP is likely to be required to evaluate swallowing within 24 hours of the doctor's order and evaluate speech and language within

72 hours. Initial daily contact notes may look something like Figure 8.2 for Enry Iggins.

Holland and Fridriksson (2001) had some suggestions for aphasia management during the early phases, which they identified as up to two to four weeks poststroke. This takes a patient through most of the subacute stage as defined here. They recommended conversational therapy (encouraging patients to talk) and counseling the patient and family regarding communicative strategies. This counseling includes providing information about aphasia and clarifying the rehabilitation process. Patients and families need to know that their perceptions and feelings are understandable and common. An SLP is also likely to introduce formal treatment activities of the type described in this and subsequent chapters. The extent of this work depends on the patient's health and motivation.

Hospitals may bill third-party payers by units of patient contact, with one unit equaling 15 minutes. Hospitals may set a goal of 22 units per day, which is considered 70 percent productivity.

Opinions have differed regarding the best time to begin individualized treatment. Wepman (1972) worried about adverse psychological reaction to intensive therapy during the acute (and subacute) period and recommended delaying language treatment until the chronic aphasic impairment becomes evident. He argued that a clinician

Short-term Goals:	Short-term Goal Summary:
Date: 3/3/03	
(1) Pt will participate in SP/L and swallowing evals	(1) Evals completed
(2) Pt will increase verbal response	(2) Object naming improved 20 to 80%
	(3) Starting to initiate conversation in PT & OT
Reviewed with patient/family:	Signature: Albyn Davis
☐ Yes ☐ No	Date: 3/7/03

Signature: Albyn Davis   Treatment Time: 3:15 – 3:45   Date: 3/3/03

Comments:

Pt able to chew solids and swallow liquids. Lang comprehension is adequate for conversation. Delayed speech initiation. Utterances very short with word-finding difficulties.

Signature: Albyn Davis   Treatment Time: 3:00 – 3:30   Date: 3/4/03

Comments:

Practiced naming family members, the Patriots football team, and talking about objects in the room. Better spirits than yesterday.

FIGURE 8.2 An example of daily patient contact notes, soon after admission to a rehabilitation unit.

should provide only a supportive psychological role during the emotionally delicate acute phase. Eisenson (1984) insisted that language therapy begin "as soon as the patient is able to take notice of what is going on and is able to cooperate in the effort" (p. 180). A neurologist agreed and wrote, "I believe that the therapy should be as intensive as the general medical situation will allow" (Rubens, 1977b, p. 1).

Some research addresses the question of whether starting time makes a difference in the efficacy of treatment. We know that a patient often makes much greater progress during the first two or three months than the next three months. An argument can be made that treatment is most effective while the brain is adjusting during the period of spontaneous recovery. In Robey's (1998) meta-analysis of 55 studies, treatment was found to be effective when started in the acute period (i.e., under 3 months postonset), postacute period (i.e., 3–12 months), and chronic period (i.e., 12 months or later). The magnitude of effect decreased over time, leading Robey to conclude that "aphasic individuals should receive treatment as early in their recoveries as is possible" (p. 181).

Because Martin had a variety of interests, his subacute treatment was designed to improve all modalities. The clinician worked on auditory comprehension and verbal expression to enhance his independence in conversation. Reading and writing were also targeted because of Martin's vocational interests in these skills. He also enjoyed reading and writing. The following goals were established, based partly on initial test performance (see Figure 3.5):

- *improve paragraph comprehension from 5/12 to 10/12*
- *increase number of words and phrase length in conversation about family and work*
- *improve sentence-level reading*
- *increase written naming from 2/10 to 7/10*

Treatment was established to be consistent with objectives but also to be conducted at a level that was likely to be successful. The clinician also considered semantic content that would be functional and interesting. Martin's wife extended two of the exercises by administering tasks at home. The initial lesson plan is shown in Table 8.13.

Chronic Phase

Entering the chronic phase of living with residual language impairment raises the following question: What happens when formal or professional treatment is over? Is aphasia treatment still available?

The answer varies depending on a patient's financial resources and type of residence. Living at home has different implications from assisted living or a nursing home where some speech and language services may still be accessible. Functional considerations in Chapter 10 become especially pertinent for the long haul. Rehabilitation hospitals may provide weekly support groups, as well as outpatient services. Volunteer-based support groups may provide a variety of communicative activities. Some aphasic individuals may become involved in training graduate students at university clinics. It is especially important that subacute management move toward preparation for life with aphasia (Lyon, 1998).

TABLE 8.13 Martin Exeter's first treatment plan.

BEHAVIORAL GOAL	TREATMENT PROCEDURE	GENERALIZATION PROBE
Improve discourse comprehension from 5/12 to 10/12	Clinician reads aloud short paragraphs from newspapers, and Martin answers questions about them; homework includes newspaper reading with Jackie	BDAE paragragph comprehension task
Increase number of words and phrase-length in conversation	Speed-naming drill; repetition drill for phrases of increasing length	Word counts and phrase-length measure from regular conversations
Improve sentence-level reading	Clinician types sentences for verification about family and current events	Clinical sentence reading test
Increase written naming from 2/10 to 7/10	Writes names of family members from photos; phonemic cues provided initially; homework includes spelling correction and sentence completion	Written naming of common objects

SUMMARY AND CONCLUSIONS

Treatment for aphasic impairment begins with an assessment to determine a patient's language problems and areas in which stimulation may address these problems. An impairment is translated into a goal. For example, if a patient is impaired in word finding, then a goal is to improve word finding. A behavioral version of this goal would be to increase number of accurate spoken naming responses to pictured objects (keeping in mind that other tasks can be used to exercise word finding). During assessment, a clinician may learn that word finding can be stimulated with a cue or by imitation. This is where treatment of word finding might begin.

Tasks are chosen to stimulate the impaired process at a high level of response accuracy. A somewhat different task may be chosen to measure whether a general objective is being met and especially for measuring generalization from the treatment. For example, treatment may be a naming task in which stimuli are supplemented with various cues and fast responses are reinforced. The measurement may be a simple naming task without cues and feedback to see if the patient is improving in naming without therapeutic assistance. In general, a treatment should be open to flexible reaction to a patient's success and demeanor, whereas a generalization probe is inflexibly controlled to be reliable.

Meta-analyses of the studies of treatment efficacy indicate that there is sufficient investigation for us to conclude that language treatment makes a difference for aphasic patients. One warning is that the treatments examined in large group studies have been atypical with respect to the managed care environment in which patients receive less treatment than the subjects received in these investigations. One positive finding is that treatment can help aphasic individuals beyond 6 months postonset and even beyond the first year. There is very little solid empirical support for the occasionally stated opinion that language treatment cannot make a difference for someone with aphasia.

Managed care has put limits on the amount of treatment. Currently we have no evidence to suggest that less treatment is less effective. Moreover, managed care has not forced a change in the fundamental principles that SLPs follow in administering language treatment. Current therapy may actually be different from many of the formally studied therapies, partly because current therapy may be more functional.

MATCHING REVIEW

Match the treatment contribution on the right with the name on the left.

____ 1. David Howard   a. originated stimulation therapy in the U.S.

____ 2. Wertz and many others   b. success principle

____ 3. Steven Small   c. reviewer of naming therapy research

____ 4. Robert Brookshire   d. semantic feature analysis (SFA)

____ 5. Richard Katz   e. compared phonological and semantic therapies

____ 6. Hildred Schuell   f. computer-assisted treatment

____ 7. Randall Robey   g. analysis of pharmacotherapy

____ 8. Boyle and Coelho   h. the VA cooperative studies

____ 9. Basso and Vignolo   i. the largest efficacy study

____10. Lyndsey Nickels   j. meta-analyses of treatment effectiveness

CHAPTER 9

TARGETING SPECIFIC DISORDERS

This chapter presents refinements of treatment for impairments. Many of the procedures are experimental in that they were provided in controlled conditions (e.g., without other therapies). Rather than thinking of therapy as being for aphasia in general, we will be thinking about therapy for specific symptoms or for diagnoses of specific cognitive impairments.

STUDYING INDIVIDUAL CASES

The efficacy of aphasia treatment may be scouted in studies of individual cases. In the clinic, a speech-language pathologist's (SLP's) minimal obligation is to measure and document a patient's progress during a period of treatment. Proving the cause of a patient's progress, on the other hand, requires a control of variables that is difficult to achieve in the usual clinical circumstance. About all a clinician can do is interpret progress occurring after six months as caused by something other than spontaneous recovery, but attributing this progress to treatment is still not a sure thing.

Single-case or **single-participant experimental designs** provide clinical investigators with a means of controlling variables in order to determine cause–effect relationships. Unlike group studies of efficacy, single-case studies enable a researcher to explore nuances of specific treatment procedures. Although clinicians have been encouraged to employ these designs while providing treatment, an adequate study usually requires external funding to pay for the time involved. Nevertheless, a general knowledge of these designs should help an SLP be a better consumer of treatment products that are purported to be efficacious.

A single-case experiment differs from a **case study.** The former institutes control of variables, whereas the latter is primarily descriptive of a patient's history and treatment. A case study may include measures taken before and after a treatment; but, without controls, conclusions about the cause of any change must be considered to be without foundation.

Like any experiment, a single-subject design consists of two components:

- manipulation of an independent variable or treatment
- a measure of a dependent variable related to a goal of treatment

A patient is said to serve as his or her own control. That is, a comparison between the presence and absence of a treatment is performed with one patient, rather than one individual (or group) receiving treatment and another individual (or group) not receiving treatment.

The strategies of single-case experimentation have been detailed in several books (e.g., Barlow and Hersen, 1984; McReynolds and Kearns, 1983), tutorials (Kearns, 1986a, 2000; McReynolds and Thompson, 1986; Willmes, 1990, 1995), and critical reviews (e.g., Fukkink, 1996). The basic strategies are compressed in Table 9.1. Single-case and group designs have given us different perspectives. Group designs have viewed treatment over the first year postonset, but single-case designs have often been applied years following onset.

One type of experiment consists of alternating phases of no-treatment (i.e., baseline) and treatment. The minimal ABA design is common (e.g., "test-treat-test"). Mitchum and Berndt (2001)

TABLE 9.1   Summary of basic single-case experimental designs.

	DESIGN	NOTATION	DESCRIPTION
Single treatment effects	Pre–post treatment	ABA	Bordering a treatment (B) with extended baselines (A)
	Alternating phases	ABAB	Alternating periods of baseline (A) and a treatment (B)
	Multiple baseline	MB	A single treatment applied sequentially to different behaviors or settings; baselines for each behavior or setting are obtained throughout the study
Comparing treatments	Alternating treatments	ATD	Two treatments given within a single day; repeated in different orders for several days
	Crossover	BCBC	Alternating treatment periods (B & C phases); in different sequences for at least two participants (e.g., BCBC vs. CBCB)

suggested that the "components of a cognitive neuropsychological treatment study" consist of the baseline, the therapy, and an outcome measure. They claimed that the "post-therapy assessment is obtained to measure changes in performance that are attributable to the intervention" (p. 560). However, an ABA design with single pre- and posttreatment measures usually fails to control for other factors occurring during the treatment phase that could contribute to a change, no matter when the therapy is provided relative to onset of stroke. Mitchum and Berndt clarified their recommendation by noting that a pattern of success and failure related to the particular treatment could be evidence for change that can be attributed to the treatment. Improving control for establishing cause–effect relationships is the reason for using other designs.

A more complete ABAB design may not be in the best interest of a client, because the most demanding experiment requires that a patient's performance be "reversed" in the second A phase to nail down causation (i.e., a return to initial baseline level). "Careful consideration must be given to the consequences of reverting to baseline for the client and those who are responsible for his or her care" (Kazdin, 1982, p. 124).

In clinical aphasiology, the more frequent strategy is a multiple baseline design. A straightforward example is Thompson and Kearns's (1981) study of a cueing treatment for naming deficit for a patient with anomic aphasia. Figure 9.1 shows that the study was actually a series of ABA designs applied sequentially to four dependent variables. The dependent variables were four different lists of words elicited in naming tasks. Two lists were from one semantic category (i.e., A_1 and B_1), and the other two lists were from another semantic category (i.e., A_2 and B_2). The cueing treatment was applied to one list and then to the other three in succession. Upward trends occurred only when treatment was instituted, indicating that the treatment had an effect, based on the small likelihood that the timing of the changes could have been caused by something else.

When comparing treatments given to a single patient, one treatment must follow another. Both alternating treatment designs (ATD) and crossover

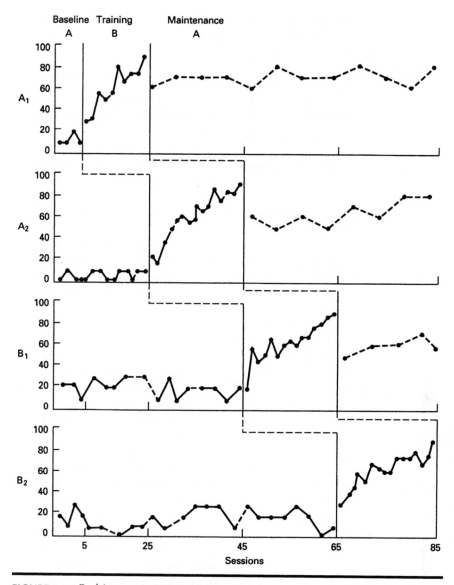

FIGURE 9.1 Probing an anomic patient's progress according to multiple baseline design. Clinicians obtained percent of naming across four sets of words during periods of baseline and treatment.

Reprinted by permission from Thomson, C, K., & Kearns, K. P., an experimental analysis of acquisition, generalization, and maintenance of naming behavior in a patient with anomia. In R. H. Brookshire (Ed.), *Clinical aphasiology conference proceedings*. Minneapolis: BRK, 1981, p. 39.

designs contain elements intended to control for sequence effects, namely, the effect that one treatment might have on another that follows.

The ATD is also known as the simultaneous-treatment or concurrent-schedule design. As in other designs, it begins with a baseline of the dependent variable. Then, the different treatments are administered on the same day (i.e., "simultaneous" treatments). Each day thereafter, the order of treatments is reversed, and the two daily sequences are randomly alternated across several days. Probes of the dependent variable are obtained for each treatment so that a graph of the treatment phase shows two sets of data (e.g., Avent et al., 1995).

Crossover designs have been commonly used in Europe to compare aphasia treatments (e.g., Springer et al., 1991). For one patient, one treatment phase (B) precedes another treatment phase (C). For another patient, the second treatment (C phase) precedes the first treatment (B phase). A study may stop at this point or continue by alternating phases. With this design, a second subject is necessary to balance sequence effects.

An important component of single-case research is that several data points should be collected across a phase, rather than simply "bordering" each phase with a pre- and posttreatment test. The goal is to determine the *trend* across a phase. A trend could be flat, upward, downward, or random variation. The problem with just two data points bordering a phase is that they could be derived from random variation and, thus, do not present conclusive evidence regarding how the patient was doing across the phase. The requirement of obtaining sufficient data points is one reason why single-case experiments are difficult to do when a clinician is strapped for time.

AGRAMMATIC PRODUCTION: EMPIRICAL TREATMENTS

Clinicians have experimented with several methods aimed at increasing the verbal productivity of patients with agrammatism. These methods can be classified according to the distinction between data-driven and theory-driven research introduced at the beginning of Chapter 4. Data-driven or empirically based therapies are derived mainly from observations of how aphasic persons respond to stimuli. Theory-driven therapies, introduced in Chapter 8 for naming, are a more recent development.

Sentence Production Program

Originally called the *Helm Elicited Language Program for Syntax Stimulation* (HELPSS) (Helm-Estabrooks, 1981), a revised version is now known as the *Sentence Production Program for Aphasia* (SPPA) (Helm-Estabrooks and Nicholas, 2000). The program is still intended to increase the syntactic variety and complexity of utterances. A few changes to HELPSS are that the number of sentence types were reduced from 11 to 8, a male gender bias was removed, and *wh*-questions were added. SPPA is generally recommended for agrammatic patients with good comprehension and a mean length of utterance of two to five words.

The procedure was modeled after a story-completion task used to elicit 14 syntactic forms in a study by Gleason, Goodglass, Green, Ackerman, and Hyde (1975). A hierarchy of structural difficulty was based on results of that study.

The story-completion format elicits sentences, and each story is accompanied by a picture. The program also consists of two broad levels for training each type of sentence. In Level A, the target phrase is included in the story so a patient can repeat it. In Level B, the patient is to complete the story with the target phrase. A response criterion of 90 percent accuracy determines movement up the sentence-type hierarchy within each level.

A couple of studies led Helm-Estabrooks and Albert (1991) to conclude that the efficacy of HELPSS has been demonstrated. These were mainly pre–post test studies showing progress in sentence production (Helm-Estabrooks, Fitzpatrick, and Barresi, 1981; Helm-Estabrooks and Ramsberger, 1986).

In early single-participant studies, HELPSS caused little stimulus or response generalization (Doyle and Goldstein, 1985; Salvatore, 1985). A similar procedure was applied successively to baselines for production of imperative transitives and intransitives (e.g., *Read a book, Stand up*), declarative transitives and intransitives (e.g., *He fixes cars, She dances*), and *wh*-interrogatives (e.g., *What is your name?*). This multiple baseline study indicated that the procedure can influence production of these sentences because of changes in each baseline that coincided with the sequential introduction of the treatment (Doyle, Goldstein, and Bourgeois, 1987).

Another study focused on measures of generalization with respect to therapies for improving sentence production (Fink, Schwartz, Rochon et al., 1995). HELPSS was administered to four nonfluent patients in three sessions per week, and each session ended with a storytelling task. The investigators examined the extent to which generalization occurred in circumstances differing from the treatment. One probe consisted of pictures and questions designed to elicit specific types of sentences. Generalization to this probe was observed, but generalization did not occur in a narrative production task.

Behavioral Treatment

In behavioral methods, sentences are elicited through modeling. One technique for lengthening utterances is called **forward chaining** in which a clinician "sequentially modeled the first two words of the target response then the remaining words of the target response, instructing the subject to repeat each portion as it was modeled" (Thompson and McReynolds, 1986, p. 198). **Reverse chaining** involves presenting all but the last word as a completion task and then eliciting an increasingly longer form by subtracting words from the carrier phrase toward the first word. In the 1980s, these methods were usually reported along with single-subject experimental designs to determine cause–effect relationships between a treatment and generalization probes.

For Kearns and Salmon's (1984) study of two cases of Broca's aphasia, the goal was to increase production of complete sentences containing the auxiliary *is* (e.g., *The boy is drinking*). Treatment consisted of imitative and spontaneous production tasks, and reinforcement was contingent upon complete sentence productions. Results for one subject are seen in Figure 9.2. Beginning with the baseline phase, probes were administered regularly to assess progress with trained and untrained auxiliary productions (upper graph). Generalization to production of a different type of sentence (lower graph) was measured with a probe of untrained copula production (e.g., *The man is a cowboy*).

Efficacy was studied with reversal of training as the second baseline phase (i.e., no training) followed by reinstatement of training. Reversal consisted of two parts. The first part was a kind of "counter-therapy." That is, agrammatic productions of previously untrained copula forms were reinforced, and the clinician ignored complete productions. In the second reversal phase, the same strategy was applied to trained auxiliary forms. After these two reversal phases, auxiliary training was resumed. The basic point was to determine if auxiliary production can be placed under a clinician's control.

The results are seen by following the trend of performance from phase to phase. Performance improved with both trained and untrained forms during the first training period, deteriorated during reversal phases, and improved again when auxiliary-*is* training was reinstated. Maintenance of progress was seen two and six weeks after termination of treatment. The treatment effect is indicated by the reversal and restoration of performance. Kearns and Salmon reported that generalization to spontaneous production was not achieved.

With four agrammatic subjects, Thompson and McReynolds (1986) compared a "direct-production" approach and an "auditory-visual" approach to training *wh*-question production (e.g., *What is he drinking?*). The former method was presumed to be a behavioral treatment, and the latter was thought to be characteristic of stimulation methods. The comparison of fundamental approaches hinged on use of single-stimulus presentation in direct-production/behavioral treatment and multimodal presentation in auditory-visual/ stimulation treatment.

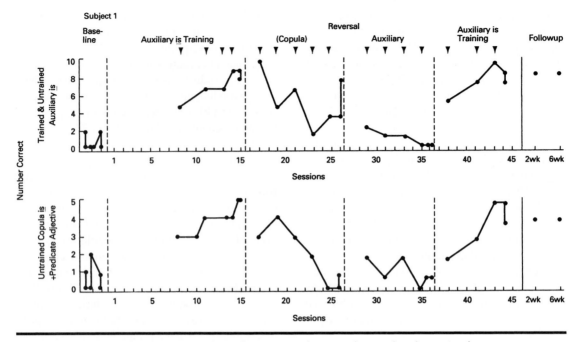

FIGURE 9.2   Results of continuous probes of correct production of trained and untrained auxiliary *is* (top) and untrained copula *is* (bottom) by one agrammatic subject. Arrows at the top mark sessions in which criterion was met for trained items. Improvement occurred for trained and untrained forms during the treatment phases.

Reprinted by permission from Kearns, K. P., & Salmon, S. J., An experimental analysis of auxiliary and copula verb generalization in aphasia. *Journal of Speech and Hearing Disorders,* 49, 1984, p.158. American Speech-Language-Hearing Association, publisher.

An alternating-treatments design was used to compare procedures. Procedures were alternated each day between morning and afternoon sessions. "To control for possible interaction effects of the two treatments, each treatment was applied to different interrogative constructions" (p. 197). The researchers found that direct production was more effective for acquisition of trained *wh*-questions, but the treatment did not generalize to untrained interrogative types.

Response Elaboration Training

Behavioral training of a few specific items was not causing generalization to untrained items. So, the clinicians decided to modify the treatment. One change was called **loose training,** which introduced flexibility in stimuli and in the response to be reinforced (e.g., Thompson and Byrne, 1984). One version is *Response Elaboration Training* (RET) developed by Kevin Kearns, who suggested that "overly structured treatment programs may actually inhibit patients from using language creatively and flexibly by severely limiting their response options" (Kearns, 2005, p. 136). He wanted to expand a patient's independence as a communicator by encouraging initiation of responses, which is often a concern in early or subacute rehabilitation. In the procedure, "the clinician shapes and elaborates spontaneously produced client utterances rather than targeting preselected response" (Kearns, 1985, p. 196). RET promotes generalization and is effective for conduction and anomic

TABLE 9.2   Steps of Response Elaboration Training (RET) for a picture of a man sweeping the floor.

RET STEPS	CLINICIAN'S STIMULUS	PATIENT'S RESPONSE	CLINICIAN'S FEEDBACK
(1) Elicit initial verbal response to picture	Line drawing of simple event (man with a broom) "Tell me what's happening in this picture."	"Man...sweeping."	
(2) Reinforce, model, and shape initial response			"Great. The man is sweeping."
(3) *Wh*-cue to elicit elaboration of initial response	"Why is he sweeping?"	"Wife...mad."	
(4) Reinforce, model, and shape the two patient responses combined			"Way to go! The man is sweeping the floor because his wife is mad."
(5) Second model and request repetition	"Try and say the whole thing after me. Say 'The man is sweeping the floor because his wife is mad'."	"Man...sweeping... wife...mad"	"Good job."
(6) After reinforcement, elicit a delayed imitation of the combined response	"Now, try to say it one more time."	"The man... sweeping because his wife... mad."	

aphasia as well (Yedor, Conlon, and Kearns, 1993).

Table 9.2 shows the steps for one stimulus item (Kearns and Scher, 1989; Kearns and Yedor, 1991). Kearns asked a patient to describe a simple event and then used modeling and shaping to encourage an expanded description. The model in step (2) is an expansion of a patient's initial response (i.e., "Man . . . sweeping"). In step (3), a *wh*-question stimulates production of additional information. In step (4), the clinician models a combination of the initial response and the subsequent response to the question. The patient practices elaborated imitations. The key is to avoid training a specific target response.

RET was introduced with a patient who had Broca's aphasia (Kearns, 1985, 1986b). Following a multiple baseline design, treatment was initiated for one set of 10 pictures and was delayed for another set. Probes for the untreated sets were taken on alternate days when treatment was not scheduled (Figure 9.3). Treatment of the first set was discontinued so it would not confound treatment of the second set. A treatment effect is observed in the upward trends of performance beginning with each treatment. The flat baselines indicate that repeated testing by itself had little effect. Some generalization occurred for a third set of pictures but did not occur for the second set before treatment was instituted. Whereas the patient had decreased in his verbal score on

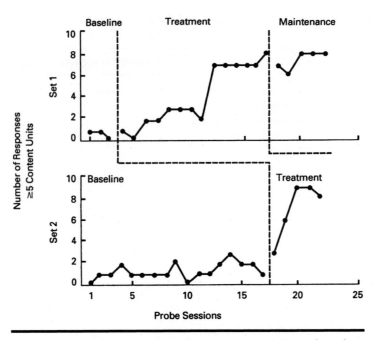

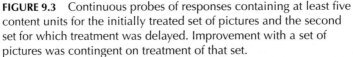

FIGURE 9.3 Continuous probes of responses containing at least five content units for the initially treated set of pictures and the second set for which treatment was delayed. Improvement with a set of pictures was contingent on treatment of that set.

Reprinted by permission from Kearns, K. P., Response elaboration training for patient initiated utterances. In R. H. Brookshire (Ed.), *Clinical aphasiology* (Vol. 15). Minneapolis: BRK, 1985, p. 199.

the PICA over the six months prior to this treatment, his score improved across this period of treatment.

More recent research has shown that RET helps to increase amount and variety of content in utterances and is useful for patients with moderate or severe apraxia of speech (Wambaugh and Martinez, 2000; Wambaugh, Martinez, and Alegre, 2001).

Verbs

Because many people with agrammatism are likely to have more difficulty producing verbs than nouns, some treatments have focused on this grammatical category. Perhaps, the first of these therapies was cueing-verb treatment or verbing

strategy (Loverso, Prescott, and Selinger, 1988). This treatment consisted of a hierarchy of tasks starting with producing an actor for a verb and culminating in producing a complete sentence when asked a question.

The centrality of verbs for sentence construction was introduced in Chapter 5 with respect to the predicate-argument information presumed to be contained in the lemma level of verb representation. Thus, it has been thought that if an agrammatic individual can retrieve verbs better, then more complete sentences should not be far behind. After all, agrammatic patients are relatively good at retrieving nouns. More recent approaches have minimized the requirement of sentence production in the therapy, emphasizing verbs and information related to them.

Fink and others (1997) employed a task centered around the verb to be used to complete a story. One example follows (p. 42):

Clinician: Someone *carried* the sofa. It was the mover. Did I say the mover *dropped* the sofa?

Patient: No, he *carried* the sofa.

Agrammatic patients improved across six sessions in the use of trained verbs and verbs that were simply "exposed" during probing.

Jane Marshall (1999a) presented the case EM for whom sentence and narrative production improved after a therapy consisting of a variety of verb-related tasks not requiring sentence production. These tasks included analyzing the semantic properties of verbs and generating a verb when given a noun. This patient may also have had some processing resources indicated by an ability to comprehend reversible sentences (also, Marshall, Pring, and Chiat, 1998).

There have been other reports of single cases receiving a verb-oriented treatment. Raymer and Ellsworth (2002) presented WR with phonological and semantic action-naming treatments. Naming of trained items improved, but there was no generalization to untrained verbs. Just stimulating action naming was associated with some generalization to sentence production. Webster, Morris, and Franklin (2005) had NS associate nouns with verbs and retrieve nouns that serve thematic roles around a verb. Again, there was poor generalization to untreated verbs, but sentences in telling the Cinderella story were much improved.

Schneider and Thompson (2003) studied seven cases with agrammatism using a relatively complex combination of crossover and multiple baseline experimental design. The crossover component accommodated a comparison between two treatments:

- *semantic verb retrieval treatment,* with extensive cueing of meaning for action naming
- *verb-argument structure retrieval treatment,* with extensive cueing of thematic roles in pictures for action naming

Schneider and Thompson obtained a familiar result of improved verb retrieval with both treatments, but little generalization to untrained verbs. Also familiar, sentence production improved even though sentence production was not stimulated directly.

Melodic Intonation Therapy (MIT)

Melodic Intonation Therapy (MIT) is based on the observation that nonfluent aphasic patients sing better than they talk. It is a carefully crafted program developed at the Boston VA Medical Center by Robert Sparks. The program has been reported in considerable detail and has been around for some time (Sparks, Helm, and Albert, 1974; Sparks and Holland, 1976). Candidates for the procedure are patients with good auditory comprehension and minimal improvement in speech production by more standard clinical procedures.

The essence of MIT is to have a patient sing an utterance. Several steps lead a patient into singing language, and then additional steps involve fading artificial melody from the production. Patients have been reported to proceed through the program successfully (Albert, Sparks, and Helm, 1973). Performance in MIT by severely nonfluent patients can be spectacular. However, reports have been elusive regarding response generalization to situations outside the context of the program. Recent results with the Persian language are more encouraging (Bonakdarpour, Eftekharzadeh, and Ashayeri, 2003).

AGRAMMATIC PRODUCTION: THEORY-DRIVEN TREATMENTS

In the 1990s, a few groups of clinical researchers began to report extensively on what they claimed are uniquely theory-driven or model-guided treatments. Actually, a theoretical basis for treatment is not entirely new; Schuell thought that therapy should be consistent with what we think aphasia is. Common therapies, based on the stimulation approach, follow the familiar assumption that aphasia is a disruption of processing, not a loss of linguistic knowledge.

Currently, investigators are capitalizing on more modern and detailed theoretical developments. Treatments are based on a diagnosis of impairment in the cognitive system or, for aphasia, in the psycholinguistic system. When applied to agrammatism, treatments are motivated by a theory of language production. A treatment might repair an impaired process or facilitate the establishment of an alternate route around the crippled process.

Externalization of Schemas

Luria (1970b) may have originated theory-motivated treatments of grammatical difficulties. He believed that agrammatic utterances are the result of difficulty with accessing structural representations. His "externalization of schemas" was intended to raise structural representation to a conscious level of awareness. He would present visual cues to grammatical categories in syntactic order, such as stick figures of agent, action, recipient. Sometimes three coins or buttons were all that was necessary. While pointing to each cue, patients magically produced a complete utterance. This cueing procedure became the basis for a more elaborate system (Davis, 1973). A patient would practice elicited sentences as the clinician gradually faded the cues.

More recent examples of cueing grammatical categories for sentence production were reported by Byng, Nickels, and Black (1994) who color coded nouns and verbs and by Walker-Batson and others (1999) who empoyed what they called a "visual retrieval language system." Patient MP, who had transcortical motor aphasia, was trained to tap in space with his left hand to facilitate sentence production. These movements were associated with colored squares on a table (Raymer, Rowland, Haley et al., 2002).

What about putting symbolic cues on a computer screen? In Philadelphia, Marcia Linebarger and her colleagues have been exploring the use of a computer to stimulate language production.

They refer to their program as the communication system (CS) or "a processing prosthesis." Speaking into a computer generates symbols on the computer screen for each word produced. The user sequences the symbols in an assembly area and then plays back the sentence. The playback provides positive and informative feedback rather than substituting for speech. Linebarger provided six agrammatic individuals with computers to take home for practice in constructing narratives. This activity was thought to help a patient access preserved linguistic knowledge, and a few individuals improved in their spontaneous spoken language production (Linebarger, McCall, and Berndt, 2004; Linebarger and Schwartz, 2005).

Diagnostic-Based Treatment

At the University of Maryland, Rita Berndt, Charlotte Mitchum, and Ann Haendiges set up a framework for refurbishing the theoretical influence on treatment of sentence production. They presented a treatment for EA, who had nonfluent aphasia and problems with phonetic aspects of speech (i.e., apraxia of speech). This case study represented a "a solution to the problem of where to focus treatment of the sentence production impairment in aphasia" (Mitchum, Haendiges, and Berndt, 1993, p. 71).

The Maryland team contrasted their approach to HELPSS which, they claimed, is "aimed exclusively at the level at which the sentence is spoken" (p. 71). They stated that the alternative is "to direct treatment at the earlier stages of the sentence production process . . . that presumably precede phonetic implementation" (p. 71). More specifically, Mitchum explored the possibility that EA was impaired in the positional level of Garrett's model of sentence production (see Figure 5.1). Yet, after extensive evaluation of EA, she concluded that she "cannot precisely identify the cause of his failure to construct an adequate sentence" (p. 85). Mitchum could conclude only that some sort of dysfunction exists prior to the selection of output modality (i.e., speech or writing).

The treatment for EA consisted of written naming of actions (i.e., verb production). The speech modality was not stimulated. Mitchum and her colleagues (1993) predicted that "If the impairments . . . affect processing components that are executed prior to the modality 'split,' . . . generalization across modalities should occur even if only one modality of output is practiced" (p. 76). They found that spoken sentence production improved following treatment of written sentence production.

Let us examine this study for a moment. The diagnosis of disorder at a level prior to the motor stage is equivalent to saying that the patient had a language disorder in addition to phonetic problems. The diagnosis had essentially the same specificity as identifying aphasia in contrast to apraxia of speech. Moreover, the cross-modal generalization achieved with the treatment is a common goal in treatments based on our understanding that aphasia is a central disorder underlying the modalities. This commentary should reassure experienced clinicians. The early theoretically motivated treatments might encourage them to reword their diagnostic base but not to change it.

Mapping Therapy

Another application of theory hinged on a more specific and controversial diagnosis. Could agrammatic production be caused by a mapping impairment? With respect to Garrett's model of production, impairment is thought to lie in the transition from the functional level of predicate-argument structure to the positional level of surface ordering and inflectional selection (Schwartz, Saffran, Fink et al., 1994). Mapping therapy is intended to repair this transitional operation.

Candidates for the procedure usually fit the following profile:

- agrammatic production (usually Broca's aphasia)
- "good" grammaticality judgment ability
- "poor" comprehension of reversible sentences, including more role reversal than lexical errors

These selection criteria indicate that identification of asyntactic comprehension is crucial for diagnosing the basis for expressive agrammatism. Moreover, the theory of mapping in comprehension contributes to the therapeutic approach (i.e., mapping thematic role interpretations onto intact structural representations).

Three research teams initially explored mapping therapy for improving sentence production (Byng et al., 1994; Marshall, Pring, and Chiat, 1993; Schwartz et al., 1994). Byng and Schwartz used the therapy to improve comprehension as well as production. Their slightly different techniques have certain fundamental common features:

- the goal of improving sentence production
- therapy tasks that do not require production (e.g., metalinguistic tasks)
- thematic role cueing similar to Luria's externalization of schemas

Similar to the semantic treatments of naming, mapping therapy is thought to stimulate a level of the sentence production process before production actually occurs. Thus, like the naming treatments, producing utterances is not a key feature of mapping therapy. Versions of this method are summarized in Table 9.3.

One difference among mapping methods is that Byng's group built a generalization stage into their therapy. This stage incorporated thematic cues to aid in the production of sentences during a PACE activity (for PACE, see Chapter 10). Other versions of mapping have not contained a generalization stage, indicating that clinicians hoped for a greater jump over the gap between the treatment and more functional sentence production.

Mapping therapy is similar to the emphasis of some verb-oriented treatments on awareness of thematic roles around a verb. Mapping therapy also emphasizes metalinguistic tasks that do not elicit utterances. In this sense, mapping therapy has been thought to tap into a mental process leading to sentence production.

Marshall and Cairns (2005) began talking about the previously reported mapping treatment of MM and verb treatment of EM as working on

TABLE 9.3 Summary of mapping therapies for improving sentence production.

INVESTIGATORS	LOCATION	TREATMENT STEPS	RESEARCH
Sally Byng Lyndsey Nickels Maria Black	Birkbeck College London	Patient sorts color coded phrases into sentence; patient describes same action (color cues); PACE therapy (color cues available)	Three cases improved in verb and sentence production
Jane Marshall Tim Pring	City Hospital London	Present simple actions on video; ask questions about agent, recipient, and action	Spontaneous production did not improve in case studied
Myrna Schwartz Eleanor Saffran Ruth Fink	Moss Rehabilitation Hospital Philadelphia	Present printed sentence; ask questions about agent, recipient, and action; patient underlines agent, recipient, and action (pens used as color cues)	Six subjects improved in comprehension and production

"thinking for speaking." This is another way of talking about working at the level of the conceptualized event or at Garrett's message level.

Movement Therapy

Cynthia Thompson and Lewis Shapiro explored a treatment modeled after a different type of theory, namely, linguistic theory of sentence structure (see Shapiro, 1997). The treatment strategy has been referred to as **linguistic specific treatment** (LST) (Thompson and Shapiro, 1994; Jacobs, 2001) or **treatment of underlying forms** (TUF) (Thompson, 2001; Thompson and Shapiro, 2005).

The clinical investigators studied the construct of *movement,* introduced in Chapter 5 (Thompson, Shapiro, Ballard et al., 1997). For example, a *wh*-question is said to be created from a declarative statement (e.g., *The woman followed the man*) by moving the direct object (e.g., *the man*) from its position after the verb to the front of the sentence (e.g., *Who did the woman follow?*). In linguistic terms, a *trace* is left behind in the position vacated by the moved noun phrase (NP), enabling us to identify *Who* as the direct object. Some type of movement characterizes most questions.

Thompson and Shapiro were interested in whether linguistic theory predicts generalization of treatment effects across baselines defined according to type of *wh*-question. Superficially, we might think that treatment of one type of *wh*-question could generalize to all other *wh*-questions. However, there are two types of movement with respect to *wh*-questions. One type of movement underlies *who* and *what* questions, and the other underlies questions beginning with *when* and *where.* Thompson and Shapiro found that treatment of *who* questions generalized to *what* questions but not to the other type of *wh*-question (Thompson, Shapiro, Tait et al., 1996). This was an instance in which a theory predicted a clinical outcome that would not necessarily have been predicted without knowledge of the theory.

Another theory-motivated feature of this research was the treatment itself. The treatment contained steps that modeled the linguistic notion of movement (although, we cannot be sure that movement is a mental process). Using cue cards with the printed words of a sentence, patients started by repeating and reading a simple sentence such as *The girl hit the boy* (akin to deep structure). The short-term goal was to help agrammatic patients produce *wh*-questions such as *Who did the girl hit?* In early steps, a patient was provided with additional cue cards including one with *who* at the end of the first sentence. Subsequent steps included moving the *wh*-cue to the beginning of the sentence. All moves led to a sequence of cues depicting the question.

Using multiple-baseline, single-case designs, Thompson's research team compared treatments of different kinds of movement. In two studies, separate treatment of *wh*-movement and NP-movement in passive sentences generalized to untreated sentences within the same movement structure. However, generalization did not extend to the other movement structure (Thompson et al., 1997; Ballard and Thompson, 1999). Similarly, object clefts and passives were trained separately with successful generalization within the structures, but generalization did not occur from one type of movement to another (Jacobs and Thompson, 2000). Thus, the different types of movement appear to possess their own processing characteristics, and we cannot expect that treatment of one type of movement will generalize to other types.

Telling the Cinderella story was used to measure generalization of these treatments to more natural narrative production, a feature of the studies that was emphasized by Jacobs (2001). Using Brookshire and Nicholas's Content Information Unit (CIU) analysis, described briefly in Chapter 6, the investigators showed that patients improved in informativeness and efficiency following various movement therapies. To enhance the social validity of these measures, naive listeners rated the narratives, but their higher ratings after treatment were not significantly different from pretreatment ratings.

Later, Thompson and others (2003) applied their complexity idea for naming treatment (Chapter 8) to the goal of improving sentence production with agrammatic aphasia. They called this strategy the *complexity account of treatment efficacy* (CATE). The treatment continued to be movement therapy or TUF, in which most steps of the activity could be easily performed. Multiple baselines followed production of complexity levels as they were not being treated and then after treatment was instituted. Results for two agrammatic participants showed that treating the complex structures first generalized to production of easier structures. However, for two other participants, treating the easiest structures first did not generalize to the more difficult structures; production of difficult structures began to improve only while being treated. The approach was also recommended for primary progressive aphasia (Thompson and Johnson, 2006).

ASYNTACTIC COMPREHENSION

Treatment of language comprehension for Broca's aphasia tends to start with sentences. General programs for sentence comprehension have consisted of manipulating length and basic structural characteristics to increase the difficulty of a task. A few clinical investigators have been evaluating treatments that may be appropriate for a cognitive impairment thought to cause asyntactic comprehension.

Externalization of Schemas

As with sentence production, Luria (1970b) attempted to improve sentence comprehension by increasing conscious awareness of syntax. Diagrams which "differ little from those used in common grammar texts" were shown in association with a spoken or printed sentence. The diagrams consisted of stick figures for actors, drawings of actions, and ideograms showing basic spatial relations. For example, *on* was represented as a ball on a plane, and *under* was represented as a ball beneath a plane.

The purpose was "to externalize the meaningful relationships implied by the constructions and compensate for the inner schemata which the patient lacks" (p. 443). Phrases like *mother's daughter* were split into parts so a patient could analyze structure. Two pictures represented the meaning of each word. A demonstrative was added for cueing the word serving as modifier (e.g., "*this* mother's daughter").

Mapping Therapy

The belief motivating mapping therapy was that asyntactic comprehension is caused by an impairment of the hypothesized mapping mechanism. Patients were assumed to have problems making conscious agent–object order decisions for reversible sentences. As indicated earlier, two research teams employed mapping therapy for improving both comprehension and production (Byng et al., 1994; Schwartz et al., 1994).

Byng (1988) found two patients who erred with reversible declarative (e.g., *The man kisses the woman*) and locative sentences (e.g., *The man is beside the woman*). She treated only locatives and measured comprehension of other types of sentences. In a treatment that was similar to Luria's externalization of schemas, comprehension was cued with a "meaning card" showing relations between noun phrases (NPs). Colors were also used to cue NP location in a sentence. One patient's progress in understanding locatives spread to untreated reversible sentence types, which Byng interpreted as repair of a mapping mechanism that contributes to comprehending all sentences.

The Maryland research team treated EA with another version of mapping therapy (Haendiges, Berndt, and Mitchum, 1996). This patient had a comprehension impairment considered to be more severe than the typical deficit in Broca's aphasia. Treatment consisted of practice with three auditory comprehension tasks. One consisted of sentence–picture verification. Another was a standard picture-choice task. In the third task, EA was instructed not to respond to the clinician's comparison of active and passive versions of one message. In all tasks, the clinician pointed out specific thematic components of a picture (i.e., agent and recipient). Because the patient's progress generalized to some untreated sentences but not others, Haendiges and her colleagues forthrightly concluded that mechanisms besides mapping were probably contributing to EA's impairment.

Comments on Theory-Driven Strategies

Most clinicians may agree with Schuell that an appropriate treatment is derived from an understanding of the nature of aphasia. The theoretical basis for stimulation treatment has been that aphasia is thought to be primarily an impairment of processing rather than a loss of linguistic knowledge. The main difference between current theory-driven treatments and the stimulation approach is that the current treatments are intended to address specific processes rather than a vague notion of processing in general.

Caramazza (1989) expressed misgivings. He suggested, "we need to ask ourselves whether we would have used a different therapeutic strategy had we had a different hypothesis about the functional lesion in the patient" (p. 395). He added that any hypothesis about the nature of deficit "is of limited use in specifying an informed therapeutic strategy because the content of our cognitive theories does not specify the modifications that a damaged system undergoes as a function of the different types of experiences with which a patient may be presented" (p. 393).

The clinical consumer of treatment ideas should ask the following questions:

• **Is the treatment really new, or is it a repackaging of an established approach?** For example, Mitchum and others' application of Garrett's production model did not carve out any new ground with respect to diagnosis or treatment. Clinicians may already be doing the theory-driven treatment. Only the rationale may be new. Thompson and Shapiro's linguistic approach led to some treatment procedures that had not been reported before.

• **Has the diagnostic basis for a treatment been validated in basic research?** Chapter 5 indicates that the diagnosis of a mapping disorder, at least, should be considered to be just one of several current explanations of agrammatism. Treatment studies might include comparisons between therapies that follow from alternative explanations of a symptom pattern (e.g., a parsing therapy vs. mapping therapy). Meanwhile, clinical investigators should do a better job of presenting their work in the context of alternative theories or explanations.

We may also be tempted to challenge theory-driven treatments regarding their efficacy. However, this would be a rather selective application of a common challenge. All treatments should be scrutinized for efficacy, and a harsh demand for efficacy in the early stages of a particular investigation risks inhibiting the discovery of new methods.

WERNICKE'S APHASIA

Wernicke's aphasia presents some unique problems for rehabilitation such as a poor "therapeutic set" (Sparks, 1978). With a lack of awareness of deficit, the patient does not appear to comprehend the reason for being in the clinic. Our expectations soon after onset should be uncertain, because some patients recover a great deal of language ability whereas others do not progress very much. Early progress in treatment may be an indication of likely overall progress.

Auditory Comprehension

Treatment of comprehension is the first step in dealing with this type of aphasia. People with frank Wernicke's aphasia are terrible repeaters; direct stimulation of production through modeling is generally unsuccessful. In a sense, we cannot enter treatment of formulation through the front door. Comprehension training doubles as a means of improving functional communication and as a means of setting up skills that can be used to gain control over expression.

The first goal is to establish a therapeutic set or, namely, consistent response to a clinician's stimulation. We may have to begin with simple modeling of a clinician pointing to a picture. The patient may be trained to point to a picture of an object in response to an environmental sound. When the patient gets the idea of listening and pointing, we begin to use words as stimuli with appropriate referents for response. Family names and photos may be used. Numbers may be readily recognized with response cards showing simple quantities. Once reliable responding is established, we sneak simple levels of word comprehension into the treatment.

Press for speech can interfere with auditory processing. We should direct attention to listening by inhibiting this tendency to talk excessively. Whitney suggested a "stop strategy" in contrast to a "go strategy" for Broca's aphasia (cited in Holland, 1977). The idea was to keep the person with Wernicke's aphasia from talking during comprehension training. An alerting signal such as a raised hand is often all that is needed to remind the patient to stop talking when the task is to listen. As comprehension improves, we look for improved recognition of jargon.

Clinicians should look out for the possibility that a patient with Wernicke's aphasia has retained some ability to comprehend single printed words. In fact, these are patients with the exceptional pattern of depression of auditory comprehension below their reading ability. Helm-Estabrooks and Albert (2004) considered this island of language clarity to be a starting point (also, Hough, 1993). Matching printed words to pictures is eventually accompanied by spoken word stimulation. Harding and Pound (1999) described their work with a 56-year-old postmaster with severe auditory comprehension impairment. They also treated semantics with pictures and printed words, including sorting tasks and picking out the word that did not belong in a series.

Mitchum and her colleagues (1995) provided mapping therapy for ML, a case who had moderate Wernicke's aphasia and who had been studied previously with other treatments. Auditory stimulation was about the same as the treatment given to EA, except that the active and passive sentence comparison was not included. Progress generalized to auditory sentences with untreated verbs and to reading sentences. Progress did not generalize to understanding longer sentences or to sentence production.

Jargon

Self-monitoring is considered to be important for getting control over unwieldy verbal expression. Jane Marshall and her colleagues in London studied four patients with a dissociation between comprehension and self-monitoring. That is, comprehension ability was good, but the patients still could not recognize their own jargon. The patients appeared to have an impairment of feedback processes (Marshall, Robson, Pring, and Chiat, 1998). Further evaluation showed that the patients could recognize neologisms when repeating words but not when naming, suggesting that the feedback problem arises when accessing semantics.

This semantically related problem led Marshall to try a semantic therapy program for naming. The treatment consisted of comprehension tasks involving associating printed words with pictures, and it was carried out for six sessions plus homework assignments. The investigators were disappointed that the patients made no progress in naming, but the patients improved in recognizing neologisms for treated items, though not for untreated items. In all, the treatment did not have a dramatic effect on the feedback mechanism.

We may have to see if repetition appears spontaneously during comprehension drills before trying intentional repetition to elicit meaningful speech. Exactly how this happens and how often it happens does not appear to have been studied systematically. Patients may get to the point where we can use standard methods of modeling, chaining, and so on. When volitional repetition begins, we can build a program for eliciting language. However, this may take months beyond the number of sessions allotted under managed care. Special funding may be needed to explore thoroughly the effects that language stimulation can have on jargonaphasia.

CONDUCTION APHASIA

Treatment studies of conduction aphasia are about as rare as studies of Wernicke's aphasia. The discovery that sentence comprehension problems are similar to those in Broca's aphasia indicates that comprehension training may be similar. In fact, tasks for making syntactic judgments and arranging words into sentences were embedded in a program to treat phonemic paraphasias (Cubelli, Foresti, and Consolini, 1988). Kearns' RET pro-

gram has also been helpful for people with conduction aphasia (Yedor et al., 1993). For targeting the definitive problems of conduction aphasia, investigators have focused on repetition or phonemic paraphasias.

Three studies were devoted to improving repetition. Reading aloud was the main activity used by Sullivan, Fisher, and Marshall (1986). During successful reading, the visual stimulus was removed so the utterance could be repeated without this cue. Peach (1987) wanted to improve sentence repetition by treating memory span. The patient started with a task of pointing to pictures in a sequence spoken by the clinician. Then, the patient was asked to repeat words in the order spoken. Repetition improved during the period of treatment. Kohn, Smith, and Arsenault (1990) concentrated on repetition as the treatment task. Usually, a level of good repetition can be established with short common sentences, and then complexity is gradually increased.

Other investigators focused on reducing phonemic paraphasias. Boyle (1989) employed a procedure in which the patient was instructed to look at a word and think about how it sounds and then read the word aloud. In Italy, Cubelli and others (1988) had clients confront phonemic–graphemic structure with a few metalinguistic tasks. In one task, the patient was shown a picture (e.g., table or *tavolo*) and cards containing each syllable of the word (e.g., *ta, vo, lo*). The patient was asked to arrange the syllables in correct order and then read the word aloud. In another task, the clinician displayed a picture (e.g., table) and a letter (e.g., E). The patient had to decide if the letter belonged to the word for the picture.

Later, Peach (1996) reported on a therapy for a patient who was initially diagnosed with Wernicke's aphasia and who then later took on some characteristics of conduction aphasia. The phonologically based procedure was centered on an oral reading task. The clinician's responses to error included having the patient write the word. If this did not improve spoken response, a phonemic error was paired with the correct sound in the beginning of another word to read. Repetition was another option for restimulation. A multiple-baseline design showed generalization to an untreated baseline rather than a sequential treatment effect on the baselines.

A patient diagnosed with reproduction conduction aphasia (see Table 5.5) received a treatment aimed at improving self-monitoring. The first phase of the treatment consisted of phoneme-discrimination tasks, and the second phase contained three levels of speech monitoring. First, the patient practiced recognizing the clinician's naming errors. Second, the patient's naming responses were played back with a tape recorder, and she had to make the same kind of judgments. The third level involved building sentences (Franklin, Buerk, and Howard, 2002).

Simmons-Mackie (2005) suggested that a variety of common clinical methods are appropriate for conduction aphasia.

ANOMIC OR MILD APHASIAS

Marshall (1987) suggested that we have paid less attention to the communicative needs of persons with mild aphasia. He advocated that we "reapportion treatment time so as to spend more hours with mildly impaired clients" (p. 70). With respect to the syndrome of anomic aphasia, the main linguistic goal is to improve word finding. Yet, good comprehension and circumlocutions frequently facilitate communicative conversation, so that functional goals may pertain mainly to the handicap caused by anomia. That is, language treatment may be motivated by social and vocational needs.

Linebaugh's (1983) *Lexical Focus* consisted of hierarchies of cueing for a convergent naming task and, for the mildest anomic aphasias, a divergent categorical word-fluency task. A hierarchy of difficulty for categories was based on "width" of exemplars in a category. That is, an easy category was *sports,* and a more challenging, narrow category was *water sports.*

Studies of cueing have had apparently contradictory results for anomic aphasia. Comparison of phonemic and semantic cues seems to depend on when cues are administered in a naming treat-

ment interaction. In prestimulation, phonemic cues were more powerful than semantic cues. For restimulation upon error, phonemic and semantic cues were about equally effective a small percentage of the time.

READING IMPAIRMENTS

Theory-driven treatments of reading are based on identifying an impaired component of the reading process (see Chapter 4). The process model and clinical analysis are centered around reading aloud or, namely, the processes leading from seeing a word to articulating a spoken response. Training may be directed at repairing the impaired component or compensating with an available alternative route. Pragmatically, we are minimally interested in *comprehension* or, namely, the activation of semantic memory upon seeing a word.

Phonological dyslexia has been diagnosed in patients with Broca's, anomic, conduction, and transcortical sensory aphasias. Key symptoms are a word superiority effect along with good word repetition, with a particular problem in reading aloud unfamiliar letter strings. Because pronunciation of unfamiliar letter strings depends on grapheme–phoneme conversion rules (see Figure 4.3), it is thought that a so-called *orthographic-phonological conversion* (OPC) mechanism is impaired.

Kendall, McNeil, and Small (1998) tried to repair the OPC for patient WT, a 42-year-old who had suffered a stroke 17 years prior to the treatment study. At the time of the study, WT had a mild nonfluent aphasia with good reading comprehension. The treatment consisted of "systematic exposure" to two conversion rules over six weeks. The rules were as follows:

- *c-rule:* when c comes before *a, o,* or *u,* it is produced as /k/; otherwise, as /s/
- *g-rule:* when g comes at the end of words or just before *a, o,* or *u,* it is produced as /g/; otherwise, as /dz/

As with most stimulation therapies for aphasia, the rules were not taught explicitly. WT practiced reading aloud words and nonwords embodying one of the rules (e.g., *cylecaber, girandole*). The clinician presented phonetic and morphological cues as restimulation upon error. Progress in treatment generalized to pronunciation of words involving other conversion rules.

Kendall's study was presented mainly to address a theoretical-clinical question rather than a functional-clinical question. We might ponder the circumstances in which an aphasic person may want or need OPC treatment when functional reading comprehension is pretty good. When does someone want to be good at reading aloud unfamiliar words? One possibility is that OPC may be important for a meticulous speller who writes letters and uses a computer.

Surface dyslexia has been found in patients with Broca's, anomic, and Wernicke's aphasias. The reading disorder differs from phonological dyslexia in that the OPC is intact. The patient pronounces nonwords and function words better than content words. With surface dyslexia, there is a strong regularity effect, and regularization errors are common (see Table 4.7). The disorder is thought to occur primarily in the graphemic lexicon or in access to it.

Several treatments have been reported for cases of closed head injury, a few with aphasia and at least one without aphasia (Weekes and Coltheart, 1996). Behrmann and Byng (1992) wanted to improve "use of the lexical procedure (via semantics) to access word-specific orthographic representations which are critical for irregular words" (p. 339). That is, the treatment was to repair the presumed impaired component rather than compensate with the alternative OPC route. For EE, who was traumatically injured due to a fall from a ladder, the treatment appeared to entail reading aloud irregular words such as *bough*. A picture (e.g., a tree) was used to help EE remember pronunciation.

Deep dyslexia has been diagnosed mainly in patients with Broca's aphasia. These patients produce many semantic paralexias when reading aloud and have a strong word-superiority effect that may be related to reading content words better than function words. Ambivalent diagnosis has been one problem with deep dyslexia, in that a disorder has been identified with OPC impairment (like phonological dyslexia) or with lexical-semantic mapping.

Marie Pierre de Partz (1986) studied a business executive who had progressed over three months after an initial diagnosis of Wernicke's aphasia (also, Bachy-Langedock and de Partz, 1989). In cognitive terms, her general goal was to repair the OPC process by using spared lexical knowledge as "a relay" between the written word and pronunciation. The treatment proceeded in three stages. First, the patient worked on associating a letter with a word and reading aloud single syllables. Then, he associated letter combinations with words. Finally, he practiced whole word reading that was focused on certain conversion rules much like Kendall's procedure for phonological dyslexia. de Partz reported that one stage was laborious, and the whole program appeared to take several months.

The relationship between diagnosis and treatment is not straightforward. Reviewers have noted that different approaches have been effective for one diagnosis, that a single approach has been effective for different diagnoses, and that a given treatment may be successful for some patients but not others with the same diagnosis. Recent reviews of reading and writing treatments include a short article by Hillis and Heidler (2005) and chapters by Beeson and Hillis (2001), Friedman (2002), and Webb (2005).

SUMMARY AND CONCLUSIONS

This chapter presented therapeutic approaches and techniques that address many of the specific symptoms and syndromes of aphasia and related language disorders. We continue to follow the fundamental principle of stimulating processes. In some instances, psycholinguistics and related cognitive sciences are being applied so treatments may be focused on more clearly defined processes. Many of the procedures are experimental and hopefully encourage an appreciation for the effort to improve rehabilitation through an understanding of language functions and an application of rigorous experimental controls.

The list of treatments for aphasia seems to be getting longer. One less daunting aspect of this situation is that familiar notions are being dressed up in new clothes. For example, we may hear the simple task of repeating words being referred to as "phonological rehearsal treatment." This relabeling may cause some communication problems between professionals, but it can also be interpreted as an attempt to connect our therapies to the scientific study of the processes we are treating. "Phonological rehearsal" provides a way of thinking about a task, but we are still more likely to write "repeated words" in daily progress notes.

MATCHING REVIEW_____

Match the treatment contribution on the right with the name on the left.
Some individuals will have more than one contribution.

_____ 1. Thompson & Shapiro   a. single-case experimental design

_____ 2. A. R. Luria   b. Sentence Production Program

_____ 3. Robert Sparks   c. RET

_____ 4. Byng, Nickels, & Black   d. MIT

_____ 5. Kevin Kearns   e. intersystemic reorganization

_____ 6. Nancy Helm-Estabrooks   f. mapping therapy

_____ 7. Marcia Linebarger   g. treatment of underlying forms

_____ 8. Marie Pierre de Partz   h. a processing prosthesis

      i. therapy for reading

      j. behavioral treatment

CHAPTER 10

FUNCTIONAL THERAPEUTICS

Repairing linguistic impairment may address communicative disability only partially. We employ several strategies to improve communication, and they generally stem from the following goals:

- maximize use of residual linguistic capacities
- develop augmentative or alternative modes of communication
- improve the role of partners and settings in facilitating communication
- maximize psychological and emotional adjustment to language impairment

As indicated in Chapter 6, the World Health Organization levels have pried the domain of aphasia rehabilitation wide open to encompass matters that stretch beyond communication, such as a person's quality of life (QoL). A group advocating social and life participation approaches to aphasia rehabilitation led the treatment presentation in the fourth edition of Chapey's (2001) text.

Some graduate students in speech-language pathology may be overwhelmed by the thought of fixing someone's quality of life. *Doesn't the social worker do that?* The SLP in the rehab hospital rushing from bedside to barium swallow may not have a patient's life participation in her plans. We may simply be recognizing the importance of language and communication to someone's QoL. However, this chapter will refer to the participation of some SLPs in unique life-affirming programs for people with aphasia.

PHILOSOPHY: THE CLINICAL–FUNCTIONAL GAP

Jeffrey Metter (1985), a neurologist, wrote a letter to *Asha* magazine in which he referred to a contra-diction between documentation of a patient's improvement in clinical tasks and his observation of no progress when conversing with the patient. The clinician observed acquisition, but Metter did not observe generalization. This distinction between clinical progress and functional progress has frustrated many clinicians. Long before managed care, we wanted to figure out ways to transfer progress in clinical tasks to a patient's daily life.

At least, researchers have wanted to see the progress in a treatment generalize to different materials used in the same activity. However, simple stimulus and response generalization has been limited with some of the treatments presented in Chapters 8 and 9. The study of naming therapy by Thompson and Kearns (1981) produced good news and bad news. The good news was that treatment had an effect on behavior. The bad news was that progress with a small list of words used in therapy was not transferring to very similar lists of words not being used in therapy. It seemed that the treatment used in the study would have to be applied to every word the patient might use in daily life.

One reason for Metter's observation may be extreme differences between the standard treatment setting and real life communicative situations. Clinical settings contain minimal distraction. Patients interact with supportive people who know what aphasia is. Repetitive drills are designed to undercut deficits and stimulate success. On the other hand, real life presents a rough road of communicative potholes for someone with language impairment. This difference might be called the "clinical–functional gap."

Looking across the gap, Busch (1993) recommended three broad functional goals that would be acceptable to Medicare:

- The patient will communicate basic physical needs and emotional status.
- The patient will engage in social communicative interactions with immediate family or friends.
- The patient will carry out communicative interactions in the community.

These goals are oriented to stimulus generalization. That is, we want to see a patient produce formally trained key phrases whenever a need arises. We want to see a patient produce behaviors in the presence of family that have been practiced with a clinician.

It has been said that clinicians would "train and hope" that clinical progress would transfer to a client's daily life (Thompson, 1989). Hope can be replaced by a bridge across the clinical–functional gap. In principle, the bridge can be built by **programming for generalization.** The steps are forged by changing stimulus conditions and response expectations in the direction of modeling real-life communicative problems. For this transition, we have used group therapies or have introduced tasks that seem important to a patient's daily life. However, Brookshire (1997) suggested that "many do not pursue generalization in a systematic way" (p. 235).

Closing the gap systematically is accomplished by bringing attributes of natural situations into the clinic and by moving the patient somewhat gradually into situations outside of the clinic. This approach has also been applied to rehabilitation for head injury: "For those who are making the transition to a home setting, guidelines establishing routines for spontaneous real-life situations should be developed and implemented prior to returning to independent living" (Starch and Falltrick, 1990, p. 28). In the words of Simmons-Mackie and Damico (1997), we make clinical conditions more "authentic."

Especially for severely impaired patients, it may be valuable to begin with standard direct procedures, focusing on a specific process in a situation free of anxiety and distraction. A patient may need to become comfortable with an awkward nonverbal strategy before trying it outside

the clinic. Later, the clinic can become more natural by encouraging the patient to deal with communicative failures.

In the previous edition of this text (Davis, 2000), the manipulation of contextual variables to bridge the gap was too metaphorical. This is a nice principle, but it sounds more like research than therapy in managed care. That said, treatment of aphasia still has a fundamental progression. We begin with a patient who is maximally dependent on the clinician for response (e.g., imitation), and we proceed in the direction of the patient's becoming independent of the clinician. Melodic Intonation Therapy is a good example of generalization programming. However, such programs have limited extension for helping a patient become maximally independent of the clinician. In real life, the clinician is not there.

Before this chapter turns to the severely impaired patient, it progresses along multiple dimensions. The setting changes from the hospital to community centers and residential settings. There is also a shift from dyadic clinical interactions to group activities. These topics are organized roughly according to the former WHO levels (Table 10.1). The literature contains recommendations that SLPs deemphasize the "medical model" and adopt a "social model" (e.g.,

TABLE 10.1 Chapter topics for functional therapeutics organized according to old WHO levels. This organization also proceeds from inpatient therapy in a rehabilitation hospital to community-based group activity.

IMPAIRMENT	FUNCTIONAL STIMULATION
Activity limitation (disability)	Compensatory behaviors Interactive therapies
Participation limitation (handicap)	Situation-specific therapies Group therapies Community reintegration Changing communities Creating communities

Simmons-Mackie, 2001; Worrall, 2000), but many SLPs still work in hospitals. An interesting problem is the extent to which an SLP in a rehabilitation hospital should and can address life participation, before the patient is actually participating again.

FUNCTIONAL STIMULATION

Our patients still want to improve the operation of impaired language processes. Maintaining this traditional objective, standard treatment exercises can be more functional than might have been indicated in the previous chapters. We may think of it as "functional repair."

Functional repair begins with the goal of maximizing the likelihood of stimulus and response generalization. That is, if a patient is failing to progress with stimuli and responses not specifically exercised in treatment, then no progress will be seen in Dr. Metter's office or at a patient's home. Brookshire's principle of aiming treatment at a process rather than a specific word or sentence is an essential first step in creating conditions that can achieve some degree of generalization. If word finding is genuinely improved, then the use of language should be better in a number of circumstances and with a wide variety of words.

In her review of generalization research, Thompson (1989) concluded that four features of treatment should maximize the possibility of transfer:

- a sufficient number of training responses
- a sufficient number of training conditions
- activities that incorporate aspects of the generalization environment
- strategies for mediating generalization

In the single-subject experiments that did not show much generalization, treatment tended to consist of drilling a small sample of language with one task.

Brookshire (1997) collapsed Thompson's suggestions under the notion of **training sufficient exemplars.** For one thing, this means training a wide variety of words within a semantic category. Instead of naming 5 foods, a patient practices naming 20 or 30 foods. It also means training a behavior in a variety of stimulus conditions; and, according to this principle, flexibility extends to participants in an interaction and in settings in a rehabilitation center. Behaviorally oriented clinicians began to present varied stimuli to elicit a particular response and accept varied responses to a particular stimulus as a strategy of "loose training" (see RET in Chapter 9).

Once we loosen our stimulation activities, we enhance functionality by molding semantic content according to a patient's world and interests. Standard or commercial materials are constructed to be familiar or appropriate for the greatest number of people. Their functionality stems from being objects and events that are common in the activities of daily living. Yet, content may also be selected to be personally relevant. What does the patient like to talk about? We can conduct "contextual inventories" to find out the unique content of a patient's life (Simmons-Mackie and Damico, 1996). Many clinicians view this ingredient as an example of applying common sense to therapy. It was given a name and an abbreviation, *Thematic Language Stimulation* (TLS) (Morganstein and Smith, 2001).

Personally relevant content is often chosen the first day of treatment. Wallace and Canter (1985) compared personal and nonpersonal content for severely aphasic persons. Personal content was defined as items pertaining to self and the immediate environment. The comparison was made for auditory comprehension (e.g., *Is your birthday in December?* vs. *Is Christmas in December?*), reading comprehension, repetition of nouns, and naming object drawings (e.g., *television* vs. *chicken*). The investigators found that personally relevant material was easier to understand than nonpersonal content. Freed, Celery, and Marshall (2004) asked patients to come up with their own semantic cues for naming common objects. For example, they asked a patient where he listens to the radio, and then the location became a cue.

Some of the cues were general (e.g., for washing dishes), but still chosen by the individual.

Our contextual inventories should also reveal activities that are common in a patient's daily life. Then, we may do a **functional analysis** of targeted situations (e.g., restaurant, airport, bridge club, sporting events). What are the basic language functions used in these situations? A situation may require some reading, some talking, or some writing. Rather than stimulating reading or writing according to a general program, stimulation could be planned to correspond to the linguistic level, semantic content, and purpose of an everyday situation or a situation that is personally relevant to the patient (e.g., Parr, 1992, 1996). Reading the phone book or street signs is functional. Reading playing cards or the box scores may be interesting. In general, we should let the patient, not a clinician's comfort, motivate the content of treatment.

COMPENSATORY BEHAVIORS

An aphasic individual should try to maximize the use of his or her residual communicative resources. These include language abilities as well as nonverbal vehicles for conveying messages.

Nonverbal modalities can be supplements to fragmentary or vague speaking or alternatives for patients with intractable expressive impairment. Severity of aphasia motivates us to attempt training alternative modes directly following principles of elicitation and programming applied to verbal behavior.

Van de Sandt-Koenderman (2004) divided many of the current alternatives into low-tech and high-tech strategies. Low-tech strategies include drawing and using communication books. High-tech strategies include using computers and other electronic devices. We will consider some low-tech strategies in this section, and will return to alternative forms of communication later in this chapter with regard to severe aphasic impairment.

Adaptive Language Strategies

There is more than one way to convey a meaning or message linguistically. In principle, when an aphasic person has difficulty constructing one linguistic form to convey an idea, another linguistic form might be attempted to convey the same general idea. Positive symptoms are indicative of spared language skills that can serve as adaptive mechanisms for conveying a message. Holland (1978) argued that it is okay for a patient to be "in the ball park, rather than pitching a verbal no-hitter."

Residual language capacities are most evident in anomic and Broca's aphasias. Patients with either type of aphasia tend to make adjustments automatically without intervention. Someone with anomic aphasia uses sentence production ability to produce circumlocutions around words that cannot be found at the moment. People with agrammatic aphasia access semantic and lexical stores to produce structurally simplified versions of an idea. Thus, saying "girl tall and boy short" is pretty close to saying that the girl is taller than the boy. The clinician's job is to reinforce meaningful circumlocution and simplification. The clinician avoids inhibiting communication by forcing a patient to shut down crucial subsystems of language production.

Also, mainly used to stimulate sentence production, a computer-assissted communication system (CS) can speak for agrammatic patients (Linebarger, McCall, and Berndt, 2004).

Communication Boards

Communication boards are often introduced early for patients with severe motor speech disorders, especially for those without linguistic or other cognitive deficits. The boards provide a means of communicating until speech or writing become functional. With minimal language impairment, words and phrases can be used freely without pictures or symbols. Pointing to letters provides flexibility for forming any word or phrase, but it is much slower. Some clinicians, however, delay use of communication boards because of a belief that they decrease motivation to speak.

Bellaire and others (1991) studied acquisition and generalization of communication board use for two patients with Broca's aphasia. The boards contained 15 line drawings of items for a coffee hour, such as social greetings, requesting food, and providing personal information. Individual treatment involved responding to requests from a clinician. Generalization training began with role-playing coffee hour situations in individual sessions, and, in the next phase, the clinician accompanied the patient to the social hour. The patients acquired requests and personal information responses but did not readily generalize use of the boards to the social setting. Instead, patients relied on vocalization or head nods that had been used before training. Also, the investigators suggested that communication boards may be more useful for individualized content that cannot be easily expressed through natural gesturing.

Gesturing and Drawing

As indicated in Chapter 6, many aphasic persons retain a capacity for gesture and drawing, whereas others are impaired. Use of these modes for communication depends on their intelligibility and a patient's willingness to use them. Patients with Broca's aphasia may spontaneously use more gesture than usual. Those with Wernicke's aphasia gesture the way they talk and may require some training if they are to clarify some of their spontaneous gestures (Le May, David, and Thomas, 1988; Smith, 1987). Drawing also may stimulate spoken word finding (Farias, Davis, and Harrington, 2006). The section on severe or global aphasia later in the chapter elaborates on the investigation of therapeutic gesturing and drawing.

INTERACTIVE THERAPIES

One step toward natural communicative conditions is to modify clinical interaction to conform to the structure of conversation. For aphasic patients, a clinician does not have to train conversational structure per se. Instead, a more natural interactive structure is an opportunity to apply communicative modalities and strategies that have been practiced in direct training. Also, patients

may increase confidence in their communicative abilities in a more natural interaction. Conversation is a collaboration between partners. A patient may come to realize that he or she does not have the sole responsibility for the success of communication.

PACE Therapy

Interaction can be modified from the basic naming task to incorporate the features of face-to-face conversation. One strategy for doing this is called **Promoting Aphasics' Communicative Effectiveness (PACE)** (Davis and Wilcox, 1985; Davis, 2005). Procedures follow four principles representing special features of conversation (Table 10.2). Any one principle may be applied in adjusting traditional tasks, but the four principles together make the interaction like conversation. PACE still is an artificial interaction which, in a progression from clinical to functional activities, falls short of real conversation.

In the new information condition, a message sender need only convey what is necessary to get the idea across. Message stimuli can be pictures of objects or events or anything else a clinician wants to explore. Turn taking removes us from a directive role and places us on equal footing with the patient. Our turns as sender are opportunities for modeling communicative behaviors that a patient is capable of using but may not be choosing. We may use direct instruction to train a communicative modality such as gesture or drawing, but in PACE we allow a client to choose modalities. Modeling shows that gesture is a reasonable option for getting the idea across.

Also, the patient can practice a few skills that are unique to conversation. One is responsiveness to a listener's attempts to interpret what the patient is trying to convey. Another skill is responsiveness to communicative failure and the use of repair or revision in trying to get a message across.

Investigators have used PACE and compared progress in different functions and have also compared PACE with another procedure with respect to the same functions. After PACE therapy for

TABLE 10.2 The four principles and essential procedures of Promoting Aphasics' Communicative Effectiveness (PACE) (Davis and Wilcox, 1985).

PRINCIPLE	DETAILS
1. The clinician and patient exchange new information.	Instead of having a picture of an object or event (called the message) in simultaneous view of the clinician and patient, a stack of message stimuli is placed face down to keep messages from the view of a message receiver. A client selects a card and attempts to convey the message on the card. The Brussels modification is to place a screen about eight inches or 20 centimeters high between the patient and clinician, and the message receiver chooses the message from options (Clerebaut, Coyette, Feyereisen, and Seron, 1984).
2. The clinician and patient participate equally as senders and receivers of messages.	This principle puts the turn-taking feature of conversation into the interaction. The clinician and client simply alternate in drawing a card and sending messages.
3. The patient has a free choice as to the communicative modes used to convey a message.	Contrary to training one modality such as gesture or drawing, the patient is left to choose the mode that is used for any message. We do not tell a client to perform in a particular way.
4. The clinician's feedback as a receiver is based on the patient's success in conveying the message.	The new information condition should make this inevitable for both participants. Our feedback should let the client know if he or she got the idea across. If we already know the message, we should respond as if we did not know.

eight patients, communicative abilities improved but not language skills, according to standard language tests (Carlomagno, Losanno, Emanuelli, and Casadio, 1991). For a patient with conduction aphasia, PACE was compared with traditional stimulation for improving naming, and more progress in naming was shown during the PACE phases of treatment (Li, Kitselman, Dusatko, and Spinelli, 1988). Avent and others (1995) compared a sentence stimulation technique with a PACE-like procedure emphasizing nonspeech modes of picture description. Results were mixed among three aphasic patients, with one favoring the "nonverbal treatment," one favoring the "verbal treatment," and the other showing no difference.

Other studies dealt with the responsiveness of patients to a clinician's modeling. Glindemann and others (1991) examined the influence of modeling names or descriptions. Patients with mild aphasia were more likely than others to switch between names and descriptions as a function of what the clinician does as sender. Greitemann and Wolf (1991) found that modeling can have an influence across verbal and gestural modalities and that the use of speech does not necessarily disappear as gesture increases. Glindemann and Springer (1995) were unimpressed with the modeling function for severe aphasia and for training compensatory communicative behavior. They recommended systematic stepwise training for this purpose. However, modeling was intended primarily to help a patient become comfortable about choosing trained modalities, and Glindemann and Springer viewed PACE as an "enrichment" of traditional treatment that motivates patients to use all available communicative options (see Davis, 2005).

Scripted Dialogues

Conversational coaching was developed by Holland (1991), who provides a patient with a short script that is slightly too difficult for the patient to produce. The patient should be able to read aloud simple sentences, but a script may also be created with few words and a few pictures. The script incorporates communicative strategies that were previously trained or suggested more directly. These strategies include "conversational management," such as asking a listener to slow down, to be discussed later in the chapter. The approach is another "bridging framework to initiate transfer of strategy use to patient-generated conversation" (p. 204).

First, the patient and clinician practice by following the script. The patient reads the script one sentence at a time. The clinician's job is to evaluate communicative effectiveness and suggest ways of conveying the information differently. The patient then may practice with another listener, often a family member. The clinician reminds the patient of strategies and sometimes coaches the listener (e.g., "If you don't understand, it's probably better to ask him to say it another way"). This activity is videotaped, and the participants get together to view and discuss it. The entire procedure may be repeated with a stranger as the listener. (Hopper, Holland, and Rewega, 2002).

A version of script training was put under the microscope of a multiple baseline experimental design for two individuals with nonfluent aphasia. These patients learned to produce the scripts naturally, and this ability generalized to some extent to novel conversation partners (Youmans, Holland, Muñoz, and Bourgeois, 2005).

Conversation as Therapy

Why not engage an aphasic patient in natural conversation? Simmons-Mackie (2001) has written about how *conversation therapy* can be part of the social approach to authentic treatment. Her method, however, is not just "having a conversation" during a therapy session. It is "goal directed and individualized" (p. 254). The SLP sets out to help a patient transfer compensatory strategies such as drawing or gesture to a conversational interaction. The patient is encouraged to use re-

sidual strategies that might have been practiced in PACE or conversational coaching.

Simmons-Mackie also encouraged the use of *scaffolded conversations,* in which the exchange of messages is supported by providing cues or facilitators with the flow of the interaction. We may quickly write a word that a participant was gesturing. Cues may be aimed at initiation of a conversational turn or conveying a message. Garrett and Ellis (1999) provided several details regarding this approach to conversation. Another activity, known as supported conversation, is a service provided at the Pat Arato Aphasia Centre, which is featured later in the chapter.

Holland (1998) was concerned that some clinicians are uncomfortable conversing with aphasic patients, and she detected a bias against conversation as a therapeutic medium. She asked "what relegates conversation to some sort of sleazy, shady, unreimbursable Neverland that must . . . follow the real goods—the therapy?" (p. 845). Chapter 6 indicated that conversation is often studied by interviewing patients. Thus, some clinicians who think they are engaged in real conversation are really engaged in something else. Holland (1998) stated that "interview models" emphasize a receiver function over a participant function, and she provided examples of the difference from a chat about "my most embarrassing moment" (p. 846):

- *interview model:* "Today we are going to talk about the most embarrassing thing that ever happened to us. Why not begin, Joe?"
- *conversation:* "You're not gonna believe what happened to me yesterday . . . Can you top this?"

LIFE PARTICIPATION

The Aphasia Center is part of the Division of Speech Pathology and Audiology at Duke University Medical Center. The center offers four basic programs:

- Treatment Groups, as a "low-cost alternative treatment"

- Community Reintegration, to assist the patient in returning to prestroke activities
- Family Support and Education, for enhancing communication among partners
- Training and Advocacy, to educate health care and community professionals

Topics in this section correspond to these types of programs, and it is good to know that they exist (Duke Health, n.d.).

Other illustrative programs are cited throughout this section. The principal architects of social and life participation approaches have been eloquent about the difficulties faced by aphasic people and their families (Lyon, 2001) and have articulated most of the strategies introduced here (Elman, 2005; Kagan, 1998; Simmons-Mackie, 2000, 2001). This text features particular group programs and community centers that have been inspired by the social and life participation concept. Let us begin, however, with preparatory activities that can be carried out in a hospital or clinic.

Situation-Specific Therapy

Role-playing provides an opportunity to induce the use of varied speech acts such as advising, warning, and arguing. A situation is created in which conflict is likely. The clinician and patient proceed to disagree over what to have for dinner or over how much to spend for a vacation.

Family members can be a part of many settings; but other partners, such as a waitperson in a restaurant, are an integral part of a particular setting. Like people, settings influence language behavior to the extent that they are familiar and demanding of the language processor. Driving a car involves reading simple signs quickly. After standing in line at the bank, we are expected to take care of business quickly.

Schlanger and Schlanger (1970) divided simulated life situations into nonstress situations such as planning a picnic and stressful situations such as going out to dinner. The stress situations could be pleasant (e.g., going out to dinner) or unpleasant (e.g., dealing with an emergency). In these activities, the client plays a role that would normally be assumed in these circumstances. For various situations, the clinician and patient begin to anticipate communicative problems and work together to figure out how a functional goal could be achieved with the patient's communicative resources.

A relatively minor shift in simple role-playing occurs when the clinician assumes the role of other persons in a communicative situation (e.g., a cab driver, a telephone operator, the minister, a waitperson in a restaurant). One characteristic of people in the community is their lack of knowledge of aphasia. By pretending to be ignorant of aphasia, the clinician can learn about the communicative failures that the patient is likely to face. Then, strategies for dealing with these failures can be developed.

In training two nonfluent patients to use symbolic gestures, Coelho (1991) first provided direct treatment in producing a gesture to a picture of a food item and then had the patient practice in a contrived restaurant. The clinician played the role of waiter, asking questions such as "What kind of sandwich would you like?" Probes for generalization included real waitresses asking similar questions in an actual restaurant. One patient generalized use of gestures to the natural setting, but a more severely impaired patient did not.

Hopper and Holland (1998) contrasted such situation-specific training with approaches, such as PACE, which are applicable to any situation. The investigators felt that managed care has moved treatment toward activities that establish functional independence in real-life tasks. They reported training two patients with Broca's aphasia to communicate over the phone in emergencies at home. Treatment consisted of the following three steps:

- describe a pictured emergency situation
- if the description was incorrect, answer *wh*-questions about components of the situation
- with the picture present, role-play the scenerio with the clinician asking "What is your emergency?"

Six pictured emergencies were trained, and four other pictures were used for a generalization probe. The patients improved over 10 sessions in responding to treated and untreated scenerios. Of course, success in communicating over the phone in a real emergency must be determined from interviews with family members.

Jacqueline Hinckley, at the University of South Florida, has referred to situation-specific role-playing as a context-based treatment approach (Hinckley and Carr, 2005). Ordering from a catalog over the telephone is one example. A few years ago, she compared this approach to the impairment-oriented treatment of Chapter 8 (called "skill based") with two groups of nonfluent aphasic patients. The two approaches appeared to lead to mixed effects not strongly related to either treatment. That is, context-based treatment was associated with improved naming but no change in scores with a functional battery (i.e., *CADL*). Nevertheless, the authors felt that they found improvements that were related to the treatments (Hinckley, Patterson, and Carr, 2001).

Group Treatment

With some group treatment, we begin to answer the question of the availability of services once third-party reimbursed hospital rehabilitation has ended. The issues include the availability of affordable services. In Chapter 8, group therapies were introduced as serving a variety of purposes (Kearns and Elman, 2001). This section focuses on groups with communicative objectives and direct involvement of a professional. For learning how to do group therapy, Elman (1999) put together an informative book on rationales and methods for a variety of approaches, and a special feature of each chapter is the frank discussion of reimbursement.

Group treatment has been supported by evidence (e.g., Wertz et al., 1981). More recently, Elman and Bernstein-Ellis (1999) compared one group receiving group treatment immediately and another group receiving the treatment on a deferred basis. While one group was receiving

the treatment, the deferred treatment group was engaged in activities not oriented to initiating conversation and conveying information. They found that increases in communication and linguistic measures were associated with receiving the group communication treatment.

Subacute hospital rehabilitation can be a setting. Graham's (1999) patients gathered in groups five days per week as a supplement to individual treatment. Basic treatment procedures were incorporated, and therapeutics were fueled by genuine empathy and peer encouragement. The procedures included conversation and simulated situations or role-playing. The ASHA-FACS (see Table 6.3) became a framework for establishing goals and defining activities. In fact, clinicians commonly used ASHA-FACS behaviors to guide construction of short-term goals.

Marshall (1999) described a program at the Portland VA Medical Center for mildly aphasic outpatients. These patients worked on solving problems related to life with aphasia. Some of the problems are listed below:

- communicating in an emergency (using identification cards)
- doctor's appointment (handling the anxiety of communicating with doctors)
- self-disclosure (telling listeners about their stroke)
- anger (dealing with the insensitivity of others)

Marshall believed that the groups increased the members' participation in life.

Other groups are conducted in university clinics, providing experiences for graduate students. Garrett and Ellis (1999) have employed scaffolded conversation in groups at the University of Nebraska. At the University of Arizona, Holland and Beeson (1999) have emphasized conversation through application of PACE therapy and role-played simulations. Students do not start off running groups alone, but participate as assistants for several weeks. Later in a term, a student may assume an increasingly bigger role in managing the group.

We have already seen that Duke University provides group therapy as a "low-cost alternative" to individual treatment. Early group treatment can be reimbursed by third parties, but services for the chronic period can be affordable for many families. Varied reimbursement strategies are suggested by Table 10.3.

Cynthia Busch (1999) has been the speech-language pathology Medicare consultant in Minnesota. She reported that, according to Medicare guidelines, "group treatment is reimbursable if the basic requirements for coverage of any speech-language pathology services are fulfilled" (p. 32). For example, the service must be necessary and accepted practice for the particular diagnosis. Documentation is vital.

At Graham's (1999) acute care hospital, group treatment was not explicitly part of the fee structure but was incorporated into the overall rehabilitation service. Early treatment was covered by Medicare Plan A or commercial insurance, and billing for long-term care was directed to Medicare Plan B, commercial insurance, or the patient (self-pay). In Graham's region, the fiscal intermediary for Medicare Plan A provided the following guidelines for obtaining re-imbursement for group therapy (Graham, 1999, p. 44):

- An SLP must be present in each session.
- Groups should be small (3–4 patients, maybe up to 6).
- Clear goals and procedures must be documented for each patient.
- Progress notes must document participation and progress.

Community Reintegration

Before going to a nearby restaurant with a group of clients, a woman with severe Broca's aphasia worked in a clinic on pointing to items on a menu as a means of ordering for herself. She pretended to order while a clinician gave her feedback. When the client got to the restaurant, she was stymied because the waitress was at the other end of the table listening for orders. While role playing might have anticipated the need to motion for the waitress to come over, there is no guarantee that role-playing and other clinical activities will anticipate everything that happens during the real thing.

TABLE 10.3   Reimbursement for group therapy in different settings, reported by chapter authors in Roberta Elman's (1999) book on group treatment. The fee structures are likely to have changed over the years.

SETTING	AUTHOR(S)	SUMMARY
Subacute hospital	Graham	Medicare Part A or B
University clinic	Garrett and Ellis	Complete and partial insurance and vocational rehabilitation (25%) Fee for service (self-pay) Local civic group donations
University clinic	Holland and Beeson	Fee for service (self-pay)
University clinic	Walker-Batson, Curtis, and others	$150 intake assessment $300 minimal semester fee
Aphasia center (nonprofit)	Bernstein-Ellis and Elman	$15 or $10 per session, or $150 "session card"
VA medical center	Marshall	No charge

After training gestures for food items, Coelho (1991) concluded that there appear to be certain aspects of real-world settings that cannot be simulated, for example, conversations stopping, persons staring, waitresses' embarrassment, all as the aphasic individual struggles to communicate, and these need to be overcome by the aphasic patient for true generalization to occur" (p. 217).

How might resumption of activities be facilitated, especially when clinicians do not have time to accompany patients outside a rehabilitation center? Jon Lyon (1992) established **Communication Partners** in which an adult volunteer from a patient's community "serves as the vehicle with which activities of the patient's choice are introduced, either at home or in the community where they naturally occur" (Lyon, Cariski, Keisler et al., 1997, p. 694).

The program has two phases. The first occurs in the clinic for six weeks. Supervised by an SLP, the volunteer and client become comfortable with each other in a variety of plausible situations. The volunteer practices several communicative strategies such as the following (Lyon et al., 1997, pp. 705–706):

- Listen for a general theme rather than specific words.
- If a spoken message is not clear, encourage use of gestures.
- If the message is still not clear, encourage the client to draw.
- Draw your best guess as to what the client is trying to say.
- Verify what you think you know every 1 or 2 minutes.

The second phase of Communication Partners is 14 weeks and consists of outside activities. In the first of two weekly sessions, the clinician assists in reviewing the previous week's activity and planning the next activity to be carried out as the week's second session. The second session involves the aphasic client and the volunteer partner and is conducted in the home or at a community site. Types of activities include a favorite from the past (e.g., gardening, card playing, grocery shopping), an activity considered but never tried before (e.g., learning computer skills), and volunteering in the community (e.g., visiting a day-care center).

For many older adults, losing the ability to drive is more distressing than losing the ability to speak. It restricts individual freedom and creates an increasing sense of dependence. Driving contributes to QoL, but it requires rapid reading of road signs for directions and street names. In the United Kingdom, Mackenzie and Paton (2003) interviewed aphasic individuals, medical practitioners, and SLPs regarding their views on returning to driving after stroke. Most of the professionals thought that driving is contra-indicated in some cases. Aphasic individuals showed some reduction in the recognition of road signs. Aphasic drivers reported driving less, more carefully, and for shorter distances. Mackenzie and Paton indicated that training in road sign recognition has definite implications for re-entry into the community.

Changing Communities

This section shifts emphasis from putting a patient in communicative contexts to changing them. It was indicated before that an aphasic individual is not solely responsible for the success of communication. In a sense, there are two kinds of adjustments that can make therapy more like real life. One, adjust the therapy. The other, adjust real life to be more like therapy. Three areas of adjustment are discussed here: caregivers, the physical environment, and reading materials.

One investigation showed that aphasic people comprehend better when their spouses make adjustments in their utterances (Linebaugh, Margulies, and Mackisack-Morin, 1984). These adjustments included increased pauses and redundancy in describing pictures. Simmons and others (1987) found that training spouses to modify their behavior led to a reduction of interruptions of their aphasic partners. More recently, training programs were reported that helped caregivers or friends improve communication with their aphasic partners (Cunningham and Ward, 2003; Purdy and

Hindenlang, 2005). Another training program for medical students made a difference in their ability to interview patients with aphasia (Legg, Young, and Bryer, 2003).

The patient may utilize strategies of **conversational management.** For example, someone with mild aphasia may not be able to process conversation at its normal rate. The aphasic person starts to get lost and is too embarrassed to say so. However, instead of allowing others to restrict his or her ability to comprehend and respond, the patient can ask people to reduce their rate of speech or repeat every now and then. Holland (1991) called these "comprehension strategies," and they included asking others to simplify or elaborate their messages.

Let us suppose a mildly impaired patient is going through a divorce and must deal with a future ex-spouse and a lawyer over the phone. In the clinic, we can play the roles of these persons so the patient can practice asking the spouse or the lawyer to explain slowly, to repeat, or to be available if a question should come up after hanging up the phone. If the spouse and lawyer cannot agree to these conditions, then perhaps the conversation should be at another time. This dress rehearsal may strengthen confidence and the likelihood that the patient will use these strategies outside the clinic.

Lubinski (2001) has been writing about **environmental language intervention.** A "communicatively impaired environment" has the following characteristics:

1. strict rules governing communication
2. few places for a private conversation
3. a staff that devalues communication between residents and between residents and staff
4. many residents with multiple problems including dementias
5. physical conditions that reduce communicative efficiency, such as linear or distant seating and poor lighting and acoustics

Clinicians should employ their diplomatic and persuasive skills to effect modifications of these conditions. New and remodeled nursing homes include spaces for private meetings with family and friends, attractive areas for social gatherings, and seating in the dining room that facilitates face-to-face interaction. Environmental language intervention may contribute to what some now call an *aphasia-friendly environment* (Howe, Worrall, and Hickson, 2004).

Changing communities to become more aphasia friendly also entails improving access to information. Worrall and her colleagues have advocated successfully for the use of **aphasia-friendly printed material** in health education literature and beyond. Aphasia-friendly formatting includes simplified text, large font, lots of white space, and helpful illustrations (Brennan, Worrall, and McKenna, 2005; Rose, Worrall, and McKenna, 2003; Worrall, Rose, Howe et al., 2005). A website may have an aphasia-friendly option (e.g., Aphasia project, http://cs.princeton.edu/aphasia/).

Creating Communities

Let us return to the question of what is available when formal treatment for aphasia has concluded. We have already considered some group therapies, especially those provided at university clinics. Another option is community centers staffed primarily by volunteers (Worrall and Yiu, 2000). There has been a stream of inspiration for the recent development of these centers, beginning with the work of Aura Kagan. Kagan inspired the social and life participation movement in the United States (e.g., Elman, 1999). Websites for community centers often refer to the social and life participation concepts as guiding their efforts. Many aphasic people and their families now have a new life inspired by their participation in these centers. The centers are listed at the website for the National Aphasia Association. The story begins in Toronto.

In 1979, Pat Arato recognized a need for a program after discharge from therapy for her husband and others. She founded an aphasia center that was eventually named for her and became part of the Aphasia Institute in Toronto. Aura Kagan became the center's director (Kagan, Black, Duchan et al., 2001; Kagan and Cohen-Schneider, 1999). The center is mentioned in Chapter 1 for its reliance on the government and fundraising for financial support. It is also recognized for its particular orientation to group activities.

A normal atmosphere is fostered at the Arato Centre by referring to aphasic participants as "members" instead of patients or clients. The program has two phases. A 12-week introductory program is for educating members and their families, improving communication, and providing psychological support. Then a 16-week program offers conversation groups, music therapy, art classes, family/caregiver groups, and other options. Volunteers, such as students interested in a rehabilitation career, serve as conversation partners.

The communication intervention has been called **supported conversation for adults with aphasia** (SCA), with a focus on severe language impairment (Kagan, 1998). SCA is based on the premise that working on the skills necessary for conversation, such as a PACE activity, is not the same as actually having an adult conversation. There are a couple other key assumptions:

- access to conversation is denied aphasic people because of a perceived lack of competence
- competence is revealed by a "communication ramp" (i.e., skilled partner) to conversation opportunities

Volunteers at the Arato Centre are trained in a workshop that includes an instructional video, role-playing, work with a group of members with severe aphasia, and an apprenticeship with experienced volunteers.

Table 10.4 contains reported characteristics of supported conversation. Kagan (1998) claimed that emphasis on "natural-sounding conversation . . . differentiates the SCA approach from other similar-sounding approaches" (p. 820), although Kagan did not identify these other approaches. Within this interactive atmosphere, aphasic members practice communicating by any means. Particular attention is given to an extensive manual of

TABLE 10.4 Reported characteristics of supported conversation with severe aphasia (Kagan, 1998).

FEATURE	DETAIL
Acknowledgment of competence	Reinforce a member's capacities
	Sound natural and adult
Revealing competence	Ensure that a member comprehends
	Ensure that a member has a response mode
	Verify a member's communicative attempt
Simultaneous use of techniques	Create natural flow and timing of modalities

pictographs used to identify conversational topics and support getting a message across.

Roberta Elman visited the Arato Centre in 1989 and decided to open the **Aphasia Center of California** in 1996. It was the first independent nonprofit organization in the United States that provides direct services to people with aphasia (Bernstein-Ellis and Elman, 1999). It is housed in a senior center in Oakland and offers several conversation groups, a support group for caregivers, reading and writing groups, and an art class.

The **Triangle Aphasia Project** (www.aphasia project.org) is located in North Carolina and offers the following programs:

- treatment groups (5–8 individuals working on communication strategies)
- home programs (needs assessment, program plan, and volunteer implementation)
- community reengagement (volunteer accompaniment to community activities)
- community training (educating community in contact with aphasic people)
- referrals and support

The professional and clerical staff consists of volunteer SLPs, retirees, and an individual with aphasia.

Mike Adler was the CEO of a global mail order company with 1,000 employees. In 1993 he suffered a stroke and aphasia. He became depressed and uncomfortable with speaking. His wife Elaine's life changed, too. She felt frustrated and helpless. They sought support from people who had a similar experience but found that professionals in their region could not direct them to a program. Wanting to help others, they investigated and discovered model support programs at aphasia centers in the United States, Canada, and England.

In 2003, Mike and Elaine created the **Adler Aphasia Center** in Maywood, New Jersey, for programs that provide social and emotional support. Like other centers, it relies on volunteers to become communication partners, computer partners, and creativity partners for art, music, and cooking. The Adlers' goal is to help aphasic people and their loved ones live a fuller life (www.adleraphasiacenter.org).

THE CHALLENGE OF SEVERE OR GLOBAL APHASIA

Severe or global aphasia is discussed here mainly because many functional therapeutic resources are required to help a patient communicate maximally (Collins, 2005; Peach, 2001). Following principles of direct stimulation, we begin with the simplest levels of language using the simplest tasks. A patient is likely to improve some in auditory comprehension, but results for verbal expression may be discouraging. Clinicians try to establish or encourage any means of communication as soon as possible.

Candidacy for Treatment

Brookshire (1997) stated that "the presence of global aphasia at one month postonset is an ominous prognostic sign." He added that "the healing effects of time apparently have little effect on the language capabilities of most patients who remain globally aphasic beyond the immediate post-onset period" (p. 247). He suggested that at least two of the following symptoms indicate that a patient

may not have the capacity to become a functional verbal communicator:

- stereotypic utterance along with severely impaired comprehension
- inability to match objects
- unreliable yes/no response to questions
- semantic or neologistic jargon without awareness and self-correction

We should note that these projections pertain to linguistic communicative capacity, not necessarily nonverbal communicative capacity. Even when improvement occurs across a period of treatment, it may have taken months or years to achieve (e.g., Samples and Lane, 1980).

Edelman (1987) suggested that lack of progress in overall language test scores may hide progress in comprehension and gesturing. Brookshire (1997) stated that a brief period of trial therapy can be indicative of whether a patient can benefit from a full treatment program, but he added that "prolonged treatment to reinstate functional verbal communication for such patients is rarely successful" (p. 248). Nevertheless, he acknowledged that new treatment programs may alter this outlook.

One study indicated that intensity of language treatment can make a difference (Denes, Perazzolo, Piani, and Piccione, 1996). Seventeen patients received treatment of auditory comprehension along with some stimulation of multiple expressive modalities in conversation. Treatment was begun around three months postonset. Nine patients received 60 sessions over a six-month period (2–3/week), and eight patients received 130 sessions over six months (5/week). More patients receiving the more intensive therapy made significant improvement.

Comprehension

Treatment of auditory comprehension can be devised according to a logical application of principles introduced in Chapter 8.

- set a reasonable functional goal
- start with a task that has a high level of accuracy

- upon meeting a criterion of success, move to a more demanding task
- measure progress toward meeting the goal

Improved comprehension can have far-reaching consequences. A goal of achieving a high level of accuracy in comprehending sentences is functional in the sense that comprehension can facilitate conversational interaction (e.g., answering another's questions). However, because treatment should begin at a level of high accuracy, it may have to begin with a task that is easier than the floor of initial assessment. For example, a word comprehension task may have two pictured choices instead of the six or eight in an aphasia test. To measure progress toward the goal, a brief test of sentence comprehension should be administered regularly. The lesson plan might look something like Table 10.5.

We should have a patient's attention for repetitive drills. In a hospital, a patient may arrive at the clinic tired from physical therapy or in a state of depressed vigilance due to trauma. Alerting signals, such as the patient's name or "Ready?" may be presented before each stimulus. Collins (1986) tried to heighten interest with playing cards in simple matching and sequencing tasks. Awareness, as well as functionality, may be heightened when the task is individualized, as in pointing to pictures of family members.

For word comprehension, several variables can be manipulated to adjust difficulty. The lexical stimulus may be repeated or presented with a printed word. Redundant verbal context might help in identifying an object. Pictures can be varied in semantic relatedness and can be supple-

mented with printed words. However, despite all of the logical manipulations that could generate a brilliant stepwise program, a patient represented by Table 10.5 should be progressing quickly out of the word-level treatment in order to meet the sentence-level goal. Stimulation should be awakening a process. If a patient is not improving over three or four sessions, then it is not likely that much repair of the language system is possible in an affordable amount of time (although there is little published data supporting this suggestion).

At a slightly higher linguistic level, four patients with severe aphasia were trained to follow simple verb–noun commands such as *take glove* and *cover fork* (Oleyar et al. 1991). The patients had AQ scores from the WAB of 19.4 to 48.8. Treatment consisted of pairing a spoken command with a model of the action. The clinician also gradually increased the time between the command and the model. Two of the four subjects responded favorably to the treatment by improving with trained commands without models and generalizing to untrained commands.

Language Formulation

Sarno and Levita (1979) noted that a few words could make a remarkable difference in someone's life over an inability to produce words. In principle, treatment begins with what a patient can do verbally; and people with global aphasia easily produce verbal stereotypes with no relation to a situation. They can be prodded into counting to ten or singing a song.

Clinicians try to harness whatever utterances are produced spontaneously. If we can get them

TABLE 10.5   A lesson plan for treating auditory comprehension for someone with global aphasia.

GOAL	TREATMENT	GENERALIZATION PROBE
Improve functional sentence comprehension from 10% to 70% accuracy	Point to pictures (2 choices) given common words and family names	10-item sentence comprehension test, including yes/no biographical questions and functional commands

under our control, then we may help a patient to produce them more appropriately and in greater variety. Helm and Barresi (1980) formalized this common practice in a program called **Voluntary Control of Involuntary Utterances.** It began with presenting the printed form of an utterance just heard. If the utterance was repeated as if read aloud, it was considered to be more volitional. If a different word was produced, a stimulus card was written for that word. No treatment was pursued for any utterance that was difficult to elicit a second time. When reading aloud and repetition elicited responses, an object picture was presented in a transition to naming tasks. Patients improved in independent testing and were reported to use some of the words appropriately in conversational interaction.

Brief trial therapy usually does not produce functional improvement in verbal behavior for patients who have global aphasia at one month post-onset. At least, clinicians can determine level of comprehension and ability to communicate non-verbally. It is more common that the clinician's primary role "is to help the family and other caregivers structure the patient's daily life environment to take advantage of the communicative abilities that the patient has retained" (Brookshire, 1997, p. 248).

Communication Boards

Severely aphasic patients may rely more on pictures for basic needs that cannot be readily expressed by pointing or natural gesturing. Severely nonfluent patients may have enough comprehension for pointing to words. Patients with more severe comprehension deficits require some training in the use of simple printed material. In the Netherlands, Visch-Brink and others (1993) train patients to use a "Language Pocket Book," which consists of word lists and pictures organized by category or situation. Part of the training includes work on conceptualization such as sorting words into functional categories. Any patient, along with frequent communication partners, may need some practice in the functional use of boards or notebooks.

Pointing behavior is a valuable communicative tool, and some real-life settings may be more communicatively accessible than others. Menus are communication boards. For ordering in a restaurant, one need only read and point to an item on the menu. Some menus have many pictures of the food. Major stores have catalogs. At home, a patient can tear out pages as a shopping list and use them for asking about the location of a product. Bus stations and travel agencies have brochures. Functional analysis of a situation includes identifying compensatory materials and strategies that are accessible in the situation.

Gesturing and Drawing

Training has been designed for pantomimic gesture (e.g., Coelho and Duffy, 1990). **Visual Action Therapy** (VAT) takes a patient through several steps involving object manipulation to train the use of pantomimic gestures (Helm-Estabrooks, Fitzpatrick, and Barresi, 1982). The program begins with matching tasks for perception and recognition of objects and proceeds to gesturing of function with the object in hand and then without the object.

If a pantomime is to replace speech as a communicative mode, it should be reasonably intelligible. Flowers and Wyse (1985) examined intelligibility of pantomimes produced by normal adults who used only their nonpreferred hand. A receiver, familiar to the sender, wrote the name of an object that was demonstrated. Subjects' gesturing was highly variable, with a 46 to 91 percent level of transparency to receivers outside of a natural situation. Like playing charades, clear pantomiming does not come naturally; but the forced-choice method probably functions like a natural situation that narrows the possible meanings. In data available for the Duffys' referential abilities test, four normal subjects were 97 percent accurate (Duffy et al., 1984).

Drawing may be attempted after traditional language treatments prove to be unsuccessful (e.g. Rao, 1995). There have been a few reports of training (Hunt, 1999; Lyon, 1995). Morgan and

Helm-Estabrooks (1987) instituted "Back to the Drawing Board" with two cases of nonfluent aphasia who copied cartoons of increasing complexity. Lyon and Sims (1989) trained "expressively restricted" patients with a wide range of overall severity of aphasia. For three months, the patients were given a cued training program. Then, transfer to communicative use was encouraged with an interactive procedure. The patients improved as a group. Holland (1995) tried to teach drawing to patients with Broca's, Wernicke's, and conduction aphasia. She encouraged self-motivated use of natural drawing abilities; but, blaming her own poor drawing skills, Holland concluded that her attempts were "notably unsuccessful."

Gestural Codes

At one time, Amer-Ind Code was enticing because it is descriptive of referents and can be used with one hand (Skelly, 1979). The iconicity of Amer-Ind and American Sign Language (ASL) has been examined according to their transparency, namely, the extent to which someone unfamiliar with the code can guess a gesture's meaning. Amer-Ind was 54 percent guessable, and ASL was 10 to 30 percent guessable (Daniloff, Lloyd, and Fristoe, 1983). From reports on training patients to use Amer-Ind, Skelly (1979) concluded that "there was almost universal dissatisfaction expressed concerning transfer from the cued retrieval/ replicative stage to self-initiated use" (p. 40).

Coelho and Duffy (1987) studied acquisition of 23 Amer-Ind signs and 14 fabricated signs. Their training method had steps for imitation, recognition, and "naming" with each gesture. The goal for the study was to develop an ability to name referents. Generalization was measured with respect to naming untrained pictures with trained gestures. The ability to acquire these signs was negligible for patients below the 35th percentile on the PICA. Those above this level increased their ability to acquire and generalize signs as a linear function of severity of aphasia.

Later, Coelho (1990) attempted training selected Amer-Ind and ASL signs. Two of his four patients were below the 35th percentile. Stages of treatment led to varying the agent (i.e., *man, woman*) with two verbs (i.e., *cook, eat*) and eight objects (e.g., *tomato, fish, egg*). Coelho concluded that "the production of sign combinations from previously acquired single signs does not occur spontaneously—that is, without training—and that even with training, at least within the context of the present experiment, the maintenance effect is weak" (p. 399).

Blissymbols, a system of pictograms, was presented to four patients with global aphasia (Johannsen-Hornbach, Cegla, Mager et al., 1985). Two patients interacted with the clinician using these symbols, and one of these patients used the system on a limited basis living with his mother. Another patient progressed enough in speaking so that Blissymbols became unnecessary (also, Funnell and Allport, 1989). Koul and Lloyd (1998) compared symbol learning by patients with "moderate global" aphasia and RHD. The training involved pointing to choices of Blissymbols in response to a spoken name. Aphasic patients were equivalent to normal controls in learning the associated pairs, whereas the RHDs recognized fewer symbols.

Purdy, Duffy, and Coelho (1994) trained 15 nonfluent patients in responding with a communication board and gestural symbols. They found that the patients did not use as many gestures in a structured conversation task as they used in direct training, and patients continued to prefer verbal over nonverbal response. Nevertheless, the investigators were particularly interested in whether the patients would spontaneously switch to one modality when an attempt with another modality failed. Patients switched modalities only 39 percent of the time, but they were successful in conveying messages 73 percent of the time when they did switch.

Contrary to the belief that gesturing inhibits speaking, gesturing may draw out verbalization when other methods fail. In one study, a gesture was paired with naming, but naming was better with gesture for nonfluent subjects, not fluent subjects (Hanlon, Brown, and Gerstman, 1990).

Rosenbek and his colleagues (1989) stated that "our assumption is that verbal expression can be improved by the appropriate pairing of performances or with the systematic use of unique sensory inputs" (p. 218). The first step of training is to teach gesture recognition. The next step involves modeling a gesture and word for imitation. If a patient should spontaneously start talking while gesturing, it is likely that the patient can benefit from other treatments for language production. The challenge is to maintain the verbal response after the gesture is faded.

C-VIC and Beyond

Speech-language pathologists have been relentless, if not heroic, in seeking a communicative mode for globally impaired patients. This effort includes the use of various shapes as symbols. Patients were trained to comprehend statements, questions, and commands constructed out of such symbols arranged in syntactic order. One team of investigators examined cut-out paper shapes that were also used to give chimpanzees a means of communicating with humans (Glass, Gazzaniga, and Premack, 1973).

Gardner and others (1976) tried a system called **Visual Communication** or VIC. Although aphasic subjects displayed a knowledge of syntactic relations, there was no sign of functional use of the system. However, such unconventional methods indicated that globally aphasic persons may have more language capacity than is usually exposed by aphasia tests (Shelton, Weinrich, McCall, and Cox, 1996).

For over a decade, a team of researchers led by Michael Weinrich at the University of Maryland developed a computerized version of Visual Communication called C-VIC. The program contains a hierarchically organized picture vocabulary that is displayed as cards on the screen. Verbs are animated to facilitate comprehension. A patient can arrange nouns around verbs without regard to syntax. A sentence looks like a row of picture cards. The clinician makes a statement on one row, and the patient responds on a second row.

Weinrich's research team used C-VIC mainly to explore the linguistic capacity of persons with global aphasia, and they found that this capacity is heterogeneous. C-VIC was found to be limited for use as an augmentative communicative device, partly because learning the system takes up to two years (Shelton et al., 1996). Two patients with severe Broca's aphasia (i.e., good comprehension) were trained to produce basic sentences with varied tense marking with C-VIC. Additionally, their spoken sentence production was improved after the training (Weinrich, McCall, Weber et al., 1995; Weinrich, Shelton, Cox, and McCall, 1997).

The programming for C-VIC has become more sophisticated and is now called *Lingraphica,* marketed by Lingraphicare (www.aphasia.com). A speech generating capacity has been added. The program contains a dictionary of over 5,000 words, each represented by icons. Once a user selects the icons, they can be turned into spoken words or sentences.

Another program for patients with severe verbal impairment is *C-Speak Aphasia,* which is conceptually based on C-VIC. Nicholas, Sinotte, and Helm-Estabrooks (2005) reported on at least six months of training five patients with severe nonfluent aphasia. Three of the patients became substantially better at conveying information with the computer than without it. The investigators found some patients simply unable to use the system for communicating and attributed this difficulty to a general cognitive deficiency in problem solving.

PSYCHOSOCIAL ADJUSTMENT

Meeting the goals of rehabilitation depends on the psychosocial adjustments by the patient and family members. Reciprocally, psychological adjustments depend on the success of communicative rehabilitation. The patient and caregivers also benefit from the good spirit of the SLP.

Clinician Characteristics

Martin Exeter's language and outlook became much improved over the first six months, and he became curious about whether he could teach again. However, memories of his rehabilitation were tarnished by an experience with one clinician. He worked with her briefly during the three-month treatment at a university in another state. One day the clinician told him that he would never get his memory back. The prediction lodged in Martin's mind as "you'll never teach again."

Rehabilitation is supported by the relationship between a clinician and a client. Rapport and trust contribute to the therapeutic process. In discussing these factors, Cyr-Stafford (1993) suggested that "the serene attitude of the knowledgeable professional who is familiar with these situations is reassuring to the person with aphasia" (p. 108). Our technical skills are not enough for a therapeutic relationship to flourish. If a patient is uncomfortable with a clinician, the patient quits. Our "people skills" are supportive of language rehabilitation.

Wulf (1979) commented on her first contact with her therapist with a "radiant smile": "And this was the first miracle speech therapy wrought for me. No word was needed—it was the magic of a look—an instantaneous rapport partly because my innermost messenger had told me that it would be that way" (p. 50). **Unconditional positive regard** creates a positive climate for therapeutic change. The influential clinical psychologist Carl Rogers (1951) defined it as "an outgoing positive feeling without reservations, without evaluations" (p. 62). Depression, frustration, and anger are allowed in the clinical setting without reservation or evaluation by the clinician.

Yet, studies have shown that patients and their families are likely to express more optimism than SLPs (e.g., Herrmann and Wallesch, 1989). An aphasic adult detects body language and prosody conveying negative attitudes. Sacks (1985) stated that "one cannot lie to an aphasic person." In a survey by Skelly (1975), patients "cited numerous subtle signs of impatience from those around them which were deeply discouraging—audible sighs, tightening of the mouth muscles, shoulder and eye movements, and drumming fingers" (p. 1141). A

few clinicians may confuse aloofness with professionalism and exude a coolness that intimidates family members.

Wulf (1979) also wrote that an SLP's rare talent is "being able to hop on anybody's wavelength and stay there until the aphasic has learned how to climb the unending tortuous crag facing him" (p. 50). In a survey of clients who evaluated attributes of a good clinician, "empathetic-genuineness" ranked second to technical skill (Haynes and Oratio, 1978). **Empathy** is a capacity to sense the feelings and personal meanings that another person is experiencing at each moment. We cannot walk in an aphasic person's shoes, but we can convey that we understand the problems created by brain damage.

Experienced clinicians are familiar with the soothing of frustration that comes with statements like "I know—you know what you want to say but just can't think of the words to say it." An SLP may be the first person to convey this understanding. A patient discovers someone who knows that he or she is not stupid and believes there is someone in the hospital who can help with the exasperation of trying to talk. A client is inclined to accept the rigors of clinical advice when he or she knows that the helper understands the problem.

Rogers (1951) advised that "it is the counselor's function to assume, in so far as he is able, the internal frame of reference of the client . . . to lay aside all perceptions from the external frame of reference while doing so, and to communicate something of this empathic understanding to the client" (p. 29). An external frame of reference includes stereotypic conceptions according to gender, age, race, or religion. Ageism, for example, may entail a fear of the elderly that interferes with addressing a client as an individual (Davis and Holland, 1981). Prospective clinical aphasiologists should evaluate their attitudes regarding these attributes so they can keep them out of clinical interactions and can attain unconditional positive regard and empathy for their patients.

A third clinician characteristic is **patience.** A family member, accustomed to a certain pace of conversation or feeling compelled to help a loved one, may jump in quickly when a patient is slow to respond. An experienced clinician, on the other hand, knows that the goal is to increase the patient's independence and allows some time for generating a response. Family members, who are used to quick cures of diseases, may become distressed over the relatively slow rate of progress that is common with stroke-related dysfunction. An experienced clinician knows that progress moves in small steps and takes some time.

Patient Adjustment

In the first three to six months postonset, a patient receives treatment in a climate of psychological adjustment. The grief response has been a model for stages of psychological adjustment to sudden language dysfunction. Tanner and Gerstenberger's (1988) four stages were denial, frustration, depression, and acceptance. Whether aphasic patients actually go through this sequence has not been clearly established (Lyon, 1998).

Denial of impairment can be a psychological defense mechanism in contrast to absence of awareness of deficit. Not all patients deny their aphasia, but, for some, it may be a patient's premorbid coping style, and it "allows patients to borrow time while they come to terms with reality" (Sarno, 1993, p. 325).

Depression, or discouragement, is common after a stroke. Depression is more common with good comprehension and nonfluent aphasia than with other types of aphasia (Starkstein and Robinson, 1988). Physicians have advised that depression may not be just a stage of coping that a patient passes through. Herrmann, Johannsen-Horbach, and Wallesch (1993) suggested that it is likely to be an unavoidable neurochemical consequence of stroke. The spectrum of poststroke depression includes *emotional lability,* which is sudden laughter or crying for no apparent reason. Treatment of severe depression or pathological crying has included antidepressant medication (Andersen, 1997).

An aphasic person thinks, "I want to be me again." Brumfitt (1993) argued that motor and communicative disabilities batter a person's **sense of self.** Holland and Beeson (1993) added that "as clinicians, we will be involved with individuals and family members as they mourn the insult to the pre-stroke identity, and as they make adjustments to the sense of self" (p. 581). Fundamental to an aphasic person's identity is his or her adulthood. Caring family members may start to treat the patient like a child, especially with respect to communicative style.

Van Eeckhout (1993) worked with patients who were artists or talented artistically. The aim was not "to spark creativity in persons with aphasia, but, rather, to revive the persons' former personality" (p. 89). One patient regained enough drawing ability with the left hand to take a job as illustrator. Another patient had Wernicke's aphasia but retained the ability to play any melody on the organ. Through continued revelation of this retained skill, the patient regained self-confidence and wrote 32 compositions since his stroke. A third patient, who was a singer and poet, received music therapy as the primary mode of communicative stimulation. Part of his therapy involved composing songs about aphasia.

Sarno (1993) reported that **social isolation** is the most frequently cited consequence of aphasia in surveys of aphasic patients, and that 70 percent believe that people avoid them because of their aphasia. Programs mentioned previously, such as Communication Partners or the Arato Centre in Toronto, were designed to relieve social isolation.

Le Dorze and Brassard (1995) interviewed patients and family members. Aphasic patients cited some of the following changes in their lives:

- *interpersonal relationships:* disruption of family relations, friction with spouse, loss of authority over children, fewer contacts with brothers and sisters, anxiety in meeting strangers
- *autonomy:* loss of employment, physical dependency, feeling of powerlessness

A patient may quickly exhibit **unproductive coping mechanisms** as a shield from impairment

(Eisenson, 1984). In interviews with 20 aphasic patients, Parr (1994) found that they employed a variety of ways of dealing with their disabilities. One patient was resigned to his impairments but pursued an active life. His relationship with his wife improved during his rehabilitation. Another patient, however, responded to his condition with "angry fatalism." He was unwilling to discuss many things about his condition, including possibilities for functional progress through rehabilitation. Patients below age 65 were more likely than older patients to take action and control in their situation.

Family Adjustment

Immediately following a stroke, the family is likely to be overwhelmed with the sense that they nearly lost a husband, wife, father, or mother. Suddenly a hospitalized life partner appears to be vulnerable to the slightest encroachment, and a skittish spouse wants to protect him or her 24 hours a day. The devoted spouse may return home only overnight, sleeping partly dressed in case there is a call from the hospital. Spousal adjustment hopefully follows a path from selflessness to a renewed sense of self, a path that may parallel the patient's progress.

Then chronic aphasia becomes a family problem, turning family dynamics upside down (Rollin, 1984). A spouse becomes annoyed with a patient's swearing, feels heightened responsibilities, becomes increasingly fatigued, and drops some favorite activities to attend to the patient (Labourel and Martin, 1993; Le Dorze and Brassard, 1995; Ponzio and Degiovani, 1993).

A patient's inability to carry out customary roles causes family members to assume new roles. Regarding traditional roles of marriage partners, a male patient may no longer be able to provide income, sign the checks, and park the car. Dahlberg noted the following: "Since I'd grown up in middle-class America, I was used to taking care of 'masculine' details. I signed into hotels, picked up the bags, gave taxi directions, and ordered in restaurants." His wife added: "I looked forward to

the time Clay would be able to do the managing again. It wasn't the physical exertion I minded as much as the loss of my female enjoyment of being 'taken care of'" (Dahlberg and Jaffe, 1977, p. 52). Michallet, Tétreault, and Le Dorze (2003) have provided detailed information from interviews regarding the life changes and coping strategies of spouses.

Porter and Dabul (1977) applied transactional analysis (TA) to helping spouses understand the situation and return to a balance. A spouse has to respond to shifts in Adult, Parent, and Child ego states by the patient. "He acts like a child." In the aphasic person, the Adult state is often weakened and turned into the dependent state of the Child. "He just sits around all day and watches TV." Childlike ego involvement dominates as impulsiveness and a continual attention to "me, me, me." The Parent state diminishes with an inability to conform to social acceptability. Other patients may exaggerate the Parent by becoming overly protective of the spouse, constantly monitoring his or her activities. We may begin to imagine the toll this takes on a spouse and children living at home. A spouse, in turn, can become overly protective of a patient.

Julianna had been notified only that her father had suffered a stroke. It did not take long for Martin to figure out that she was considering leaving school to be with him and help out at home. She was afraid he was going to die, and so she hovered over him and pampered him as if he were an infant. He tried to assure her with his ability to squeeze a rubber ball, and he did not want to feel guilty about interfering with her life. She felt better after having a chance to see his early progress, and she returned to school the next semester. Later, they would communicate regularly through e-mail, which became part of Martin's self-imposed rehabilitation.

Peter was having a difficult time adjusting. He was living at home and could sense his mother's frustrations, although she tried to make everything seem normal. Maybe that made it harder than it already was for him to talk about it. Every-

one was feeling his or her way. Peter had to help out more around the house, doing some of the repairs and yardwork that he and his father used to do together. His life was changing and he did not like it, but he would not say anything for fear of appearing to be selfish.

Zraick and Boone (1991) found that spouses develop different attitudes toward their aphasic spouse than "control spouses." The investigators used an attitude assessment technique called Q-methodology in which spouses sorted and ranked 70 attributes according to what was most and least representative of the aphasic person. In general, spouses had more negative attitudes than controls, indicating that spouses' attitudes had changed after onset. The most prevalent perceived characteristics of the impaired spouse were *demanding* and *temperamental* in contrast to *mature* and *kind* for controls. Least prevalent characteristics for the clinical group included *sexy, mature,* and *intelligent.* Spouses of nonfluent patients had more negative attitudes than spouses of fluent patients, which, in part, could have been due to the more frequent presence of hemiplegia in the nonfluent group.

Jackie's sense of loss did not last long, once she realized that Martin was safe and could communicate in some ways. Others had real tragedies to deal with. She felt she still had a partner and realized that it would be better for both of them if she cultivated those feelings and showed them often. She did not have to learn to park the car or pay the bills. She and Martin had tried to balance or share roles. She knew about the finances and did not have to scramble to figure them out.

Jackie also tried to find out as much information as she could about stroke and aphasia. She read several pamphlets and books. She did Google searches on the Internet and found information on sites for medical schools and professional associations. She shared some of the information with Julianna and Peter. She brought print-outs to Martin's clinicians. She also found information on therapy procedures that were promoted as

being promising. Because Martin was a professor, Jackie knew to ask if the data at a website was peer reviewed. Over time she learned that she did not have to anticipate every need, and she and Martin became equals again.

Probably the best source of support was a group of family members and aphasic people that met once a month at Martin's hospital. Jackie met wives who had been through the same experience. They shared stories. They laughed. Each meeting had a social time and a formal presentation either by a professional or by a member of the group. She and Martin would go together. He was inspired by seeing others like him talk before the group about a family vacation or a particular problem.

The program at the University of Arizona has included separate voluntary support groups for family members (Holland and Beeson, 1999). These groups are run at various times by clinical psychologists, clinical psychology interns, or social workers. As new members join the group, the more experienced ones share stories of conquering difficulties. Each member discovers that he or she is not alone.

Support groups may have one of the follow sponsors:

- The **American Heart Association** sponsors "Stroke Clubs" that include persons with varied problems (Sanders, Hamby, and Nelson, 1984).
- The **National Aphasia Association,** founded by Martha Taylor Sarno at Rusk Institute of Rehabilitation Medicine in New York City, is promoting community awareness and encouraging the creation of support groups specifically for aphasic persons and their families (www.aphasia.org).
- The **Aphasia Hope Foundation** (www.aphasiahope.org) is a nonprofit organization founded in 1997, and includes a website that provides information for stroke survivors and caregivers, including a forum where anyone can have questions answered by a panel of

professionals. The foundation also lobbies Congress for research funding.

DOCUMENTING FUNCTIONAL OUTCOME

Unless a clinical procedure (e.g., using a phone) is identical to a functional objective (e.g., to improve using the phone), the functional outcome of a treatment is documented with a generalization probe or a report from a family member that the patient is doing something new. A generalization probe is a measure of progress toward an objective. It is not a measure of performance in a treatment. For example, if a goal is "to carry out communicative interactions in the community," then we document observations of communicative interactions in the community.

According to Busch (1993), clinicians should document significant functional change in patient performance for Medicare. The meaning of "significant" can be unclear. Citing the official guidelines, Busch said that it refers to a "measurable and substantial" increase in the patient's level of communication" compared to the level of communication when treatment began. The requirement was not intended to refer to a percentage of improvement on a specific language task.

Holland (1998) suggested that while "third-party intermediaries like to see numbers . . . they have never told us what to count" (p. 846). She added that, besides our "professional obsession with counting linguistic units," we can count "sociolinguistic units of conversation, such as ideas encoded, topics maintained . . . repairs completed, messages transmitted and so forth" (p. 846).

A fairly straightforward approach to documenting social change is to compare what a patient can do before and after therapy. Before therapy, the clinician records specific activities that a patient has discontinued due to stroke or other brain injury. After therapy, the clinician records which of these activities the patient now pursues. For example, a patient may have stopped working after a stroke but, after therapy, has returned to work. Lyon recorded specific activities that were initiated during treatment and then were continued after treatment concluded. These activities included grocery shopping, attending a Stroke Club, maintaining a bank account, participating on a church committee, volunteering at a day-care center, and so on (Lyon et al., 1997).

Social validation is a component of single-subject experiments. It pertains to whether progress reaches "the demands of the social community of which the client is a part" (Kazdin, 1982). Thompson and Byrne (1984) used a probe called a *novel social dyad* to observe production of trained social conventions. The dyad was a five-minute conversation in a "comfortable, non-treatment room" with an unfamiliar person (i.e., undergraduate students). The clinicians also gave the probe to two normal adults as a standard for interpreting peak levels of progress reached by aphasic patients. The wide range of scores exhibited by the controls exposed a problem with interpretation of natural progress: "We really don't know what patients are supposed to do when they go out into the real world because we don't always know what non-brain-damaged people do" (p. 142).

Sarno (1993) urged that we look into using **quality of life** measures (see Chapter 6). In a study of functional progress over a five-month period, Lyon and his colleagues (1997) found no progress with respect to the Boston Exam and the CADL. However, significant change was detected with two nonstandard questionnaires related to goals of the treatment. One measure was a "Communication Readiness and Use Index" that questioned a client's comfort, confidence, and skills when conversing with family members or strangers. The other was a "Psychological Well-Being Index" regarding life satisfaction and general comfort with self and others.

Minimally, reimbursement systems rely on pre- and post-treatment estimates of functional status, especially with the FIM. The American Speech-Language-Hearing Association has developed their own **National Outcomes Measurement System** (NOMS) (Mullen, 2003). An early version of this system was published in a book edited by Carol Frattali called *Measuring Outcomes* *in Speech-Language Pathology* (see Gallagher, 1998).

An essential characteristic of functional outcome is that it should represent a real and meaningful change in a patient's life. This is what Dr. Metter was looking for. There can be a perception of dishonesty in advertising the effects of a language treatment program with a picture-naming score without evidence of change at home. Scherzer (1992) argued that "only successful results will convince politicians that long-term rehabilitation is worth investing in. Therefore, we have to be very careful and absolutely honest in our statements, not exaggerating good results and not venturing out with over-optimistic predictions" (pp. 102–103).

MARTIN'S CONCLUSION

During his rehabilitation, Martin Exeter was receiving encouragement from colleagues in the Netherlands and Belgium. They had been keeping in touch over e-mail. His colleagues were familiar with specialists in aphasia who, in turn, were accustomed to integrating aphasic people into social situations. In Europe, conferences on rehabilitation commonly included professionals and aphasic people. Psycholinguists suggested to Martin that he give an updated version of his speech at a meeting of rehabilitation specialists, many of whom were interested in his specialty of cognitive processing.

At the first hint of resurrecting his speech, Martin refused to consider it seriously because he did not think he could do it. He had not thought much about teaching during the months of arduous work on basic linguistic skills. Although some of his self-imposed treatment involved typing simple letters and other things on his computer, these abilities did not immediately translate into a desire or an attempt to write an article or a lecture. A small paragraph would take hours, especially after editing for spelling errors, grammatical mistakes, and empty words. For e-mail, he would have to compose in his word processor and then import the letter into his e-mail system. All of *this effort was tiring. He could only do a little at a time.*

Eventually Martin's friends suggested that he seek advice and further help from an SLP who was teaching on his campus. Neither he nor his colleagues in the Psychology Department had known much about the Department of Communicative Disorders, which, with hindsight, seemed strange considering that both departments were teaching about cognition and language. Nevertheless, Martin made an appointment with the faculty member who was teaching the aphasia course, Dr. Norma Johnson.

Collegiality and a mutual distaste for pomp quickly put Martin and Norma on a first name basis. After talking with him for a few minutes, Norma recognized that his aphasia was a relatively mild form. She knew that he had retained his knowledge and his recall. He described the circumstances of his stroke and explained his specialty in psychology. He also spoke of frustration in following conversation that seemed too fast for him, especially in a social group when the topic turned to politics. He needed some advice on managing other people in conversations, but his main problem appeared to be a lack of confidence in his ability to convey messages.

Norma was careful. Initially she wanted to see what Martin could do with respect to his area of expertise. She asked him to define basic concepts about memory and describe some memory experiments. Because writing was time-consuming and probably embarrassing in front of her, she gave him a list of terms to define on his computer at home. Martin was surprised when she concluded later that giving the lecture in Belgium was a reasonable goal. He would have to be patient. Writing would always be slow. He may not be ready for this year's conference, but maybe next year. She thought to herself that giving the lecture would be therapeutic in the long run.

Norma gave Martin some assignments and met with him occasionally to assess his work. He practiced writing in steps from definitions to explanations to a structured argument. They talked about the organization of a good lecture. He wrote outlines at home and then showed them to Norma. She found that her main task was to prove to him that his writing was good enough, even though it took time. She pointed out moments in their conversations that sounded like a strong part of a speech. "Just say that in Brussels," she said. Meetings with Norma decreased in frequency. He did speak to her class about his experiences with aphasia. Nine months after their first meeting, he practiced presenting a formal lecture to her.

If she were reporting to an insurance company, Norma would have documented Martin's initial status as "mild aphasia" and "currently not working as a lecturer in psychology." The initial goal was to become a lecturer. Later, documentation of progress would have been that he gave a one-hour lecture to her class.

*Meanwhile, Martin and Jackie were met at the airport in Brussels by one of his psycho-*linguistics colleagues, who drove them to what sounded like the "Marmalade Hotel." When they got there, it turned out to be a Ramada Hotel. Because their flight had been delayed in London, they had only a couple of hours to unpack and rest before a dinner in the city with other hosts and speakers. After dinner, he and Jackie returned to their room where he practiced reading the manuscript, like that night three long years before.*

The next day their host took them to the conference location, which had a long lobby with a glass front and colorful mosaics on the opposite wall inside. In the enormous lecture hall everything was red. Every seat had headphones. Looking up, Martin saw glass booths where interpreters would work. He whispered to Jackie that it felt like the United Nations. Yet, it also felt like Norma Johnson's classroom. When he was introduced, he picked up his outline and left the manuscript at his seat. He walked to the podium with ease. He was ready to get started.

SUMMARY AND CONCLUSIONS

Communicative treatment for aphasia is aimed at helping a patient maximize the capacity to comprehend and convey messages through any means. Functionality comes with the use of communicative capacity in real-life situations. The contexts interacting with the language system are internal and external to a patient. The internal contexts roughly consist of the patient's world knowledge, belief system, and emotional state. The external contexts consist of settings and other people. These contexts suggest a menu of variables that clinicians consider in providing a functional or pragmatic treatment program.

A great deal of functional or pragmatic treatment does not repair damaged language processes or teach something new. Instead, it reduces fear. We walk patients to the end of the diving board and ask them to "look down." It increases confidence in the use of retained capacities or of processes repaired as a result of stimulation. With confidence comes participation. For severely impaired patients, a clinician's job is to determine communicative capacities and then maximize confidence in and opportunities for their accepted use.

MATCHING REVIEW_____

From Chapters 1–10, match the acronym or abbreviation on the right with its best association on the left.

_____	1. quick standardized assessment	a. NAA
_____	2. a grammatical morpheme	b. QoL
_____	3. documentation of syndrome	c. WAB
_____	4. a professional	d. BOSS
_____	5. linguistic treatment for sentences	e. BEST
_____	6. picture of cortical activity	f. fMRI
_____	7. score of aphasia severity	g. TIA
_____	8. CN-oriented assessment battery	h. PALPA
_____	9. ethnographic method	i. AQ
_____	10. emergency clot buster	j. BNT
_____	11. warns of thrombosis	k. CA
_____	12. treatments supported by evidence	l. PACE
_____	13. target for rehabilitation	m. ASHA-FACS
_____	14. information and support organization	n. TUF
_____	15. word-finding assessment	o. TDH
_____	16. payment in managed care	p. EBM
_____	17. communication stress	q. SLP
_____	18. functional scale	r. PPS
_____	19. linguistic theory of agrammatism	s. tPA
_____	20. turn-taking therapy	t. ING

CHAPTER 11

RIGHT HEMISPHERE DISORDERS

In 1974, Associate Supreme Court Justice William O. Douglas suffered a stroke in the right side of his brain (Gardner, 1982). Because he could talk and write, he appeared to recover rapidly. He checked himself out of rehabilitation and was anxious to resume work, claiming his weakened left arm was injured in a fall. Upon returning to the Court, he insisted he was the Chief Justice. In court "he dozed, asked irrelevant questions, and sometimes rambled on." After being asked to resign, "he came back to his office, buzzed for his clerks . . . asked to participate in, draft, and even publish his own opinions separately; and he requested that a tenth seat be placed at the Justices' bench" (p. 310).

For a long time, persons with nondominant or right hemisphere strokes were not referred to speech-language clinics, because their primary disorders are related to nonverbal cognitive systems and they do not display the word-finding and grammatical deficits associated with aphasia. Now, these patients may be referred for the following reasons:

- The patient has a swallowing problem or motor speech deficit.
- Someone with an old right-hemisphere infarct has recently suffered a left-hemisphere stroke.
- The patient has communicative difficulties.

Justice Douglas' rambling talk and failure to appreciate situations might have put him in the third category.

At least two clinical aphasiologists have been prominent in the study of **right hemisphere dysfunction** (RHD) or *right hemisphere syndrome.* Penelope Myers of the Mayo Clinic and Connie Tompkins of the University of Pittsburgh have studied the pragmatic language problems of these patients and have provided extensive analysis of the literature (e.g., Myers, 1999, 2001a; Tompkins, 1995). Myers and Tompkins assisted Margaret Lehman-Blake in reviewing the medical charts of 123 individuals with RHD. Only 45 percent of the patients had been evaluated by a speech-language pathologist (SLP) (Lehman-Blake, Duffy, Tompkins et al., 2003).

Because this chapter begins a set of three dealing with cognitive-communicative disorders, it begins with an introduction to clinical neuropsychology that is relevant for the three chapters. General clinical assessment is followed by segments about the primary cognitive impairments of RHD along with secondary implications for linguistic and communicative functions. The third broad topic of this chapter is the pragmatic language difficulties of RHD. The final topic covers various aspects of rehabilitation.

CLINICAL NEUROPSYCHOLOGY

Because of its important role in assessing the effects of neuropathologies, let us become more familiar with *clinical* neuropsychology. It is a specialized area of practice in clinical psychology and, thus, is different from *cognitive* neuropsychology. Initially, psychologists applied tests used for the evaluation of neurologically intact populations to the assessment of neurologically impaired populations. A chronology of neuropsychological assessment and its origins is shown in Table 11.1.

Unofficial guidelines for training have been published (Bornstein, 1988a, 1988b). A clinical neuropsychologist should be licensed or certi-

TABLE 11.1 Chronology of the development of clinical neuropsychological test batteries, from the early period of applying tests constructed for normal children and adults to a more recent period of tests intended for neurologically impaired populations.

	ASSESSMENT	DESCRIPTION	REFERENCE
1900s	Stanford-Binet Intelligence Scale	Terman's revision of the first intelligence test (in France) at Stanford University; some use with brain-damaged patients	Terman and Merrill (1937)
1930s	Weisenburg and McBride	First comparison of aphasic patients to normals with standardized tests	Weisenburg and McBride (1935)
1940s	Wechsler-Bellevue Scale	Developed at Bellevue Hospital in New York City; used in hospitals during World War II	
	Armed services test batteries	Screening of newly enlisted personnel; origin of some neuropsychological tests	
1950s	Wechsler Adult Intelligence Scale (WAIS)	Refinement of Weschler-Bellevue Scale; became the core neuropsychological test	
1970s	Halstead-Reitan Neuropsychological Test Battery	6–7 hours of tests, including the WAIS; standardized for neuropsychological evaluation	Reitan and Wolfson (1993)
	Mini-Mental State Exam (MMSE)	Brief standardized screening evaluation	Folstein, Folstein, and McHugh (1975)
1980s	WAIS-R	Revision of WAIS	
	Luria-Nebraska Neuropsychological Battery	Controversial standardization of Luria's informal clinical tests	Golden, Hammeke, and Purisch (1980)
1990s	Cognistat	Bedside screening taking 20–30 minutes	Kiernan and others (1987)
	WAIS-III	Second revision	Wechsler (1997a)
2000s	WAIS-IV	In development; tryout research	

fied as a psychologist in the state where he or she practices. The American Board of Professional Psychology (ABPP) certifies clinical psychologists and recognizes specialty certification by the American Board of Professional Neuropsychology (ABPN) established in 1981. The credential is called a *diplomat in clinical neuropsychology.*

Qualifications is one issue addressed by Stern (1995) in an article advising attorneys on how to conduct a direct examination of a neuropsychologist in a trial. For example, someone with traumatic brain injury may be seeking compensation from a defendant. Stern explained that the neuropsychologist compares test findings to the patient's academic, vocational, medical, and psychiatric records to estimate the effect of injury on cognition and personality and on social and emotional behavior. State jurisdictions vary as to whether a neuropsychologist is allowed to render opinions regarding the status of the brain and its relationship to function. However, many states do permit a clinical neuropsychologist to discuss, for example, the function of the frontal lobe, how it can be injured, and what the residual impairments are likely to be.

Probably the most common comprehensive battery for brain-damaged patients is the **Wechsler Adult Intelligence Scale,** now in its third edition as the **WAIS-III** (Wechsler, 1997a; see also, Kaufman and Lichtenberger, 1999). The battery has maintained its basic structure (Table 11.2), but three subtests have been added, partly to beef up assessment of working memory and processing speed. The WAIS-III is divided into verbal and performance scales. Three main scores consist of the Full Scale IQ (FSIQ), and the VIQ and PIQ for the verbal and performance sections. The difference between the VIQ and PIQ, called the *discrepancy score,* is of interest when someone has unilateral brain damage. A patient with left hemisphere damage is likely to have a lowered VIQ relative to the PIQ, and someone with right hemisphere damage is likely to present the reverse (Hom and Reitan, 1990). Several studies have shown that any discrepancy occurs more for men than for women, who tend to have little difference between the VIQ and PIQ, no matter

TABLE 11.2 Subtests of the Wechsler Adult Intelligence Scale (WAIS-III). The verbal and performance sections have been interpreted as corresponding roughly to left hemisphere and right hemisphere functions. New subtests are in boldface.

VERBAL (VIQ)		PERFORMANCE (PIQ)	
Subtest	*Description*	*Subtest*	*Description*
Information	Answer questions about knowledge generally available in the United States	Digit Symbol	Using a key of number–symbol pairs, write the paired symbol beneath the numbers in 90 secs (i.e., a speed test)
Comprehension	Answer questions requiring common sense, reasoning, and proverb interpretation	Picture Completion	Tell what is missing from pictures of common objects or scenes
Arithmetic	Complete verbal math problems (i.e., story problems)	Block Design	Using colored blocks, reproduce a pattern shown by examiner or in pictures
Similarities	Explain what a pair of words has in common	Picture Arrangement	Arrange cartoon pictures in a sequence that tells a story
Digit Span	Repeat number sequences forward and backward	Object Assembly	Assemble parts into an object; scored for time and accuracy (optional timed test)
Vocabulary	Verbally provide the meanings of increasingly difficult words	**Symbol Search**	Rapidly find target symbol in a group
Letter–Number Sequencing	Read alternating letters and numbers in order	**Matrix Reasoning**	Pattern completion; like Raven's CPM (p. 251)

which side of the brain is damaged (e.g., Sundet, 1986).

One new subtest, called Matrix Reasoning, has its origins in Raven's (1938/1965) *Progressive Matrices,* which are familiar to SLPs as a nonverbal predictor of intelligence with a long history of use with aphasic patients. One segment of Raven's test, called the Coloured Progressive Matrices (CPM), has the patient figure out geometric patterns in order to identify a missing piece. Kertesz and McCabe (1975) discovered that people with moderate-to-mild aphasia were comparable to those with RHD. Aphasic patients with severe comprehension deficit were substantially deficient with the CPM.

Clinical psychologists begin with the WAIS when using the **Halstead-Reitan Neuropsychological Test Battery** (Reitan and Wolfson, 1993). This battery contains the WAIS and additional tests of attention, rhythm, and thinking. A personality inventory and an aphasia screening test are also included. Reitan's company has provided a computerized *Neuropsychological Deficit Scale* for facilitating interpretation of raw scores. Other software transforms scores into an image of the probable site of lesion.

A clinical neuropsychologist can choose from several tests for specific cognitive functions; the total array can be appreciated only by seeing a handbook covering the landscape (e.g., Lezak, Howieson, Loring, Hannay, and Fischer, 2004; Snyder and Nussbaum, 1998; Spreen and Strauss, 1998). Some of the specific tests are introduced here in the last three chapters.

In her review of records for patients with RHD, Lehman-Blake and others (2002) found that deficits of attention, perception, memory, and reasoning were reported most frequently (i.e., more than 60 percent of the cases). These areas of difficulty run the gamut of cognition, except for language processing. Subsequent analysis indicated that these diagnoses tended to be made by clinical neuropsychologists and others.

Speech-language pathologists tended to be the professionals who would identify deficits of prosody and interpersonal interaction (Lehman-Blake et al., 2003). Such communication difficulties had

been noted in fewer than 20 percent of the patients' charts. Overall, the investigators concluded that the same deficit may be viewed differently by different professionals and that other professionals do not tend to recognize communication deficits in patients with right hemisphere stroke. Also, SLPs are trained to see certain cognitive problems as communication disorders. There does not seem to be a consensus on what constitutes a right hemisphere syndrome (Myers, 2001b).

Considering the occasional variation of research findings appearing later in this chapter, one apparent issue is the basis for selection of cases for research participation or retrospective chart reviews. Some disagreement has arisen as to whether selection should be neurologically oriented based on a range of RH lesion sites (Brady, Armstrong, and Mackenzie, 2005) or cognitively oriented based on an area of deficit (Myers, 2001b). The investigator's choice may influence the extent to which a deficit is found. Also, findings may differ depending on whether participants had been referred to rehabilitation. Brady and her colleagues (2005) noted that in Scotland very few people with RHD are referred for communication assessment. Resolution of the issue may come in the form of valuing each approach for a particular purpose and interpreting results within the context of the selection method.

AWARENESS OF DEFICITS

Justice Douglas's insistence on continuing his Supreme Court duties indicates either a lack of awareness or a denial of disability. McGlynn and Schacter (1989) distinguished among phenomena associated with unawareness. The term **anosognosia** refers to a lack of awareness or recognition of disease or disability. Clinicians have used other terms such as *lack of insight* or *imperception of disease.* In general, patients are unable to become aware of a neurological dysfunction. A different problem is the **denial of impairment,** which is a psychological defense mechanism; a patient who is strictly in denial is considered to be capable of awareness of deficit.

Anosognosia is usually observed as lack of awareness of paralysis. For example, a patient with left hemiplegia makes plans to play golf (Tompkins, 1995). However, unawareness of right hemiplegia by LHDs is rare (Cutting, 1978). Pendley and Ramsberger (1996) created a six-point scale to measure self-awareness of task performances with respect to self-correction behavior and response to a clinician's questions. They found that RHDs were impaired relative to a normal control group and that self-awareness was not correlated with actual task performance.

Myers (2001a) described a patient who will "deny a need for rehabilitative services, refusing to take his physical limitations seriously . . . He may talk about returning to work next week, yet be unable to transfer himself from bed to wheelchair" (p. 809). Another patient may not recognize his paralyzed limbs as his own. Myers suggested that this behavior is part of a disorder called left neglect, which is presented next. Symptoms appear to overlap diagnoses.

LEFT NEGLECT AND READING

We may see a patient who is "only half made-up, the left side of her face absurdly void of lipstick and rouge" (Sacks, 1985, p. 74). Neglect of one-half of space is caused by damage in the parieto-temporal region. It is more frequent and/or obvious after RHD, so that **left neglect** is more common than right neglect. Patients with posterior RHD bump into things on their left, leave food on the left side of the plate, dress only the right side, and draw only the right side of an object. Left neglect was noted in 63 percent of the cases reviewed by Lehman-Blake and others (2003).

Clinical detection of left neglect includes a **crossing out test** of marking lines through circles scattered about a page. A person with left neglect crosses out circles on the right, ignoring the circles on the left. Severity of neglect is measured by the number of omissions. With lines scattered about a page, called the **line cancellation test,** Plourde and others (1993) showed that some RHDs have severe neglect and others have no or very mild

neglect, with very few in between. Most patients with LHD exhibited no or mild neglect.

In a **line bisection test,** a patient is asked to mark the center of a horizontal line. Someone with left neglect marks to the right of midline. Patients with severe neglect perform this task differently than those with mild neglect. Patients with mild neglect vary their mark slightly as line length and position vary, but those with severe neglect mark the line at a consistent distance from the right end (Koyama, Ishiai, Seki, and Nakayama, 1997).

Manipulation of visuospatial attention is demonstrated with a *cued line-bisection test* in which some lines have letters at the right end, others have letters at the left end, and other lines have letters at both ends (Harvey, Milner, and Roberts, 1995). Patients are instructed to name the letter cues, called "anchors," and then bisect a line in the middle as accurately as possible. There is a bias toward the cued end, even for people without neglect. Harvey was interested in the effect of these cues for patients who already have a tendency to bisect to the right. Unilateral left cues decreased the extent of rightward error as if "dragging" attention leftward. Unilateral right cues did not increase the rightward error. This study provides a hint as to how patients with RHD are trained to compensate for left neglect.

Anosognosia for hemiplegia could be construed as being a symptom of left neglect. However, neglect and anosognosia do not necessarily occur together, and some patients with neglect are aware of their problem (McGlynn and Schacter, 1989). A double dissociation between left neglect and anosognosia for paralysis was demonstrated among 97 patients with RHD (Bisiach, Vallar, Perani et al., 1986). Thirty-two of these patients had little or no neglect to account for substantial anosognosia, whereas four patients ignored the left side of the body but were fully aware of motor impairment.

Neglect is thought to be a disorder of selective or focused attention and, thus, is often called *hemi-inattention.* Focusing attention is managed by "special-purpose" attentional systems in specific functional systems. That is, we have a spatial attention mechanism and an auditory attention mechanism. The visual attention mechanism is like a spotlight with an adjustable beam.

Posner discovered that *covert attention,* or the cognitive spotlight, is impaired, rather than overt, shifts of eye movement (Posner, Walker, Friedrich, and Rafal, 1984, 1987). In Posner's theory, there are three stages in shifting covert attention:

1. disengagement from a current focus
2. moving attention to a target
3. engagement of the target

A right parietal lesion prohibits disengagement from a current focus in the right visual field. Visual cues are thought to facilitate disengagement, permitting movement of the internal spotlight to information in the left field (see Arguin and Bub, 1993).

A sense for the internal spotlight was provided by Bisiach and others (1981) in Milan, Italy. In the clinic they asked patients with RHD to imagine the familiar Piazza del Duomo, a large square commanded at one end by a 600-year-old cathedral. Asked to report buildings on each side, patients could report buildings on the right but not on the left. Intact stored structural description of the neglected buildings was exhibited when the patients imagined the piazza facing the opposite direction. Now, the previously neglected buildings were reported from the right side, whereas the previously reported buildings were ignored.

An indication that spatial attention is a special system occurs with American Sign Language (ASL). One RHD patient "correctly uses the left side of signing space to represent syntactic relations, despite her neglect of left hemispace in non-language tasks" (Klima, Bellugi, and Poizner, 1988, p. 323).

Right-hemisphere damaged individuals with or without clinically diagnosed neglect drove through a wheelchair obstacle course in the courtyard of a rehabilitation center. Obstacles were folding chairs on either side of corridors, and errors were recorded as direct hits or sideswipes. Both groups sideswiped more chairs on the left than the right, and subjects with obvious neglect made more direct hits than those without obvious neglect. All RHDs also made more errors than LHDs who had to steer mainly with the nondominant hand. Some RHDs were taught to scan the course before starting and while driving. The training reduced their direct hits but not their sideswipes (Webster, Cottam, Gouvier et al., 1988).

An SLP should watch for the influence of neglect when evaluating language. Neglect can affect any test requiring the scanning of a visual array. Word comprehension errors disappeared for many RHDs when investigators controlled for neglect of the left side of picture displays (Gainotti, Caltagirone, and Miceli, 1983). The clinician can arrange pictures vertically to the right side or can verbally cue a patient to shift gaze leftward.

Both left hemianopia (see Chapter 2) and left neglect interfere with processing stimuli in the left hemispace. The former is a sensory impairment affecting the ability to see left of center and can be referred to as "field-cut." These patients are aware of the problem and on their own try to compensate with eye movement. Left neglect, on the other hand, is an attentional impairment. "Patients fail to report stimuli in the neglected area, not because they cannot see them, but because they do not *notice* them" (Myers, 1999, p. 30). These patients are often unaware of the problem and have to be prompted to compensate.

One method for distinguishing a left field-cut from left neglect is to have the patient direct gaze to the left (putting formerly left objects into the center or right field) and then to the right. If an apparent field-cut disappears upon shifting gaze back to the right, then the problem is neglect. However, if the patient still cannot report objects in the left field, then the disorder is hemianopia which "moves with the eyes" (Myers, 1999).

"A *rose* is a *rose* or a *nose*" (Patterson and Wilson, 1990). Some people with RHD misread the beginning of words (Riddoch, Humphreys, Cleton, and Ferry, 1990). Other patients omit or misread words on the left side of a page. Some patients have both types of problems (Ellis, Flude, and Young, 1987; Young, Newcombe, and Ellis, 1991). Misreading the left side of words or the left side of a page are symptoms of **neglect dyslexia,** also classified as a peripheral dyslexia. Rare cases of right neglect dyslexia with LHD have been reported (e.g., Warrington, 1991).

One test is to present words that can still be words when the first letter is omitted or substituted (e.g, *blight*). Case VB understood targets according to the errors (e.g., *blight* as "light"), indicating that the impairment was in an early point in the process, such as perception or recognition. Of the errors, 66 percent were clear left-side errors, usually substitutions of the first one or two letters irrespective of word length (e.g., "slain" for *train,* "pillow" for *yellow*). A patient may have many more errors reading orthographically legal nonwords than real words (Arguin and Bub, 1997).

Cubelli and Beschin (2005) wondered how patients with left neglect would deal with the last syllable stress marking used in Italian for distinguishing between words such as *papa* for pope and *papà* for *dad.* Six patients read lists of words and nonwords with or without the accent mark, and they exhibited the neglect effect in which most errors were the deletion of the initial letter. Three patients were better reading accented words. One had the opposite effect, and two showed no difference. Thus, patients with left neglect have different patterns regarding the right-sided accent marking, with some being aided by it. In fact, there are very subtle variations of neglect dyslexia (Hillis, Newhart, Heidler et al., 2005).

Are words in the neglected space processed at an automatic level? This question was addressed with a priming task in which the prime was a pictured object (e.g., a bat) presented 400 msec before a semantically related target (e.g., *ball*) (McGlinchey-Berroth, Milberg, Verfaellie et al., 1993). A twist in this study was that the prime was shown in either the left or right visual field. To avoid stimulus-biased attentional adjustments, a nonsense drawing was always presented in the other field. Four patients with left neglect displayed normal semantic priming with primes presented to either field. Thus, neglect was thought to be a disruption of controlled or intentional processing.

What is the effect of left neglect on "reading" American Sign Language? Patient JH was partially deaf since birth and learned ASL in a residential school for the deaf. He was working for an aircraft manufacturer when he suffered a stroke in his right hemisphere. Corina, Kritchevsky, and Bellugi (1996) compared his lateralized sign identification with object recognition. His recognition of objects was strongly affected by neglect, but recognition of signs was not affected. This dissociation is another demonstration that the visuospatial modality per se is not as significant functionally as the system underlying use of the modality. For JH, the intact left hemisphere's linguistic system appears to have overridden the visual attention deficit.

VISUOSPATIAL ORIENTATION

Persons with RHD suddenly find it difficult to find their way around, especially in the unfamiliar maze of hospital corridors. With **topographic disorientation,** a patient fails to orient to the immediate environment. The patient also has difficulty reading maps, remembering familiar routes, and learning new ones. This disorder can be attributed to an inability to recognize landmarks, but it also occurs when object recognition is preserved (Ellis and Young, 1988). Lehman-Blake and others (2003) found orientation problems in 43 percent of their reviewed records. This type of disorientation is identified to contrast with *geographic disorientation,* in which a patient relates to immediate surroundings but fails to conceptualize general locale.

Topographic disorientation can differ in subtle ways depending on the precise location of damage in the posterior right hemisphere. One site of lesion can cause a "way finding" problem in familiar and novel environments, whereas another site of lesion can cause difficulty orienting mainly in novel environments such as the hospital (Nyffeler, Gutbrod, Pflugshaupt et al., 2005).

The appearance of disorientation occurs with "false memories" in which a patient asserts the existence of two or more places with the same attributes but only one of them exists in reality. Patterson and Mack (1985) reported a case with RHD who described several hospitals in the area where he lived that were similar to his rehabilitation hospital. One was a "floating hospital." It is as if a real place is duplicated in the patient's mind. The problem is known as *reduplicative paramnesia.*

CONSTRUCTIONAL SKILLS

Impairments of visuospatial motor functions, such as drawing or building something, are called **constructional apraxia.** The most common clinical test is a drawing task. Copying figures is preferred over drawing on command, because the former is less influenced by cultural variations. RHDs have lower scores than LHDs on the shape copying subtest of the PICA. In other tests, a patient may be asked to draw a clock, house, or flower. Clinical neuropsychologists may present a Picasso-like abstraction called the Rey-Osterrieth figure to be copied. The block design subtest of the WAIS is also used as a test of constructional skill.

First let us consider motor impairments that might interfere with constructional abilities. Anteriorly damaged RHDs are likely to have left hemiparesis, but the unimpaired right side is usually preferred for writing and drawing. Also, limb apraxia is relatively rare with RHD. Estimates vary from no patients with this disorder (DeRenzi et al., 1969) to 27 percent (Duffy and Duffy, 1989), whereas 68 percent of LHDs may be impaired. This variation is probably due to inconsistent criteria for diagnosing impairment of praxis. Regardless of criteria, we can say that RHDs are less likely than LHDs to have praxic interference with visuospatial skills.

Early comparisons of RHDs and LHDs showed the opposite hemispheric asymmetry regarding constructional apraxia. There was a higher prevalence of constructional apraxia in RHDs than LHDs (e.g., Arrigoni and DeRenzi, 1964). In a study of drawing objects from memory, RHDs had lower recognizability scores than LHDs (Grossman, 1988). In other studies, the

two groups turned out to be similar regarding the presence of drawing defiency, with a 30 to 40 percent prevalence in each group (e.g., Arena and Gainotti, 1978; Carlesimo et al., 1993). Patients with copying deficit have particular difficulty with three-dimensional figures such as a cube (Griffiths, Cook, and Newcombe, 1988).

RHDs and LHDs differ in qualitative features of their drawing deficits. For example, RHDs neglect the left side of a figure and are more likely to have poor spatial relationships among parts. LHDs draw more deliberately, overly simplify drawings, and preserve spatial relationships among parts (Gainotti, and Tiacci, 1970). In drawing a person, RHDs are disorganized and embellish with extraneous detail (Swindell et al., 1988). Gardner (1982) described RHDs' artistry as "fragmented and disconnected drawing, whose parts, while often recognizable, do not flow or fit together into an organized whole" (pp. 322–323). In general, parietal RHDs draw details incoherently, whereas parietal LHDs omit details in a coherent structure.

What is the effect of RHD on the use of ASL, especially the spatially configured syntactic component? In one study, three RH-damaged signers were impaired in comprehension of syntax but not other components of the language. However, they were "flawless" in production of syntactic and other features of ASL (Poizner et al., 1987). Better production than comprehension is one of those exceptions to the typical pattern for aphasia (see Figure 1.1), which indicates that the comprehension problem was due to something other than language disorder. Problems with visuospatial perception may interfere with comprehension of ASL. Otherwise, like hearing individuals, RHD spares fundamental aspects of the use of a language.

PROBLEMS WITH SOUND

Right-hemisphere-damaged individuals are generally normal in recognition of common sounds (Faglioni, Spinnler, and Vignolo, 1969; Spinnler and Vignolo, 1966). Like visual object agnosia,

agnosia for environmental sounds usually occurs with bilateral damage (Bauer and Rubens, 1985).

Persons with severe aphasia may have normal nonverbal sound recognition or have a severe auditory agnosia along with the language comprehension deficit (Faglioni et al., 1969; Varney, 1980). Difficulties may be related to verbal mediation. Riege and others (1980) found that aphasic patients with impaired word comprehension were normal in recognizing sounds that would be difficult to label (i.e., bird calls). Auditory agnosia does not seem to be connected to language dysfunction. When it occurs in aphasic persons, it is a distinct disorder that is an "accident of location" of lesion.

The right temporal lobe seems to be responsible for storing and activating familiar melodies. When neurosurgeons used tiny electrodes to stimulate this region, the patients reported hearing an orchestra or a choir (Penfield and Perot, 1963). Sacks (1985) described an elderly woman with a right temporal infarction. In the early months after her stroke, she woke up to hearing familiar songs even though she was nearly deaf and no radio was on. She would ask "Is the radio in my head?" Sacks called this a "musical epilepsy."

Sidtis and Volpe (1988) detected that RHDs were impaired in pitch pattern perception but not speech perception, whereas aphasic patients had difficulty with speech but not tones. A problem with music after an RH stroke, called **amusia,** is focused on melody rather than lyrics. It is also called *music agnosia* (Peretz, 2001). In one study, LH damage caused more problems in recognizing music with familiar lyrics than RH damage. However, RHDs did worse than LHDs in recognizing music without commonly known lyrics such as "Hail to the Chief" (Gardner and Denes, 1973). This study indicated that familiar lyrics are encoded when listening to melodies, a mental skill that helps RHDs but hinders LHDs (see Winner and von Kardyi, 1998).

Imitation of rhythm tapping is part of the Boston Exam for aphasia. People with RHD and LHD have been shown to differ with respect to **pitch** and **rhythm.** Early research indicated that pitch processing is more susceptible to RH damage and, to a lesser degree, rhythm processing is more susceptible to LH damage (Shapiro, Grossman, and Gardner, 1981). Years later, Alcock and her colleagues (2000) compared RHDs and LHDs with perception and production tasks. Production was tested for single-note production (pitch), singing melodies, and manual and oral rhythm production. RHDs were impaired in all three areas of perception but only slightly with pitch and rhythm. They were distinctively impaired producing pitch and melodies, especially those without well-known words. LHDs with aphasia were slightly impaired in discriminating melodies and were distinctively impaired in rhythm production. So far, it appears that pitch and rhythm differentiate RHD and LHD more clearly with production than with perception.

The *Seashore Rhythm Test* (SRT) is incorporated in the Halstead-Reitan battery. It requires patients to discriminate between pairs of musical beats. In clinical circles, it was believed that this test is sensitive to unilateral RH damage. However, two studies have shown that LH- and RH-damaged groups do not differ with the SRT (Karzmark, Heaton, Lehman, and Crouch, 1985; Sherer, Parsons, Nixon, and Adams, 1991). RHDs do appear to have more difficulty than LHDs on the less frequently used *Seashore Tonal Memory Test* (STM), in which patients are asked to discriminate between pairs of three- to five-note melodies (Karzmark et al., 1985).

Prior, Kinsella, and Giese (1990) compared RHDs and LHDs with respect to a small battery of music tests. The tests included perception of pitch and rhythm variation in familiar and unfamiliar tunes, as well as production tasks involving imitated tapping and singing familiar and unfamiliar songs. Results were mixed, as comprehensive impairments occurred with LHD and RHD. Both groups were impaired in imitative tapping and singing familiar tunes. LHDs were more impaired than RHDs in rhythm perception and singing unfamiliar melodies.

The French composer Maurice Ravel was stricken by Wernicke's aphasia. He continued to recognize melodies, but was no longer able to compose. He could not read notes or perform from a score (Gardner, 1982). Although individuals with aphasia can have a music-processing impairment, generally people with aphasia retain purely musical competencies; whereas RH damage causes problems with melodies while retaining the ability to deal with symbolic codes (Botez, Botez, and Aube, 1980).

What about the sound of a person's voice? Two tasks have been used to study *speaker recognition* in brain-damaged people. One was a discrimination test in which patients were asked to tell if two voices were the same or different. The other task involved recognizing famous voices (Van Lancker, Kreiman, and Cummings, 1989). Impairment of discrimination or recognition was called **phonagnosia.** Temporal lobe damage in either hemisphere caused voice discrimination deficit. Impaired recognition of famous voices was associated with right parietal lobe damage. Even globally aphasic persons were able to recognize the voices of Johnny Carson or John F. Kennedy.

EMOTION AND PROSODY *Skipped*

The neurology of emotion is a complex interaction of systems. It is a feeling in the gut of limbic and autonomic nervous systems and is a message recognized in cognitive cortex. Both hemispheres have been shown to contribute to emotional qualities of behavior, but the RH is dominant (Silberman and Weingartner, 1986). Persons with RHD may display a flat affect or indifference that often accompanies left neglect (Gainotti, 1972). Based on measures of skin response, heart rate, and respiration, RHDs demonstrated **hypoarousal** to tactile stimulation (Heilman, Schwartz, and Watson, 1978) and emotional pictures (Morrow, Vrtunski, Kim, and Boller, 1981). In their chart review, Lehman-Blake and others (2003) found a diagnosis of "hyporesponsive" in about 40 percent of the cases. Myers (2001a) has identified hypoarousal with a reduction of alertness or attention to surroundings.

Recognition and expression of emotion are important ingredients of meaning exchanged in communicative interactions. In the clinical literature, any clinical test may be said to address emotion broadly, or investigators consider it useful to focus on emotion conveyed through facial expression, speech intonation, or the semantic content behind words. A deficit across all vehicles would be a strong case for a central impairment of emotion.

For cognitive testing, patients are usually examined for recognition of primary emotional expressions in faces, such as happiness, sadness, and anger. RHDs have been found to have difficulty recognizing and remembering facial expressions and recognizing the emotional significance of pictured situations (Cicone, Wapner, and Gardner, 1980; Dekosky, Heilman, Bowers, and Valenstein, 1980; Weddell, 1989). Dissociation of autonomic and cognitive systems was indicated when hypoarousal did not necessarily co-occur with deficient recognition of facial emotion (Zoccolotti, Scabini, and Violani, 1982).

People with LHD and RHD demonstrated deficits in identifying emotional words and sentences, but the deficit in RHDs was more pronounced (Borod, Andelman, Obler et al., 1992). A later study indicated that subcortical damage may be necessary to produce an emotion-recognition deficit. Ten RHDs and ten LHDs participated in three recognition tasks (half of each group had subcortical in addition to cortical lesions). Emotive sentences conveyed sadness (e.g., *I'm going to miss you when you leave*), happiness (e.g., *I can hardly believe I passed the test*), and anger (e.g., *I want you to stop harassing me*). The same emotions were presented with facial expressions and with prosody in another task. Response for all tasks was pointing to words representing each emotion. Participants with only cortical lesions performed these tasks without difficulty. Participants with additional subcortical lesions had deficits with one exception. Only the RHD subcortical group was impaired in recognizing emotion of facial expressions (Karow, Marquardt, and Marshall, 2001).

With respect to expression of feeling, Gainotti (1972) described some patients with RHD as having a flat affect, perhaps indicative of hypoarousal. Facial reactions of RHDs were inaccurate in response to pictures of familiar people, pleasant and unpleasant scenes, and unusual photographic effects (Buck and Duffy, 1980). The expression of emotions appears to be unrelated to recognition of emotion (Borod, Koff, Perlman-Lorch, and Nicholas, 1986). Blonder and others (1993) compared RHDs and LHDs during interviews along with their spouses in their homes. Facial expressions were videotaped. The RHDs demonstrated less facial expressivity than the LHDs, particularly with respect to smiles and laughter.

RHD and LHD transform mood differently with respect to positive or negative valence of emotion or mood. RHDs tend to joke and laugh excessively, a change in a "positive" direction. Aphasic LHDs can be depressive and may cry excessively (Gainotti, 1972). In one study, depression was greatest with anterior LHD. Some RHDs react to cartoons with excessive hilarity, and others are unresponsive (Gardner, Ling, Flamm, and Silverman, 1975). Posterior RHDs may be more depressed than anterior RHDs, who can be "unduly cheerful" and apathetic about their disorders (Robinson, Kubos, Starr et al., 1984). Prevailing mood may be related to awareness of deficit.

Along with facial expression, we express our emotions through the intonation or prosody of our speech. Is the disorder of hypoarousal manifested in the sound of a patient's voice? Does the cognitive impairment of recognition occur with auditory input as well as in the look on others' faces? Furthermore, can emotional and linguistic prosody be dissociated by focal brain damage?

A disorder called **aprosodia** has been diagnosed in RHDs. Like classifying aphasias, Ross (1981) proposed that there are receptive and expressive forms of this deficit associated with posterior and anterior lesions, respectively. Some patients speak in a flat intonational contour or monotone (e.g., Ross and Mesulam, 1979). Some patients are deficient in identifying emotional tone

in mundane sentences, detected in tasks requiring pointing to a happy, sad, or angry face (Heilman, Bowers, Speedie, and Coslett, 1984; Schlanger, Schlanger, and Gerstman, 1976; Tucker, Watson, and Heilman, 1977). Much more recently, Pell (2006) compared RHDs and LHDs with three emotion-recognition tasks. LHDs had difficulty recognizing emotion conveyed in linguistic meanings, whereas RHDs had a more pervasive deficit for recognizing emotional prosody.

Linguistic prosody includes stress and juncture markers of meaning and sentence structure. A few investigators have pursued the question of whether affective and linguistic prosody can be dissociated in RHD. Some studies indicated that RH damage spares linguistic prosody in receptive and expressive tasks. RHDs comprehended lexical stress normally (e.g., *blackboard, black board*), and most had no problem producing lexical stress (Behrens, 1988; Emmorey, 1987). They produced contrastive stress when answering "who did what" questions. Others could read aloud declarative sentence contours (Cooper, Soares, Nicol et al., 1984).

Other researchers found somewhat surprising problems with linguistic prosody. Using a reading task, Shapiro and Danly (1985) concluded that RHDs have deficits in producing sentence contours as well as affective prosody. Bryan (1989) found RHDs, especially with parietal lesions, who were impaired in comprehending and producing lexical stress (e.g., *con*vict, con*vict*) and discriminating and recognizing sentence contours. Behrens (1989) studied a wider variety of sentence contours with a different task (i.e., story completion). Her RHDs were deficient for producing declaratives and yes/no questions but had no problem with imperatives and *wh*-questions. A deficit for syntactic contours may only be partial.

The study of linguistic prosody expanded when Walker and her colleagues (2002) looked at lexical stress, sentence-type contours, and the use of pauses to clarify syntactically ambiguous sentences. An example of the syntactic ambiguity follows:

(1) The boy said the girl is fat.
  (a) The boy said, the girl is fat.
  (b) The boy, said the girl, is fat.

The two possible interpretations are indicated by the commas in 1a and 1b. The task was to point to the picture that goes with the sentence. LHDs were significantly worse than RHDs for all three types of prosody. The study supported the expected double dissociation when RHDs proved worse than LHDs in recognizing emotional prosody.

Baum and Dwivedi (2003) felt that Walker's off-line tasks provided an incomplete view of prosody in syntactic processing, especially because structural assignment probably occurs long before a person points to a picture. Baum and Dwivedi used garden-path sentences very much like those used in psycholinguistic studies of syntactic parsing. One example follows:

(2) The workers considered the last offer from the management was a real insult.

Prosody (or inserting *that* after the first verb) would disambiguate the sentence. A cross-modal priming task was used to determine if prosody facilitates the assignment of structure. Unlike Walker's results, both LHDs and RHDs showed deficits relative to controls.

Investigators have looked for a logical double dissociation, namely, that RHD involves a deficit of emotional but not linguistic prosody and LHD involves a deficit of linguistic but not emotional prosody. So, researchers began to compare linguistic and affective prosody with both RHDs and LHDs (e.g., Walker et al., 2002). In an investigation of comprehension, Pell and Baum (1997) found neither group to have a deficit for emotional prosody. LHDs had a problem with linguistic cues. Also, acoustic analysis showed that RHDs and LHDs utilized duration, fundamental frequency, and amplitude to produce affective and linguistic cues (Baum and Pell, 1997). These researchers could not support previous claims that impairments in comprehending or producing affective tone are common features of RHD.

Geigenberger and Ziegler (2001) used three receptive prosody tasks to compare relatively large groups of RHD and LHD patients. For emotional prosody, participants were asked to identify a general positive or negative feeling in utterances. For pragmatic prosody, they reacted to appropriate and inappropriate prosodic cues for conversational turn taking. For linguistic prosody, they comprehended sentences containing emphatic stress. Both clinical groups displayed receptive deficits for prosody, with RHDs performing worse. Patterns of deficit distinguished the groups. RHDs had more problem with emotional and pragmatic prosody. LHD aphasic participants were impaired in the linguistic task and unimpaired in the more pragmatic tasks, providing a clearer dissociation between emotional and linguistic prosody in the traditionally predicted direction. Turn-taking prosody was a fairly unique feature of the study.

There have been a few attempts to review and analyze the research. Based on studies conducted through the 1990s, Baum and Pell (1999) concluded that LH-stroke, not RH-stroke, can cause an impairment in the comprehension and production of linguistic stress. However, both LHD and RHD may include a deficit in processing emotional prosody, probably for different reasons. Partly because methods have been inconsistent, a clear double dissociation has not been demonstrated consistently. Wunderlich, Ziegler, and Geigenberger (2003) suspected that difficulties with LHD may be attributed to the reliance on explicit tasks rather than their prosody abilities. Comparing implicit and explicit processing may present a different picture.

Seddoh (2002) wrote an essay that was critical of the use of linguistically established notions of prosody and intonation in relation to emotion and language. One problem is that researchers have used the terms *intonation* and *prosody* interchangeably, whereas it is more correct to consider intonation to be an element of prosody. The present discussion has probably been guilty of this error. A bigger problem is that researchers have failed to recognize an overlap between emotional and linguistic intonation. Thus, attempts to make a distinction between language and emotion may have to be reconsidered. Let us wait and see if Seddoh's instruction improves future study.

SPEAKER MEANING

The pragmatics of language use, especially in conversation, entails an exchange of speaker meanings (Chapter 6). That is, communication involves transmitting a message in the mind of a sender to the mind of a receiver. Instead of "message," authors may refer to a **communicative intention** (e.g., Sabbagh, 1999). Figuring out the message or intent necessarily involves relating a linguistic form to an external or internal context. These principles inform the construction of an experiment that addresses pragmatic language use (e.g., nonliteral meanings and/or contextual manipulation). Furthermore, explanations draw from the same theories used to account for regular language processing. That is, the same mind is used. For example, a person is still activating meanings stored in a semantic network.

This section starts with comprehension of single words. Some studies focus on RHD in comparison to matched neurologically intact controls. As introduced early in Chapter 4, this comparison allows for determination of deficits. Other studies consist of comparisons between RHDs and aphasic LHDs, allowing for determination of whether the deficit is a unique component of the RHD syndrome.

Metaphor is an example of nonliteral meaning that can be studied simply at the word level. The study of metaphor comprehension began with presentation of phrases like *heavy heart* and *colorful music*. Aphasic subjects chose nonliteral meanings more often than literal meanings and scoffed at absurd literal options. RHDs often exhibited the opposite pattern. They could paraphrase intent of the phrases but still chose pictured literal meanings more often than aphasic patients (Winner and Gardner, 1977). In another study, idioms were more difficult to comprehend than novel sentences, whereas LHDs again displayed the opposite pattern (Van Lanker and Kempler, 1987).

Clinical researchers also examined connotative or suggestive meaning. When choosing the most similar pair of words in a triad (e.g., *loving-hateful-warm*), RHDs relied on denotation (e.g., *loving-hateful*) more than connotation (e.g., *loving-warm*). In contrast, aphasic LHDs relied on connotation more than denotation. Normal controls used both meaning components (Brownell, Potter, Michelow, and Gardner, 1984). Later, Brownell wondered if this is a fundamental semantic problem (Brownell, Simpson, Bihrle, Potter, and Gardner, 1990). He compared performance with his connotation triads and a similar semantic task. RHDs were still more impaired in the connotation task, whereas LHDs were equally impaired in both tasks (also, Schmitzer, Strauss, and DeMarco, 1998).

Following up Brownell's first study of word triads, Tompkins (1990) wondered if metaphoric interpretation varies as a function of automatic and effortful levels of processing. She employed a semantic priming task in which a lexical decision target (e.g., *sharp*) was preceded by a metaphoric prime (e.g., *smart*), literal prime (e.g., *dull*), or an unrelated prime (e.g., *warm*). Unlike the dissociations found by Brownell, both related primes facilitated target recognition for RHDs and LHDs. Tompkins argued that the divergence from Brownell's findings was related to his use of a strategic task. RHDs were able to access nonliteral meaning automatically. Impairment may exist in controlled operations for choosing pictures or giving definitions.

A study in Montreal returned to Brownell's method but had a different result. The main task consisted of word triads arranged vertically. Participants were asked to choose the word most similar in meaning to the target in the middle (e.g., *vulgar, DIRTY, rag*). One option was a metaphoric meaning, and the other was a semantic associate of the literal meaning (e.g., *grossier, MALPROPRE, chiffon*). The investigators concluded that both RHDs and LHDs were impaired for metaphor processing. The article is unclear as to the operational definition of impairment, but perhaps we can assume that participants tended to choose the literal meaning. Lack of a double dissociation is inconsistent with Brownell's finding that only the RHDs had this result. Because RHDs had a metaphor deficit, the researchers in Montreal concluded that this syndrome may include a difficulty with semantics (Gagnon, Goulet, Giroux, and Joanetter, 2003).

Myers (1999, 2001a) has cited two explanations of the preference for literal meaning. Both explanations presume that the problem is an impaired ability to manage alternative meanings (i.e., literal and nonliteral). One explanation is **activation theory,** which suggests that people with RHD have difficulty (or are slow) activating multiple meanings, especially those more distant to the initially activated concept. The other explanation is **suppression theory,** in which patients fail to inhibit the activation of possible meanings, which then interferes with selection of the meaning that is appropriate for a situation. These theories are different. The former proposes a reduction of meaning activation, and the latter proposes an excess of meaning activation. These theories were developed to account for other pragmatic phenomena, but, for now, let us look at a study of suppression theory that may have implications for metaphor comprehension.

Tompkins and her colleagues (2000) used an auditory semantic priming task to test the suppression theory. Instead of metaphor, they presented semantically ambiguous words which, like metaphor, carry multiple meaning. In the task, the prime was a short sentence ending in either an ambiguous word (e.g., *seal*) or a similar unambiguous word (e.g., *dolphin*). Primes were followed by a target at either a short (175 msec) or long interval (1,000 msec). Participants made judgments as to whether the target was related to the meaning of the preceding sentence. The following are examples of the stimuli:

(3a) He trained the *seal.*   *tighten*
(3b) He trained the dolphin.

The sentence was constructed to favor activation of the dominant meaning (i.e., a sea creature). The target represented the nondominant meaning, so

the correct response was *no* (see also Tompkins, Lehman-Blake, Baumgaertner, and Fassbinder, 2002).

The response should take longer with the ambiguous prime (3a) than with the unambiguous prime (3b) if multiple meanings are activated and interfere with the target decision. This would occur at the short interval because multiple activation is an automatic phenomenon. Suppression of inappropriate meanings is a more controlled operation requiring some time. It should show up at the longer interval with equivalent response times between the conditions. Tompkins compared 40 RHDs to 40 matched controls. Contrary to controls, the RHDs maintained a longer response with ambiguous primes at the longer interval (i.e., 1,000 msec). This indicated that multiple meanings were interfering with the judgment decision and, thus, the RHDs failed to suppress alternate meanings when given time to do so. A faulty suppression function was applied to the explanation of excessive literalness.

Metaphors can be spoken with sentences so a speaker's intent differs from sentence meaning. Other examples of this difference include **indirect requests** and **sarcasm.** In lieu of studying statements made in real situations, investigators present hypothetical situations called "vignettes" and patients make judgments about a target statement often presented at the end of the vignette. In one study, short vignettes ended with a conventional indirect request (e.g., "Can you . . . ?") or a request worded to favor literal interpretation (e.g., "Are you able to . . . ?") (Weylman, Brownell, Roman, and Gardner, 1989). Both vignettes established situations in which the most appropriate response was to indirect meaning, so the study would examine use of linguistic context. RHDs were impaired relative to normal controls but still could use context to comprehend an indirect message.

RHDs also answered questions about vignettes that ended with one person praising or deriding another about a good or poor performance (e.g., golfing) (Kaplan, Brownell, Jacobs, and Gardner, 1990). Patients were given information about whether the characters liked or disliked each other. The closing comment could be interpreted literally or sarcastically (e.g., *You sure are a good golfer*). RHDs were accurate when conclusions were literally true. Yet, when conclusions were literally false, RHDs had difficulty detecting sarcasm based on the characters' relationship. Patients thought a sarcastic positive statement makes a person feel better, indicating a reduced sensitivity to beliefs and desires of others (i.e., taking another person's point of view).

Tompkins and others (1994) saw the sporting acceptance of sarcasm as requiring revision of an initial interpretation, and they wondered if this heightened demand on processing is related to working memory capacity. To understand this notion of inference revision, let us examine two versions of a short story presented to patients:

(4a) Nan invited her new neighbor, Mark, to a party.
      He told hilarious stories and everyone enjoyed listening.
      Nan's husband said to her, "Good decision. He's really fun to have around."
(4b) Nan invited her new neighbor, Mark, to a party.
      He told boring stories and no one enjoyed listening.
      Nan's husband said to her, "Good decision. He's really fun to have around."

Story 4a was congruent in that the second and third sentences convey a positive mood, whereas 4b was incongruent in that the second and third sentences are inconsistent with respect to mood. Yet, the incongruent story is coherent when the husband's comment is interpreted as sarcasm (thus, requiring revision of an initial interpretation).

Rounding out the experiment, Tompkins presented a simpler story in a third condition. Comprehension was tested with yes/no questions after each story, and working memory capacity was also measured. Results showed that incongruent sarcasm was more difficult to comprehend than the other stories for all groups. For RHDs, working memory had its highest correlation with the incongruent condition. The investigators concluded that inference revision is especially strenuous for people with RHD.

DISCOURSE

With their clinical test of discourse comprehension (see Chapter 6), Nicholas and Brookshire (1995a) found that RHDs recalled main ideas better than details and explicit information better than implied information. However, aphasic patients and normal controls had the same pattern of ability, indicating that this strategy of assessment may not detect differences between brain-damaged groups. This section presents other approaches to the examination of discourse comprehension.

Brownell (1988) contrasted RHDs with aphasic persons according to a simple but powerful framework. He suggested that "aphasic patients often appear to understand more of a conversation or story than one would expect given their impairments with words and sentences, and RHD patients appear to understand less than one would expect given their intact linguistic skills" (p. 249). Early characterizations of RHDs were that they "miss the point" of proverbs and narratives and tend to "wander from the point" when telling a story.

Comprehension

Two investigations focused on inferring relations between propositions. McDonald and Wales (1986) presented items involving spatial (5a) and nonspatial (5b) inferences.

(5a) The bird is in the cage.
      The cage is under the table.
      TEST: The bird is under the table.
(5b) The woman held the little girl's hand.
      Her daughter was only 3 years old.
      TEST: The woman held her daughter's hand.

After hearing the two statements and engaging in a brief distractor task, patients were tested as to whether they had heard a statement before. RHDs matched normal controls by recognizing true inferences as often as true facts (e.g., *The cage is under the table*).

Another study exposed a deficit. Patients made true/false judgments about sentence pairs (6).

(6)   Barbara became too bored to finish the history book.
      She had already spent five years writing it.
      TRUE/FALSE TEST: Barbara became bored writing a history book.

RHDs made more errors with inferences than with factual statements, indicating a deficiency in combining information between sentences (Brownell, Potter, Bihrle, and Gardner, 1986).

Online investigations have concentrated on the **bridging inference,** which is generated to establish a cohesive relationship between sentences. Beeman's (1993) study provides an example:

(7)   George left the bathtub water running.
      George cleaned up a mess in the bathroom.

The bridge is the inference that the water overflowed. Beeman embedded such statements in stories told to participants in a cross-modal priming task. The stories were built to examine other aspects of narrative comprehension, but let us focus on bridging inference. As participants listened to a story, they made visual-lexical decisions for words that were related or unrelated to the inference (e.g., *overflow*). If participants activated the inferred concept, they would have been primed for the related target. RHDs responded more slowly to inference-related targets, whereas controls were facilitated for the related targets. Beeman concluded that RHDs fail to activate concepts necessary to build the bridge, which became known as the activation theory.

Tompkins decided to conduct a similar study. Her main purpose was to compare Beeman's activation theory with her suppression (or "multiple activation") hypothesis. Tompkins simplified the stories and employed a strictly auditory task in which the target word was presented after the last sentence. Example (8) shows the last two sentences of a story about Roger going to a lake for a swim:

(8)   Roger did not know that there was a lot of glass there.
      The lifeguard came running when Roger called for help.

Whereas one target pertained to the bridging inference that Roger stepped on the glass (e.g., *cut*), a twist to this study was that another target was semantically related to the second sentence only (e.g., *drown*). The failed activation hypothesis was rejected, because RHDs were primed by the presumed activation of bridging inferences in this simpler task. Tompkins's suppression hypothesis was also not strongly supported, because the alternate target was not primed by the last sentence. Apparently the bridging inference dominated interpretation of the final sentence, and alternative meanings were suppressed (Tompkins, Fassbinder, Lehman-Blake et al., 2004).

Beeman's and Tompkins's studies are instructive for showing how online investigation of inference generation can be done. In general, the evidence for activation theory and suppression theory is mixed. We should be sympathetic, because the online investigation of inference processing is relatively new for clinical populations. More substantive reasons for the mixed results are suggested later.

Jokes were among the first devices used to study the detection of coherence in stories. A conclusion becomes a punch line because of surprise relative to expectations in the body of a joke and because of its coherence relative to a theme (Brownell, Michel, Powelson, and Gardner, 1983). After hearing the body of a joke, patients selected a conclusion from choices containing a punch line, a suprising nonsequitur, and two coherent conclusions (e.g., 9). When RHDs fail to choose the punch lines, do they err in favor of surprise or coherence?

(9)   BODY: The neighborhood borrower approached Mr. Smith on Sunday afternoon and

asked if Mr. Smith would be using his lawn-mower. "Yes, I am," Smith answered warily. The neighborhood borrower then replied:
CORRECT: "Fine, then you won't be need-ing your golf clubs. I'll just borrow them."
SURPRISE: "You know, the grass is greener on the other side."
NEUTRAL COHERENCE: "Do you think I could use it when you're done?"
SAD COHERENCE: "Gee, if I only had enough money I could buy my own."

Asked to pick the funny conclusion, RHDs chose the punch line 60 percent of the time. Normal controls got the joke 81 percent of the time. Therefore, RHDs were deficient but not devoid of a sense of humor. In their errors, they chose surprise over coherence. Later, this study was expanded by using cartoons and adding a humorless story condition, and the results were similar (Bihrle, Brownell, Powelson, and Gardner, 1986). Both studies were considered to indicate that RHDs have a problem with the coherence feature of a narrative.

A few studies addressed sensitivity to over-all structure of a discourse. RHDs had difficulty arranging sentences into a story (Delis, Wap-ner, Gardner, and Moses, 1983) and sequencing frames of cartoons (Huber and Gleber, 1982). In one study, the crucial thematic statement for a story was put at its usual position at the beginning or at an unusual position at the end. Patients were tested for recalling main ideas (Hough, 1990). For normal controls, there was no effect of delaying the theme. However, RHDs scored much better when the theme was early than when the theme was delayed. Hough decided that these subjects were "unable to utilize the macrostructure as an organizer in apprehending the paragraph" (p. 271). Another possibility is that RHDs recognize com-mon macrostructure, and exceptions create hard-ships for processing narration.

Interpreting Situations

People with RHD have difficulty recognizing emotion or humor in a pictured scene, whereas aphasic patients do not have this problem (Cicone

et al., 1980; Gardner et. al., 1975). In one study, patients were asked to group pictures accord-ing to a theme such as despair or love (Myers, Linebaugh, and Mackisack-Morin, 1985). Some themes, such as hugging, were considered to be explicit. Other themes were implicit, such as love. Unlike aphasic patients, RHDs had more difficulty sorting according to implicit themes than explicit themes. This pattern indicated that RHDs have a problem with inferring the nature of situations when it is not concrete or obvious.

Another indication of impaired situational in-ference came from a content analysis of descrip-tions of the Cookie Theft picture. Myers (1979) looked for literal content (e.g., a woman) and interpretive concepts (e.g., "She is the mother"). RHDs produced fewer interpretive concepts than normal. When cartoon sequences were used to elicit stories, RHDs omitted inferences that fill in transitions between pictures (Joanette et al., 1986).

Tompkins (1995) warned that we could go overboard in anticipating that people with RHD will be insensitive to situations. Stemmer, Gir-oux, and Joanette (1994) examined the ability to produce direct requests (e.g., "Turn down the radio") and indirect requests (e.g., "I can't con-centrate") when presented with contexts calling for one type or the other. RHDs were sensitive to context in that they did not produce direct com-mands in situations in which an indirect request was appropriate.

Discourse Production

Eisenson (1962) characterized extended verbal expression with RHD as "empty." This charac-terization was supported by content analyses that demonstrated reduced informativeness of description or narration (Joanette, Goulet, Ska et al., 1986). Trupe and Hillis (1985) found some patients to be verbose, whereas others exhibited a paucity of utterance.

As indicated in Chapter 6, the assessment of discourse production has two key elements, namely, the method of eliciting a sample and the method of analysis. We can elicit discourse without analyzing the features that make it coherent. The study of discourse with RHD has been quite varied. Characteristics of the research are compared to the study of closed head injury in the next chapter. In the study of RHD, picture elicitation has been used more often than spontaneous conditions. Narrative has been the most frequently studied type of discourse, and information or content analysis has been used more than cohesion or macrostructural analyses (Davis, O'Neil-Pirozzi, and Coon, 1997).

Trupe and Hillis (1985) found some RHDs were overly literal and focused on detail in picture description. The following example is the beginning of a lengthy description of the Boston Exam's Cookie Theft picture:

> *Well, it's on 8½ x 11 inch paper overall covered by plastic. Looks like it may have been done with drawing pens and India ink on white paper. It's less than 20 pound paper. Else you wouldn't have used black to keep it from shining through . . . (p. 94)*

As indicated earlier, RHDs have been said to wander from the point or theme when telling stories. In several studies, autobiographical stories and story retelling included event-sequence errors, confabulations, digressions, and embellishments (Gardner, Brewnell, Wapner, and Michelow, 1983; Myers, 1979; Rivers and Love, 1980; Trupe and Hillis, 1985). RHDs varied widely in script production; some were tangential, and others terminated too soon (Roman, Brownell, Potter et al., 1987). Patients were compared with normal controls in telling a story from a short video, and they were deficient in cohesion and number of episodes told to a naive listener (Uryase, Duffy, and Liles, 1991). On the other hand, Bloom and others (1995) found that RHDs were not deficient in telling stories with respect to completeness, logic, and having a beginning, middle, and end.

Aware of some of the early research on storytelling, a group of neuropsychologists decided to try out a different scoring system for the Logical Memory subtest of the *Wechsler Memory Scale* in which a patient is asked to recall two short stories

(Webster, Godlewski, Hanley et al., 1992). The system consisted of scores for recalling essential thematic information and nonessential details and for producing intrusion errors. RHDs recalled a normal number of essential propositions but recalled fewer details and produced significantly more idiosyncratic intrusions than controls and LHDs.

Indications of possible difficulties come from a study that included telling a story from a cartoon (Davis et al., 1997). The cartoon, called the "Flower Pot Story," shows a man walking his dog when a falling flower pot hits him on the head. He gets angry and storms into the building where the pot came from. After rapping on a door, a female culprit appears. She is nice to his dog, and he tips his cap without mentioning the bump on his head (Huber and Gleber, 1982; also Snow, Douglas, and Ponsford, 1995). Here are a couple of versions from individuals with RHD:

> *It looks like the man is out walking his pet dog, and it looks kinda like he's lost, and he's looking for help. So he goes banging on one of the doors, and a lady opens her door, and out runs her pet. Looks like he's asking her for directions, and she gives 'em to him. (pp. 202–203)*

> *The first one it looks like he's returning home with a stray dog. He takes him in. The third one. Fourth one, he's banging on the door. Fifth one, he's giving the dog a bone. Sixth one, he seem to be pleased with him. And the dog is taking off with his bone. (p. 204)*

The first one is a good story with a theme, characters, motivated events, and related resolution. Yet, it is the wrong story with an incorrect detail about the pet. The second version is also the wrong story and has inaccurate details and less logical coherence than the first story. Pictures are treated as independent entitites.

Davis was concerned that patients might have had problems with interpretation of visual stimuli. Patients were more accurate when retelling a story told to them. Myers and Brookshire (1994) compared visual and inferential complexity of pictures, and found that complexity had little influence on information content. Bloom and others (1993) presented picture sequences that had an emotional theme (i.e., a pet gets hit by a car), a visuospatial theme (i.e., moving a box from a chair), or a procedural/neutral theme (i.e., how to fry an egg). Instead of measuring content, they looked for certain pragmatic features of the stories (e.g., topic maintenance, conciseness). Emotional content impaired RHDs' discourse and seemed to facilitate aphasic discourse.

Marini and her colleagues (2005) compared story retelling and cartoon elicitation across the levels of discourse analysis (i.e., within-sentence linguistics, between-sentence cohesion, and overall coherence). RHDs were compared to LHDs without aphasia. Difficulties appeared only for the RHDs with cartoon elicitation, supporting the general idea that RHD involves impairment in generating a narrative from visual information.

The general point is that our picture of RHDs' discourse may depend on our choice of methods of elicitation and analysis. We should be hesitant about forming a diagnostic opinion from one task or one story.

Interview and Conversation

Kennedy (2000) studied eight adults with RHD in a *first-encounter conversation* with a stranger, according to a framework used by Kellermann and others (1989). Kennedy wondered if a problem with suppression of irrelevant information would appear in conversation. A conversation was thought to occur in three phases: initiation, maintenance, and termination. Kellerman identified high- and low-frequency topics, called "topic scenes," for each phase in conversations between college students. For example, hometowns and people in common were the most frequent topics in the maintenance phase of a first encounter, whereas books, vices, and religion were among the least frequent topics. The college students were a good frame of reference for Kennedy's study, because her middle-aged adult controls introduced the same topics.

In addition, because interviewing is a frequent clinical interaction, Kennedy's instructions to participants are of interest:

- *For the RHD participants:* "I would like you to meet someone that you have not met before . . . This is not an interview, so she doesn't have a list of questions to ask you . . ."
- *For the SLP partner:* "This is not an interview. Converse as you would with anyone you have met for the first time. Allow the participant to initiate topics . . . Do not take notes . . ." (p. 76)

The experimental particpants did not differ from controls in number of topics contributed. One-fourth of the RHDs' topics were coded as off-list or misplaced, and most of these could be accounted for by one RHD participant. Four of the RHDs produced more off-list and misplaced topics in the termination phase; these participants had difficulty terminating the interaction, especially after their partners attempted termination. Any problem with suppression was evident mainly at the end of conversations. Some RHDs could not be easily distinguished from the controls. In another study, however, RHDs had difficulty deciding whether a speaker should refer to a third party formally (e.g., *Mr. Smith*) or informally (e.g., *Bob*) (Brownell, Pincus, and Blum, 1997).

Brady and her colleagues (2003, 2005) in Scotland could not find consistent or widespread differences between RHDs and control participants in topic coherence or management. There was minimal tangential utterance. Their study of 17 patients included interviews, procedural discourse, and picture description. Brady considered their results to be a striking contrast to other literature that had created the impression that veering off topic is common in RHD. These investigators acknowledged that their findings could be a function of the participant selection bias that was mentioned earlier in this chapter.

Humor is one fuel for energizing and maintaining social interaction. Heath and Blonder (2005) wondered if the laboratory findings of

Brownell and others might be observed in natural settings. The researchers compared people with RHD and LHD in semistructured interviews, and then independent raters coded humor events. The raters did not come up with a problem in the participants with RHD, but spouses rated the patients as being different in the telling of funny stories following their strokes. Ability to decode prosody was also related to the spouses' ratings of change. Heath and Blonder interpreted these mixed results as pointing to limitations of their interview rating methodology, rather than a lack of evidence for humor reduction in RHDs' interactions at home.

WHAT IS RHD SYNDROME?

A few years ago, Myers (2001b) posed this question and noted that our clinical efforts "are hampered by the lack of a definition and a universally accepted label for these deficits—one that is not solely dependent on lesion location" (p. 913). She was prompted to contemplate this problem because Yves Joanette and Ana Ansaldo (1999) of the University of Montreal had proposed that the communicative deficits of RHD be collectively called "pragmatic aphasia." Let us come back to this later.

We may feel compelled to come up with a single label befitting the various communicative dysfunctions of RHD, because we are accustomed to thinking of RHD in monolithic terms. This chapter reinforces this idea to some extent. Yet, experimental results have been inconsistent, especially regarding inferencing. One person with an RH stroke may have a problem with inferencing, but another may not (e.g., Lehman-Blake and Lesniewicz, 2005), and this variability along with small participant groups can lead to different results among studies. Also, there is the problem of selecting RHDs to participate in studies, and experiments vary with respect to types of inference, stimulus materials, and procedures. What appears to be a contradiction may actually reflect the notion that the impact of a deficit depends on the situation.

One orientation to explaining communicative deficits of RHD is **theory of mind** (ToM). Originally proposed as a theory of autism, ToM is the ability to infer another person's mental states. Facial expression and prosody are cues to a person's mental state, so that RHD may include a weakened ToM (e.g., Brownell, Griffin, Winner et al., 2000; Martin and McDonald, 2003). Others refer to a problem with detecting a speaker's intent (e.g., Sabbagh, 1999). The failure to take the point of view of another has usually been identified in off-line studies, such as one that demonstrated a difficulty with recognizing the beliefs of one character about another when telling lies or ironic jokes (Winner, Brownell, Happé et al., 1998).

Another orientation is to find a processing impairment. Processing hypotheses include **activation theories** (either too much or not enough), and we have seen that they are tested with online experiments (i.e., Beeman, 1993; Tompkins et al., 2004). This paradigm has also been inconsistent in exposing a disorder. In general, we may not have to choose between ToM and activation hypotheses, because they may be addressing two levels of the same thing, one at a conscious strategic level and the other at the subconscious automatic level.

So, what is RHD syndrome? Actually there may be no such thing, just as there is no one LHD syndrome. The real issue probably lies with identifying different RHD syndromes. This means finding consistently co-occurring patterns of symptoms caused by focal neuropathology, and then figuring out the common thread that is the main clue to diagnosing the underlying cognitive dysfunction. The absence of clear answers simply means that we are witnessing the early stages of the study of a difficult problem.

Does it help to call the communication problems of RHD "pragmatic aphasia"? Myers (2001b) noted that this label was chosen based on three assumptions: that aphasia is a language disorder, that pragmatic skills are inherent to language, and that communication disorders of RHD are pragmatic. She thought that the first and third assumptions are acceptable but the second is debatable, if we are to think of pragmatics as a language system interacting with context. Thinking of this interaction as inherent to language (second assumption) seems to twist basic concepts into an unfamiliar shape. Another way of accepting a notion of pragmatic aphasia would be to change our definition of aphasia (or of language, or of pragmatics). The idea certainly stimulated some thought.

CLINICAL ASSESSMENT

A speech-language clinician might begin evaluating someone with an RH stroke by administering familiar tests of language ability that were designed for assessing aphasia. Our standard language tests assess mostly word- and sentence-level abilities. Another perspective is that "RHD patients are most often nonaphasic in that they can normally process most words and sentences in isolation" (Brownell, 1988, p. 248).

Aphasia Batteries

The *Western Aphasia Battery* (WAB) was given to 53 nondominant-hemisphere-damaged patients

(Kertesz, 1979). This mostly RHD group had an average Aphasia Quotient (AQ) of 92.9, which is slightly beneath the cut-off score of 93.8 for language impairment but well above the 53.5 average for stroke-induced aphasia. Many were normal, but others were somewhat below the cut-off.

On the *Porch Index of Communicative Ability* (PICA), RHDs had an average overall score of 13.03 compared with 11.12 for an aphasic group (Wertz and Dronkers, 1994). Porch and Palmer (1986) produced conversion tables according to the subtest categories. Table 11.3 displays a few scores at the same percentile levels for RHDs and aphasic LHDs, indicative of the general severity levels of each group. As severity of deficit increases, the difference between aphasia and RHD becomes more pronounced. A difference in auditory comprehension does not appear until severe overall impairment (25th percentile). A difference in verbal expression becomes pronounced at a higher level (50th percentile) favoring the RHDs.

TABLE 11.3   Response levels from 94 right-hemisphere-damaged patients (Porch and Palmer, 1986) compared with 357 left-hemisphere-damaged aphasic patients (Porch, 1981) at percentiles determined for each group. Copying shapes is subtest F, in which RHDs have lower scores than LHDs.

		OVERALL	AUDITORY COMPREHENSION	VERBAL	WRITING	COPYING SHAPES
90th	RHD	13.99	15.00	14.59	13.21	13.8
	LHD	14.04	15.00	14.35	13.18	14.5
75th	RHD	13.47	15.00	14.24	11.94	12.8
	LHD	12.89	15.00	13.50	11.05	14.0
60th	RHD	12.95	14.87	13.92	10.66	12.1
	LHD	11.71	14.60	12.30	9.23	13.3
50th	RHD	12.60	14.80	13.73	9.82	11.7
	LHD	10.89	14.25	10.77	8.22	13.0
40th	RHD	12.34	14.66	13.45	8.90	11.2
	LHD	9.96	13.60	8.90	7.33	12.4
25th	RHD	11.32	14.15	12.56	7.50	9.9
	LHD	8.38	11.70	6.04	6.29	11.1
10th	RHD	9.33	11.30	10.30	5.63	7.3
	LHD	6.15	8.05	3.75	4.98	8.0

Above the 60th percentile, RHDs' spoken language falls in the normal range.

Also in Table 11.3, comparative deficit is reversed for the nonverbal test of copying shapes (subtest F) in which RHDs have lower scores. Their drawing difficulty is especially striking, considering that these patients are not likely to have paralysis of their preferred (right) hand, whereas many aphasic people attempt to draw with their weakened preferred (right) hand.

In general, RHD does not allow patients to escape difficulty with some language-related activities, especially when overall dysfunction is severe and the language system is challenged. Some patients will score below an aphasia test's cut-off for language impairment that some might say is diagnostic of aphasia. However, we should be reminded of a point in Chapter 3 stating that we do not allow a test to do our diagnosing for us. Someone with RHD makes mistakes on language tasks for reasons other than having a language disorder or aphasia, and the reader should have identified these reasons in this chapter.

Assessment of RHD

Myers extended the use of established assessments by providing methods for measuring severity and recovery. One method was applied to descriptions of the Cookie Theft picture that comes with the Boston Exam. She divided information units into literal and interpretive concepts and developed a scoring system (Myers, 1999, pp. 182–183). The assessment is to distinguish whether a patient produces literal concepts to the exclusion of interpretive concepts. It can also identify an increase in the number of interpretive concepts for documenting recovery.

Another of Myers's embellishments was for a test of copying a scene that consists of a simple house, a fence, and trees to the left and the right (Myers, 1999, pp. 161, 185). For measuring left neglect, she provided a *copy-scene scoring system* whereby a patient gets a point for each detail of the drawing. The drawing is structured so that the four objects span the page, and the scene and

each object have a midline for comparing details produced from the left and the right.

A few SLPs produced assessments of communication for RHD patients in the 1980s, during the early stage of the study of this population. Perhaps the first is the *Rehabilitation Institute of Chicago Evaluation of Communication Problems in Right Hemisphere Dysfunction* (RICE), which was modified for a second edition (Halper, Cherney, and Burns, 1996). Its *Pragmatic Communication Skills Rating Scale* consists of 10 four-point ratings for nonverbal and verbal communication (e.g., facial expression, turn taking, topic maintenance). Another scale addresses awareness of illness, attention, orientation, and recent memory.

Soon after, the *Right Hemisphere Language Battery* (RHLB) was published, now also in a second edition (Bryan, 1995). The test assesses lexical-semantic comprehension, inference generation, and comprehension of metaphor and verbal humor. Other components are for production of emphatic stress and conversational discourse. Italian researchers used the test to study effects of aging on pragmatic skills (Zanini, Bryan, De Luca, and Bava, 2005). Independent investigators studied patients with RH tumors. They found no difference between RHDs and controls preoperatively and no difference for the patients pre- and postoperatively. The investigative authors decided that they could not recommend the RHLB for diagnosis of deficit or measuring recovery (Thomson, Taylor, Fraser, and Whittle, 1997b).

The *Mini Inventory of Right Brain Injury* (MIRBI-2) first appeared in 1989 (Pimental and Knight, 2000). It is a screening for primary cognitive impairments and pragmatic abilities with affective language, humor, and metaphor. It should take 25 to 30 minutes to obtain severity of deficit in these areas. The second edition has more reliability and validity data. Although the test did not change, the rationale was updated to reflect current trends.

Two psychologists developed the *Right Hemisphere Communication Battery* (RHCB) (Gardner and Brownell, 1986). It contains 11 subtests distributed within four parts: Humor (Pictorial Humor, Verbal Humor, Humor Production),

Emotion (Prosody), Nonliteral Language (Indirect Requests, Pictorial Metaphors, Verbal Metaphors, Inferences), and Integrative Processes (Sarcasm, Alternative Word Meanings, Narrative Comprehension). A Hebrew adaptation was given to 27 RHDs, 31 LHDs, and 21 age-matched controls. The only subtests distinguishing RHDs and LHDs were Indirect Requests and Verbal Metaphors, and it was the LHDs who did worse. Scores also correlated with scores on the WAB, although more strongly with the Cortical Quotient (CQ) than the Aphasia Quotient (AQ) (Zaidel, Kasher, Soroker, and Batori, 2002).

Zaidel, Kasher, and others' results pose some problems for the RHCB and, perhaps, other batteries for the RHD population. Although the research forming the basis for the RHCB had shown deficits for RHDs, the test may not tap into problems unique to RHD. The test may more likely be a measure of general cognitive functions performed by the LH as well as the RH.

TREATMENT

Treatment for RHD is an underdeveloped territory (Lehman-Blake, 2005). Authors tend to recommend research paradigms that *may* be applied according to the logic of familiar aphasia treatment principles. Actual case demonstrations are published infrequently, and efficacy studies are rare. According to the logic of rehabilitation, each problem area of RHD should be treated in two ways:

- stimulation/facilitation of an impaired process
- teaching compensatory strategies to bypass an impairment

We should recall that compensatory strategies capitalize on a patient's retained abilities, and RHDs retain language abilities. Therefore, compensatory strategies are often verbal/linguistic. Also, whereas common sense is inherent to aphasia therapy, limited precedent forces us to rely more on this clinical tool for treatment of RHD.

Clinical aphasiologists continue to emphasize improvement in communicative functions and strive to select activities that are important in an individual patient's daily life (i.e., a patient-centered approach). Anita Halper, Leora Cherney, and Martha Burns have been particularly active in the Chicago area in developing treatment methodology for RHD (Halper, Cherney, and Burns, 1996; Cherney and Halper, 1999). However, this section is guided mainly by Myers's (1999) recommendations.

Awareness, Orientation, and Attention

A patient should be aware of a communication problem in order to make sense of a referral to an SLP. However, the literature does not contain many suggestions for improving awareness of deficit. We do not force someone to receive treatment. A number of people with RH stroke are aware of difficulties. Some seek rehabilitation. We tend to provide treatment for those who want it. Myers (1999) has addressed mildly impaired patients who become aware of a problem, such as mechanical prosody, once it is defined for them.

An SLP is likely to be involved in providing language-oriented stimulation and compensatory aids for disorientation (see Chapters 12, 13). Improving orientation is important for a patient's **safety,** which is a vital concern in anyone's rehabilitation. Clocks, calendars, and schedules are prominent in rehabilitation facilities. Hospital staff is trained to remind patients of the date and time. Cherney and Halper (1999) wrote about orientation groups for patients with RHD during acute and subacute rehabilitation.

Myers (1999, 2001a) has recommended treatment of all aspects of attention (see Table 12.5). Her principal sources come from cognitive rehabilitation of traumatic brain injury, especially treatments developed by Sohlberg and Mateer. Treatment of attention is covered in the next chapter (see Table 12.10).

Left Neglect and Reading

Stimulation treatment for neglect dyslexia is likely to begin with treatment of left neglect in general. Straightforward application of assessment tasks includes some practice with crossing out items in an array. *Leftward search-and-find activities* are designed to encourage subconscious perception of left space. A patient is asked to locate certain colored cubes in a small array. The idea is to set up a simple condition for volitional attention without external cueing, which Myers (1999) believed increases the likelihood of generalization. Another suggestion is the use of *contiguous stimuli* for picture description or search and find. These stimuli are coherent only across the midline, to the left and right (e.g., a couple holding hands). A patient is likely to realize that recognition requires shifting attention leftward. For reading, patients read aloud words and sentences that make sense only with leftward attention.

Compensatory aids are cues that encourage leftward scanning, although Myers (2001a) was not enthusiastic about this strategy for restoring attention. She noted that "verbally cuing the patient to look to the left or highlighting stimuli on the left . . . rarely translates into an internal self-cue" (pp. 811–812). Nevertheless, if attention improves slowly, compensatory cues may be helpful. For reading, *anchors* such as colored lines or arrows may be placed on the left side of a page. Letters or numbers may be printed to the right and left of text, and the patient is occasionally told to read the letter or number. Some patients may resort to tricks, such as "imagine a little green man on my shoulder, tapping me to remind me" (Andrewes, 2001).

Prosody

Myers (1999) explained that a mildly impaired patient may have a vague sense that he or she does not sound like him- or herself. We should spend some time educating and counseling the patient and family regarding the role of prosody in communication and the fact that the patient's flat tone and affect are due to the stroke rather than indifference. A heightened awareness can lead to some changes by family members that compensate for the patient's difficulties.

Regarding comprehension deficits, families can be advised to identify their own moods and emotions verbally and, perhaps, use more words with emotional meaning (e.g., saying "I am happy" in addition to sounding and looking happy). Drills might be attempted, beginning with a pitch discrimination task, then identifying melodies and listening to sentences for meaningful pitch variation (e.g., questions versus statements).

Regarding production deficits, patients may follow the advice given to families with respect to verbal identification of feelings. Restorative practice may begin with imitation of emotionally expressed neutral sentences. Sentences may represent an emotion in their wording, and a patient must express the emotion with prosody. A higher-level activity consists of reading a story in which the patient identifies and conveys the moods and emotions of the characters. This activity is likely to overlap with working on inference and narrative coherence. A patient could follow a script for a play. Acting the parts is analogous to role-playing situations in which certain emotions are common.

Leon, Rosenbek, Crusian and several others (2005) used a single-case experimental design to study the treatment of expressive aprosodia in three cases with RHD. The study was reported in a Veterans Administration research journal. The researchers compared two treatments of emotional prosody. One was an imitative treatment that started with repeating a clinician's model. The other was a cognitive-linguistic treatment in which the participant produced intonation based on other cues, including the emotion's name and a picture of the facial expression. In both procedures, all stimulus information was systematically removed in steps. The study documented "modest to substantial" positive treatment effects. The comparison between treatments was mixed but seemed to favor the imitative treatment.

TABLE 11.4   Examples of inference and discourse tasks (Myers, 1999).

SKILL	TASKS
Inference generation	Create titles for pictures or stories Provide the ending to a story Tell what a cartoon story is about Discuss the meaning of a painting
Integration/organization	Arrange objects by categories Identify fragmented objects Work puzzles Arrange pictures or sentences into a story

Discourse and Inference

There are many overlapping aspects to working with discourse. We can focus on the organization of narrative, which often has to be inferred. The patient can figure out the global theme of a news story through thinking of a headline, or generate a news story when given a headline. The patient can contemplate the implicit meaning of a Rockwell drawing. The patient can work on recognizing and explaining what is funny about a cartoon or written joke. A few suggestions are listed in Table 11.4.

Although the status of activation theories is uncertain, Myers (1999) had some suggestions for either increasing activation or suppressing unwanted meanings. Investigators were particularly worried about the ability to suppress an initial interpretation that turns out to be inappropriate for the context. So-called *activation tasks* are intended to stimulate the generation of alternate meanings. One example is to have a patient provide two meanings for semantically ambiguous words, such as *bank*. So-called *suppression tasks* are intended to stimulate inhibition. A task would be to have a patient produce a single meaning for an ambiguous word as quickly as possible, particularly words for which two meanings are equally common.

Some therapy consists of explicit work on conversation. In aphasia treatment, conversation is an authentic context in which to build confidence in language skills or adaptive strategies. The same principle may be followed for generalization of task-related improvements of prosody. On the other hand, components of a conversation, such as turn taking or staying on topic, also become targets of treatment. Cherney and Halper (1999) reported on how this is done in groups. Therapy begins with identifying turns and topic maintenance in videotaped conversations. The next chapter touches upon conversational management a little more with closed head injury.

RECOVERY AND OUTCOMES

We should anticipate that general characteristics of recovery with RHD follow the path that is typical for stroke, namely, a period of sometimes impressive spontaneous recovery for a few weeks or months, followed by a slowing of the rate of progress. However, we do not have a picture of changes in key communicative functions with RHD. It is unclear as to whether the tests for communication deficits in RHD are built for measuring recovery in the way that the PICA and WAB were constructed for aphasia.

The study by Thomson and others (1997b) hinted that the *Right Hemisphere Language Battery* (RHLB) may have difficulty detecting a patient's progress.

Although little outcome research has been reported for RHD, experienced clinicians tend to recommend using currently available tests and scales for documenting general functional status and quality of life (QoL) (Chapter 6). SLPs specializing in the right hemisphere also borrow from the cognitive rehabilitation of traumatic brain injury (TBI), partly because areas of deficit are similar (Chapter 12). Both RHD and TBI involve problems with self-awareness and attention, and both have difficulties with the pragmatic use of language. Outcome for TBI is often documented with respect to return to school or work; although the RHD population is older, we may resort to a similar approach. Is the individual functioning independently at home? Has the individual returned to work?

Odell and others (2005) noted that studies of rehabilitation outcomes with RHD tend to focus on the relationship between left neglect (or hemi-inattention) and outcome. Patients with left neglect have had lower outcomes than those without neglect (e.g., Cherney, Halper, Kwasnica et al., 2001). Odell examined Functional Independence Measures (FIMs) administered at the discharge of 101 persons with RHD. The patients received treatment in a rehabilitation unit of a community hospital. The investigators looked at the relationship between some common predictive factors (e.g., initial severity, age) and different aspects of outcome (e.g., amount of gain, final functional status, discharge placement). Neglect was not a significant predictor of any outcome measure. The strongest predictors were initial severity and age. Motor items showed more recovery than cognitive items but were also more severely impaired.

SUMMARY AND CONCLUSIONS

Right hemisphere dysfunction (RHD) is actually an umbrella term for numerous cognitive impairments that may or may not co-occur with each other. In this chapter, we had brief encounters with problems of self-awareness, visuospatial attention, orientation to immediate surroundings, constructional skills, melody processing, and emotion processing. Some language difficulties are a direct manifestation of these disorders (e.g., neglect dyslexia, emotional aprosodia). Pragmatic language deficits, especially with inferencing and managing conversation, point to cognitive difficulties in taking the perspective of others and activation of alternative meanings.

The recognition of communication disorders with RHD may create an expectation that these patients would be referred to SLPs more

often than they are. Rehabilitation hospitals may refer all stroke cases to the SLP for swallowing evaluation and to ensure personal safety before discharge. A patient's nonchalance and the mysteries of RHD may make some SLPs reluctant to check for communication problems. Yet, the research is beginning to suggest a fairly reliable list of possible treatment goals, when the patient is willing.

The absence of real rehabilitation stories is troubling. We might be more confident with a substantial and expanding body of case studies illustrating how it went with particular clients. How was awareness dealt with? Did family members make the client participate? What was the setting of treatment? What were the pitfalls? What was the outcome? How was it paid for?

MATCHING REVIEW_____

Match the contribution on the right with the name on the left.

____ 1. David Wechsler

____ 2. Hiram Brownell

____ 3. Penelope Myers

____ 4. Connie Tompkins

____ 5. Bisiach in Milan

____ 6. Marc Pell and Shari Baum

____ 7. Margaret Lehman-Blake

____ 8. Leora Cherney and Anita Halper

____ 9. Karen Bryan

____ 10. Yves Joanette

a. metaphor, jokes, and sarcasm

b. the RICE and group therapy

c. suppression theory

d. medical chart retrospective

e. left neglect

f. "pragmatic aphasia"

g. perception of prosody

h. copy-scene scoring system

i. WAIS

j. *Right Hemisphere Language Battery* (RHLB)

CHAPTER 12

TRAUMATIC BRAIN INJURY

It was kind of a freak accident. I was on a motorcycle and I didn't have my helmet buckled. I just put it on, you know, and didn't buckle it. I was comin' down the road, and there's like an island in the road, you know, there was an island with two telephone poles in the middle, and I bounced off both those poles. Bounced off and flew forty feet through the air and lost my helmet in the meantime. And my brains were leaking out on the ground, and then I got to the hospital, and I was in a coma for four months. I was supposed to croak but I didn't. I fooled them all.

Traumatic brain injury (TBI) impairs cognitive functions that have a wide reach. These general cognitive systems include attention, memory, and a resource management capacity called the executive system. After 18 years of examining 2,500 head injured cases, Hagen (1981) sorted them into three general diagnostic categories:

- residual cognitive impairment without language dysfunction
- disorganized language secondary to cognitive impairments
- predominant language-specific disorder, or aphasia

These possibilities indicate that the speech-language pathologist (SLP) has an important role in the evaluation of persons with head injury. It can cause aphasia or, like right hemisphere dysfunction (RHD), can cause language difficulties that are expressions of other cognitive impairments. The clinician's job is to figure out which is which.

HEAD TRAUMA

Traumatic brain injury is the most common cause of death under age 38 in the United States. The most typical head-injured person is male, single, of lower socioeconomic status, who has a high school education or less (Anderson and McLaurin, 1980; Cooper, 1982). More than half are caused by motor vehicle accidents (MVAs). Falls are the next major cause. The most common contributing factor is alcohol use, and most injuries occur in summer or fall. In one study, 12 percent of head injuries were precipitated by interpersonal violence, and most of these were self-inflicted or stemmed from domestic problems (Rimel and Jane, 1983).

If the human skull is placed on the ground and weight is slowly piled on, it can support three tons (Rolak, 1993). Nevertheless, violent forces can damage the skull, and the brain can be damaged without harm to the skull. Head injuries have been broadly classified according to whether the skull is displaced, meninges are torn, or cortex is violated. A traditional and still common approach is to distinguish **open** (i.e., penetrating) from **closed** (i.e., nonpenetrating) head injuries. Mechanisms of injury are quite variable (Table 12.1).

Large samples of war-related open head injuries revealed a great deal about cerebral dysfunction. Small caliber weapons provided Luria (1970b) with "cleanly punched out" lesions to study. Investigations followed World War I (Goldstein, 1942), World War II (Luria, 1966; Newcombe, 1969; Russell and Espir, 1961), and the Vietnam war (Mohr, Weiss, Caveness et al., 1980). High-velocity injuries from modern weapons can be quite devastating, causing extensive *laceration* (i.e., tearing) of brain tissue. Low-velocity traumas are like closed head injuries, except for the laceration of brain tissue when skull fracture is severe.

TABLE 12.1   Classification of head traumas.

TYPE	DEFINITION	SUBTYPE	DESCRIPTION	CAUSES
Open	Skull fragments penetrate brain tissue	High velocity	Projectiles perforate or pierce the skull, bringing hair and skin with them	Gunshots Explosions
		Low velocity	Concentrated blunt trauma causing skull fracture rather than perforation	Blows to head MVAs
Closed	Foreign substances do not penetrate brain tissue	Acceleration	Unrestrained head struck by moving object or moving head strikes stationary object	Blows to head Falls MVAs
		Nonacceleration	Fixed head struck by moving object	Blows to head

Most of this chapter is devoted to **closed head injury** (CHI) because it is a common form of trauma in a civilian population and its consequences are unique compared to dysfunctions presented in previous chapters. Table 12.1 distinguishes acceleration and nonacceleration injuries. The latter are usually much less severe than acceleration traumas. Nonacceleration causes *contusion* (i.e., bruising) of the brain's surface at the point of impact, called impression trauma.

The **primary effects** of acceleration traumas occur at the moment of impact. Linear acceleration causes both contusion at the point of impact (i.e., *coup* injury), and contusion opposite the point of impact (i.e., *contrecoup* injury). Angular acceleration, on the other hand, creates more twisting forces on the brain and usually produces more severe injuries.

In either case, violent movement against the sharp bony floor of the skull damages the "orbital" underside of the **prefrontal area** (see Figure 1.3) and the **anterior temporal lobes.** Neuropsychologists identify particular cognitive deficits or "syndromes" with damage to each of these regions. Because the lateral walls and roof of the skull are smooth, laceration is uncommon in the superior frontal lobes and the parietal and occipital lobes. In addition, twisting or stretching forces cause **diffuse axonal injury** (DAI). This stretching (or "shearing") of white fiber tracts within the cerebrum and brain stem occurs more with high speed traffic accidents than with blows or falls.

The brain's responses to such trauma are called **secondary effects.** Accumulation of fluid (i.e., edema) over the first few hours causes swelling and intracranial pressure. Because of laceration of blood vessels, a variety of hemorrhages can occur. Reduced pulmonary output can reduce blood flow to the brain, causing some ischemic damage. Widespread embolism can occur within hours. Sometimes secondary effects are dominant, such as when a person is conscious for a while before lapsing into unconsciousness.

THE TRAUMA UNIT

When a hospital is notified that a trauma patient is on the way, the beepers of the Trauma Team are activated simultaneously for a trauma code. All members not occupied with patient responsibilities proceed immediately to the booth in the emergency room for trauma patients. The trauma surgery attending physician is the team leader. The team includes the senior trauma surgery resident, resuscitator, airway manager, procedure residents, primary nurse, nurse assistant, and X-ray technician.

On the resuscitator's count of three, the team and paramedics transfer the patient from a transport litter to a gurney. The nurse assistant removes the patient's clothing and obtains vital signs. The resuscitator directs the team to establish an airway and an access to intravenous fluids. The oropharynx and nasopharynx are suctioned for blood, secretions, and foreign matter. When the patient is stabilized, the senior resident confers with the team leader and resuscitator regarding an evaluation plan, which includes a CT scan. An unstabilized patient is taken immediately to an operating room. Depending on the nature of trauma, the surgeon evacuates subdural hematomas and/or repairs the skull and removes foreign matter.

A patient may be classified as a "talker" or "nontalker" in the emergency room. A nontalker is assessed for state of arousal. Pupils are checked for size and reaction to light. A thumb pressed next to an eyebrow might elicit a motor response. Is respiration abnormal? Does eye gaze respond to commands? The aroused or talking patient is questioned for awareness of surroundings.

Around 25 percent of head-injured people are nontalkers at hospital admission (Rimel and Jane, 1983). Loss of consciousness, or **coma,** is usually attributed to diffuse axonal injury. Acute care decisions are based partly on depth of coma, which is commonly assessed with the *Glasgow Coma Scale* (GCS) (Jennett and Teasdale, 1981). Ratings are obtained for eye opening, motor response, and verbal behavior. The maximum "coma score" is 15. Depth and duration of coma are indicators of

severity of injury (Table 12.2). A critical decision path for multiple trauma patients may specify that a medically stable patient with a GCS less than 12 should get a CT scan before surgery.

Ylvisaker, Szekeres, and Feeney (2001) described the ensuing chain of service settings, which is similar to those for stroke. After initial stabilization in the emergency room, patients are transferred to intensive care for a short time. Then, they may move to a neurological care ward where they may receive early rehabilitation, or, depending on the size of the hospital, they may proceed to the hospital's rehabilitation facility where they receive more intensive therapies. Following inpatient rehabilitation, the individual is discharged to home and may continue treatment as a outpatient or may participate in a community support group.

NEUROPSYCHOLOGICAL ASSESSMENT

The neuropsychological assessments mentioned in the previous chapter and others introduced in this chapter comprise a vast army of tests that can be brought to bear on the problems of TBI (e.g., Sohlberg and Mateer, 2001). Only a small number are likely to be used by an SLP. Let us begin with broad assessment of cognition, with more specific tests to follow in sections on attention, memory, and other functions.

Richardson (2000) reviewed several studies of the *Wechsler Adult Intelligence Scale* (WAIS) given to patients with closed head injury (CHI) and found variation in Full Scale IQs among the groups, from 76.3 in one study to 98.0 in another. In the middle, a sample of 263 cases had a mean Full Scale IQ of 83.0, with a Verbal IQ of 85.8, and a Performance IQ of 81.3 (Cullum and Bilger, 1986), which is indicative of a general finding that the performance section is more deficient than the verbal section (Crawford et al., 1997). With the recovery that is common with CHI, individuals often approach normal or average IQ within two years (Table 12.3).

For a quick test of cognition, the ***Neurobehavioral Cognitive Status Examination*** (NCSE)

TABLE 12.2 Bases for estimating severity of traumatic brain injury (Hannay and Levin, 1989; Jennett and Teasdale, 1981).

	GCS SCORE	DURATION OF COMA
Mild	13–15	Less than 20 minutes
Moderate	9–12	
Severe	8 or less	More than 24 hours

TABLE 12.3 Comparison of 20 persons with closed head injuries (CHI) and 20 matched controls on selected subtests of the WAIS-R. The CHIs had severe injuries at least 18 months prior to testing (Schmitter-Edgecombe, Marks, Fahy, and Long, 1992).

		CHI	CONTROLS
Full Scale IQ		95.60	102.80
Verbal IQ	Arithmetic	9.10	9.90
	Similarities	9.35	10.30
	Digit span	9.40	11.35
	Vocabulary	8.40	10.25
Performance IQ	Digit symbol	7.80	12.05
	Block design	10.20	11.40

or **Cognistat** is designed to assess intellectual functioning in five ability areas (i.e., language, construction, memory, calculation, and reasoning/judgment). It takes 20 to 30 minutes to administer to cognitively impaired patients (Kiernan, Mueller, Langston, and Van Dyke, 1987). Although recommended for elderly individuals, it may be better suited for younger adults because of its difficulty relative to other brief screening tests mentioned later in Chapter 13 (Nabors, Millis, and Rosenthal, 1997).

Cited mainly in speech-language pathology literature, SLPs developed two tests of cognition for head injury. One is the *Scales of Cognitive Ability for Traumatic Brain Injury* (SCATBI), which contains 41 subtests for perception, orientation, organization, recall, and reasoning. Administration can take 10 to 45 minutes depending on which tests are given (Adamovich and Henderson, 1992). The other is the *Brief Test of Head Injury* (BTHI), which is a screening test that, like Cognistat, can be administered at bedside in 20 to 30 minutes. It contains more subtests for language, such as reading comprehension and naming (Helm-Estabrooks and Hotz, 1990).

For overall functional measurement, the FIM or FIM+FAM are commonly used in rehabilitation

settings at admission and discharge in the manner described in Chapter 6. In a study of 965 patients with CHI, seen in several rehabilitation settings, the physical and cognitive sections were found to be reliable (Hawley, Taylor, Hellawell, and Pentland, 1999). The **Disability Rating Scale** (DRS) seems to combine the Glasgow Coma Scale and the FIM (Rappaport, Hall, Hopkins et al., 1982) and is described later in the chapter.

The **Rancho Los Amigos Scale** (RLA) has been a popular rating of cognition and behavior (Table 12.4). Researchers often use the RLA to identify the severity of deficit in experimental participants. A participant may have had a severe head injury but, at the time of the study, may have a mild overall deficit at RLA level VII. The scale is sometimes a frame of reference for characterizing phases of recovery.

COMPUTERIZED ASSESSMENT AND MTBI

An automobile accident may cause a **mild traumatic brain injury** (MTBI) which is an insult to the head, resulting in a temporary alteration or loss of consciousness for less than 20 minutes. The Glasgow Coma Scale (GCS) rating would be in the 13 to 15 range, and usually there would be no findings with neuroimaging. The hospital stay is likely to be no more than 48 hours. MTBI is a common hazard in many sports, such as football, boxing, and skiing. It may result in subtle cognitive deficits known as *postconcussion syndrome* (PCS) (Barth, Broshek, and Freeman, 2006). Although PCS rarely includes serious speech or language disorders, sports neuropsychologists have been developing an approach to screening for cognitive difficulties known generally as *computerized response time-based assessment.*

Precedents for this screening appeared in the mid-1980s, initially at the University of Virginia. Investigators took a different approach to the study of mild head injury called the Sports as a Laboratory Assessment Modal (SLAM). Instead of comparisons to control groups, football players were compared before and after a season with a 15-minute battery of traditional tests. By the

TABLE 12.4 Rancho Los Amigos Scale of cognitive-behavioral function (Hagen, 1981). Only a few characteristics of each level are shown, rendering this summary insufficient for using the RLA.

LEVEL	GENERAL RESPONSE	DEFINITION SUMMARY
I	No response	Unresponsive to all stimuli
II	Generalized	Nonpurposeful, inconsistent, or gross response to stimuli; may have delayed response to pain
III	Localized response	Responses related to stimuli but inconsistent; responds to some commands
IV	Confused—agitated	Bizarre behavior, incoherent utterance, short attention span, uncooperative
V	Confused—inappropriate, nonagitated	Follows simple commands, affected by complexity of task, better attention span, has difficulty learning new things
VI	Confused—appropriate	Remote memory returning, recent memory still deficient, some goal direction
VII	Automatic—appropriate	Oriented in familiar situations, improved but shallow recall of recent activities, lacks insight and judgment
VIII	Purposeful—appropriate	Capable of new learning, remote and recent memory good, poor stress tolerance; supervision not needed

end of the decade, research expanded to the Ivy League colleges and the University of Pittsburgh. In 1993, a neuropsychological evaluation program for professional sports started with the Pittsburgh Steelers (Lovell, 2006). The goal was to develop a protocol for quickly identifying PCS and determining whether a player should return to a contest (i.e., return-to-play guidelines). Premature return to play can result in a serious outcome known as *second impact syndrome* (SIS).

One of the resultant computerized tests is called **CogSport** (Collie, Maruff, Darby et al., 2006). It consists of five tasks: simple reaction time, choice reaction time, sustained attention, working memory, and new learning. The stimuli for each task are familiar playing cards that appear on a computer screen. A common test strategy is to measure simple reaction time before and after testing to assess fatigue and provide a baseline for evaluating response times for the more cognitively demanding subtests. An advantage of

brief computerized testing is that large numbers of individuals can be examined simultaneously at one sitting. Also, a battery can be easily administered with a handheld computer on the sideline during a contest.

ATTENTION

Impaired attention/concentration is the factor found to be most responsible for difficulties with the WAIS (e.g., Crawford et al., 1989). Attention is multifaceted. Some aspects overlap with working memory and resource allocation. Attention is also multileveled in that it exists from a very gross level of awareness to skillfully trained concentration on a single event. Each aspect can be problematic and is summarized in Table 12.5. Sohlberg and Mateer (2001) included *alternating attention* in their list of components, which others may consider to be a way of managing divided attention. There are clinical assessments that are

TABLE 12.5 Levels and types of attention. Selective and divided attention are discussed later in the chapter.

LEVELS AND TYPES	FUNCTION	ASSESSMENT
Arousal	State of consciousness; primitive wakefulness	Gross motor response to sensory stimulation
Awareness	Assumes arousal; from stupor to clear perception of surroundings	Answer questions
Selective attention	Focus; resistence to distraction; managing limited resources by selection	Two stimuli or tasks; response to one (e.g., dichotic listening)
Sustained attention	Vigilance or concentration; maintaining focus on one stimulus for a period of time	A series of stimuli and response to one
Divided attention	Allocating limited resources to multiple processes or tasks	Two stimuli or tasks; response to both (dual task paradigms)

said to emphasize one aspect of attention, but it is difficult to test one component without others being involved. Some tests are said to be used for, let us say, focused attention but still require concentration.

Cortical arousal to any environmental stimulus depends on the reticular activating system in the brain stem (see Figure 1.3), and damage to this system is thought to cause the comatose state. Once a patient is aroused or conscious, levels of awareness vary from stupor (or "obtundation") to alertness. An alert patient can still be distractible, or can have difficulty focusing attention. Degree of arousal is measured with the Glasgow Coma Scale (GCS), and awareness is assessed with questions about personal identity and surroundings.

Selective or focused attention is thought to be managed by connections between the thalamus and prefrontal cortex, called the *thalamofrontal gating system* (Trexler and Zappala, 1988). These structures are vulnerable to the forces of CHI. Ponsford and Kinsella (1992) studied a group with severe CHI just one to three months postinjury. The researchers presented several color-naming tasks. One consisted of printed names of colors in different colors, so that the word *red* might be printed in blue. This is called the Stroop interference task. The color name could be a distraction when the task is to name the color of the print (i.e., *blue*). CHIs were slower but as accurate as controls, indicating that focused attention was intact in the Stroop task.

For focused attention, according to Sohlberg and Mateer (2001), clinical neuropsychologists may use the new Symbol Search subtest in WAIS-III (Table 11.2) or the ***Trail Making Test*** (TMT) (Reitan and Wolfson, 1995). In the TMT, the simpler Part A consists of randomly displayed, circled numbers that must be connected in sequence. Part B looks like Part A but contains circled numbers and letters that must be connected in alternation and in sequence.

For assessment emphasizing sustained attention, a patient may be asked to concentrate on a boring task for 20 or more minutes (Sohlberg and Mateer, 2001). In Ponsford and Kinsella's (1992) study, participants watched lights go on and off and pressed a button whenever a target light appeared. The CHI group was again slower but not less accurate than controls, and performance did not deteriorate over the time of the task (also, Parasuraman, Mutter, and Malloy, 1991). With the WAIS, the Digit Symbol subtest has been used as a measure of concentration, and it produced the largest deficit with CHI shown in Table 12.3.

Divided attention is thought to be evaluated with the new Letter-Number Sequencing subtest of WAIS-III, which entails alternating focus. Schretlen's auditory ***Brief Test of Attention*** (BTA) presents lists of alternating letters and numbers, increasing in length from 4 to 18 units, via audiocassette. Form N for numbers asks patients to ignore the letters and count the numbers. Form L poses the reverse problem for letters. The challenge is to ignore certain units while counting the others (Schretlin, Bobholz, and Brandt, 1996).

The ***Test of Everyday Attention*** (TEA) consists of eight tasks for assessing varied aspects of attention (Robertson, Ward, Ridgeway, and Nimmo-Smith, 1994, 1996). Its simulations include finding symbols on a map and in a telephone book, and tracking various stimuli associated with an elevator. Also, Sohlberg and Mateer (2001) have an **Attention Questionnaire** that asks patients to rate the frequency of general problems in everyday life, such as "my mind keeps wandering" or "difficult to pay attention to more than one thing at a time" (p. 155).

MEMORY

A common tool is the **Wechsler Memory Scale** (WMS), which contains seven subtests (Table 12.6). The sum of subtest scores is called the Memory Quotient (MQ). Performance on the WMS is not necessarily related to overall intelligence. A case whose frontal lobe was penetrated by a billiard cue was impaired on this memory test but had a Full Scale IQ of 123 (Kapur, 1994). The MQ has been criticized for representing memory as an odd variety of cognitive functions. Also, the test is heavily weighted on verbal abilities and immediate memory skills. The WMS-III is an update (Wechsler, 1997b).

Traditional clinical tests of memory have an unclear relationship to theories of memory. Our survey of the study of aphasia has given us some idea of the distinction between working memory (WM) and long-term memory (LTM). By now we should also be sensitive to the corresponding distinction between process and the stable storage of knowledge. Processes, constrained by WM, make contact with knowledge in LTM. These processes are involved in the *acquisition* of new information and the *activation* of old or stored information whenever it is needed for a task. Basic investigation of CHI has been sensitive to these and other distinctions in a multidimensional memory system.

Short-Term and Working Memory

The Digit Span subtest of the WAIS has exposed a deficiency of short-term buffer capacity in patients with CHI (see Table 12.3). A patient can be left with only a short-term memory (STM) deficit six months after injury (Van der Linden, Coyette, and Seron, 1992). Duration of short-term retention can be studied with a **continuous recognition**

TABLE 12.6 Subtests of the Wechsler Memory Scale (Wechsler, 1945).

SUBTEST	DESCRIPTION
I. Personal and current information	Give age, birthdate, and current and recent public officials
II. Orientation	Answer questions about time and place
III. Mental control	Say alphabet, count by fours
IV. Logical memory	Provide immediate retelling of two short stories
V. Digit span	Count forward and backward, slight difference from WAIS subtest
VI. Visual reproduction	Demonstrate immediate recall of three designs
VII. Associate learning	Demonstrate recall of related and unrelated word-pairs

memory task. For example, a series of drawings may be presented and some are repeated. As each drawing appears, a subject reports if the drawing is "new" or "old" (i.e., like one seen before). In a study of adolescents with CHI, Hannay and Levin (1989) found that short-term recognition memory varied as a function of severity of injury. Those with mild head injuries performed like normal controls, whereas moderately and severely injured subjects were impaired.

Another method for testing duration of retention in STM consists of placing a few seconds between a subspan series of digits and the recall test. Also, a subject is asked to count backwards during the interval in order to minimize rehearsal of the list. One version of this paradigm is the *Portland Digit Recognition Test,* which has been used to determine if financial incentives influence the measurement of cognitive deficit in mildly head-injured people (Binder, 1993). A group seeking compensation was compared to a group not seeking compensation. CHI was caused by falls, motor vehicle accidents (MVA), and timber cutting or sawmill accidents. The no-compensation group was superior to the compensation-seeking group, which is consistent with the possibility that the compensation-seeking group was exaggerating memory deficits or malingering (also, Trueblood and Schmidt, 1993).

Many studies, including the studies of attention mentioned earlier, have led to identifying "mental slowness" or **slow information processing** as a fundamental consequence of head injury. Pronounced deficit in the Digit Symbol subtest of the WAIS is a clinical indication of this problem.

Sternberg's (1975) classic *short-term memory scanning* procedure provides a more precise picture of processing speed and style. The new Symbol Search subtest in the WAIS-III appears to have been modeled after the Sternberg procedure.

The Sternberg task is a short-term recognition test in which response time is measured. A short series of digits (i.e., within memory span) is presented, followed immediately by a test digit. Subjects indicate if the test digit was in the preceding list. Researchers vary the length of the digit series to determine scanning speed and type of search (i.e., terminating at recognition or exhaustive no matter when the match is found). The task was given to severe CHIs who were at least 18 months postinjury (Schmitter-Edgecombe, Marks, Fahy, and Long, 1992). Again, the subjects with CHI were slower than controls, but they scanned exhaustively and made matching decisions like the controls.

Long-Term Memory

Head-injured patients experience two types of difficulty:

- **retrograde amnesia** involves forgetting memories acquired *before* injury (e.g., "remote memory")
- **anterograde amnesia** involves forgetting experiences occuring *after* injury (e.g., "recent memory")

The time periods of the original memory formation are illustrated in Figure 12.1. Although anterograde amnesia involves recent memories of just a

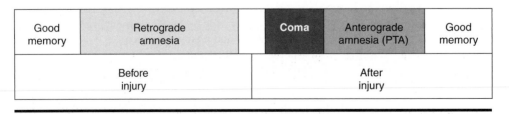

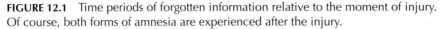

FIGURE 12.1   Time periods of forgotten information relative to the moment of injury. Of course, both forms of amnesia are experienced after the injury.

few previous hours, the clinical reference to recent memory is not the same as working memory. The information to be recalled should have been consolidated into LTM according to theories of the memory system.

Severity of retrograde amnesia increases as the memory gap extends further into the past. Any experiment or clinical assessment must delve into memories acquired prior to injury. Depending on a patient's age, an interview may explore recollections from contemporary life, early adulthood, and childhood (e.g., Van der Linden, Bredart, Depoorter, and Coyette, 1996). Memory for impersonal world events might be quizzed with questions organized according to periods of time (e.g., Beatty, Salmon, Bernstein, and Butters, 1987). During recovery, the amnesic gap shrinks toward the time of injury. A mild gap comprises 30 minutes prior to injury and is usually long lasting.

One formal assessment for retrograde amnesia is the *Autobiographical Memory Interview* (AMI), a test of "personal remote memory" (Kopelman, Wilson, and Baddeley, 1989). It is a semistructured interview that focuses on three time periods of a patient's life. Each recollection is scored for amount of information and vividness. In general, anyone's memory of the distant past is spotty, and an evaluator should check with a family member or friend for a substantiating source.

Anterograde amnesia, along with disorientation, is a significant component of what is widely known as **post-traumatic amnesia** (PTA). With anterograde amnesia, the patient does not remember meeting hospital staff or what was for breakfast earlier that day. The patient also experiences retrograde amnesia, but day-to-day recording of postinjury events is more prominent and problematic. PTA appears after regaining consciousness and usually lasts much longer than the duration of coma. It is said to end when a patient "remembers today what happened yesterday and does not begin each day with a blank mind" (Jennett and Teasdale, 1981, p. 89). A brief assessment is the *Galveston Orientation and Amnesia Test* (GOAT) (Levin, O'Donnell, and Grossman, 1979). Eight

of its 10 questions assess orientation to person, place, and time. The other two questions ask a patient to recall the first memory after the injury and the last memory before the injury.

Claudia Osborn (1998) was a physician and teacher at New York University. She was riding a bicycle when she was struck by a car and sent flying through the air. She was initially diagnosed as having postconcussive syndrome, a mild head injury. Nevertheless, she insisted on returning to work where other doctors had to remind her of things such as having seen a patient earlier in the day. She forgot appointments. Visiting one patient, she asked, "Where's her chart?" Her intern replied, "You have the chart in your hand" (p. 37).

Because anterograde amnesia involves information that should be acquired after the injury, research has commonly consisted of new learning procedures. One example is a paired-associate learning task (Schacter and Graf, 1986). A list of unassociated word pairs is presented for a subject to study (e.g., *window-reason*). Then, recall or learning is tested two ways. An **explicit test** consists of presenting the first word (e.g., *window-*) to see if the paired word is remembered. A subject is aware that memory is being tested. Prior to the explicit test, the subject is also given a word-stem completion task that can be done without prior exposure to the list (e.g., *rea____*). Performance on this test could be affected by priming or, namely, by the facilitating effect of prior experience. By seeing if the subject completes stems from the list more accurately or faster than stems not in the list, this turns out to be an **implicit test** of list learning.

The terminology for this distinction varies (Table 12.7). However, results are fairly consistent. Schacter and Graf found impairment with explicit testing but not with implicit testing. Implicit recall also indicates that new information can be acquired and retained for a while. The impairment lies in effortful retrieval processes. Yet, there is also a stimulus encoding problem mainly in the first year postinjury and the problem with distractibility. Both can make it difficult to acquire new information.

TABLE 12.7 Different terminology for two levels of the memory test. The terms tend to identify different aspects of the same thing (Levin, Goldstein, High, and Williams, 1988; Schacter and Graf, 1986).

LEVELS OF RECALL TEST	DEFINITION
automatic, covert, implicit, incidental	Without awareness that prior learning or memory is being tested; "unconscious"
effortful, overt, explicit, intentional	With awareness that prior learning or memory is being tested; "conscious"

Can the nature of these amnesias be pinpointed with respect to features of the memory system? Are retrograde and anterograde amnesias different cognitive disorders? Two main issues have been considered. One is whether people with CHI have a characteristic difficulty with one type of information storage, such as semantic or episodic memory. The other question pertains to whether the impairment is a disappearance of information from long-term storage or is a disruption of processes that make contact with preserved long-term storage.

Several cases have been presented to address the question of whether memory deficit is specific to one type of information. Gene, who suffered a severe head injury in a motorcycle accident, was one of these cases (Schacter, 1996). He could not recall day-to-day events and could not remember specific events from any period in his life. He could not recall motorcycle trips with his friends or a train derailment near his home. Yet, he could remember facts such as the floor plan of his childhood home and names of friends and schools. He could discuss the nature of his work prior to injury but could not recall events that had occurred while on the job. He could tell how to change a tire but could not recall ever having changed one. The deficit was with episodic memory, not semantic memory. Based on the study of Gene and other cases, Schacter (1996) suspected that event-specific knowledge is episodic and more general levels of autobiographical knowledge are recorded in semantic memory.

Assuming pretraumatic memories were acquired normally, then retrograde amnesia can be either a destruction of stored memories or a retrieval problem. The spontaneous gradual return of remote memories is indicative of preserved storage and a damaged retrieval mechanism. By itself, however, this does not account for the retrieval of memories of the distant past better than memories of the more recent past (Squire, 1987).

Functional Memory

Do laboratory tests predict everyday memory? This question was posed by Sunderland, Harris, and Baddeley (1983) in a comparison between self-reports of everyday memory and a variety of experimental and clinical tests (e.g., continuous recognition, story recall, and paired-associate learning). Also, a group about three months after injury was compared to a group between two and eight years postinjury. Patients and their relatives filled out questionnaires for rating the frequency of occurrence of memory errors over the previous few weeks. They also took home booklets that contained checklists regarding the same 35 items for indicating whether the memory failure occurred each day for seven days.

The 35 items in the questionnaires and checklists were selected according to five categories. Here are some examples that might inform any work with a patient's memory:

Speech

- Forgetting the names of friends or relatives or calling them by the wrong names.

- Forgetting something you were told a few minutes ago. Perhaps something your wife or a friend just said.
- Forgetting to tell somebody something important. Perhaps forgetting to pass on a message or remind someone of something.
- Repeating a story or joke you have already told.

Reading and Writing

- Forgetting what the sentence you have just read was about and having to reread it.
- Finding yourself unable to follow the thread of a story. Losing track of what it is about.

Faces and Places

- Forgetting where you have put something. Losing things around the house.
- Failing to recognize television characters or other famous people by sight.
- Getting lost or turning in the wrong direction on a journey or walk you have often been on.

Actions

- Forgetting to do some routine thing that you would normally do once or twice in a day.
- Starting to do something, then forgetting what it was you wanted to do. Maybe saying, "What am I doing?"

Learning New Things

- Finding yourself unable to remember the name of someone you met for the first time recently.
- Forgetting to keep an appointment.

Sunderland and his colleagues found that the relatives' questionnaire correlated with 6 of 14 test performances for the long-term head-injured group but not for the recently injured group. The patients' questionnaire did not correlate with any of the laboratory tests. The results reflect the instability of memory in the first few months after injury and indicate that formal tests may not be predictive of everyday memory, at least, in the way that everyday memory was assessed in this study.

This type of research motivated creation of the **Rivermead Behavioural Memory Test** (RBMT), which can be given by "qualified speech therapists" (Wilson, Cockburn, and Baddeley, 1985). It is used to predict the status of everyday memory. Subtests entail learning someone's name, finding an object that has been hidden from view, recalling a route, and recalling a sequence of actions. It includes evaluation of *prospective memory,* in which a patient is asked to remember to do something at a prearranged time or signal (i.e., "remember to remember"). Research indicates that the RBMT is predictive of functional independence in the community (Wilson, Baddeley, Cockburn et al., 1989).

Memory and Sense of Self

What is the impact of amnesia on an individual's sense of who he or she is? A severe retrograde amnesia can have devastating consequences. Schacter (1996) commented on the aftermath of Gene's motorcycle accident: "A life without any episodic memory is psychologically barren . . . Nothing much happens in Gene's mind or in his life. He has few friends and lives quietly at home with his parents . . . he thinks little about the future. It does not occur to him to make plans . . ." (pp. 149–150). Another patient could not remember most of what happened in his life prior to a bilateral thalamic stroke, but he could remember details about his service in the navy during World War II nearly 50 years before (Hodges and McCarthy, 1993). In fact, his identity became so attached to that period that he came to believe that he was still in active service and would have to return to his ship soon.

EXECUTIVE FUNCTIONS

"Action disorganization" is caused by an impairment of the central executive component of working memory (Baddeley, 1986). Shallice (1988) called it a Supervisory Attentional System (SAS). Although a central executive is occasionally associated with any aspect of WM (e.g., Van der Linden et al., 1992), it usually refers to the management of resources in dual-tasks and in the performance of multiple actions. Tasks used to assess the executive appear to be related to success at work.

The general assumption is that simple routine or highly skilled actions are carried out quickly and efficiently in the automatic processing mode. The executive system, on the other hand, is thought to be invoked intentionally for novel or difficult actions or when errors occur in routine actions. It regulates attentional resources to reach a goal. Let us assume that a goal is to get to work. According to Duncan (1986), executive function starts with *goal lists* such as taking a shower, getting dressed, and eating breakfast before going to work. An *action list* is the mental operations and overt actions engaged in meeting these goals. *Self-monitoring* or means-ends analysis compares current states and goal states, ensuring that goals are being met.

Another depiction of the executive includes other components, all of which are thought to be a reponsibility of the frontal lobes (Norman and Shallice, 1986):

- *initiation and drive:* activating a cognitive system
- *inhibition:* stopping behavior
- *task persistence:* maintaining behavior
- *organization:* structure of actions
- *generative thinking:* creativity and flexibility
- *awareness:* self-monitoring and modification

Sohlberg and Mateer (2001) identified some symptoms of deficit in each of these components, namely:

- does not go to the grocery when the refrigerator is empty
- shops impulsively
- does not get all items on a shopping list
- does not use aisle headings

- does not think of a substitute for an unavailable item
- is not concerned about a need for groceries

These components also appear under the heading of *problem solving,* which begins with initiating a solution. Claudia Osborne (1998) was returning home from rehabilitation one day in hectic Manhattan. Standing on a curb, she froze. "My thinking was on hold, my mind blank" (p. 61). She called it *flooding,* when her mind is overwhelmed, her thinking slows down, and she becomes mentally stuck.

Impaired executive control produces what is known as **dysexecutive syndrome.** Executive control applies to any information-processing domain, and the syndrome should be manifested in a wide variety of tasks. The *Wisconsin Card Sorting Test* (WCST) (Grant and Berg, 1948) is often used to test executive function. It is said to test abilities to identify abstract categories and shift cognitive set. The WCST contains 64 cards depicting one to four colored shapes. Patients must determine a sorting strategy according to a criterion that an examiner has in mind (e.g., color or shape) and that is deduced from the examiner's feedback (i.e., "right" or "wrong"). Once a patient uses one criterion consistently, the examiner changes the criterion.

In one study, CHIs exhibited fewer sorts and more perseverative errors than normal controls on the WCST (Gansler, Covall, McGrath, and Oscar-Berman, 1996). In general, patients have difficulty shifting response sets and evaluating their performance.

The *Behavioral Assessment of the Dysexecutive Syndrome* (BADS) is explicitly intended to test executive functions of planning and problem solving (Wilson, Alderman, Burgess et al., 1996). The BADS consists of six subtests:

- *Temporal Judgment:* predict duration of events
- *Rule Shift Cards:* similar to card-sorting tests
- *Action Program:* remove a cork
- *Key Search:* search for lost keys
- *Zoo Map:* plan a route to visit six sites at a zoo

- *Six Elements:* schedule time for six tasks in 10 minutes

Perhaps because most tasks are relatively easy, Sohlberg and Mateer's (2001) experience has been that BADS is insensitive to mild cognitive deficit.

PERSONALITY AND BEHAVIOR

After a boat accident while on a family vacation, Alan Forman went through "an extreme disinhibited phase" described by his wife Cathy (Crimmins, 2000). He threw things and called the nurses "bitches" and "assholes." Professionals refer to this as a social skills deficit.

The person with CHI appears to have taken on a different personality. There is an absence of self-regulation. The patient becomes easily agitated and embarrassingly impulsive. These **challenging behaviors,** according to Sohlberg and Mateer (2001), may be reactive factors associated with feelings of loss and frustration. The patient "acts in ways that appear selfish, rude, or otherwise unmindful of others" (p. 338). These behaviors may be piled on to the natural distress of sudden disability and are disruptive of attempts at rehabilitation.

Neuropsychologists have tried to document the life-altering effects of disability. Stambrook and others (1991) administered self-report questionnaires to obtain perspectives of patients and their spouses. One questionnaire addressed emotional, psychological, and physical problems. Another measured extent of emotional distress. A third questionnaire measured social and free-time activities and negative social behaviors. Stambrook compared CHIs and a group with spinal cord injury. Moderately impaired CHIs and spinal cord injured patients were equivalent on all measures. Severely impaired CHIs were distinctive in being more bewildered, depressed, and hostile than the other groups. Wives rated the severe CHIs as being more belligerent, helpless, and withdrawn than the others.

Denise was 42 years old when her truck was broadsided by a bigger truck. When she arrived at rehabilitation, she had no energy for therapy. She was bored and surly, and she preferred to stay in bed. She was always adjusting her neck brace, and she was impatient. "Why are you asking all these questions? I'm 24." From the halls, she could be heard screaming for no apparent reason. After four items of the SLP's testing, she shouted "I'm overloaded right now!" With the SLP's easy and steady tone, Denise calmed down but could not continue with the assessment. The goals for the first week of her rehabilitation were to tolerate the presence of her therapist and to interact for 20 minutes without agitation.

Two weeks later, Denise was in physical therapy joking around with the therapists and her husband, who was on his cell phone telling his friends how well she was doing. "We take so much for granted," he was saying. She stood three times for three minutes each and then got dizzy. With support, she walked five feet. Denise turned, smiled, and declared, "OK. The bitch is back."

Often therapists are patient and wait until early agitation disappears. Sometimes the clinical neuropsychologist calls in a major assessment. The **Minnesota Multiphasic Personality Inventory** (MMPI) is part of the Halstead-Reitan battery and is the most widely used objective personality measure (Hathaway and McKinley, 1951). It is a 566-item true/false questionnaire requiring sixth grade reading skills. Answers contribute to 4 *validity scales* (i.e., test-taking competency) and 10 *clinical scales.* Interpretation of the clinical scales is based on a pattern of scores that can be related to normal control subjects and diagnostic groups of psychiatric patients. Neuropsychologists are careful to avoid blind psychiatric interpretation without taking medical conditions into consideration.

Marsh (1999) reviewed other assessments targeting social skills. One was the *Simulated Social Interaction Test* (Curran, 1982). It provides an initial assessment for identifying situations in which a patient has difficulty. The test procedure consists of the evaluator describing a situation in which a confederate makes a response. The patient's response to the confederate is rated. The wide range of interpersonal problems includes criticism, anger expression, conflict with a relative, and more.

INSIGHT (AWARENESS)

Patients are often unaware of their behavior or personality changes, an anosognosia that is linked to frontal lobe damage (McGlynn and Schacter, 1989). Whereas family members become stressed by a patient's anxiety and bad temper, the patient denies such disturbances. Persons with CHI also may not complain of physical disabilities. Neuropsychologists say that patients have a **posttraumatic insight disorder** that is observed as an underreporting of the severity of impairments (also, referred to as "unawareness").

Dr. Osborn's friend Marcia knew that Claudia was different, but Claudia insisted on returning to work soon after the accident. At work, she had trouble following conversations. She recognized that a particular conversation was difficult, but she did not recognize that she could not follow conversations in general. "My family perceived my problems more clearly than I did" (Osborn, 1998, p. 32). After another doctor told her that she had a "moderately severe head injury" and insisted she have therapy before returning to work, she declared, "I still know medicine . . . It's only the little pieces causing trouble." When asked what she meant by "the little pieces," Claudia replied, "Memory problems, according to them" (p. 40).

Several studies show that patients with mild or severe head trauma often underestimate memory impairments (McGlynn and Schacter, 1989). They realize their memory is worse but are not aware of the severity of deficit. Family members feel that the memory impairment is more serious than the patient does (e.g., Van der Linden et al., 1996). Patients with more LH damage are more likely to report memory problems than patients with more RH damage. A patient might admit to a slight memory problem when questioned but still insist that returning to work is a realistic goal. Some training of compensatory strategies may be accompanied by an increase of self-awareness in

the training tasks, but this more realistic estimate of deficit sometimes does not carry over to the work setting.

Investigators found that CHI patients at six months postinjury continued to underreport severity of deficits. Other patients with CHI demonstrated greater insight at one year and at two to three years postinjury (Godfrey, Partridge, Knight, and Bishara, 1993). However, improved insight was accompanied by increased emotional dysfunction. Depression and anxiety were found to be less in the first six months postinjury than later, and these problems peak between 7 and 12 months after injury (Lezak and O'Brien, 1988). The delayed onset of depression may be the result of a gradually increasing awareness of impairments. In general, patients may be difficult to engage in rehabilitation during the first year because of unrealistic treatment goals, while a later challenge is the negative reaction to an emerging understanding of impairment (see Prigatano and Klonoff, 1998).

LANGUAGE

At the beginning of this chapter, Hagen (1981) was cited for suggesting that CHI in some cases causes cognitive disorders without language problems and in other cases causes aphasia or language problems that are secondary to cognitive disorders. Wertz (1985) referred to the secondary deficits as "language of confusion" (e.g., McDonald, 1993). Let us begin our examination of language with results of clinical tests.

Clinical Tests and Diagnosis

What proportion of CHIs have aphasia? Heilman, Safran, and Geschwind (1971) administered an unspecified aphasia examination to 750 patients with CHI and concluded that only 2 percent had aphasia (also, Schwartz-Cowley and Stepanik, 1989). Fifty patients were studied elsewhere, and they had minimal deficits on language tests except for 40 percent who had naming difficulties (Levin, Grossman, and Kelly, 1976). Among Heilman's

13 diagnosed with aphasia, 9 had anomic aphasia and 4 had Wernicke's aphasia. Hartley and Levin (1990) said that acute CHIs can display language behavior similar to Wernicke's aphasia, which evolves to anomic-like aphasia as orientation improves.

Sarno, Buonaguro, and Levita (1987) examined 25 CHIs nearly four months after injury with four tasks from a standard aphasia battery. The tests consisted of naming, sentence repetition, word fluency, and the Token Test of sentence comprehension. The patients were impaired in all tasks to levels found in stroke-related aphasia. Sarno decided that they had found "parallel aphasias which characterized both CHI and CVA aphasic patients" (p. 336). Earlier, Sarno (1980) had concluded that 32 percent of a head-injured group had aphasia whereas others had a "subclinical aphasia" with no apparent deficit in conversation but still an impairment in word fluency.

Thirty Italian severe CHIs received an Italian translation of a German test for aphasia plus some more naming tasks and tests of other cognitive functions (Luzzatti, et al., 1989). Sixteen participants had unilateral lesions according to CT scan. On the aphasia test, CHIs scored in the range for mild language deficit. Of 18 participants classified as aphasic, 11 were diagnosed as having Broca's aphasia according to test criteria. However, presence of dysarthria influenced classification of six of these nonfluent cases.

Porch identified three **bilateral signs** with respect to performance on the PICA:

1. a visual-auditory reversal with either auditory subtests higher than the visual object matching subtests
2. high verbal ability near levels of receptive modalities
3. unusually low copying in subtests

To examine the validity of this diagnostic aid, Bernstein-Ellis and others (1985) gave the PICA to 15 cases of traumatic brain injury. The patients had deficits in all areas of language function, but statistical analysis showed a unique pattern. Visual matching was worse and writing sentences was better for patients with TBI than for those with stroke-related aphasia. Yet, the bilateral signs did not distinguish traumatic injury. Ten of the head-injured patients showed one sign, five showed two signs, and none displayed all three.

These studies indicate that some patients with CHI exhibit deficits on language tests. The studies also leave an impression that clinical investigators differ with respect to diagnosing these deficits as aphasia. However, even if everyone agrees on what aphasia is, findings are going to differ when one sample size is 750 and another is 25. One sample may have more predominantly unilateral lesions than another. Yet, there is an impression that "language of confusion" has been diagnosed as aphasia or, at least, as "subclinical" aphasia. Holland (1982) did not mince words: "If the language problems seen in closed head injured patients don't look like aphasia, sound like aphasia, act like aphasia, feel, smell or taste like aphasia, then they aren't aphasia" (p. 345).

A debate over diagnosis of aphasia has implications for treatment. Sarno and others (1987) concluded that "the traditional language rehabilitation approaches implemented with CVA aphasic patients are appropriate for the management of aphasia in CHI patients as well" (p. 336). On the other hand, Holland (1982) stated that CHI patients "will not be terribly responsive to the traditional methods by which we have come to treat aphasia" (p. 345). This apparent disagreement dissolves if we agree that CHI is not a homogeneous neurological condition and is similarly diverse in its consequences. It is possible that CHI patients with secondary language deficits may not be responsive to traditional aphasia methods, whereas CHI patients with aphasias caused by more focal insults may be responsive to these methods.

In general, SLPs have been avoiding aphasia testing for patients with CHI, because language-specific disorders are rare (e.g., Body and Parker, 1999). People with CHI have language difficulties induced by cognitive impairment and pragmatic difficulties with the use of language, neither of which are addressed by traditional tests for aphasia.

Language Comprehension

The experimental study of language comprehension with CHI is a barren landscape compared to the study of aphasia caused by stroke. To examine lexical contact with semantic memory, Haut and others (1991) presented a unique priming task in which subjects made rapid judgments about whether a second word is a member of the semantic category of the first word. The subjects with CHI were primed, indicating that semantic organization was preserved both before and after one year postonset. However, the patients were also slow. This result is consistent with Schacter's clinical observation of preserved semantic memory (while access to episodic memory is impaired) and is consistent with the robust finding that CHI reduces the speed of information processing in working memory.

Patients with CHI were compared with patients with stroke-related aphasia on Caplan's Thematic Role Battery introduced in Chapter 4 (Butler-Hinz, Caplan, and Waters, 1990). The battery tests "final interpretation" of various canonical and noncanonical sentence structures and employs the enactment strategy of manipulating toy animals. Pattern of difficulty among sentence types was similar between groups. However, French-speaking clinical groups differed in that the stroke group had more severe impairment than the CHI group; English-speaking clinical groups did not differ in severity of deficit. The French stroke group was more impaired than the other three groups, attributed mainly to the small size of each group. The similarity of pattern led the investigators to conclude that LH stroke and CHI cause qualitatively similar sentence comprehension impairments.

One lesson of Chapter 5 was that we should delay conclusions about the nature of disorder until we have a body of online research that taps into ongoing sentence processing. Tyler (1985) reported some unusual online studies of DE who, at age 16, was involved in a motorcycle accident and apparently had a secondary occlusion in the left internal carotid artery. There was no evidence of RH damage. Apparently DE's main disorder looked, sounded, and acted like aphasia, as his Boston Exam indicated that he was "a typical Broca's agrammatic patient." Tyler began her studies around 13 years after the accident.

With the word-monitoring procedure, Tyler initially examined "global" capabilities without a clear relationship to a particular comprehension mechanism. DE was handed a word on a card (e.g., *church*) and was instructed to press a button as soon as he heard it. Tyler presented normal sentences (1a), anomalous sentences that retained syntactic form (1b), and scrambled utterances without syntactic or semantic sense (1c).

(1a) Everyone was outraged when they heard. Apparently, in the middle of the night some thieves broke into the *church* and stole a golden crucifix.

(1b) Everyone was exposed when they ate. Apparently, at the distance of the wind some ants pushed around the *church* and forced a new item.

(1c) They everyone when outraged heard was. Of middle apparently the some of the into the broke night in thieves *church* and crucifix stole a golden.

In such studies of linguistic violations, the normal processor slows down in the vicinity of errors. DE's response also slowed down as semantic sense and syntactic form were stripped away. He was unlike normals, however, by not responding with increasing speed as the location of target words was changed from left to right in anomalous sentences like 1b. Tyler diagnosed this absence of word-position effect as an impairment in detecting the syntactic structure of these sentences.

A second word-monitoring experiment was more focused, as Tyler examined sensitivity to violations of verb-argument relations. The target word was placed in either a correct context (2a), a selection violation after verbs that take a direct object (2b), or a strict subcategorization violation after verbs that do not take a direct object (2c).

(2a) The crowd was waiting eagerly. The young man grabbed the *guitar* and . . . [one more clause].

(2b) The crowd was waiting eagerly. The young man drank the *guitar* and . . . [one more clause].

(2c) The crowd was waiting eagerly. The young man slept the *guitar* and . . . [one more clause].

Slowed response in the vicinity of verb-argument violations indicated that DE was sensitive to verb-argument structure. The longest response was for subcategorization violation (2c). Tyler suggested that DE retained this lexically driven capacity, so that difficulties with anomalous sentences in the first experiment had to be because of a problem with some other aspect of syntax.

Later, Tyler (1989) focused on anomalous sentences to see if DE could detect phrase-level structural violations (called "local" violations). A baseline condition contained a target word in a normal phrase (3a). Then, word-order violations were placed in the same location as in 3b.

(3a) An orange dream was loudly watching the house during smelling lights because within these signs /a slow *kitchen*/ snored with crashing leaves.

(3b) An orange dream was loudly watching the house during smelling lights because within these signs /slow very *kitchen*/ snored with crashing leaves.

Tyler also located the target word early or late in the sentence; again, DE did not have the normal position effect (replicating the result in 1985). He also had the normal pattern of slowing down when there was a local structural violation late in the sentence. This result, along with his verb-argument, ability, led Tyler to conclude that DE could assign structure at a local level and was, in fact, dependent on this level of syntactic processing.

Language Production

When CHI causes linguistic impairments, "anomia is the primary linguistic deficit reported" (Hartley and Levin, 1990, p. 356). Boles (1997) found that patients with TBI and Alzheimer's disease make more visual misperception errors than stroke patients with aphasia (e.g., "can" for *drum*). In discussing misnaming, Holland (1982) argued that impaired language behavior need not be indicative of aphasia. Errors with CHI may be perceptually based or confabulatory.

As with RHD, deficit is most frequently evident in word fluency tasks. Several investigators studied CHI with a letter fluency task (e.g., Gruen, Frankle, and Schwartz, 1990; Wertz et al., 1986). Lohman and others (1989) found that the number of words produced per letter increased as Rancho Los Amigos (RLA) cognitive level increased from V to VII (see Table 12.4). These investigators also found substantial reductions in words produced for nine categories such as clothes, furniture, and birds. Typicality of words was unusual for only two categories, which is again consistent with the retention of fairly good semantic organization.

Another component of the Halstead-Reitan battery is the **Thurstone Word Fluency Test** developed in 1938 (see Pendleton, Heaton, Lehman, and Hulihand, 1982). In this short test, a patient is asked to produce words to a couple of letters; the main difference from other tests is that the response is in writing. Pendleton's research team administered the test to several neurologically impaired groups, comparing effects of localized and diffuse lesions. They found that letter fluency is disrupted by any type or location of damage. Frontal and LH damage produced more difficulty, but the test did not discriminate frontal and diffuse lesions.

Crowe (1992) wanted to see if frontal lobe syndromes behave differently on the FAS letter-fluency test. All groups had reduced levels of response, despite the impaired impulse control of the orbitofrontal group (mainly CHIs). The CHIs produced more uninhibited responding, such as random neologisms, than a medially damaged group consisting of a variety of neuropathologies.

Word-finding deficits may translate into information deficiencies in discourse. Ehrlich (1988) elicited picture descriptions from severe CHIs at various times postonset. A standard content analysis showed no difference from normal controls in syllables per minute and number of content units produced. However, the clinical group produced fewer content units per minute.

Glosser and Deser (1991) studied interviews with nine patients at RLA Levels V to VII. The CHIs produced paraphasias but did not produce more indefinite or generic words than normal controls. The patients made some syntactic errors and had some grammatical omissions but spoke at a normal level of syntactic complexity.

PRAGMATICS AND DISCOURSE

Holland (1982) suggested that "it is in the area of language pragmatics that aphasia and head injured language most vividly contrast" (p. 347). We may suspect that anterograde amnesia and either apathy or disinhibition would affect interpersonal interactions. Retrograde amnesia and dysexecutive syndrome may influence storytelling.

Discourse Comprehension

Skye McDonald of Sydney, Australia, has conducted a variety of experiments to examine the pragmatic use of language with TBI. Like the study of RHD, the comprehension of sarcasm seemed to be a good vehicle for examining instances in which literal meaning of an utterance differs from the speaker's intent and, thus, for studying the status of theory of mind in persons with CHI. There is some neuroimaging evidence that frontal lobes are important for forming a representation of the intentions or beliefs of others (e.g., Gallagher and Frith, 2003).

McDonald and Pearce (1996) studied a clinical group of 10, six with severe closed head injury, three with open head injury, and one with an anterior hemorrhage. Their common characteristic was frontal lobe damage. McDonald first asked participants to read snippets of a conversation (see examples 4 and 5) and then answer questions about what Mark and Wayne meant.

(4a) *Mark:* What a great football game.
(4b) *Wayne:* So you are glad I asked you.

(5a) *Mark:* What a great football game.
(5b) *Wayne:* Sorry I made you come.

We should be particularly interested in Mark's intent in the second example (5a) where he must have really thought it was a lousy football game. The head-injured group could comprehend literal meaning (i.e., sincere intent) but had difficulty with sarcastic intent. The same results were found when speakers provided sarcastic prosody. The type of error was mainly literal interpretation of remarks like 5a. In the same report, five of seven patients had difficulty interpreting the emotion conveyed with semantically neutral utterances. Together, these experiments indicated that some individuals with frontal lobe damage have a pragmatic problem with nonliteral interpretation.

There were some problems with McDonald and Pearce's task, such as its sparse context. Channon and others (2005) decided to try a slightly different approach that entailed making a distinction between direct and indirect sarcasm. An example (6) is shorter than the stimuli used in their study.

(6)   Alex removes two thoroughly burned pieces of toast from a toaster. Mary arrives, and Alex asks with a puzzled expression, "Am I a good cook?"
   (a) Direct sarcasm: "The best cook in the world."
   (b) Indirect sarcasm: "I'll hire you in my restaurant."

Direct sarcasm requires a simple inference, whereas indirect sarcasm requires a longer inferential chain for comprehension (i.e., additionally, cooks in restaurants need to be good) and is not necessarily the direct opposite of a literal expression. Channon presented more informative complex scenarios to a larger group of 19 with CHI. They were poorer in comprehending both types of sarcastic remarks relative to sincere literal remarks. In another task, the CHIs had a similar problem with interpreting ironic actions of characters (e.g., Alex served Mary a burnt meal that he had spent the day preparing. Mary ate all her meal and took a second helping).

The type of error is detected in these studies by asking participants to explain the meaning of target statements. Contrary to McDonald and Pearce's results, errors were mostly a variety of incorrect nonliteral interpretations and few literal interpretations (i.e., Alex is a great cook). This showed that the CHIs had some appreciation for nonliteralness but still had difficulty with processing the inference. Also, the difficulty across tasks was evidence for a general deficit in theory of mind (i.e., inferring another's beliefs or intentions) as opposed to a problem using social knowledge which is specific to the exchange of remarks.

Martin and McDonald (2003) crafted a hefty essay that explored three theories of pragmatic impairments observed with autism, RHD, and CHI. There are pros and cons regarding each theory. A key point, however, applies to many areas of clinical investigation including discourse production in the following section. Martin and McDonald worried about overly narrow theoretical perspectives in the context of differences among methodologies aimed at a general problem, such as pragmatic comprehension. The risk is that a perspective can be the product of a method and have limited explanatory value because not all methods have been enlisted to solve the problem.

So, Martin and McDonald (2005) compared two of the three explanations of pragmatic comprehension impairment in a study of the comprehension of ironic jokes. The task was adapted from Winner and others' (1998) study of RHD. One theory of pragmatic dysfunction is the theory of mind deficit. The other theory is the impairment of executive function. The role of executive function is thought to pertain to the ability of listeners to adjust interpretations according to context. The theories were evaluated with theory of mind (ToM) tasks and tests of executive functioning, and Martin and McDonald looked for associations between these tests and irony comprehension. Although CHIs were impaired on most tasks, there was no correlation between ToM tasks and joke comprehension, nor between certain executive tasks and joke comprehension. Tests of inferen-

tial reasoning were correlated, however, a further indication that a general process of inferencing is the problem.

Nicholas and Brookshire (1995a) commented on the dearth of research on discourse comprehension with CHI. They gave their *Discourse Comprehension Test* to a group with TBI, and these patients performed similarly to RHDs and aphasic patients. If there is a special influence of attention deficit or other primary impairments on this level of language comprehension, asking about main ideas and details in stories does not seem to tap into it. Testing recall with these test materials may be more demanding, but performance with details and main ideas does not appear to differentiate injury from normalcy (Kennedy and Nawrocki, 2003).

Discourse Production

A few investigators, such as Carl Coelho at the University of Connecticut, have specialized in the study of CHI. Others have specialized in the study of RHD. As a result, research has had broadly differing styles according to the discourse elicited and the analysis employed (Table 12.8). The study of CHI has relied less on pictures to elicit discourse and has utilized more cohesion analysis and less information analysis. A standard comprehensive strategy for assessing discourse production across clinical groups has not yet materialized. However, a broad multitask approach was initiated by Snow, Douglas, and Ponsford (1995).

In an unpublished dissertation, Wyckoff reported that CHIs produced a deficient number of cohesive ties and had an additional problem with accuracy when telling stories (cited in Mentis and Prutting, 1987). Hartley and Levin (1990) analyzed Wyckoff's data and decided that it contained three general profiles:

- confused discourse soon after injury, containing frequent inaccuracies, repetitions, and revisions
- cohesive discourse that is accurate but sometimes wordy or inefficient

TABLE 12.8 Characteristics of discourse research through 1994 in 13 studies of CHI and 21 studies of RHD. Some totals are over 100% because investigators often used more than one procedure (Davis et al., 1997).

	N	DISCOURSE TYPE	STIMULUS/TASK	ANALYSIS
CHI	13	8% description 38% narration 46% conversation	62% spontaneous 38% picture elicitation	23% information, content 54% cohesion 31% macroanalysis 31% conversational
RHD	21	33% description 57% narration 14% conversation	29% spontaneous 52% picture elicitation	48% information, content 14% cohesion 29% macroanalysis 10% conversational

• impoverished discourse with short utterances, little cohesion, and limited content

Published studies contain different conclusions. For example, Mentis and Prutting (1987) assessed cohesion for three patients at or above RLA Level VII. Subjects made high scores on a test for aphasia, and syntax was judged to be preserved. Subjects engaged in 10 minutes of conversation with a familiar partner, described their work or rehabilitation program, and produced routines (e.g., how to play a sport or bake a cake). The subjects used fewer cohesive ties than normal controls for description and routines. Glosser and Deser (1991) found nine CHIs to be unimpaired in referential cohesion. Glosser and Deser studied lower levels of function (V–VII), limited discourse to interviews, and looked for ties only within the preceding three "verbalizations."

Liles, Coelho, Duffy, and Zalagens (1989) compared elicitation procedures with four CHIs at RLA Level V and above. Two stories were elicited with pictured stimuli. One story was told after viewing a 19-frame filmstrip. The other story was told about a Norman Rockwell painting that remained in view during narration. Two CHIs were deficient in cohesion, and all CHIs presented cohesive styles that differed according to condition. While viewing the Rockwell painting, CHIs decreased pronoun reference and increased lexical cohesion relative to telling stories from memory.

The diminished cohesion was attributed to the requirement of translating a static representation into a dynamic series of events.

At the level of macrostructure, Liles and others (1989) studied completeness of narrative structure with respect to the presence of an initiating event, actions, and a consequence marking the attainment of goal. Three of four subjects produced no complete episodes for telling a story from a Rockwell painting. The report did not say whether CHIs deviated from story structure in any particular way.

Other studies have compared levels of discourse. Glosser and Deser (1991) studied thematic coherence by judging topic maintenance through an entire discourse. CHIs were distinctly impaired, contrary to their good cohesion and sentence form. Deficit was described as being greater for "global" coherence than for "local" cohesion. In a study by Coelho, Liles, and Duffy (1991), two patients with CHI displayed opposite patterns of ability. One had poor cohesion but good story structure. The other had poor story structure but good cohesion. Over 10 years later in a study of five patients who had been in motor vehicle accidents, Hough and Barrow (2003) found a "dissociation" between local and global coherence, with impairment of the global level reflected in thematic coherence. The exception in Coelho's study could be due, in part, to a difference between a measure of thematic coherence and his analysis of story structure as representations of global level formulation.

Coelho (2002) has continued to accumulate narrative transcripts. His work is interesting for the size of his groups (i.e., 55 CHIs and 47 non-brain-injured) and the attempt to cover multiple levels in analysis (i.e., within-sentence, cohesion between sentences, and story grammar). The only omission appears to be some sort of indicator of global thematic coherence. In this study, CHIs differed from the controls in all measures. Cohesion and story grammar were better for story retelling than for story generation, indicating the latter is more likely to expose difficulties.

Davis's study of narrative elicitation and retelling with RHDs was also conducted with a small group of individuals with CHI (Davis and Coelho, 2004). It may be one of a few examples of the same method being applied to the two populations.

Two patients at the RLA Level VII told the Flower Pot story quite differently (see Chapter 11). One gave the following fairly accurate version:

(7) "Looks like the guy got hit on the head with a flower pot, and he's probably swearing or something. He's gonna go up and paste the guy one. He's banging on the door, and the woman goes up, 'Oh, nice doggie.' And he's all sucked in. And he's showin' her the bump on his head. She gave the dog a bone."

Technically, *the woman* has no antecedent in the narration as an instance of signaling lexical co-reference. Also, the order of the last two events is reversed. However, this is a rather picky analysis of a fairly good story compared with another patient when telling the story from memory:

(8) "The apartment of the Mrs. Jones or Mr. Jones each waving his cane up her, cause he was watering the plants and fell out the window."

Conversation

As indicated in Table 12.8, conversational interactions have been investigated much more frequently with CHIs than RHDs. Some of these interactions are bolstered by a series of planned questions, which Snow, Douglas, and Ponsford (1995) called "semi-structured conversation." In general, the studies give us more ideas on how to assess functional communication. Some clues about what to look for come from the test of everyday memory presented earlier in the chapter. Head injured patients are asked if they forget things they were just told or forget what they had just said, perhaps repeating a recent story or joke.

Dr. Osborn's experience illustrates the influence of attention impairment and lack of insight on discourse comprehension and conversation. When she returned to work unaware of her impairments, she could not stay focused on the presentations by residents. "I lost track of the conversation . . . I faked understanding because I couldn't believe I didn't understand" (Osborn, 1998, p. 32).

Coelho and his colleagues (1993) compared five mildly aphasic patients with five CHIs at the highest RLA level in conversations on topics of the patients' choosing. Both clinical groups had difficulties initiating and sustaining conversation, and it was difficult to discern differences between them. Their communication partners had to assume more communicative burden than in control interactions between two neurologically intact partners (e.g., topic and turn initiation). The CHIs were described as especially subdued or requiring prompting to talk.

Later, Coelho, Youse, and Le (2002) had developed a larger sample of 32 CHIs in 15-minute conversational dyads with a clinician. Some results were similar to the earlier report. Compared to 43 hospital employees, the CHIs deviated in taking responsibility for initiating topics. The clinician had to ask more questions and introduce more topics when talking to the patients. Also, the CHIs produced information that did not contribute to the flow of conversation. For example, a patient would embark on tangents as if a topic made him think of something about himself.

In New Zealand, psychologists examined interactions with a significant other and an opposite-sex stranger (Marsh and Knight, 1991).

CHIs were more than 18 months postinjury. These clinical patients and significant others engaged in problem-solving tasks requiring them to reach a consensus. Interaction with the stranger was conducted in the guise of a social break in which the stranger took a seat next to the patient and asked, "How has everything been going this morning?" The interactions were evaluated with the *Behaviorally Referenced Rating System of Intermediate Social Skills* (BRISS) developed by Wallander and others (1985). In the problem-solving interactions, verbal communication was hampered by word-finding problems, lack of coherence, and the use of inappropriate expressions. With the opposite-sex partners, CHIs were passive and appeared disinterested.

McDonald investigated the pragmatic sensitivities of two cases who had been in motor vehicle accidents. She was especially interested in the influence of the disinhibition syndrome associated with frontal lobe damage. As indicated earlier in this chapter, the syndrome includes disorganization and poor impulse control or self-regulation.

In one study, McDonald (1993) isolated a component of conversation by having the two patients explain how to play a game to a naive listener who was blindfolded. She wanted to examine the ability to meet the informational needs of a listener, and she developed ratings based on Grice's maxims of conversation. For example, the maxim of quantity states that a speaker will say no more or less than is required. Scales classified whether there was too much or too little repetitiveness and detail. Both subjects were disorganized and ineffective in the task. One was repetitive, and the other had too little detail. Cohesion was not a problem, but statements were irrelevant or badly sequenced, making instructions very confusing.

McDonald and van Sommers (1993) focused on the use of polite indirect requests. They presented various situations verbally and asked the two subjects how they would respond (e.g., asking a stranger for the time, asking to borrow a car, hinting that you want to leave a dinner party). The subjects appeared to appreciate the situations but had difficulty formulating requests indirectly. At-

tempts at indirect requests ended up being more impulsively direct than those of control subjects. The investigators concluded that "impaired problem-solving ability and poor behavioural control also disrupt normal social communication skills" (p. 313). Later, they had similar findings with a group of 15 patients mostly with CHI (McDonald and Pearce, 1998).

Diagnosis with Discourse

Snow, Douglas, and Ponsford (1997) were concerned about the selection of control groups or norms for the diagnosis of deficit. For example, should 7 be considered to be deficient? In Snow's study, 26 TBIs were compared to two groups. One was a slightly older group of orthopedic patients who were similar demographically to the head-injured group. The other control was a somewhat younger group of university students considered to be demographically dissimilar from the clinical group. The TBI group differed from the students but not from the orthopedic group in productivity and content measures. The TBI group differed from both control groups with respect to a pragmatic measure (e.g., topic maintenance, situational appropriateness).

Thus, with some measures, identification of "deficit" depends on our frame of reference. Sociolinguistic variations need to be explored more before we settle on a normative basis for diagnosing discourse disorders. Moreover, several studies have shown that the appearance of deficits depends on the task and measurement.

Youse, Coelho, and others (2005) performed discriminant function analyses for comparing CHIs and non-brain-injured adults in the production of narrative and conversational discourse. Their first goal was to determine whether discourse performance is diagnostic of CHI. The statistics were successful in identifying CHI 70 percent of the time for narratives and 77 percent of the time for conversation. Then, Youse and Coelho turned their attention to those who had been misdiagnosed. These CHIs and controls overlapped considerably with respect to the same measures that had discriminated others initially. They concluded that the use of discourse measures for diagnosis continues to be risky. One reason may be the variability of discourse behavior among those without brain injury.

A related issue is whether discourse ability is managed directly by the executive system, so that observation of discourse can help to identify executive dysfunction or, reciprocally, so that executive dysfunction can be presumed to lie at the heart of discourse difficulties. Some literature seems to assume that someone with CHI is impaired in the executive system or that this impairment is responsible for narrative difficulties. Martin and McDonald (2005) provided evidence that executive ability is not related to difficulty in comprehending sarcasm and irony.

COGNITIVE REHABILITATION

Speech-language pathologists have built upon the pioneering work of Yehuda Ben-Yishay (1980), George Prigatano (1999), Barbara Wilson (1987), and certainly others, in part, by integrating principles of clinical aphasiology with cognitive rehabilitation (e.g., Adamovich, Henderson, and Auerback, 1985; Chamberlain, Neumann, and Tennant, 1995; Gillis, 1996; Hartley, 1995; Johnstone and Stonnington, 2001; Ponsford, Sloan, and Snow, 1995; Sohlberg and Mateer, 2001; Ylvisaker, Szekeres, and Feeney, 2001). Rehabilitation in the United States has been supported on a large scale by the National Institute on Disability and Rehabilitation Research (NIDRR) with a data-collection program called the Traumatic Brain Injury Model System (TBIMS). An additional boost was provided by passage of the federal Traumatic Brain Injury Act of 1996.

These days we find few clinicians focusing only on direct treatment of impairments, and most clinicians are employing strategies that combine the targeting of impairment and the training of compensatory strategies, all with functional activities and within a realistic milieu. Hartley (1995) staunchly advocated functional adaptation and compensation, "not restoration of function." Yet,

she still recommended restorative procedures for some problems.

Mark Ylvisaker and others (2001) claimed that traditional rehabilitation proceeds in one direction. It starts with minimizing impairment (i.e., restorative), proceeds to reduction of activity limitation (i.e., disability), and concludes with increasing participation (i.e., minimizing the handicap). Instead, Ylvisaker preferred what he called a *contextualized, everyday, routine-based approach,* which proceeds in the opposite direction, beginning with participation and concluding with an attention to impairment that emphasizes internalization of compensatory strategies. Thus, this is not a literal reversal, as indicated by the stages summarized in Table 12.9. We would not start to treat attention deficits at the end of rehabilitation. Nevertheless, Ylvisaker provided one challenging take on the prevalence of instituting functionality and authenticity as soon as possible. Simply put, we should "actively facilitate generalization from the start of treatment" (Sohlberg and Mateer, 2001, p. 137).

Coma Management

A few specialists acknowledge a controversial treatment generally known as *coma stimulation therapy* (or coma arousal therapy), which need not be conducted by an SLP. Multiple approaches have been devised (e.g., multisensory, familiar routines, and structured stimulation). They are supported with complex neurological rationales and animal studies, but evidence of efficacy for humans is hard to find. The purpose is to improve responsiveness to environmental events (e.g., Chamberlain et al., 1995; Gillis, 1996).

The general procedure consists of 10- to 15-minute intervals of stimulation and passive motion exercise to prevent muscle atrophy. The procedure is similar to the *Glasgow Coma Scale.* Senses are stimulated with smells, tastes, and touch. The sensations may be related to daily activities such as drinking coffee or brushing teeth. There may be a progression from unisensory to multisensory stimulation. Eager to do whatever they can, family

TABLE 12.9   Stages of cognitive rehabilitation, which are drawn loosely from Table 33-11 in Ylvisaker, Szekeres, and Feeney (2001).

STAGES	THERAPEUTIC SUPPORT	SAMPLE GOALS
Early	Maximum	• increase alertness • improve focus • increase recognition of people and objects • improve basic communication
Middle	Moderate	• increase duration of attention • improve recent memory (with prosthetics) • improve organization of functional tasks • improve organization of discourse • improve awareness of deficits
Late	Minimum	• increase independent use of compensatory strategies and aids • decrease reliance on cues for organization • improve language functions related to vocational and avocational goals

members or caregivers may be trained to perform these simple tasks.

Challenging Behaviors and Fatigue

Rehabilitation cannot proceed on all cylinders until (a) posttraumatic amnesia (PTA) has passed and the patient recognizes the therapist and can remember goals and strategies, and (b) acute agitation subsides, as illustrated by the case of Denise earlier in this chapter. Alan Forman's story is instructive. "Nurse Megan . . . doesn't cringe when he yells obscenities at her or throws food" (Crimmins, 2000, p. 87). It was helpful for Alan and his wife Cathy to realize that this rudeness was the result of brain injury and was certainly not Alan's natural personality.

Intervention may be necessary when the challenging behaviors persist and time for rehabilitation is running out. Strategies include altering the environment to minimize irritants, counseling caregivers, and providing behavioral treatments that reinforce good behavior and discourage bad behavior. However, "the ultimate goal . . . is internalized self-regulation of behavior" (Sohlberg and Mateer, 2001, p. 360). This begins by training individuals to become more aware of their behavior, leading to monitoring and evaluating their own behavior.

Instituting therapeutic measures may also be stalled by a patient's fatigue in combination with the lack of initiation associated with executive dysfunction as well as some depression. A general lack of energy or extreme lethargy is a common consequence of brain damage, particularly, traumatic injury (Stoler and Hill, 1998). Fatigue may be dealt with through medication, dietary modifications, and a mid-day nap. Compensatory strategies also include rationing time for strenuous activities and reducing distracting stimulation. Feelings of strength and cognitive energy should return with recovery, encouragement and patience from caregivers, and successes in treatment.

Insight (Awareness)

Do we remember Dr. Osborn's return to work too soon? A patient's cognitive rehabilitation can proceed smoothly with a heightened awareness of the impairments caused by the head injury. Sohlberg and Mateer (2001) advised that an *awareness-enhancing program* is likely to benefit patients who have a little recognition that some abilities have changed and who have sufficient cognitive resources to integrate information. It is not likely to benefit patients who have an intense global unawareness and weak cognitive resources.

An awareness-enhancing program begins with an educational approach by reviewing the client's medical records and providing information about the nature of deficits. Structured exercises allow the individual to experience difficulties that may await when leaving the hospital. Eventually, the client should be asked to predict performance on a particular task and then compare actual performance with the prediction.

Orientation and Attention

Management for low-level attention (e.g., arousal, alertness) is usually instituted *after* a patient comes out of a coma and while the patient is experiencing problems with orientation and attention during PTA. According to Ylvisaker and others (2001), goals of increasing alertness or arousal are important in the early stage of rehabilitation, and procedures should emphasize stimulation and managing the environment as opposed to anything that requires new learning or puts demands on memory.

Although there is some spontaneous diminishing of PTA, clinicians should still help patients orient to personal identity, time, and place. Orientation programs are similar to those that might be instituted for RHD or dementias. Training begins immediately postcoma with **passive drills** consisting of repeating orienting information and pointing out cues that are posted on the bulletin board and walls of a patient's room. Large clocks and calendars, names of hospital staff, and other reminders are part of a rehabilitation center's décor. **Active orientation training** consists of activities aimed at recognition of people, place, and time (e.g., Hartley, 1995).

Various approaches to treating attention are organized around the forms of attention. Perhaps the most well-known system is **Attention Process Training** (APT) by Sohlberg and Mateer (1987), which is now available on computer software. A skeleton view is provided in Table 12.10. General tasks are modeled after basic assessment procedures and are aimed at a process stripped of any functional identity. In principal, they exercise a cognitive process that is used in any real-life activity.

The patient should identify meaningful problems: "I cannot concentrate when preparing dinner because of the noise of the children playing.

TABLE 12.10 Treatment of attention in language- and communication-related activities, mainly following Sohlberg and Mateer's (2001) *Attention Process Training* (ATP).

GOALS		PROCEDURES	
		General	*Functional*
Focused	Decrease response to distraction	Crossing-out task with distracting designs	Conversation in a busy physical therapy gym
Sustained	Increase duration of concentration on a simple task	Raise hand whenever a digit is heard in a list	Read newspaper for increasing lengths of time
Alternating	Improve allocation of attention to multiple stimuli	Crossing-out task with letters, then numbers	Conversation about news simultaneously on TV
Divided	Improve ability to perform two tasks at once	Sustained-attention activity along with a simple computer task	Read a newspaper while listening to music; later asked about each

I forget ingredients or parts of the meal. I get frustrated and blow up at the children" (Sohlberg and Mateer, 2001, p. 156). The approach to this problem is multifaceted: practice elements of the task (e.g., recall recipes, prepare meals in quiet, gradually increase artificial distractions); anticipate and discuss difficulties; when at home, manage the environment by having the children play somewhere else while dinner is being prepared. Sohlberg and her colleagues (2000) felt that the effectiveness of APT was demonstrated in structured interviews where clients reported changes in specific real-life situations (e.g., "I can drive and listen to music").

Memory

Let us consider basic memory rehabilitation briefly, because we shall reconsider memory and apply some of the basics when dealing with language and communication. Two general approaches parallel work with other disorders, including aphasia. Treatment may be oriented to restoration of memory or compensation for the reality of memory deficit. With CHI, we consider retrograde and anterograde amnesias for treatment. Relatively less emphasis is placed on improving remote episodic memory, but we keep track of its progress. More emphasis is placed on anterograde amnesia as it contributes to the patient's functioning in the here and now. Although the conditions for rehabilitation are more favorable when PTA appears to be over, certain compensatory strategies are instituted early.

A logical restorative tactic is to use *memory drills* or the repetitive practice of remembering lists and other things, suggesting that, according to Sohlberg and Mateer (2001), "memory can be strengthened as if it were a mental muscle" (p. 177). Although Sohlberg and Mateer have found no empirical support for memory drills, they have also found numerous computer programs and workbooks devoted to them. Another possibility is commonly taught to neurologically intact people who want to improve their memory. A *mnemonic strategy* is an internal self-cueing

technique that entails associating important information with a visual image or some other link, but there is little indication that using mnemonics in the clinic generalizes to real life for head-injured individuals.

Clinicians have had some success with training **prospective memory,** which is remembering to do something in the future, such as taking medication or shaving. Prospective memory has practical implications, and Sohlberg and Mateer's *Prospective Memory Process Training* (PROMPT) appears to generalize across contexts and tasks (Raskin and Sohlberg, 1996; Sohlberg, White, Evans et al., 1992). The basic task is to carry out a target activity in a specified number of minutes (e.g., in five minutes, go open the door). So, how do we train someone to carry out the task? Training invokes the following variables:

- gradually increase the interval between request and execution
- start with a simple one-step task, then make the task more complex
- introduce self-cues such as an alarm
- introduce a distracting task during the time interval

The prospective memory task should also model real-life target tasks such as returning a phone call, shutting off an appliance, or paying the bills.

Rehabilitation specialists have become interested in a couple of learning techniques:

- **spaced practice,** which entails gradually increasing the interval between tasks or trials (also referred to as spaced rehearsal or spaced retrieval)
- **errorless learning,** or using tasks and cues so that the client makes no mistakes

Errorless learning (Baddeley, 1992) is conspicuously similar to the success principle in aphasia rehabilitation. We shall return to these concepts in the management of dementias (Chapter 13).

Compensatory strategies tend to be preferred and are incorporated into ostensibly restorative tasks, such as prospective memory activities. These strategies consist of the use of **external**

memory aids, because the individual with CHI cannot rely on his or her memory alone. All of us use memory aids such as calendars and shopping lists. We just do not usually need them for remembering to shower or turn off the stove. Examples for the patient include lists, memory notebooks, environmental props, alarms, pocket electronic devices, and paging systems in computers (Hersh and Treadgold, 1994; Sohlberg and Mateer, 1989). Some time is spent in the clinic for training to remember to use the memory aids, and caregivers are alerted that the individual should be using them. Establishing awareness of memory difficulty is important, because the individual must recognize a problem when it occurs or, even better, anticipate a problem before it occurs.

Remote memories (i.e., retrograde amnesia) may be targeted incidentally in topics for group interaction that form the core of some communication or community-based rehabilitation programs. Sohlberg and Mateer (2001) suspected that retrograde amnesia involves both episodic and semantic memory to some degree. Conceptual knowledge becomes a component of domain-specific training, when we are working within an *avocational* interest or a vocational problem. Perhaps the most common activity devoted to individualized remote memories is the creation of an *autobiography,* which may consist of a scrapbook, written memoir, résumé, or pages in a memory book.

Dysexecutive Syndrome

Rehabilitation of the executive system addresses components of function and dysfunction, namely, initiating, planning, organizing, and executing (Table 12.11). Like the general tasks for treatment of attention (Table 12.10), some precedents have consisted of assessment procedures, such as the Tower of London puzzle of transferring rings across pegs (Cicerone and Giacino, 1992). More functional activities include tasks of daily living (e.g., doing laundry, paying bills, making a reservation, going somewhere) or work activities (e.g., using a computer, ordering supplies).

TABLE 12.11 Elements of an activity for executive functions.

Initiation	• treatment of challenging behaviors and fatigue • set up reminders
Planning	• articulate the goal • anticipate subgoals and steps • use calendars and notes • get help from caregivers
Organizing	• sequence the steps (organizational aids) • simplify the task • organize the environment for a task • self-monitoring (look for and correct mistakes)

Treatment emphasizes the use of organizing aids as well as environmental structuring and supports (e.g., Hartley, 1995; Sohlberg and Mateer, 2001; Ylvisaker et al., 2001).

Group Therapies

Rita Gillis (1999b) noted that group therapy is widely employed for cognitive rehabilitation. "In many facilities, group therapy is the only format used" (p. 143). Criteria for selecting members include (a) choosing those with a deficit shared by all and (b) limiting numbers so enough professional staff are available in case a member becomes verbally or physically unruly. Gillis also distinguished between two types of groups. *Therapy in a group* may be arranged for economic reasons and consists of a cognitive therapy administered to several people at one time. It is as if we are providing individual therapies in sequence or simultaneously. *Group therapy,* on the other hand, is conducted because its interactions are a means to achieve communicative and social goals that only a group can provide. There are certain familiar recommendations, such as encouraging group members to establish their own goals and plan their own programs. Both types of groups are common for CHI.

Groups oriented around particular cognitive functions are conducted in different stages of recovery and tend to have a "therapy in a group" structure. Gillis (1999b) described an *orientation group* that is helpful in addressing and monitoring the early PTA phase. Another early intervention theme is *attention*. One category of activities is to present lists or lots of information and have members listen for a target item. This may produce some motivating friendly competition (also, Table 12.10). *Organization and memory groups* tend to be offered in later recovery and/or for higher level patients.

Discourse and Conversation

Here is where the SLP's role is most dominant. As with RHD, pragmatic theory and pragmatic assessments certainly give us some direction for coverage in treatment. Yet, one reason for doing research is to see if people with CHI have particular pragmatic difficulties that may help us narrow our focus for assessment as well as treatment. Three general targets stand out:

- theory of mind or the ability to take the perspective of another for making inferences
- global or thematic coherence of discourse-level formulation
- conversational management and social skills

Regarding perspective taking, the clinician may borrow situations from the research on sarcasm and irony and then discuss them with the client. For each of these areas, we consider restorative and compensatory strategies, often operating in tandem. Also, certain components of functional communicative treatment for aphasia and RHD are applicable, such as conversation therapies and situation-specific role-playing.

Telling a story might not be considered to be the most useful activity per se, although it may be an important activity in some families. Conversation is often about the story told in a movie. Storytelling can also be a means by which the SLP contributes to team rehabilitation of attention and

TABLE 12.12   The correspondence of narrative behavior and structure to the basic elements of executive functions.

Initiation	Start to tell a story
Planning	Goal is to tell a story (What is a story?) Elements (Who? Where? When?)
Organization	Initiating event (What gets a story started?) Episode sequence (What happens? In what order?) Conclusion (Happy ending?)

executive disorders. This task requires sustained attention. It has an identifiable structure, and Table 12.12 is suggestive of question cues for helping a patient tell stories initially in view (e.g., cartoon sequences), then in a recall activity of retelling a story, and finally in telling a favorite story from recent memory (the day before) or long-term memory (childhood).

Although conversation and role-playing have a general similarity to aphasia treatment, the problems and objectives are different. Some of the cognitive difficulties that have been found to interfere with conversational interaction are noted in Table 12.13. An individual session may be designed to focus on one or two of these problems. An overarching objective is to increase self-awareness. Awareness activities include viewing oneself on videotape, looking for what is good as well as for what might interfere with the smooth exchange of information.

The clinician and patient should agree on specific objectives, such as improving concentration on a topic or reducing the number of interruptions. Some treatment may consist of instruction and discussion concerning the components of a conversation, which should heighten awareness of aspects of everyday interaction that had previously been taken for granted. Then, we want to see if this work generalizes to real-life situations by role-playing phone skills, a job interview, or conflict resolution with a family member or fellow employee. Favorite real-life group activities

TABLE 12.13   Target problem areas for treatment of conversation.

Controlling emotions	Disruptive turn interruptions
Focusing attention	Not listening to conversational partner
Sustaining attention	Unexpected topic shifts
Recent memory	Forgetting topic-related experiences
Executive initiation	Not starting a conversation Not raising a new topic Not taking a turn
Thematic coherence	Off-topic, tangential talk
Theory of mind	Missing the point of others

can be anticipated with a game of poker or a simulated group tour of an art gallery.

Genuine group therapy is devoted to communicative and social skills. Adamovich (2005) recommended several types of groups that may be incorporated into a single, ongoing communication group. Her groups were for interpersonal interaction, social skills, empathic abilities, personal and social adjustment, and life skills. Peers in a group may encourage initiation of speaking turns. Groups are a good place to work on reducing the impulsivity of talking out of turn.

Community Reintegration/Re-entry

Community re-entry programs provide the boost for achieving **long-term goals** of cognitive rehabilitation (Fraiser and Clemmons, 1999). These programs address social skills and complex cognitive functions such as executive organization and problem solving. They are often conducted in groups and by rehabilitation teams, and Gillis (1999a) provided detailed guidelines for conducting and evaluating re-entry groups. Much of the work of community re-entry is conducted in the community and has some similarities to Jon Lyon's Communication Partners program for aphasia (Chapter 10).

The demographics of people with TBI dictate that **return to work** is a frequent individual goal and an indicator of successful rehabilitation outcome (Penn and Jones, 2000). At the Office of Vocational Rehabilitation (OVR) in Pennsylvania, Alan Forman was advised that the goal of community re-entry is not necessarily to return to one's old job but rather to find a way to contribute to society (Crimmins, 2000). However, Alan wanted to return to his job at a bank.

Vocational rehabilitation offers **supported employment** in which a rehabilitation counselor, or *job coach,* works with the individual and employer (Wehman, Bricout, and Targett, 1999). OVR partially funded Alan's counseling through a community training program. Bill Gardner, a graduate student in neuropsychology, was Alan's job coach. The bank agreed to allow Alan to work part-time. Bill came to Alan's house three days a week, four hours each day. In the beginning, Alan had to work on selecting, initiating, and completing work-related tasks. Bill also had to help Alan with strategies for managing irritability and impulse control which, among other things, drained Alan's energy. Cathy Crimmins's book about Alan is an instructive cautionary tale.

One strategy for aphasia suggested in Chapter 10 is to change communities or change real life. In other words, we can change what is authentic. A job coach negotiates with employers to make accommodations. In Sydney, Australia, SLPs evaluated a program for improving police recruits' service encounters with people with TBI. The service encounters consisted of telephone inquiries before and after a six-week training program for the recruits. Training included education about TBI and role-playing. The investigators found that the prospective police officers improved in establishing the nature of the inquiry and providing information. The callers with TBI were better at staying on topic (Togher, McDonald, Code et al., 2004).

Several organizations provide support for patients and families and education for employers and police officers (Table 12.14). The Brain Injury Association of America (BIAA) successfully advocated for reauthorization in 2000 of the Traumatic Brain Injury Act of 1996. The original

TABLE 12.14 Organizations providing support for research and people with TBI.

ORGANIZATION	DESCRIPTION	WEBSITE
Brain Injury Association of America (BIAA)	Advocacy and support for brain-injured people and their families (chartered affiliates in most states)	www.biausa.org
Traumatic Brain Injury Model System (TBIMS)	National data-gathering center, supporting a variety of programs at 16 rehabilitation centers in the United States (many are university affiliated)	www.tbindc.org
Center for Outcome Measurement in Brain Injury (COMBI)	Resource for information on measures; includes details about particular outcome scales	www.tbims.org
National Resource Center for Traumatic Brain Injury (NRC for TBI)	Provides information for professionals, brain-injured people, and family members	www.neuro.pmr.vcu.edu

legislation provided for state-based grant programs to improve the care of persons with TBI. In addition, the Traumatic Brain Injury Model System (TBIMS) coordinates innovative research at 16 sites on all aspects of care and contributes results to the TBI National Data Center at the Kessler Medical Rehabilitation Research and Education Center (e.g., Sherer, Sander, Nick et al., 2002). One of the 16 sites is Spaulding Rehabilitation Hospital in partnership with Harvard Medical School and other hospitals in Boston. Planned studies include the use of fMRI as a predictor of outcome and the evaluation of various measures and tests.

RECOVERY AND OUTCOMES

In this final section, we examine cognitive recovery, functional outcome, prognosis, and the influence of rehabilitation. For characterizing functional outcomes, researchers and clinicians have relied on general scales, judgments of psychological status, or whether the individual has returned to school or work (Richardson, 2000).

There are different portrayals of phases of recovery, and one of these is shown in Table 12.15.

Post-traumatic amnesia lasts longer than one day in all severe head injuries. Conclusion of PTA is identified when a patient begins to remember day-to-day events and conversations from a few hours earlier. In more than 90 percent of cases, this phase lasts more than a week; and more than four weeks in 60 percent (Jennett and Teasdale, 1981). The longer PTA lasts, the more difficult it is to recognize when it ends. Identification of the end of PTA can be one or two weeks off.

The WAIS has been used to measure cognitive recovery beyond PTA. Becker (1975) tested 10 head-injured patients two weeks after their accident and then 10 to 11 weeks later. IQ-matched controls were also retested for the same interval. The head-injured patients improved significantly, but so did the controls, indicating that test-related improvement over about three months can be attributed to practice or experience with the test. Bond and Brooks (1976) administered the WAIS to 40 patients at three-month intervals up to two years postinjury. Most recovery occurred in the first six months. Verbal IQ returns to normal levels before Performance IQ, consistent with the greater severity of deficit with Performance IQ (e.g., Mandelberg and Brooks, 1975). Aphasia assessments

TABLE 12.15   Phases in recovery from closed head injury (CHI) (Cripe, 1987).

PHASE	DESCRIPTION	TREATMENT ORIENTATION
Coma	Loss of consciousness lasting hours to months	
Posttraumatic amnesia (PTA)	Beginning when consciousness is regained and ending when a patient can remember day-to-day events	Assistance with attention and orientation; complex cognition is avoided
Rapid recovery	Significant progress over three to six months depending on severity	Focus on basic skills; minimize unrealistic expectations
Long-term plateau	Persisting residual deficits; progress is painstakingly slow	Emphasis on adjusting to disabilities

have substantiated observations that basic language functions recover fairly impressively within six months postinjury (e.g., Levin, Grossman, Sarwar, Meyers, 1981; Luzzatti et al., 1989).

Two general scales have been used. The **Glasgow Outcome Scale** (GOS) offers general levels defined by severity of disablement and amount of social support required (Jennett and Bond, 1975; see Richardson, 2000 for a review). A sketch of the categories follows:

- *Death*
- *Persistent vegetative state:* unresponsive
- *Severe disability* (conscious but disabled): dependent for daily support
- *Moderate disability* (disabled but independent): can work in a sheltered environment
- *Good recovery:* resumption of normal life despite mild deficits

If we compare this scale to the PICA's multidimensional scoring (Table 3.2), we may get the feeling that the GOS is more of a classification guide than a measure. The other scale, the **Disability Rating Scale** (DRS), was introduced earlier in this chapter (Rappaport et al., 1982; Fryer and Haffey, 1987). It consists of eight general ratings for eye opening, communication, motor response, feeding, toileting, grooming, level of functioning, and employability. It was compared to the FIM+FAM and Glasgow Outcome Scale and was determined to be more likely to document improvement than the GOS.

Investigators have also turned to proxy reports of outcomes, which most frequently consist of family members' perceptions of how a head-injured individual is doing. Brooks and others (1986) asked relatives about changes between one and five years postinjury. They were most worried about slowness, memory, irritability, and temper. Concentration and memory problems got worse. Individuals were forgetting what they were doing in the middle of a task or losing track of what they were saying in conversations (also, Brooks, McKinlay, Symington, 1987).

What is the status of an individual 13 years postinjury? Dawson and Chipman (1995) conducted a survey of 454 persons with TBI; 66 percent still needed assistance for some daily living activities, 75 percent were unemployed, and 90 percent were unhappy with social integration. Ponsford and others (1999) studied outcomes of over 1,220 patients followed between 2 and 10 years after injury. One-third still needed support for shopping, finances, and home maintenance, whereas over 90 percent had attained independence performing more basic activities of daily living. Around 50 percent were working by two years postinjury, but many did not sustain their employment. Only 45 percent had returned to favorite leisure activities. More than half were depressed and anxious, and many of these were socially isolated (also, Johnson, 1998).

Duration of PTA has been used as an indicator of severity of head injury and as a predictor of recovery. There is some evidence that recovery to normal levels of cognitive function within six months to a year is predicted by PTA of under six weeks. If PTA lasts longer than three months, outlook is not promising. Investigators have tended to be more interested in predicting return to work than a level of cognitive function (e.g., Prigatano, 1999).

In a follow-up study of 134 cases of severe head injury based on proxy reports, Brooks and others (1987) found that **communication deficits** were significant predictors of failure to return to work. As it was for Claudia Osborn, family members reported difficulties with conversation. The following list highlights the other most frequently supported predictors of returning to school or work (Boake, Millis, High et al., 2001; Crepeau and Scherzer, 1993; MacMillan, Hart, Martelli et al., 2002; Ruff, Marshall, Crouch et al., 1993; Sherer, Sander, Nick et al., 2002):

- preinjury substance abuse history
- age (young adult more likely than older adult)
- information processing speed
- executive function ability
- early neuropsychological test performance

In other research, WAIS Performance IQ (not Verbal IQ) was a strong predictor of returning to work or school (Ip, Dornan, and Schentag, 1995). Measures of early severity of injury (e.g., PTA) and time postinjury were not related (also, Crepeau and Scherzer, 1993).

Technically correct efficacy data appears to be rare. Evidence supporting rehabilitation consists mainly of follow-up outcomes for large rehabilitation programs or several pre–post assessments of specific treatment procedures for individual patients, with some small group studies in between. The state of the science was demonstrated by Carney, Chestnut, and others (1999) in a review process that started with over 3,000 articles that might have something to say about cognitive rehabilitation. Eventually, 600 seemed to address the key question of whether cognitive rehabilitation affects outcomes. Only 32 of these satisfied criteria for a good study. Only 15 included a control group. Only six measured real-life outcomes.

Hall and Cope (1995) provided general support for cognitive rehabilitation. They reviewed 28 studies published between 1984 and 1994. Acute rehabilitation reduced post–acute rehabilitation by two-thirds. Post–acute rehabilitation (e.g., outpatient programs) was beneficial for functional outcomes even after a reasonable period for spontaneous recovery. There is some evidence that early intervention is more effective than later intervention (e.g., Rappaport, Herrero-Backe, Rappaport et al., 1989).

For SLPs, Coelho, DeRuyter, and Stein (1996) sampled studies that addressed general rehabilitation programs and specific training for attention, memory, executive functions, and social skills. These studies provided documentation of improvements. The investigators also gathered their own retrospective outcome data from five inpatient rehabilitation programs across the United States. The average length of stay was 46.3 days, ranging from 32.5 to 58.4 days (or about two months). Most patients demonstrated improvement with functional status measures. An average of 84 percent were discharged to home, and 11 percent were discharged to long-term care facilities.

SUMMARY AND CONCLUSIONS

Cases with closed head injury (CHI) can be quite different from cases with stroke. The condition of the damaged brain is quite different. Cognitive impairments can also be quite different. Furthermore, the needs of a younger population with CHI differ from an older population with stroke. CHI has direct impact on parents, brothers, and sisters, whereas stroke has direct impact on spouses and children.

Young people with CHI have deficits of attention, episodic memory, learning new information, and behavioral organization. Sometimes their personalities seem to change as they become irritable or impulsive. Some seem to be unconcerned or unmotivated. On the other hand, older adults with stroke can concentrate for long periods, remember their past, absorb new information, and structure their daily routines. They tend to maintain their prestroke personalities and have normal reactions to sudden disability. Many are highly motivated to improve their language abilities. Thus, CHI presents a special challenge for rehabilitative teamwork among neuropsychologists, psychologists, and speech-language pathologists.

Except for the cases in which a focal trauma causes a nearly classic aphasia, a striking difference between the effects of stroke and CHI is the level of residual or chronic language ability. People with CHI are likely to be able to retrieve words and formulate fluent sentences. Many have such mild and subtle impairments that they seem ready to return to school or work. Upon returning, some succeed but many fail because of demands that exceed their concentration or patience. Their communicative difficulties appear in the organization of discourse and in pragmatic aspects of conversation related to primary cognitive impairments.

An SLP's contribution to rehabilitation primarily consists of assessing and treating the communicative consequences of cognitive impairments. Both assessment and treatment take into consideration the impact of communication and participation limitations on a young adult's educational and vocational objectives. Again, treatment is consistent with the two fundamental approaches to aphasia and right-hemisphere dysfunctions, namely, stimulation for treatment of impairments and training of compensatory strategies to bypass impairments.

MATCHING REVIEW

Match the contribution on the right with the name on the left.

_____ 1. McKay Sohlberg and Catherine Mateer

_____ 2. Alan Forman

_____ 3. Yehuda Ben-Yishay

_____ 4. Daniel Schacter

_____ 5. Barbara Wilson

_____ 6. Skye McDonald

_____ 7. Carl Coelho and Kathleen Youse

_____ 8. Rita Gillis

_____ 9. Chris Hagen

_____ 10. Mark Ylvisaker

a. chapter for SLPs in Chapey's book

b. sarcasm and theory of mind (ToM)

c. RLA scale

d. discourse production and conversation

e. *Where is the Mango Princess?*

f. Attention Process Training (APT)

g. memory research

h. cognitive rehabilitation pioneer

i. memory rehabilitation and several tests

j. group therapies

CHAPTER 13

DEMENTIAS

Thomas DeBaggio, a journalist and coauthor of books about growing herbs, wrote, "I am alone and I can hear water running somewhere in the house. I don't remember going to the bathroom. Who else turned on the water?" (DeBaggio, 2002, p. 5). A few months after his 57th birthday, he was diagnosed as having Alzheimer's disease.

Dementia is a general category of cognitive dysfunction with many causes. In the past, the term was associated with the idea that the dysfunction sweeps across the entire domain of cognition. Dementias are now considered to be a "group of disorders" with "multiple cognitive deficits" (American Psychiatric Association, 1994). This chapter introduces a few causes of dementia, but, for the purpose of attaining an understanding of the cognitive-communicative impairments and rehabilitation, it focuses on Alzheimer's dementia.

DIAGNOSIS AND ASSESSMENT OF DEMENTIA

In 1992, the Agency for Health Care Policy and Research, part of the U.S. Public Health Service, sponsored a panel of experts to develop a clinical practice guideline on screening for Alzheimer's and related dementias. A diagnosis of dementia is based on a focused history, a focused physical examination, informant reports, and a mental status evaluation. The general criteria for diagnosis are briefly as follows (Fields, 1998):

- is a change from a previous level of cognitive function
- occurs without a disruption of consciousness
- is sufficient to influence daily functioning
- cannot be explained by situational stress
- may result from a variety of conditions, some reversible

More specifically, doctors want to see if the dementia represents an early stage of Alzheimer's disease or another form of dementia (e.g., Ballard, 2000). "However, doctors do not routinely screen people for dementia or cognitive impairment . . . primary care doctors routinely miss the diagnosis" (Dash and Villemarette-Pittman, 2005, pp. 16, 17).

A clinical neuropsychologist may administer a comprehensive evaluation. Thomas DeBaggio (2002) was given the National Adult Reading Test (NART), the WAIS-R, and the WMS-R. He complained that "it was numbing and took about six hours" (p. 15). The NART was developed in the United Kingdom and consists of 50 irregular words to pronounce (Nelson and O'Connell, 1978). For an American version, Schwartz and Saffran replaced words that were unfamiliar to Americans (e.g., Grober and Sliwinski, 1991). Combined with other information, it has contributed to estimating intelligence either premorbidly or without having to give an entire WAIS (e.g., Crawford, Parker, Stewart et al., 1989). DeBaggio's estimated premorbid IQ was 124. The results of his assessment showed that his postonset IQ was 91, and his memory test scores indicated severe impairment.

The most widely used screening test for cognitive deterioration is the *Mini-Mental State Examination* (MMSE) (Folstein, Folstein, and McHugh, 1975). It is commonly employed to identify participants in cognitive and linguistic research. The MMSE is a 10-minute bedside assessment of six areas, namely, orientation for date and location, "registration" (repeating three words), concentration (counting backward by sevens), short-term or recent memory (repeating the previ-

TABLE 13.1 A sample of frequently mentioned brief tests and scales measuring mental status, presented roughly in chronological order.

ABBREVIATION	TITLE	DESCRIPTION	REFERENCE
DS	*Blessed-Dementia Scale*	Coverage similar to FIM; deficit increases with scores from 0–28	Blessed et al. (1968)
MMSE	*Mini-Mental State Examination*	10-minute bedside test of six cognitive areas	Folstein, Folstein et al. (1975)
DRS	*Dementia Rating Scale*	Series of quick tasks; introduced in 1976	Mattis (1988)
GDS	*Global Deterioration Scale*	Detailed descriptions of seven levels	Reisberg, Ferris et al. (1982)
CDR	*Clinical Dementia Rating Scale*	Another subjective rating	Hughes, Berg et al. (1982)
ADAS	*Alzheimer Disease Assessment Scale*	21 items; *ADAS-Cog* is the 11 items for cognition	Rosen et al. (1984)
Cognistat (NCSE)	*Neurobehavioral Cognitive Status Examination*	Found more sensitive to dysfunction than other short tests	Kiernan et al. (1987)
ACE	*Addenbrooke's Cognitive Examination*	30-minute test for detecting early stage Alzheimer's dementia	Dudas et al. (2005)
MiniCog	*MiniCog Rapid Assessment Battery*	Borrows established tests of cognition; used on a PDA	Shephard and Kosslyn (2005)

ous three words), language (naming, following instruction), and visuospatial (copying shapes). The best score is 30. The MMSE has been criticized for being sparse, and a longer version was created in which each of the six areas is expanded (Ashford, Kumar, Barringer et al., 1992).

There are several other brief tests and rating scales. Some of the scales were created for drug research, and most of them can be found on the Internet. The evening news may trumpet a new test that identifies a dementia in 10 minutes. However, mental status tests are not by themselves diagnostic. They are used to document deficits that may lead to a diagnosis and to monitor the course of impairment over time (Table 13.1).

The **Global Deterioration Scale** (GDS) consists of seven levels with Level 1 representing no cognitive decline and Level 7, very severe cognitive decline (Reisberg, Ferris, de Leon et al.,

1982). Level 2 and Level 3 are identified with mild cognitive decline. Diagnosis of dementia begins with Level 4 (Table 13.2). The GDS is supported by two other scales, namely, the *Brief Cognitive Rating Scale* (BCRS) and the *Functional Assessment Staging Test* (FAST), which focuses on the last area of the BCRS (Reisberg, Ferris, and Franssen, 1985).

TABLE 13.2 MMSE and GDS scale definitions of severity levels ("stages"). MMSE scores are commonly used to describe severity of deficit in experimental participants.

STAGE	MMSE SCORE	GDS LEVEL
Mild	20–26	4
Moderate	10–19	5
Severe	< 10	7

At Addenbrooke's Hospital, University of Cambridge (UK), physicians and psychologists have been developing a battery called ***Addenbrooke's Cognitive Examination*** (ACE) (Dudas, Berrios, and Hodges, 2005). This test takes about 30 minutes to evaluate orientation, attention, memory, verbal fluency, language, and visuospatial ability. Validation began in the mid-1990s. The ACE detected dementia in 82 percent of mild cases, whereas the MMSE detected dementia in 51 pecent (Mathuranath, Nestor, Berrios et al., 2000). Another study was designed to determine if the ACE is predictive of whether patients with questionable dementia will progress to Alzheimer's disease. Of 31 patients with apparent dementia, 11 progressed to Alzheimer's disease within 24 months. Prediction was considered to be possible with the ACE and an MRI showing atrophy in the medial temporal region (Galton, Erzinclioglu, Sahakian et al., 2005).

What about a quick self-assessment that could be used anywhere? The ***MiniCog Rapid Assessment Battery*** (MRAB) is a software package in development at the Kosslyn Laboratory at Harvard University (Shephard and Kosslyn, 2005). It was originally designed for astronauts who would wear the testing device on their wrists in space (i.e., "a blood pressure cuff for the mind"). More generally, the *MiniCog* can be administered with a handheld PDA (e.g., PalmPilot) or a desktop computer. It is intended to provide an "early warning" for someone who is suffering from stress-related deficits that may affect performance. The battery assesses nine cognitive functions with established tasks, and each takes about two minutes to complete.

ALZHEIMER'S DISEASE

In Frankfurt, Germany, in 1906, Alois Alzheimer wondered about the progressively deteriorating memory of a patient known as Frau Auguste D. Following her death, the young physician performed an autopsy and discovered some unusual tangles and a "peculiar substance" spread over the entire cortex that others later said was neuritic plaques (Shenk, 2002).

Until the 1950s, Alzheimer's disease (AD) was thought to be a rare affliction of middle age (i.e., 40 to 65 years), whereas "senile dementia" was thought to be a condition of old age that is simply a severe form of normal aging. Then, Neumann and Cohn (1953) found plaques and tangles in the brains of elderly individuals. They established that Alzheimer's disease causes dementia at any age and, therefore, that dementia in old age can often be the result of a disease rather than a manifestation of aging.

Two types of nerve cell stains expose the hallmark co-occurrence of tangles and plaques. The Congo red stain reveals **neurofibrillary tangles,** which are triangular and looped fibers located within nerve cell bodies. The tangles appear early in the disease and contain a protein called *tau.* The silver stain detects granular deposits and remains of degenerated nerve fibers called **neuritic plaques** located outside of neurons. The plaques contain a beta-amyloid protein and are often called amyloid plaques. Together these two pathologies cause death of brain cells (or neuron loss) (Dash and Villemarette-Pittman, 2005).

Location of pathology expands as the disease spreads. It begins with the tangles in the **hippocampus,** a structure within the temporal lobe that is important for memory. It then infiltrates frontal, parietal, and temporal lobes (Petersen, 2002). Tangles are pronounced in the *inferior temporal lobe* and accumulate in the *parieto-temporal juncture.* Studies of cerebral blood flow and metabolism reveal bilateral reduction in parietal and posterior temporal lobes. There can be more hypoperfusion in one hemisphere than in the other hemisphere in early stages. This concentration of pathology results in fairly specific impairments, especially of memory and language in the early stage.

Alzheimer's disease causes dementia, but what causes AD? In the decade of the 1990s, there was an intense debate over whether plaques or tangles hold the key to understanding the nature of AD. In 1999 at an international conference in Taos, New Mexico, John Hardy of the Mayo Clinic advocated the "amyloid cascade hypothesis," which claimed that plaques are closer than tangles to the root of AD. "Most Alzheimer's re-searchers—probably some 80 percent—had come to embrace this line of thinking . . ." (Shenk, 2002, p. 152). On the other side of the debate was Allen Roses who, although not at the meeting, was employed by a large pharmaceutical company at the time. He believed that tangles, or tau, are mainly responsible for the disease.

Earlier, at Duke University in 1992, Roses had discovered that the presence of a variant of a gene called *apolipoprotein E* (ApoE) in chromosome 19 increases the risk of developing AD. Whereas mutations of genes in other chromosomes are linked to AD diagnosed before the age of 65, inheriting a variant of ApoE, called ApoE4, increases the likelihood of developing the late-onset form of AD. Some believe that the presence of ApoE4 along with worsening memory is a predictor of the disease.

Once thought to be rare, Alzheimer's disease is now recognized as the most frequent cause of dementia in adulthood, probably responsible for over 50 percent of cases. A history of AD is summarized in Table 13.3. The long period of dated terminology, such as *presenile dementia* and *senile dementia,* coincided with the time in which cognitive problems after age 60 were considered to be simply old age. Use of the term *senile* and its variants has been dwindling rapidly but has still lingered. Labels for specific versions of Alzheimer's disease are becoming common:

- *early-onset Alzheimer's disease,* before age 65, like Thomas DeBaggio
- *familial Alzheimer's,* in multiple members of the same family
- *sporadic Alzheimer's,* in only one member of a family

Informative introductions to Alzheimer's disease include one published by the Mayo Clinic (Petersen, 2002) and another published by the American Academy of Neurology (Dash and Villemarette-Pittman, 2005).

TABLE 13.3 History of Alzheimer's disease and dementia (e.g., Gillick, 1998; Shenk, 2002).

YEAR	EVENT
1906	Alois Alzheimer finds plaques and tangles in a patient's brain
1910	Alzheimer's mentor Emil Kraepelin mentions "Alzheimer's disease" in his *Handbook of Psychiatry*
1953	Neumann and Cohn recognize Alzheimer's disease as a pathology that can occur in middle and late adulthood
1975	*Mini Mental State Examination* (MMSE) introduced
1979	First board meeting of the Alzheimer's Disease and Related Disorders Association (now the Alzheimer's Association); Mace and Rabins begin distributing handmade copies of *The 36-Hour Day.*
1984	Diagnostic criteria for probable Alzheimer's disease established by NIH-NINCDS
1987	Omnibus Budge Reconciliation Act mandating comprehensive evaluation in long-term care
1994	President Reagan diagnosed with Alzheimer's disease
1996	FDA approval of Aricept; developing *Addenbrooke's Cognitive Examination* (ACE) at Cambridge, UK
2001	Medicare funding for AD rehabilitation authorized; *MiniCog* in development at Kosslyn Laboratory, Harvard University

Also, following the persnickety logic in Chapter 1 (Table 1.5), let us try to differentiate reference to disease from reference to the resulting dysfunction. In this chapter, the abbreviation **AD** is used for Alzheimer's disease (the neuropathology), and **DAT** is used for dementia of Alzheimer's type (the dysfunction). This type of dementia may also be labeled *probable dementia of Alzheimer's type* (pDAT) and, of course, presumes a diagnosis of AD.

OTHER CAUSES OF DEMENTIA

The pattern of an individual's dementia depends on etiology. Pathologies may be classified as progressive or nonprogressive, or, as nonreversible or reversible (Table 13.4). Alzheimer's disease is one of several progressive and irreversible neuro-

pathologies with a gradual onset and relentless deterioration.

Primary location of pathology is another basis of classification, and researchers refer to cortical or subcortical dementias. For example, AD is concentrated in the cerebral cortex, whereas pathology in Parkinson's disease is concentrated beneath the cortex. We may hedge with phrases like "primarily located" because white matter pathology has been found with AD, and frontal lobe hypometabolism has been detected in some subcortical pathologies.

What if it's not Alzheimer's? asked Lisa and Gary Radin (2003) in their book about **frontotemporal dementias** (FTDs). This category of dementias can have different causes, including Pick's disease. Histology includes tangles that are different from those with Alzheimer's disease, and

TABLE 13.4   Neuropathologies that cause dementias.

	DIAGNOSIS	SITE OF DAMAGE	DISEASE PROCESS
Progressive	Alzheimer's disease	Bilateral parietal and temporal lobes (including hippocampus)	Accumulation of neuritic plaques and neurofibrillary tangles
	Lewy Body disease	Frontal and temporal lobes; basal ganglia	Protein deposits (i.e., Lewy bodies) in neuronal cells
	Frontotemporal dementia (FTD)	Frontal lobe degeneration; more temporal lobe atrophy than in Alzheimer's disease	Absence of plaques; presence of tau protein ("Pick's bodies")
	Parkinson's disease	Subcortical dementia; substantia nigra in the brain stem	Cell loss reducing production of the neurotransmitter dopamine
	Huntington's disease	Subcortical dementia; caudate nucleus of the basal ganglia	Inherited atrophy of the caudate
Nonprogressive	Vascular dementia (including multiple infarcts)	Any location	Arteriosclerotic reductions of blood supply (accumulated small ischemic strokes)
	Herpes simplex viral encephalitis (HSVE)	Medial temporal areas extending into orbitofrontal regions; usually bilateral	Infection causing acute necrosis, edema and hemorrhage; sometimes evolves to coma in 2–3 days

it does not include the amyloid plaques characteristic of AD. Personality change is an early sign of FTD, such as inappropriate disruptive behavior that is likely to lead to psychiatric evaluation (Cooke, DeVita, Gee et al., 2003; Davis, Price, Moore et al. 2001; Hodges, Patterson, Ward et al.,1999; Snowden, Neary, and Mann, 2002).

Lewy body disease occurs alone, or it can occur along with around 20 percent of cases with AD. Lewy bodies are abnormal protein deposits that progressively destroy brain cells. They are widespread throughout the cerebral cortex and hippocampus, but they are also found in the brain stem. Thus, a person may have a symptom complex that appears as if it were a combination of Alzheimer's and Parkinson's diseases. Problems with focusing attention and memory usually appear before the rigidity and tremors of motor dysfunction (e.g., McKeith, Fairbarn, Perry et al., 1994). Also, around 30 percent of people with Parkinson's disease eventually develop dementia.

With **reversible dementias,** the cause can be treated to restore normal or nearly normal cognitive function. The most frequent causes are depression, alcohol abuse, and drug toxicity. Depression is common in the elderly and often ignored (i.e., "underdiagnosed"). Also common in the elderly is *polypharmacy* or the simultaneous use of multiple medications, which can promote declining intellectual function. Medications with cognitive side effects include anticholinergics such as Elavil and Benadryl, narcotics such as Vicodin and Percocet, and sedatives such as Xanax and Valium (Dash and Villemarette-Pittman, 2005).

DEMENTIA OF ALZHEIMER'S TYPE

Because some causes of dementia are treatable and because there is no *definitive* diagnostic criterion for AD short of autopsy, diagnosis is usually a painstaking process of elimination of other possible causes. The **NINCDS-ADRDA criteria** for diagnosis of *probable Alzheimer's dementia* were developed at the National Institute of Neurological and Communicative Diseases and Stroke–Alzheimer's Disease and Related Disorders Association (McKhann, Drachman, Folstein et al., 1984). These criteria are commonly used for selecting experimental participants. This type of dementia is considered seriously when there are two or more declining functions from the following list areas (or memory impairment and one other area of impairment):

- language (e.g., misnaming)
- memory (e.g., forgetting appointments)
- orientation (e.g., getting lost in familiar settings)
- judgment (e.g., not wearing a coat in freezing weather)

Also, Alzheimer's dementia is likely in the absence of depression, multiple infarcts, alcoholism, malnutrition, or other conditions that produce similar symptoms. An MRI may appear normal in the early stage, whereas atrophy is noticeable in later stages (also, Blacker, Albert, Bassett et al., 1994).

In the study of cognition and language with dementias, experimental participants are usually identified according to both the NIH criteria and MMSE scores. Healthy control participants are usually matched according to age and education. Because more women than men have AD, most participant groups have many more women. In addition, investigators often note the following common shortcomings in their experiments (e.g., Price and Grossman, 2005):

- Focus on mild and moderate deficits minimizes generalization to more severe impairment.
- Diagnosis is not confirmed by autopsy.
- Sample sizes are relatively small (e.g., 8 to 10 participants with AD).

Stages

For Burton Wheeler's (2001) wife, "there was no evident trigger, no first domino" (p. 3). ". . . it is not uncommon for a patient to already be in the early phase of AD by the time a family member first feels memory lapses are an actual problem"

(Dash and Villemarette-Pittman, 2005, p. 20). The onset of Alzheimer's dementia is invariably identified with the date of diagnosis, because the actual beginning of the disease cannot be determined. Early warning signs include forgetting things more often, becoming confused about time and place, having erratic changes in mood, changing in personality, and having difficulty finding words.

"Researchers are attempting to clarify the boundaries between what we consider the effects of normal aging and the onset of Alzheimer's disease" (Petersen, 2002, p. 31). A transitional area between normal aging and AD is termed **mild cognitive impairment** (MCI) and is assigned the Level 3 in Reisberg's GDS scale. MCI is characterized primarily by recent memory impairment that is greater than what we would expect for the individual's age. Other cognitive skills will begin to decline at a faster rate than those of people without MCI but at a slower rate than those with a diagnosis of AD. People with MCI may never progress to Alzheimer's disease but do have an increased risk for it (Peterson, Smith, Tangalos et al., 1993).

The course of Alzheimer's disease is a continuum of changes usually parsed into three stages of functional deficits (Table 13.5). The individual in *Stage I* conducts household chores carelessly but can follow established routines. Conversation contains some word-finding difficulty. *Stage II* is characterized by an increasing burden on family members, as a spouse becomes a parenting caregiver. Memory impairments are more obvious and disruptive. Shoes are put on before socks. There is frequent pacing and staring into space. Sensory and motor deficits arise after the early and middle stages. Neuromotor disability appears in terminal *Stage III*. The individual sits motionless in a corner and becomes totally dependent on others for tasks of daily living. When discussing someone with DAT, clinicians often identify if they are referring to an "early stage" or "late stage" condition.

Short-Term and Working Memory

MacDonald and others (2001) found that persons with mild or moderate DAT were not much worse than matched controls with the standard forward digit span test of short-term memory. Thus, simple STM does not appear to decline in the early to middle stages of DAT. To address working

TABLE 13.5 Stages in the progression of dementia of Alzheimer's type (DAT).

	OTHER TERMS	INTELLIGENCE	PERSONALITY	LANGUAGE
Stage I	Early Mild	Forgetful Disoriented Careless	Apathetic Anxious Irritable	Usually comprehends Vague words in talk Naming may be impaired Word fluency impaired Good repetition
Stage II	Middle Moderate	Recent events forgotten Math skills reduced	Restless	Comprehension reduced Paraphasias, jargon Irrelevant talk Naming becomes wordy Poor self-monitoring
Stage III	Late Severe	Recent events fade fast Remote memory impaired Family not recognized Incontinence		Becomes unresponsive Becomes mute

memory, MacDonald preferred a *digit-ordering* task in which participants repeat randomly presented digits (e.g., 7-2-4-9-1) in ascending numerical order (e.g., 1-2-4-7-9). This task requires a mental conversion process in addition to simple retention. Scoring is based on number of correct trials, not the span of digits recalled. Persons with "questionable dementia" were similar to controls, but those with mild or moderate DAT were significantly worse than controls in digit ordering. These results are similar to performance with the more common test of backward digit span that is part of the *Wechsler Memory Scale.*

Episodic Memory

Daniel Schacter (1996), who has written a great deal about memory impairments, played two rounds of golf with Frederick, who was in the early stage of AD. It was a test. One round was on a familiar course, and the other on an unfamiliar course. Frederick could still play, indicative of retention of procedural memory. He also retained perfect use of golf strategy and terminology, considered to be indicative of intact semantic and lexical stores. He chose the right club, knew who should putt first, and evaluated slopes on the green before putting. However, he forgot the shots he had just hit. He could not remember where his ball went after being the first to tee off, that is, when there was a delay between hitting and walking to the ball. Unlike most golfers in the clubhouse, he could not recall a single shot from the round. Frederick had a specific problem with episodic memory.

We began to learn about the neurological basis of episodic memory from HM, who underwent a bilateral medial temporal lobectomy in 1953 at the age of 27 in order to relieve intractable epilepsy (Scoville and Milner, 1957). To this day, HM's memory and language have been thoroughly investigated (e.g., Milner, Corkin, and Teuber, 1968; Skotko, Andrews, and Einstein, 2005). Two years after the surgery, HM scored a Full Scale IQ of 112 on the WAIS, but he did not recognize hospital staff who were treating him and forgot when

he had recently eaten a meal. Besides his anterograde amnesia, he also had retrograde amnesia for events several years prior to his operation. Like the association of Broca's area and speech nearly a century before, it is thought that HM provided the first direct evidence that the medial temporal lobe, the hippocampus in particular, plays an important role in memory.

We have learned that Alzheimer's disease usually begins in the hippocampus. This structure is thought to be responsible for sorting the parts of new memories and then reassembling them for recall. MRI studies have demonstrated substantial neuron loss with atrophy in the hippocampus (e.g., Galton et al., 2005). Later we shall consider a related deficiency in the production of acetycholine (ACH), a neurotransmitter in the region of the hippocampus that is also important for memory.

Semantic Memory

Semantic memory is the long-term storage of general conceptual knowledge and is widely presumed to contain the meanings of words. When there is a deficient semantic memory, more specific issues arise pertaining to whether there is a problem with storage (i.e., degraded conceptual representations) or with the processes of activation or access (e.g., Hodges, Salmon, and Butters, 1992). Furthermore, there is the question of whether word-finding difficulty is related to any one of these deficiencies of semantic memory.

Some researchers have employed effortful tasks to study semantic memory. Bayles, Tomoeda, and Rein (1996) relied on the repetition of short phrases that were meaningful (e.g., *remote tropical isle*), improbable (e.g., *personal burlap rug*), or meaningless (e.g., *quiet pencil jacket*). Mild and moderate participants with DAT used their semantic knowledge to maximize their repetition ability. Another effortful task consists of giving definitions. Two studies showed that people with DAT produce definitions that are not quite as good as elderly controls. The investigators concluded that there may be a subtle degradation of semantic memory (Garrard, Lambon Ralph, Patterson et al.,

2005) or that the metalinguistic task is too challenging to consider slight difficulty to be a deficit (Astell and Harley, 2002).

In previous chapters, semantic priming was presented as a means of studying the automatic activation of meaning for word comprehension. Researchers may also be thinking about semantic memory per se. An advantage of this method over effortful clinical procedures is that the content and structure of semantic memory can be examined with minimal conscious manipulation by an experimental participant.

Initial studies of semantic priming with mild-to-moderate Alzheimer's dementia produced mixed results, according to a meta-analysis by Ober and Shenaut (1995). People with DAT had normal semantic priming when studies tapped into automatic processing with short stimulus onset asynchronies (SOAs) (e.g., an SOA of 250 msec), indicating that they maintained a normal semantic structure. A surprising **hyperpriming** occurred when studies allowed for controlled strategic processing, such as with long SOAs (e.g., 1,000 msec). Hyperpriming is a priming effect that is larger for the experimental group than for a control group, indicating that people with mild DAT engage in extra mental effort when given time to do so. Ober and Shenaut's own study was consistent with their meta-analysis (Shenaut and Ober, 1996). In another study, hyperpriming occurred in a comparison of picture and word primes with a long SOA of 600 msec that was reported as a 250 msec prime duration and a 350 msec offset–onset interval (Margolin, Pate, and Friedrich, 1996).

Findings regarding semantic priming may depend on the type of relationship between the prime and target used in the experiment. For example, an associative relationship (e.g., *cottage-cheese*) is based on common experience, and categorical associates (e.g., *peach-plum*) are related to the conceptual structure presumed to characterize semantic networks. One study found that participants with DAT were primed for associates but not for categorical relationships (Glosser, Friedman, Grugan et al., 1998).

In a study of 10 participants with a range of DAT, Bell, Chenery, and Ingram (2001) examined two principal variables that previous researchers studied only partially. Automatic and controlled processing was differentiated through manipulation of the SOA and the proportion of related prime–target pairs. Another difference of method was the use of a neutral prime to detect facilitation by a semantically related prime and inhibition by an unrelated prime. This study produced some new differences from controls. The group with DAT produced no priming when strategies were discouraged with a low relatedness proportion, and they exhibited **hyperfacilitation** when relatedness proportion was high. Automatic priming in the latter condition indicates that semantic memory is fairly intact. There still may be some impairment of automatic activation, but people with DAT may resort to some access strategies when recognizing a high proportion of related word pairs.

Depression

Apathy, not forgetfulness, was the first sign of trouble for Burton Wheeler's (2001) wife. He wrote, "She became listless; the brightness of her eyes dimmed. She lost interest in going to concerts, plays, and movies. Her enthusiasm for travel vanished" (p. 3). Depression occurs at a higher rate among people with Alzheimer's dementia than among older adults without DAT.

Depression in the elderly can be easily mistaken for Alzheimer's dementia. People who appear to have DAT but really have only depression are said to have **depressive pseudodementia.** In fact, people with depressive pseudodementia are considered to be different from those who are simply depressed, because the former resemble DAT on cognitive testing. Physicians recommend that older adults with depression be evaluated regularly for cognitive decline and that people with AD be evaluated regularly for depression (Dash and Villemarette-Pittman, 2005).

The *Geriatric Depression Scale* (another GDS) is one respected screening measure for depression in older adults (Yesavage, Brink, Rose et al., 1982). It was originally a 30-item question-naire that was reduced to 15 items, and it has been translated into many languages. The GDS is in the public domain and can be completed on the Inter-net. Some of the items follow:

- Have you dropped many of your activities or interests?
- Do you feel happy most of the time?
- Do you often feel helpless?
- Do you think that most people are better off than you are?

LANGUAGE WITH ALZHEIMER'S DISEASE

As speech-language pathologists, let us hone in on some of the language research with Alzheimer's dementia. Some patients appear to have aphasia, usually mixed with other cognitive deficits. Most studies have been done with mild-to-moderate dementia. People with mild dementia correspond to early-stage DAT, and those with moderate dementia correspond to those with mid-stage DAT. People with early-stage dementia are able to participate in some of the most sophisticated experiments.

Comprehension

Let us first consider comprehension of sentences according to the common clinical task of sentence–picture matching. Rochon, Waters, and Caplan (1994) presented a wide range of syntactic struc-tures to 23 individuals with early-stage DAT. They found that these participants comprehended five of nine structures normally. Difficulty was not re-lated, however, to syntactic complexity but was, instead, related to the number of propositions in a sentence. Later, we shall consider Rochon and others' concern for the influence of the task used to assess sentence comprehension. Other research has shown signs of slight decline in the early stage (Bickel, Pantel, Eysenbach et al., 2000).

Using an implicit indicator of comprehension, MacDonald and her colleagues (2001) studied 11 persons with mild-to-moderate DAT (MMSE

16–24). First, they found that the group with DAT had a deficit in making grammaticality judgments. Then the participants engaged in a cross-modal task, in which the investigators measured time to read aloud a word that either appropriately or in-appropriately completed a spoken sentence. The group with DAT was just as quick as matched controls in reading the appropriate word relative to the inappropriate word, leading to the conclu-sion that the implicit task was needed to show that individuals with DAT have a normal ability to un-derstand sentences.

MacDonald's experiment came close to de-tecting comprehension as it occurred. As discussed in Chapters 4 and 5, researchers have considered it necessary to supplement familiar off-line tests of sentence comprehension with online experiments that tap into comprehension "in real time." Also, off-line tasks are more effortful and take up more room in working memory than online tasks. Thus, simple processes are difficult to target with off-line tasks that are complicated by a variety of pro-cesses contributing to performance of the task.

Murray Grossman, at the University of Penn-sylvania, has directed a series of studies of lan-guage comprehension with dementia, including some with Parkinson's disease (Lee, Grossman, Morris et al., 2003). Price and Grossman (2005) had 15 individuals with mild-to-moderate DAT (ave MMSE 21.7) engage in a word-monitoring task that tapped into processing within a sentence. Semantic and syntactic aspects of verbs were examined, namely, semantically oriented infor-mation about actions and their agents and syntac-tically oriented information about whether a verb can take a recipient (i.e., transivity). This was a subtle look at whether people with DAT have defi-cits of semantics or syntax.

In each trial, participants first heard a target word and then the sentence. They pressed the space bar on a computer keyboard when they heard the target (e.g., *through*). The target ap-peared either immediately following the violation or downstream a few syllables, so that immedi-ate effects could be differentiated from delayed effects. In the examples, 1 contains semantic (or thematic) violations, and 2 contains syntactic (or transivity) violations.

(1a) *immediate:* The [turtles/birds] crawl *through* the dry grass toward . . .

(1b) *delayed:* The [turtles/birds] crawl through the dry grass *toward* . . .

(2a) *immediate:* The jury [listens/listens lawyer] *quietly* for more . . .

(2b) *delayed:* The jury [listens/listens lawyer] quietly for *more* . . .

Like healthy matched controls, the group with DAT was sensitive to transivity by more quickly recognizing the immediately positioned target word (2a) when it followed appropriate wording than when it followed inappropriate wording. When the target was positioned downstream (2b), however, the appropriateness difference was absent. Unlike healthy matched controls, the group with DAT was insensitive to thematic appropriateness both immediately and downstream (1a, 1b). This result reinforced the view that people with early DAT are more impaired for semantics than for syntax. Price and Grossman favored the view that some of semantic network storage has been degraded, contrary to the semantic priming studies.

Price and Grossman (2005) also studied 14 individuals with frontotemporal dementia (ave MMSE 22.6). The group with FTD differed from the group with DAT by being insensitive to both thematic and transitive agreements when the target word was positioned immediately (i.e., semantics and syntax). The investigators noted that this broader deficit cannot be attributed to task-related resource demands because of the automaticity of the word-monitoring task.

A familiar question regarding any communication disorder is whether working memory has anything to do with a language comprehension deficit. Waters, Caplan, and Rochon (1995) followed their sentence comprehension study with one in which 14 patients with mild or moderate DAT remembered digits presented while doing the sentence–picture matching task. The experimental participants were more affected than matched controls by the digit load, leading the researchers to conclude that "they have reduced working memory capacity for language" (p. 22). Later Waters and her colleagues (1998) employed a variety of picture-matching formats, from single picture verification to choosing among three pictures. Again, there was no evidence of a syntactic deficit. Difficulty arose with a combination of listening to sentences with two propositions (e.g., a horse kicked an elephant, the elephant touched a dog) and choosing a picture from an array. Processing demands of the task seemed to cause the problems.

Let us return to the study by MacDonald and her colleagues (2001). They showed that processing demands are related to performance on sentence comprehension tasks. The digit-ordering task introduced earlier was correlated with performance on the grammaticality judgment task but not the word-naming test of implicit comprehension. MacDonald suspected that the implicit task supported the retention of syntactic processing. Difficulty with grammaticality judgment exposed a deficiency of working memory that influences the particular task being used rather than pure sentence comprehension.

In moving on to discourse comprehension, let us first examine the ability to connect pronouns to antecedents across sentences. MacDonald and her colleagues (2001) used the same cross-modal word-naming procedure to study sensitivity to pronouns. Participants heard short stories concluding with a compatible or incompatible pronoun, such as the following:

(3) The children loved the silly clown at the party. The show was very funny. During the performance, the clown threw candy to *him/ them.*

Patients with DAT and healthy controls were sensitive to pronoun appropriateness, indicating that the correct antecedent was reactivated at the end of the story. However, the experimental participants did not have as strong an effect, indicating that people with DAT process pronouns less effectively. Also, contrary to the single sentence task, digit-ordering scores were correlated with cross-modal naming of pronouns. This correlation indicated that pronoun processing across a short story is more demanding of working memory for people with dementia.

Welland, Lubinski, and Higginbotham (2002) administered the *Discourse Comprehension Test* (Brookshire and Nicholas, 1993) to persons with mild or moderate DAT. Both groups of DAT scored significantly worse than matched intact controls, but the mild and moderate stage participants unexpectedly scored the same. Those with DAT had the same pattern of performance as the controls, namely, better scores for recalling main ideas than details and better scores for recalling explicit content than implicit content. Not surprisingly, deficient comprehension was highly correlated with a measure of episodic memory. The comprehension test has a strong episodic memory component, as it entails answering questions about a story just heard.

Word Finding and Retrieval

People with DAT say that they have trouble remembering words or names. Is this difficulty like aphasia, in which the impairment is one of accessing the mental lexicon rather than a degradation of lexical or conceptual knowledge? Let us consider traditional clinical tasks of naming and word fluency and then attempts to relate word finding to semantic memory.

To have a sense for word finding in clinical terms, let us consider results with the *Boston Naming Test* (Nicholas, Obler, Au et al., 1996). Persons with mild DAT were only somewhat different from age- and education-matched older controls, but naming deficit was pronounced with moderate DAT (Table 13.6). Another naming test was used to analyze changes in naming over a two-year period (Cuetos, Gonzalez-Nosti, and Martinez, 2005). There was a considerable reduction in naming accuracy. Type of error changed from semantic errors to "I don't know" responses.

TABLE 13.6   Alzheimer's dementia scores on the *Boston Naming Test* (Nicholas et al., 1996).

	MEAN	RANGE
Younger controls	57.4	52–60
Older controls	51.5	34–59
Mild DAT	45.7	33–54
Moderate DAT	26.5	13–42

Naming in nonbiological categories (i.e., clothing, furniture, tools) seems to be more affected in DAT than naming in biological categories (i.e., animals, fruits, vegetables). The problem with nonbiological naming was associated with DAT, because patients with other dementias did not have the same dissociation, and the difficulty with the nonbiological category worsened with increased severity of DAT (Whatmough, Chertkow, Murtha et al., 2003).

In the study by Whatmough and others (2003), words acquired early in life were more resistant to deterioration. Substantial research indicates that **age of acquisition** is an influential variable in various tasks involving access to lexical memory (Zevin and Seidenberg, 2002). Researchers in Canada have examined two interacting factors. *Cumulative frequency* is how often a word is encountered, and one approach to research is to compare popular and rare words. *Frequency trajectory* refers to when a word is learned or the variation of word frequency over a lifetime, and one approach is to compare dated words (e.g., *hep-cat*) and contemporary words (e.g., *homophobia*).

In the Toronto research, Westmacott and others (2004) presented a variety of tasks that tapped into the temporal gradation of semantic and lexical knowledge. The tasks relied on 480 names of famous people classified according to the period of time when they became famous. The tasks included speeded reading of names, classification of names, matching last names to first names, matching movies to actors, and reading and recognition of vocabulary from different periods. All patients with mild-to-moderate DAT showed temporally graded abilities. Names and words from the remote past were better preserved than recent names and words. One year later, the period of deficit extended back further in time.

Caza and Moscovitch (2005) concentrated on cumulative frequency and frequency trajectory with a simple lexical decision task, which is indicative of lexical activation. Participants with DAT (MMSE 18 or more) did not have a trajectory effect but did have a cumulative frequency effect. Therefore, age-of-acquisition effects may be more likely to appear with tasks involving word retrieval rather than simply accessing a word.

Word fluency may be an effective screening test for dementia according to Hopper and Bayles (2001), but just about any brain damage affects this divergent word-finding ability. Hough and Givens (2004) compared common categories (e.g., furniture, birds) and goal-directed categories (e.g., things to take on a picnic). Results were consistent with previous studies of word fluency. Participants with DAT produced examples of categories, and people with moderate dementia were less accurate than those with mild dementia. More atypical responses were produced with moderate DAT than mild DAT. Use of response strategies (e.g., clustering) was also weakened, even in mild DAT. However, type of category was not a factor. Hough (2004) also studied word fluency with Parkinson's disease.

Deficits with DAT have been more severe for semantic categories than letters (e.g., Barr and Brandt, 1996; Crossley, D'Arcy, and Rawson, 1997). The greater problem with semantic categories and the nature of responses has led to the frequent conclusion that degraded semantic memory is responsible for word fluency in DAT. Yet, Diaz and others (2004) noted that the many studies of word fluency have relied on highly overlapping materials. The so-called FAS test for letters is well-known, and most studies of letter fluency have employed these letters. For semantic fluency, most studies have relied on the categories of animals, fruits, and vegetables. Therefore, Diaz worried that the semantic-letter difference may

not be true for all categories, and he suggested that category size may also be a factor.

Diaz and his colleagues examined category size with the common categories for semantic fluency (i.e., animals, fruits, vegetables) and letter fluency (i.e., F, A, S). For example, the animal category in common knowledge is likely to have many more exemplars than the vegetable category, and a letter is likely to have many more exemplars than many semantic categories. Using some sophisticated mathematics, the researchers estimated that the deficit with DAT was larger for the larger categories, indicating, at least, that category size may overlap with type of category as a factor in word fluency. Diaz recommended that future studies include a wider variety of semantic and letter categories.

Can naming difficulties be related to changes in semantic memory? Astell and Harley (1998) were interested in whether the basic problem could be a degradation of semantic memory or a problem involving access of semantic memory (i.e., meaning) or lexical memory (i.e., words). They presented word-comprehension tasks and a naming task to 12 individuals with moderate-to-severe DAT (MMSE 4–18). The experimental participants did much better with comprehension than naming. Contrary to previous studies, related naming errors were not predominantly general category names (i.e., superordinates), and the types of errors were similar to previous studies of healthy adults. These investigators concluded that the naming deficit in DAT is mainly a processing problem of retrieval. Other error analyses cast doubt on semantic knowledge deficit as the basis for word-finding problems (Moreaud, David, Charnallet et al., 2001; Nicholas et al., 1996).

Semantic memory and naming have been investigated extensively in the United Kingdom by John Hodges and Karalyn Patterson of Cambridge and Matthew Lambon Ralph of Manchester. Semantic memory was assessed with a definitions task mentioned earlier in this chaper (Garrard et al., 2005). They studied participants with mild DAT (MMSE 20–25) and moderate DAT (MMSE 14–19). The participants with significant word-finding deficit were in the moderate stage. The ability to name pictures was related to the number of attributes accessed when giving definitions. The results also indicated that the more specific or distinctive the definition, the more appropriate the naming response was likely to be. Therefore, naming ability was related to the quality of semantic memory, at least, as measured by an effortful task.

When tip-of-the-tongue (TOT) states were induced, individuals with a range of DAT (MMSE 8–22) were unable to produce information about the word, unlike elderly controls. This was indicative of a serious deficit in accessing the lexicon. The people with DAT produced semantically related errors, indicating access to the appropriate region of semantic memory. The investigators speculated that the impairment was the weakening of connections between semantic and lexical stores (Astell and Harley, 1996). The inability to retrieve lexical information differs from the ability of many people with aphasia to retrieve some information about a word.

Sentence Production

Research over the years has led to the broad characterization of language production with mild-to-moderate DAT as declining mainly in the area of semantics, whereas phonology, morphology, and syntax (or morphosyntax) remain well preserved (e.g., Appell et al, 1982; Kempler, Curtiss, and Jackson, 1987). These individuals tend to hold on to a fluent conversational ability long after the initial diagnosis. In terms of general linguistic categories, lexical retrieval begins to decline early, whereas syntactic features of utterances become problematic at later stages (Bates, Harris, Marchman et al., 1999).

Small, Kemper, and Lyons (2000) asked 13 people with mild-to-moderate DAT to repeat sentences of varying complexity very much like the sentences used by Caplan and Waters in their research (Chapter 4). We may recall that people with aphasia distinctly favor canonical over noncanonical sentences; however, the participants with DAT

had no clear canonicity effect. Separate tests of verbal working memory correlated with sentence repetition, leading the investigators to conclude that working memory constraints hindered sentence repetition with DAT.

Elizabeth Bates and her colleagues (1999) analyzed descriptions of short, animated films of simple actions. The first procedure was *free description* to a neutral cue of "now," and the second procedure was *probed description* in which participants were cued to describe from the recipient character's point of view in order to elicit passive sentences. Bates analyzed the passivisation and structural complexity of descriptions by 16 people with mild-to-moderate DAT (ave MMSE 20.4). In these constrained conditions, she found simplification of structure and reliance on certain common forms. Bates concluded that people with DAT do have syntactic deficiencies in the early stages that may reflect a difficulty in accessing forms much like difficulties in accessing words.

The role of the verb has been of great interest in clinical sentence production research. Kim and Thompson (2004) compared a group with moderate-to-very mild DAT (MMSE 13–26) to a group with agrammatism on noun and verb naming, sentence completion, and narrative production. For each group, Kim and Thompson compared syntactic and semantic complexity of the verbs, the latter having to do with the level of elaboration in their semantic representations. The syntactic characteristic of verb argument structure influenced those with agrammatism (see Chapter 5) but not those with DAT. On the other hand, semantic complexity of verbs affected the DAT group but not the agrammatic group. The authors considered that these results add to the mounting support for a deficit of semantic representations in Alzheimer's dementia.

One problem with the broad linguistic characterization of areas of language ability is the disagreement among linguists and psycholinguistics as to where certain types of words belong. Are some closed-class words semantic and others grammatical? Some believe that pronouns are closed-class words (more syntactic), and others believe that pronouns are open-class words (more semantic). So, Altmann and her colleagues (2001) decided to modernize the classification of errors produced in a spontaneous speech task and a constrained production task. In particular, they paid attention to pronouns as separate from grammatical closed-class words (e.g., articles, auxiliaries).

Altmann found that the nature of the task influenced the errors produced by 10 individuals with mild-to-moderate DAT (MMSE 18–22). The spontaneous speech task consisted of conversation about familiar topics. The constrained production task involved presenting a card showing a transitive verb and two nouns, and participants were asked to make up a grammatical sentence containing these words. In spontaneous speech, individuals with DAT simply produced more of the type of errors that were produced by matched healthy adults. On the other hand, the experimental participants had difficulties performing the constrained production task. Most errors were with grammatical closed-class words. Almost no errors occurred with pronouns and open-class words. Three of these participants were nearly agrammatic. The investigators concluded that morphosyntax (e.g., grammatical closed-class words) is deficient with DAT, but the deficit is more salient in a constrained production task.

Speech and writing may be different, having something to do with the deliberate pace of writing. "Some days it seems I live in two worlds," wrote DeBaggio (2002), ". . . gasping as words slip through my lips with effort and imprecision . . . In the other, slower world where I write on paper or directly on the computer, vocabulary is more fluid and I often surprise myself . . ." (p. 180).

Discourse and Conversation

A few studies of discourse production have relied on information analysis, such as counting small information units (e.g., Arkin and Mahendra, 2001). Giles, Patterson, and Hodges (1996) elicited spoken descriptions of the Cookie Theft from DAT patients, and they were particularly inter-

ested in whether production of information units and syllables would distinguish early or minimal dementia from healthy adults. In a somewhat exceptional application of the MMSE, "minimal" DAT was identified with relatively high scores of 24 to 29. Mild DAT was identified as MMSEs of 14 to 23, which extends into moderate dementia (see Table 13.2). Minimal DAT was distinguished with respect to the total number of information units produced.

Research demonstrated some differences between writing and speech. Oral and written descriptions of the Cookie Theft were elicited in a study of 22 persons with DAT and an average MMSE of about 19 (Croisile, Ska, Brabant et al., 1996). Oral descriptions were longer but were as informative as written texts. In general, participants with DAT produced fewer words than healthy controls. Consistent with other findings, syntax was relatively preserved but simplified to some extent. Participants with DAT produced more implausible details, especially in written descriptions. The investigators concluded that inappropriate intrusions and reduction of subordinate clauses made written descriptions of the Cookie Theft more sensitive to the presence of dementia than oral descriptions.

Some analysis has reached into the discourse level. In a comparison of stimulus types, a picture of a bank robbery was accompanied by the instruction "Tell me the story that you see," which is more likely to elicit a narrative than asking for a description (Duong, Giroux, Tardif et al., 2005). The single picture was compared to elicitation with a seven-picture story of a car accident. The narratives were analyzed at three general levels from lexical production to the formulation of transitions between story elements. The researchers identified participants as having mild to moderate DAT with respect to GDS levels 3 and 4. However, the analysis failed to differentiate half of the DAT participants from healthy controls, perhaps partly because the GDS level 3 denotes mild cognitive impairment rather than dementia.

Introduced in Chapter 6, conversation analysis (CA) was employed by Watson and others

(1999) to analyze 10 conversations between persons with DAT and strangers. The experimental participants had a fairly wide range of dementia, including some with moderate-to-severe impairment. Conversation analysis targeted trouble indicators, repair trajectories, repair types, and success of repairs. Results indicated that the unimpaired partners shouldered much of the burden of indicating trouble and initiating repairs. Some inappropriate repair behavior by those with DAT, such as veering off topic, was accepted by partners, apparently to preserve the self-esteem of the experimental participants.

MEDICAL TREATMENTS

Another story can be found in the development of drugs for Alzheimer's disease. The plot is driven by science, the pharmaceutical industry, the federal regulatory system, and the public. In the early 1970s, scientists discovered the deficiency in acetycholine (ACH). In 1986, William Summers published a study extolling the effectiveness of a new drug, called tacrine, to boost the production of ACH. The scientific community was skeptical of the investigator's credentials and the study itself, which was completed on only 14 participants. The outcome measures were questioned, and the data appeared to be mainly anecdotal. The Food and Drug Administration (FDA) accused Summers of misrepresentation.

Nevertheless, word got out, and an anxious public was impressed with the possibility that a wonder drug could improve memory. They vilified the FDA "as heartlessly impeding the relief of suffering and demanded the immediate release of tacrine" (Gillick, 1998, p. 132). Hate mail sent to the director of the FDA illustrates the conflict between an "activist public" that wants any promising new drug immediately and a deliberate regulatory agency that seeks to protect the public.

The Tacrine Collaborative Study Group was formed; their results, reported in 1992, were promising but also reinforced previous findings of damaging side effects. Another study of a stronger dose for a longer period prompted the FDA

to approve tacrine in 1993. However, two of the authors were employees of the pharmaceutical company that made tacrine, and 70 percent of the participants had dropped out of the study because of the same side effects, namely, liver toxicity or gastrointestinal problems of nausea, vomiting, and diarrhea. Tacrine also proved to be taxing on a patient and caregiver, because it had to be taken four times per day.

Tacrine has been replaced by three FDA-approved drugs that have a similar mechanism of action on the brain. The goal of boosting ACH is achieved by inhibiting the action of cholinesterase, a chemical that breaks down ACH across the synapse. Thus, the drugs are classified as "cholinesterase inhibitors." The first, approved in 1996, goes by the increasingly familiar trade name **Aricept** (donepezil). Its mechanism is the same as tacrine but without the liver toxicity side effect, and it is taken only once a day. More recently approved drugs include Exelon in 2000 and Reminyl in 2001.

In 2003, the FDA released a drug with a different mechanism for use in the United States. Namenda (memantine) prevents excessive production of glutamate, which, in proper amounts, is a neurotransmitter that is important for learning and memory. The drug also has few side effects and is taken twice per day. In 2005, various clinical trials were underway for the investigation of Namenda used in combination with any of the three cholinesterase inhibitor drugs (Dash and Villemarette-Pittman, 2005).

Soon after his diagnosis, DeBaggio (2002) was prescribed Aricept and experienced its gastrointestinal side effect. His doctor also prescribed over-the-counter **vitamin E** soft gels and ibuprofen. Vitamin E is an "antioxidant," which combats toxic side effects of the body's defense mechanisms. One study showed that a group taking a substantial amount of vitamin E had delayed institutionalization or death compared to a group taking a placebo. The American Academy of Neurologists has recommended its use. However, there has been no evidence that vitamin E retards intellectual deterioration. Scientists are still investigating the value of vitamins C and B, as well as vitamin E. Alternative treatments include the herbs gingko biloba and lemon balm, and an alleged memory boosting dietary supplement called huperzine (hupA). We can keep up with new possibilities by simply doing a Google search for "Alzheimer's news."

COMMUNICATIVE ASSESSMENT

With respect to traditional language batteries, results have been reported with the *Western Aphasia Battery* (WAB). In one study, all 25 patients with Alzheimer's dementia were below the Aphasia Quotient's 93.8 cut-off for aphasia. We do not know the stage of these cases, because MMSE scores or other measures of mental status were not reported (Appell, Kertesz, and Fisman, 1982). Later, a discriminant analysis showed that the WAB had difficulty identifying those with Alzheimer's dementia relative to others with stroke-related aphasia (Horner, Dawson, Heyman, and Fish, 1992).

In addition to the general tests and scales reviewed earlier in the chapter, dementia-oriented tests and scales for language and communication have been developed by SLPs. Any evaluation begins with a check of hearing and vision and of hearing aids and glasses.

At the University of Arizona, Kathryn Bayles and Cheryl Tomoeda (1993) developed probably the best-known assessment of mild-to-moderate deficit, namely, the *Arizona Battery for Communication Disorders of Dementia* (ABCD). The battery consists of 14 subtests addressing the following five areas of cognition:

- linguistic expression
- linguistic comprehension
- verbal episodic memory
- mental status
- visuospatial construction

An SLP can compute summary scores, which are converted for determining the status of the five cognitive areas. Hopper and Bayles (2001) suggested that the Story Retelling subtest of the

ABCD is an effective screening tool. A second battery was developed for middle- and late-stage DAT. The *Functional Linguistic Communication Inventory* (FLCI) consists of 10 components covering everyday language and communicative behaviors and takes less than 30 minutes to administer. Tasks include greeting, naming, comprehending signs, and reminiscing (Bayles and Tomoeda, 1994).

In addition to tests, scales for communicative abilities have appeared. Caregiver and self assessments are employed for *Communication Adequacy in Daily Situations* (CADS) (Clark and Witte, 1995). It relies on five-point frequency scales for 26 items of functional communication. For moderate-to-severe dementia, the *Pragmatic Assessment of Communication—Dementia* (PAC-D) allows SLPs to rate the adequacy of communicative behaviors with 10 common objects (England, O'Neill, and Simpson, 1996).

COGNITIVE INTERVENTIONS

Regarding the fundamental orientations that have driven rehabilitation for other disorders, we can assume that restoration of function is an unrealistic goal for progressive dementias until medical discoveries reverse the tide. However, some temporary restoration is attempted through stimulation. Compensatory strategies comprise the main orientation to cognitive intervention. People with DAT may receive clinical assistance in a variety of settings (Table 13.7). Some facilities combine all the components of independent retirement living, assisted living, and nursing home care. "The most appropriate facility for someone with advanced and terminal stages of the disease would be a nursing home with a dedicated Alzheimer's care program" (Dean, 2004, p. 246).

The first or "archetypal" approach was called **Reality Orientation,** which is thought to have begun in U.S. Veterans Administration Hospitals in the 1960s. Reality Orientation consists of the repetitive presentation of date, time, and place, which are posted in residents' rooms, rehearsed with hospital staff, and rehearsed again in group

TABLE 13.7   Settings of Alzheimer's care programs (Dean, 2004; Petersen, 2002).

Retirement homes with assisted-living programs	Has licensed personal care programs along with independent living; often for couples when one has early stage or mild AD
Assisted-living facilities (ALFs)	Usually smaller than retirement homes; provide health care for those who need assistance in daily living; includes community living spaces
Licensed residential-care home	A home setting for a maximum of six residents with moderate to severe AD; provides basic care but not skilled nursing
Alzheimer's dedicated-care facility	Currently rare, larger residential-care facility for severe-stage AD
Nursing homes	Provides skilled medical care for those in a wheelchair or those who are bedridden; often the "final stop" for someone in advanced or terminal stage

meetings. Its notoriously rigid implementation led to a reduction of popularity in the 1980s, but more sensitive remnants of the program continue in rehabilitation and residential settings as components of cognitive stimulation and other approaches (Spector, Orrell, Davies et al., 2001).

Efficacy of Intervention

Let us first consider the question of whether cognitive and communicative treatments are helpful. Moore and others (2001) demonstrated that a memory training program improved recognition and recall. Another program, called procedural memory stimulation, trained 13 activities of daily living (e.g., personal hygiene, telephone, dressing) for one hour per day, five days per week, for three weeks. A group with an average MMSE of 20 showed significant improvement over an untrained control group in the time it took to complete the activities (Zanetti, Zanieri, Di Giovanni, et al., 2001).

Again at the University of Arizona, Arkin (2001) studied student-administered training in a community-based program. She compared two groups with an MMSE range of 15 to 29. The individual with the near-maximum MMSE score was diagnosed with dementia using another scale and also had an ApoE genetic test profile with a high

probability of AD. Both groups received physical fitness and volunteer work sessions, but one group received additional memory and language exercises for two semesters (28 weeks). The cognitive training group improved in a few of the measures, whereas the other group did not improve in the measures.

In Dallas, Texas, Chapman and her colleagues (2004) evaluated a two-month cognitive stimulation program with 54 mild-to-moderate AD patients (MMSE 12–28) who were receiving donepezil (Aricept). Roughly half the patients received the functional program along with donepezil, and the other half received donepezil alone. The stimulation treatment consisted of discussions and some homework. After 12 months, the stimulation–donepezil group was performing better on discourse and quality of life measures. The authors concluded that "this study adds to growing evidence that active cognitive stimulation may slow the rate of verbal and functional decline and decrease negative emotional symptoms" when combined with medication (p. 1149).

Many group and single case studies have indicated that rehabilitation services can be helpful, especially for mild-to-moderate DAT (Lawton and Rubinstein, 2000). Also, earlier diagnosis means that more people have an opportunity to benefit from the treatments that are effective during the early stage. Because of these advances, the Bush administration authorized Medicare coverage for the treatment of AD in 2001, including speech-language therapies.

Memory Strategies

Memory problems impact conversation. Individuals do not remember what was just said and do not remember a topical event that occurred the previous week. One principle of memory training, introduced in Chapter 12, has been adopted for memory practice. **Spaced retrieval training** (SRT) requires recall of material at increasing intervals between presentation and test/recall and, conversely, includes shortening the interval when there is recall failure (Brush and Camp, 1998; Camp, 2006). Let us suppose we tell an individual that lunch is going to be chicken salad and soup. We ask her to repeat it. Then a few seconds later, we ask her what is for lunch. If she is correct, we ask again a couple minutes later, and so on. SRT has produced favorable results in naming therapy for aphasia (Fridriksson, Holland, Beeson et al, 2005).

In articles and video presentations, Bayles has alerted SLPs to the value of basic memory theory for providing comprehensive compensatory strategies (e.g., Hopper and Bayles, 2001). Her principles have been conveyed in various ways. Here we will consider a few of them.

One of Bayles's recommendations is to **reduce demands on episodic memory.** In conversation, this means avoiding requests to retrieve experiences from memory and, instead, stating the possibilities for easier recognition (e.g., yes/no response). Bayles recommended stimulating spared stores such as procedural memory (e.g., Zanetti et al., 2001). Also, *external memory aids,* like those suggested for traumatic brain injury, support long-term memory generally.

Michelle Bourgeois (1992; 2006) at Florida State University has studied the use of a "memory wallet" as an external aid. A memory wallet is a 25-page book of pictures and sentences pertaining to memory failures determined from a question-naire completed by the family. Each page contains one sentence and a related picture or photograph. The book is intended to help sustain conversations with caregivers. In Bourgeois's research, nursing home residents with varied dementias were trained in three or four sessions to use memory wallets in conversations with nursing assistants. Results showed an increase in factual utterances by residents and a reduction of non-facilitative behavior by nursing assistants. Non-facilitative behavior was reduced further with additional training of the nursing assistants, and turn taking became more balanced (Hoerster, Hickey, and Bourgeois, 2001). Spaced retrieval is also useful in training with the memory wallet (Bourgeois, Camp, Rose et al., 2003).

Another one of Bayles's recommendations is to **support working memory.** Limitations of working memory lead to forgetting previous utterances in an exchange, forgetting the topic of a conversation, and being susceptible to distraction. In principle, support comes from reducing distractions, writing down a topic or important information, and keeping statements short and simple.

A third suggestion from Bayles is **to provide stimulation and environments to evoke positive memory, emotion, and action.** This refers broadly to programs of activity and environmental management in nursing homes and other facilities. On any day, we can visit one of these facilities and find residents being entertained with music or being involved in art, crafts, or gardening. The setting is sunlit and cheerful. A few nursing homes have created "50s environments" in which the décor is reminiscent of the time when residents were young adults.

Field trips are common, and some are extensions of art therapy. Museums have been opening their doors to people with Alzheimer's disease. For example, small groups with mild-to-moderate dementia pay weekly visits to the Museum of Modern Art in New York City and the Museum of Fine Arts in Boston. Individuals are encouraged to say whatever comes to mind about the art works, and caregivers have noticed increased energy and talkativeness after the visits.

Language and Communication

Language-oriented therapies begin with word finding. In France, Ousset and others (2002) provided a "Lexical Therapy" for a group with mild DAT, and they compared them to a group that received occupational therapy. The lexical therapy consisted of naming from definitions and reading narratives. Half of the definitions were from the narrative and half were not. The therapy was assessed with a pre–post naming test with some of the items from the narratives, others from the non-narrative definitions, and others that were not part of the treatment. Ousset found significant improvement for the lexically treated group only for the treated items, leading to the conclusion that people with mild DAT can benefit to some extent from a contextually rich naming therapy.

One common objective of lexically oriented treatment is to improve people recognition and naming through the practice of face–name associations. **Errorless learning** has been applied to such tasks (e.g., Clare, Wilson, Carter et al., 2001). In Chapter 12, it was suggested that minimizing mistakes is essentially the same idea as the principle of success that is so essential to stimulation treatment for aphasia. Accuracy is maximized by using the most familiar materials, providing plenty of cues, and repeating the successes.

Arkin and Mahendra (2001) reported on an "easy-to-use" but detailed informational analysis of discourse that helped them to re-evaluate the two treatment groups mentioned earlier. The experimental language intervention was conducted during physical fitness workout sessions for persons with DAT living in various settings in the community. The treatment consisted of a variety of tasks intended to activate semantic memory. The tasks included free and prompted descriptions of Norman Rockwell paintings, associations to evocative words, and proverb completion and interpretation. Another group was stimulated with informal conversation during their fitness class. There was no difference between the groups on most discourse measures, indicating that the fitness program was enough for maintenance of discourse abilities.

The Breakfast Club is a conversational group for nursing home residents with DAT. It centers around planning, preparing, and eating a breakfast. The clinician uses a 10-step program for facilitating interpersonal communication with visual cues, conceptual associations, and questions with two-choice answers to support memory. Santo Pietro and Boczko (1997, 1998) compared this group with a pared down discussion group in which the clinician provided a topic and questions were open ended. The Breakfast Club displayed many more improvements in language and functional independence than the other conversational group, indicating that the type of conversation group can make a difference.

Hopper and Bayles (2001) explained Medicare reimbursement for speech-language therapy provided to people in skilled nursing facilities. The main approach is **functional maintenance therapy** (FMT) based on a functional maintenance plan (FMP). The FMP consists of evaluation and a short-term diagnostic treatment program for patients who demonstrate a potential for improvement. Brief trial therapy is usually justified, and the program is likely to be carried out by caregivers trained by SLPs who prescribe the treatment. Educating caregivers may be reimbursable.

Caregiver Training

"Initially, I refused to believe my wife was suffering from dementia. Something was wrong, yes, but she was too perceptive, too alert for such an illness" (Wheeler, 2001, p. 3). Acceptance is a tough state to reach. Arkin (2001) noted that a community-based program in Arizona is called Elder Rehab, "because some participants and/or their families do not acknowledge an Alzheimer's disease (AD) diagnosis or prefer not to be publicly identified with AD" (p. 273).

Caregivers find themselves struggling with "the 36-hour day" (Mace and Rabins, 1999). Information is plentiful to guide and support family members and residential staff (e.g., Dean, 2004;

Gruetzner, 2001; Schulz, 2000), including those who have maintained a sense of humor (Smith, Kenan, and Kunik, 2004). However, in writing about his wife's Alzheimer's disease, Burton Wheeler (2001) expressed his discomfort with the term "caregiver." "It implies to me a constancy and stability . . . I wish I were capable of such behavior, but I'm not" (p. 1). He added, "Most mornings I crawl out of bed slowly. Not only slowly, but painfully. I'm in my mid-seventies" (p. 2).

The following is a sample of general recommendations for caregivers (Dash and Villemarette-Pittman, 2005; Mace and Rabins, 1999; Petersen, 2002):

- Educate yourself regarding DAT.
- Get appropriate medical care for your loved one.
- Make sure your loved one's legal documents are complete.
- Keep the impaired person active but not upset.
- Take care of yourself.
- Plan ahead.
- Solve problems one at a time.
- Share the burden.
- Join a support group.

Some of these strategies are important for relieving the stress of adjusting to a new life. Support includes a "caregiver's bill of rights" and a caregiver stress test (Dean, 2004).

For SLPs, Danielle Ripich, now president of the University of New England in Maine, developed the FOCUSED caregiver communication program. It is organized around seven strategies for successful communication: Face to face, Orient to topic, Continuity of topic, Unstick blocks, Structured questions, Exchange of turns, and Direct short sentences. The program is divided into modules with guidebooks to use in small-group training. Caregivers are encouraged to ask yes/no questions instead of open-ended questions, which has become a fairly consistent recommendation. In addition, a series of videotapes for indepen-

dent learning by caregivers has been developed (Ripich, 1996; Ripich, Ziol, and Lee, 1998; also, Bourgeois, Schulz, Burgio et al., 2002).

At the University of British Columbia, Jeff Small has been examining the interactions between caregivers and people with DAT. In one study, he compared what caregivers thought they were doing to support conversation with what they were actually doing and how successful they were. What should get our attention is that the study targeted 10 communication strategies frequently recommended by SLPs and others, so that this complex study has implications for caregiver-training programs. In general, caregivers perceived themselves as following certain recommendations but were not actually employing them (Small, Gutman, Makela et al., 2003).

In Small's study, the use of simple sentences was the most effective strategy that caregivers both thought they were using and were actually using. Encouraging the use of yes/no questions has been integral to some training programs. Most of the caregivers' questions were this type, and yes/no questions were relatively effective. Another successful strategy was to reduce distractions, and a frequent strategy was to avoid interrupting the patient. On the other hand, slowing the rate of speech and repeating verbatim were infrequently used and often ineffective for communication. Also, caregivers rarely encouraged circumlocution for conveying information.

Later, Small and Perry (2005) thought that focusing on the general question type is insufficient for considering the various demands that conversation places on memory. An additional dimension is the type of memory storage that is tapped by questions. Semantic questions address basic conceptual information (e.g., What is this thing?). Episodic questions address autobiographical events (e.g., What did you eat for dinner yesterday?). As indicated by the example, episodic questions can be subclassified as to whether the event occurred recently or occurred in the remotely distant past (e.g., Where did you go to college?).

TABLE 13.8   Some resources on Alzheimer's disease for professionals and caregivers.

RESOURCE	WEBSITE	DESCRIPTION
Alzheimer's Association	www.alz.org	Main support and advocacy organization
Alzheimer's information	www.alzinfo.org	Information source
ALZwell Caregiver Support	www.alzwell.com	From MedicineOnline: "Information and vent page for caregivers of loved ones with Alzheimer's Disease or other memory impairment."
Geriatric Resources, Inc.	www.geriatric-resources. com	Company specializing in caregiving resources and services for those suffering from Alzheimer's Disease
theforgetting.com	www.randomhouse. com/features/forgetting	News about the disease, inspired by Shenk's (2002) book

Looking at these various types of memory demands, Small and Perry (2005) studied conversations between 18 caregivers and spouses with mild or moderate AD (MMSE 12–27). Contrary to previous studies, caregivers asked open-ended questions as often as yes/no questions. Communication was more successful when the questions tapped into semantic memory than episodic memory, which is a result that is consistent with what we know about the nature of memory deficit in AD. There were many more episodic questions about recent information than about remote information. Small and Perry were surprised by this result, considering the recent memory impairment in AD, but the researchers defined *recent* as events "within the last few months" (p. 129) rather than just in the past few minutes or hours. The pattern of question asking did not differ according to the stages of AD assessed in this study.

A variety of assistance is available for families (Table 13.8). The **Safe Return Program,** administered by the Alzheimer's Association, assists individuals who are at risk for wandering from home and getting lost. It provides identification bracelets or pendants with an identification number and a hotline number. It also maintains a national database in case a loved one is missing. The database includes a photograph and contact information.

SUMMARY AND CONCLUSIONS

The main theme of this chapter is the study and treatment of progressive dementias, with a concentration on Alzheimer's disease. Included are stories about discovering the nature of this devastating disease and about developing drugs for improving memory. A great deal of research has focused on semantic memory, language comprehension, and word finding for naming and discourse. Cognitive rehabilitation contains a heavy dose of linguistic and communicative activity, and language is often used in compensatory strategies to support weakened memory systems. Speech-language pathologists provide training and support for caregivers who must cope with immense challenges that increase over time.

MATCHING REVIEW_____

Cognitive rehabilitation across chapters 11 and 13. Match a disorder category on the right with an item on the left.

_____ 1. hyperpriming

_____ 2. neglect dyslexia

_____ 3. expressive aprosodia

_____ 4. executive dysfunction

_____ 5. hippocampus

_____ 6. Skye McDonald

_____ 7. activation theories

_____ 8. MiniCog

_____ 9. Sohlberg and Mateer

_____ 10. Kathryn Bayles

_____ 11. Reality Orientation

_____ 12. spaced retrieval training (SRT)

_____ 13. external memory aids

_____ 14. memory wallets

_____ 15. vocational re-entry groups

a. right hemisphere dysfunction (RHD)

b. closed head injury (CHI)

c. dementia of Alzheimer's type (DAT)

d. two or more of the previous choices

REFERENCES

Adamovich, B. B., & Henderson, J. A. (1992). *Scales of Cognitive Ability for Traumatic Brain Injury* (SCATBI). Chicago: Riverside.

Adamovich, B. B., Henderson, J. A., & Auerback, S. (1985). *Cognitive rehabilitation of closed head injured patients: A dynamic approach.* Boston: Little, Brown.

Adamovich, B. L. B. (2005). Traumatic brain injury. In L. L. LaPointe (Ed.), *Aphasia and related neurogenic language disorders* (3rd ed., pp. 225–236). New York: Thieme.

Adams, M. L., Reich, A. R., & Flowers, C. R. (1989). Verbal-fluency characteristics of normal and aphasic speakers. *Journal of Speech and Hearing Research, 32,* 871–879.

Ahlsén, E., Nespoulous, J-L., Dordain, M., Stark, J., Jarema, G., et al. (1996). Noun phrase production by agrammatic patients: A cross-linguistic approach. *Aphasiology, 10,* 543–559.

Akmajian, A., Demers, R. A., Farmer, A. K., & Harnish, R. M. (2001). *Linguistics: An introduction to language and communication* (5th ed.). Cambridge, MA: MIT Press.

Albert, M. L. (1976). Short-term memory and aphasia. *Brain and Language, 3,* 28–33.

Albert, M. L., & Obler, L. K. (1978). *The bilingual brain.* New York: Academic Press.

Albert, M. L., Sparks, R., & Helm, N. A. (1973). Melodic intonation therapy. *Archives of Neurology, 29,* 130–131.

Alcock, K. J., Wade, D., Anslow, P., & Passingham, R. E. (2000). Pitch and timing abilities in adult left-hemisphere-dysphasic and right-hemisphere-damaged subjects. *Brain and Language, 75,* 47–65.

Alexander, M. P., Fischette, M. R., & Fischer, R. S. (1989). Crossed aphasias can be mirror image or anomalous: Case reports, review and hypothesis. *Brain, 112,* 953–973.

Alexander, M. P., Naeser, M. A., & Palumbo, C. L. (1987). Correlations of subcortical CT lesion sites and aphasia profiles. *Brain, 110,* 961–991.

Al-Khawaja, I., Wade, D. T., & Collin, C. F. (1996). Bedside screening for aphasia: A comparison of two methods. *Journal of Neurology, 243,* 201–204.

Altmann, L. J. P., Kempler, D., & Anderson, E. S. (2001). Speech errors in Alzheimer's disease: Reevaluating morphosyntactic preservation. *Journal of Speech, Language, and Hearing Research, 44,* 1069–1082.

American Psychiatric Association (1994). *Diagnostic and statistical manual of mental disorders* (4th ed.). Washington, DC: American Psychiatric Association.

Andersen, G. (1997). Post-stroke depression and pathological crying: Clinical aspects and new pharmacological approaches. *Aphasiology, 11,* 651–664.

Anderson, D. W., & McLauren, R. L. (Eds.). (1980). Report on the national head and spinal cord injury survey conducted by NINCDS. *Journal of Neurosurgery* (Suppl.) 1–43.

Anderson, J., Gilmore, R., Roper, S., Crosson, B., Bauer, M., et al. (1999). Conduction aphasia and the arcuate fasciculus: A reexamination of the Wernicke-Geschwind model. *Brain and Language, 70,* 1–12.

Anderson, J. R. (1983). *The architecture of cognition.* Cambridge, MA: Harvard University Press.

Andrewes, D. (2001). *Neuropsychology: From theory to practice.* Hove, UK: Psychology Press.

Ansaldo, A. I., Arguin, M., & Lecours, A. R. (2002). The contribution of the right cerebral hemisphere to the recovery from aphasia: A single longitudinal case study. *Brain and Language, 82,* 206–222.

Ansell, B. J., & Flowers, C. R. (1982). Aphasic adults' use of heuristic and structural linguistic cues for sentence analysis. *Brain and Language, 16,* 61–72.

Appell, J., Kertesz, A., & Fisman, M. (1982). A study of language functioning in Alzheimer patients. *Brain and Language, 17,* 73–91.

Arena, R., & Gainotti, G. (1978). Constructional apraxia and visuoperceptive disabilities in relation to laterality of cerebral lesions. *Cortex, 14,* 463–473.

Arguin, M., & Bub, D. (1993). Modulation of the directional attention deficit in visual neglect by hemispatial factors. *Brain and Cognition, 22,* 148–160.

Arguin, M., & Bub, D. (1997). Lexical constraints on reading accuracy in neglect dyslexia. *Cognitive Neuropsychology, 14,* 765–800.

Arkin, S. (2001). Alzheimer rehabilitation by students: Interventions and outcomes. *Neuropsychological Rehabilitation, 11,* 273–317.

Arkin, S., & Mahendra, N. (2001). Discourse analysis of Alzheimer's patients before and after intervention: Methodology and outcomes. *Aphasiology, 15,* 533–569.

Arrigoni, G., & DeRenzi, E. (1964). Constructional apraxia and hemispheric locus of lesion. *Cortex, 1,* 170–197.

Arvedson, J. C., McNeil, M. R., & West, T. L. (1985). Prediction of Revised Token Test overall, subtest, and linguistic unit scores by two shortened versions. In

R. H. Brookshire (Ed.), *Clinical aphasiology* (Vol. 15, pp. 57–63). Minneapolis: BRK.

Ashcraft, M. H. (1989). *Human memory and cognition.* Gleview, IL: Scott, Foresman.

Ashcraft, M. H. (1994). *Human memory and cognition* (2nd ed.). New York: HarperCollins.

Ashford J. W., Kumar, U., Barringer, M., Becker, M., Bice, J., et al. (1992). Assessing Alzheimer's severity with a global clinical scale. *International Psychogeriatrics, 4,* 55–74.

Astell, A. J., & Harley, T. A. (1996). Tip-of-the-tongue states and lexical access in dementia. *Brain and Language, 54,* 196–215.

Astell, A. J., & Harley, T. A. (1998). Naming problems in dementia: Semantic or lexical? *Aphasiology, 12,* 357–374.

Astell, A. J., & Harley, T. A. (2002). Accessing semantic knowledge in dementia: Evidence from a word definition task. *Brain and Language, 82,* 312–326.

Avent, J. R., Edwards, D. J., Franco, C. R., Lucero, C. J., & Pekowsky, J. I. (1995). A verbal and non-verbal treatment comparison study in aphasia. *Aphasiology, 9,* 295–303.

Bachy-Langedock, N., & de Partz, M-P. (1989). Coordination of two reorganization therapies in a deep dyslexic patient with oral naming disorders. In X. Seron & G. Deloche (Eds.), *Cognitive approaches in neuropsychological rehabilitation* (pp. 211–248). Hillsdale, NJ: Lawrence Erlbaum.

Baddeley, A. D. (1986). *Working memory.* London: Oxford University Press.

Baddeley, A. D. (1992). Implicit memory and errorless learning: A link between cognitive theory and neuropsychological rehabilitation? In L. R. Squire & N. Butters (Eds.), *Neuropsychology of memory* (2nd ed., pp. 309–314). New York: Guilford Press.

Baker, E., Blumstein, S. E., & Goodglass, H. (1981). Interaction between phonological and semantic factors in auditory comprehension. *Neuropsychologia, 19,* 1–15.

Ballard, C. (2000). Criteria for the diagnosis of dementia. In J. O'Brien, D. Ames, & A. Burns (Eds.). *Dementia* (2nd ed., pp. 29–40). London: Arnold.

Ballard, K. J., & Thompson, C. K. (1999). Treatment and generalization of complex sentence production in agrammatism. *Journal of Speech, Language, and Hearing Research, 42,* 690–707.

Bamber, L. (1980). *A retrospective study of language recovery in adult aphasics.* Unpublished thesis, Memphis State University.

Barlow, D. H., & Hersen, M. (1984). *Single case experimental designs: Strategies for studying behavior change* (2nd ed.). New York: Pergamon.

Barr, A., & Brandt, J. (1996). Word-list generation deficits in dementia. *Journal of Clinical and Experimental Neuropsychology, 18,* 810–822.

Barth, J. T., Broshek, D. K., & Freeman, J. R. (2006). Sports: A new frontier for neuropsychology. In R. J. Echemendía (Ed.), *Sports neuropsychology: Assessment and management of traumatic brain injury* (pp. 3–16). New York: Guilford Press.

Bartha, L., & Benke, T. (2003). Acute conduction aphasia: An analysis of 20 cases. *Brain and Language, 85,* 93–108.

Bartha, L., Mariën, P., Poewe, W., & Benke, T. (2004). Linguistic and neuropsychological deficits in crossed conduction aphasia. Report of three cases. *Brain and Language, 88,* 83–95.

Barton, M. I. (1971). Recall of generic properties of words in aphasic patients. *Cortex, 7,* 73–82.

Basso, A. (1992). Prognostic factors in aphasia. *Aphasiology, 6,* 337–348.

Basso, A. (1996). PALPA: An appreciation and a few criticisms. *Aphasiology, 10,* 190–193.

Basso, A. (2005). How intensive/prolonged should an intensive/prolonged treatment be? *Aphasiology, 19,* 975–984.

Basso, A., Capitani, E., & Moraschini, S. (1982). Sex differences in recovery from aphasia. *Cortex, 18,* 469–475.

Basso, A., Capitani, E., & Vignolo, L. A. (1979). Influence of rehabilitation on language skills in aphasic patients: A controlled study. *Archives of Neurology, 36,* 190–196.

Basso, A., Lecours, A. R., Moraschini, S., & Vanier, M. (1985). Anatomo-clinical correlations of aphasias as defined through computerized tomography: Exceptions. *Brain and Language, 26,* 201–229.

Basso, A., Razzano, C., Faglioni, P., & Zanobio, M. E. (1990). Confrontation naming, picture description and action naming in aphasic patients. *Aphasiology, 4,* 185–196.

Bastiaanse, R., Bosje, M., & Franssen, M. (1996). Deficit-oriented treatment of word-finding problems: Another replication. *Aphasiology, 10,* 363–383.

Bastiaanse, R., Edwards, S., & Kiss, K. (1996). Fluent aphasia in three languages: Aspects of spontaneous speech. *Aphasiology, 10,* 561–575.

Bastiaanse, R., & Jonkers, R. (1998). Verb retrieval in action naming and spontaneous speech in agrammatism and anomic aphasia. *Aphasiology, 12,* 951–969.

Bastiaanse, R., & Thompson, C. K. (2003). Verb and auxiliary movement in agrammatic Broca's aphasia. *Brain and Language, 84,* 286–305.

Bates, E. A., Chen, S., Tzeng, O., Li, P., & Opie, M. (1991). The noun-verb problem in Chinese aphasia. *Brain and Language, 41,* 203–233.

Bates, E. A., Friederici, A. D., & Wulfeck, B. B. (1987a). Comprehension in aphasia: A cross-linguistic study. *Brain and Language, 32,* 19–67.

Bates, E. A., Friederici, A. D., & Wulfeck, B. B. (1987b). Grammatical morphology in aphasia: Evidence from three languages. *Cortex, 23,* 545–574.

Bates, E. A., Friederici, A. D., Wulfeck, B. B., & Juarez, L. A. (1988). On the preservation of word order in aphasia: Cross-linguistic evidence. *Brain and Language, 33,* 323–364.

Bates, E. A., Harris, C., Marchman Wulfeck, B., & Kritchevsky, M. (1999). Production of complex syntax in normal ageing and Alzheimer's disease. *Language and Cognitive Processes, 10,* 487–539.

Bates, E. A., & Wulfeck, B. (1989). Comparative aphasiology: A cross-linguistic approach to language breakdown. *Aphasiology, 3,* 111–142.

Bauer, R. M., & Rubens, A. B. (1985). Agnosia. In K. M. Heilman & E. Valenstein (Eds.), *Clinical neuropsychology* (2nd ed., pp. 187–241). New York: Oxford University Press.

Baum, S. R. (1988). Syntactic processing in agrammatism: Evidence from lexical decision and grammaticality judgement tasks. *Aphasiology, 2,* 117–136.

Baum, S. R. (1989). On-line sensitivity to local and long-distance syntactic dependencies in Broca's aphasia. *Brain and Language, 37,* 327–338.

Baum, S. R. (1997). Phonological, semantic, and mediated priming in aphasia. *Brain and Language, 60,* 347–359.

Baum, S. R. (2001). Contextual influences on phonetic identification in aphasia: The effects of speaking rate and semantic bias. *Brain and Language, 76,* 266–281.

Baum, S. R., Daniloff, J., Daniloff, R., & Lewis, J. (1982). Sentence comprehension by Broca's aphasics: Effects on suprasegmental variables. *Brain and Language, 17,* 261–271.

Baum, S. R., & Dwivedi, V. D. (2003). Sensitivity to prosodic structure in left- and right-hemisphere-damaged individuals. *Brain and Language, 87,* 278–289.

Baum, S. R., & Pell, M. D. (1997). Production of affective and linguistic prosody by brain-damaged patients. *Aphasiology, 11,* 177–198.

Baum, S. R., & Pell, M. D. (1999). The neural bases of prosody: Insights from lesion studies and neuroimaging. *Aphasiology, 13,* 581–608.

Baumgaertner, A., & Tompkins, C. A. (2002). Testing contrasting accounts of word meaning activation in Broca's aphasia: Experiences from a cross-modal semantic priming study. *Aphasiology, 16,* 397–412.

Bayles, K. A., & Tomoeda, C. K. (1993). *The Arizona Battery for Communication Disorders of Dementia.* Tucson, AZ: Canyonlands.

Bayles, K. A., & Tomoeda, C. K. (1994). *The Functional Linguistic Communication Inventory.* Tucson, AZ: Canyonlands.

Bayles, K. A., Tomoeda, C. K., & Rein, J. A. (1996). Phrase repetition in Alzheimer's disease: Effect of meaning and length. *Brain and Language, 54,* 246–261.

Beatty, W. W., Salmon, D. P., Bernstein, N., & Butters, N. (1987). Remote memory in a patient with amnesia due to hypoxia. *Psychological Medicine, 17,* 657–665.

Beauchamp, T. L., & Childress, J. F. (1994). *Principles of biomedical ethics* (4th ed.). New York: Oxford University Press.

Becker, B. (1975). Intellectual changes after closed head injury. *Journal of Clinical Psychology, 31,* 307–309.

Beeman, M. (1993). Semantic processing in the right hemisphere may contribute to drawing inferences from discourse. *Brain and Language, 44,* 80–120.

Beeson, P. M., & Hillis, A. E. (2001). Comprehension and production of written words. In R. Chapey (Ed.), *Language intervention strategies in adult aphasia* (4th ed., pp. 572–595). Baltimore: Lippincott, Williams & Wilkins.

Beeson, P. M., Holland, A. L., & Murray, L. L. (1997). Naming famous people: An examination of tip-of-the-tongue phenomena in aphasia and Alzheimer's disease. *Aphasiology, 11,* 323–336.

Behrens, S. J. (1988). The role of the right hemisphere in the production of linguistic stress. *Brain and Language, 33,* 104–127.

Behrens, S. J. (1989). Characterizing sentence intonation in a right hemisphere-damaged population. *Brain and Language, 37,* 181–200.

Behrmann, M., & Byng, S. (1992). A cognitive approach to the neurorehabilitation of acquired language disorders. In D. I. Margolin (Ed.), *Cognitive neuropsychology in clinical practice* (pp. 327–350). New York: Oxford University Press.

Bell, E. E., Chenery, H. J., & Ingram, J. C. L. (2001). Semantic priming in Alzheimer's dementia: Evidence for dissociation of automatic and attentional processes. *Brain and Language, 76,* 130–144.

Bellaire, K. J., Georges, J. B., & Thompson, C. K. (1991). Establishing functional communication board use for nonverbal aphasic subjects. In T. E. Prescott (Ed.), *Clinical aphasiology* (Vol. 19, pp. 219–228). Austin, TX: Pro-Ed.

Ben-Yishay, Y. (Ed.). (1980). *Working approaches to remediation of cognitive deficits in brain damaged persons.* New York: New York University Medical Center.

Beretta, A., Piñango, M., Patterson, J., & Harford, C. (1999). Recruiting comparative crosslinguistic evidence to address competing accounts of agrammatic aphasia. *Brain and Language, 67,* 149–168.

Berger, P. E., & Mensh, S. (2002). *How to conquer the world with one hand . . . and an attitude.* Merrifield, VA: Positive Power.

Bergner, M., Bobitt, R. A., Carter, W. B., & Gilson, B. S. (1981). The Sickness Impact Profile: Development and final revision of a health status measure. *Medical Care, 19,* 787–805.

Berman, M., & Peelle, L. M. (1967). Self-generated cues: A method for aiding aphasic and apractic patients. *Journal of Speech and Hearing Disorders, 32,* 372–376.

Berndt, R. S., Haendiges, A. N., Mitchum, C. C., & Sandson, J. (1997). Verb retrieval in aphasia. 2. Relationship to sentence processing. *Brain and Language, 56,* 107–137.

Berndt, R. S., Haendiges, A. N., Mitchum, C. C., & Wayland, S. C. (1996). An investigation of nonlexical reading impairments. *Cognitive Neuropsychology, 13,* 763–802.

Berndt, R. S., Mitchum, C. C., & Haendiges, A. N. (1996). Comprehension of reversible sentences in "agrammatism": A meta-analysis. *Cognition, 58,* 289–308.

Berndt, R. S., Mitchum, C. C., Haendiges, A. N., & Sandson, J. (1997). Verb retrieval in aphasia. Characterizing single word impairments. *Brain and Language, 56,* 68–106.

Berndt, R. S., Mitchum, C. C., & Wayland, S. (1997). Patterns of sentence comprehension in aphasia: A consideration of three hypotheses. *Brain and Language, 60,* 197–221.

Berndt, R. S., Wayland, S., Rochon, E., Saffran, E., & Schwartz, M. (2000). *Quantitative production analysis: A training manual for the analysis of aphasic sentence production.* Hove, UK: Psychology Press.

Bernstein-Ellis, E., & Elman, R. J. (1999). Aphasia group communication treatment: The Aphasia Center of California approach. In R. J. Elman (Ed.), *Group treatment of neurogenic communication disorders: The expert clinician's approach* (pp. 47–56). Boston: Butterworth Heinemann.

Bernstein-Ellis, E., Wertz, R. T., Dronkers, N. F., & Milton, S. B. (1985). PICA performance by traumatically brain injured and left hemisphere CVA patients. In R. H. Brookshire (Ed.), *Clinical aphasiology* (Vol. 15, pp. 97–106). Minneapolis, MN: BRK.

Berthier, M. (1999). *Transcortical aphasias.* Hove, UK: Psychology Press.

Bickel, C., Pantel, J., Eysenbach, K., & Schröder, J. (2000). Syntactic comprehension deficits in Alzheimer's disease. *Brain and Language, 71,* 432–448.

Bihrle, A. M., Brownell, H. H., Powelson, J. A., & Gardner, H. (1986). Comprehension of humorous and nonhumorous materials by left and right brain damaged patients. *Brain and Cognition, 5,* 399–411.

Binder, L. M. (1993). Assessment of malingering after mild head trauma with the Portland Digit Recognition Test. *Journal of Clinical and Experimental Neuropsychology, 15,* 170–182.

Bird, H., Howard, D., & Franklin, S. (2000). Why is a verb like an inanimate object? Grammatical category and semantic category deficits. *Brain and Language, 72,* 246–309.

Bird, H., Howard, D., & Franklin, S. (2001). Noun-verb differences? A question of semantics: A response to Shapiro and Caramazza. *Brain and Language, 76,* 213–222.

Bisiach, E., Capitani, E., Luzzatti, C., & Perani, D. (1981). Brain and the conscious representation of outside reality. *Neuropsychologia, 19,* 543–551.

Bisiach, E., Vallar, G., Perani, D., Papagno, C., & Berti, A. (1986). Unawareness of disease following lesions of the right hemisphere: Anosognosia for hemiplegia and anosognosia for hemianopia. *Neuropsychologia, 24,* 471–482.

Black, F. W., & Strub, R. L. (1978). Digit repetition performance in patients with focal brain damage. *Cortex, 14,* 12–21.

Blacker, D., Albert, M. S., Bassett, S. S., Go, R. C., Harrell, L. E., et al. (1994). Reliability and validity of NINCDS-ADRDA criteria for Alzheimer's disease. The National Institute of Mental Health Genetics Initiative. *Archives of Neurology, 51,* 1198–1204.

Blessed, G., Tomlinson, B. E., & Roth, M. (1968). The association between quantitative measures of dementia and of senile change in the cerebral gray matter of elderly subjects. *British Journal of Psychiatry, 114,* 797–811.

Blomert, L., Kean, M-L., Koster, C., & Schokker, J. (1994). Amsterdam-Nijmegen Everyday Language Test: Construction, reliability and validity. *Aphasiology, 8,* 381–407.

Blomert, L., Koster, C., van Mier, H., & Kean, M-L. (1987). Verbal communication abilities of aphasic patients: The everyday language test. *Aphasiology, 1,* 463–474.

Blonder, L. X., Burns, A. F., Bowers, D., Moore, R. W., & Heilman, K. M. (1993). Right hemisphere facial expressivity during natural conversation. *Brain and Cognition, 21,* 44–56.

Bloom, M., & Fischer, J. (1982). *Evaluating practice: Guidelines for the accountable professional.* Englewood Cliffs, NJ: Prentice-Hall.

Bloom, R. L., Borod, J. C., Obler, L. K., & Gerstman, L. J. (1992). Impact of emotional content on discourse production in patients with unilateral brain damage. *Brain and Language, 42,* 153–164.

Bloom, R. L., Borod, J. C., Obler, L. K., & Gerstman, L. J. (1993). Suppression and facilitation of pragmatic performance: Effects of emotional content on discourse following right and left brain damage. *Journal of Speech and Hearing Research, 36,* 1227–1235.

Bloom, R. L., Borod, J. C., Obler, L. K., Santschi-Haywood, C., & Pick, L. (1995). An examination of coherence and cohesion in aphasia [abstract]. *Brain and Language, 51,* 206–209.

Blumstein, S. E. (1973). *A phonological investigation of aphasic speech.* The Hague, Netherlands: Mouton.

Blumstein, S. E., Burton, M., Baum, S., Waldstein, R., & Katz, D. (1994). The role of lexical status on the phonetic categorization of speech in aphasia. *Brain and Language, 46,* 181–197.

Blumstein, S. E., Byma, G., Kurowski, K., Hourihan, J., Brown, T., et al. (1998). On-line processing of filler-gap constructions in aphasia. *Brain and Language, 61,* 149–168.

Blumstein, S. E., Cooper, W. E., Goodglass, H., Statlender, S., & Gottlieb, J. (1980). Production deficits in aphasia: A voice-onset time analysis. *Brain and Language, 9,* 153–170.

Blumstein, S. E., Cooper, W. E., Zurif, E. B., & Caramazza, A. (1977). The perception and production of voice-onset time in aphasia. *Neuropsychologia, 15,* 371–383.

Blumstein, S. E., Katz, B., Goodglass, H., Shrier, R., & Dworetsky, B. (1985). The effects of slowed speech on auditory comprehension in aphasia. *Brain and Language, 24,* 246–265.

Blumstein, S. E., Milberg, W., Dworetzky, B., Rosen, A., & Gershberg, F. (1991). Syntactic priming effects in aphasia: An investigation of local syntactic dependencies. *Brain and Language, 40,* 393–421.

Blumstein, S. E., Milberg, W., & Shrier, R. (1982). Semantic processing in aphasia: Evidence from an auditory lexical decision task. *Brain and Language, 17,* 301–315.

Blumstein, S. E., Tartter, V. C., Nigro, G., & Statlender, S. (1984). Acoustic cues for the perception of place of articulation in aphasia. *Brain and Language, 22,* 128–149.

Boake, C., Millis, S. R., High, W. M., Jr., Delmonica, R. L., Kreutzer, J. S., et al. (2001). Using early neuropsychologic testing to predict long-term productivity outcome from traumatic brain injury. *Archives of Physical Medicine and Rehabilitation, 82,* 761–768.

Bock, K., & Levelt, W. (1994). Language production: Grammatical encoding. In M. A. Gernsbacher (Ed.), *Handbook of psycholinguistics* (pp. 945–984). San Diego, CA: Academic Press.

Body, R., & Parker, M. (1999). The use of multiple informants in assessment of communication after traumatic brain injury. In S. McDonald, L. Togher, & C. Code (Eds.), *Communication disorders following traumatic brain injury* (pp. 147–174). Hove, UK: Psychology Press.

Boles, L. (1997). A comparison of naming errors in individuals with mild naming impairment following poststroke aphasia, Alzheimer's disease, and traumatic brain injury. *Aphasiology, 11,* 1043–1056.

Boller, F., & Vignolo, L. A. (1966). Latent sensory aphasia in hemisphere-damaged patients: An experimental study with the Token Test. *Brain, 89,* 815–830.

Bonakdarpour, B., Eftekharzadeh, A., & Ashayeri, H. (2003). Melodic intonation therapy in Persian aphasic patients. *Aphasiology, 17,* 75–95.

Bond, M. R., & Brooks, D. N. (1976). Understanding the process of recovery as a basis for the investigation of rehabilitation for the brain injured. *Scandanavian Journal of Rehabilitation Medicine, 8,* 127–133.

Booth, S., & Perkins, L. (1999). The use of conversation analysis to guide individualized advice to carers and evaluate change in aphasia: A case study. *Aphasiology, 13,* 283–203.

Booth, S., & Swabey, D. (1999). Group training in communication skills for carers of adults with aphasia. *International Journal of Language and Communication Disorders, 34,* 291–309.

Borkowski, J. G., Benton, A. L., & Spreen, O. (1967). Word fluency and brain damage. *Neuropsychologia, 5,* 135–140.

Bornstein, R. A. (1988a). Entry into clinical neuropsychology: Graduate, undergraduate, and beyond. *Clinical Neuropsychologist, 2,* 213–220.

Bornstein, R. A. (1988b). Guidelines for continuing education in clinical neuropsychology. *Clinical Neuropsychologist, 2,* 25–29.

Borod, J. C., Andelman, F., Obler, L., Tweedy, J., & Welkowitz, J. (1992). Right hemisphere specialization for the identification of emotional words and sentences: Evidence from stroke patients. *Neuropsychologia, 30,* 827–844.

Borod, J. C., Carper, J. M., & Naeser, M. (1990). Long-term language recovery in left-handed aphasic patients. *Aphasiology, 4,* 561–572.

Borod, J. C., Fitzpatrick, P. M., Helm-Estabrooks, N., & Goodglass, H. (1989). The relationship between limb apraxia and the spontaneous use of communicative gesture in aphasia. *Brain and Cognition, 10,* 121–131.

Borod, J. C., Goodglass, H., & Kaplan, E. (1980). Normative data on the Boston Diagnostic Aphasia Examination, Parietal Lobe Battery, and the Boston Naming Test. *Journal of Clinical Neuropsychology, 2,* 209–215.

Borod, J. C., Koff, E., Perlman-Lorch, M., & Nicholas, M. (1986). The expression and perception of facial emotion in brain-damaged patients. *Neuropsychologia, 24,* 169–180.

Botez, M. I., Botez, T., & Aube, M. (1980). Amusia: Clinical and computerized scanning (CT) correlations. *Neurology, 30,* 359.

Bottenberg, D. E., & Lemme, M. L. (1991). Effect of shared and unshared listener knowledge on narratives of normal and aphasic adults. In T. E. Prescott (Ed.), *Clinical aphasiology* (Vol. 19, pp. 109–116). Austin, TX: Pro-Ed.

Bottenberg, D. E., Lemme, M. L., & Hedberg, N. L. (1987). Effect of story content on narrative discourse of aphasic adults. In R. H. Brookshire (Ed.), *Clinical aphasiology* (Vol. 17, pp. 202–209). Minneapolis, MN: BRK.

Bourgeois, M. (1992). Evaluating memory wallets in conversations with patients with dementia. *Journal of Speech and Hearing Research, 35,* 1344–1357.

Bourgeois, M., Camp, C., Rose, M., Blanche, W., Malone, M., et al. (2003). A comparison of training strategies to enhance use of external aids by persons with dementia. *Journal of Communication Disorders, 36,* 361–378.

Bourgeois, M., Schulz, R., Burgio, L., & Beach, S. (2002). Skills training for spouses of patients with Alzheimer's disease: Outcomes of an intervention study. *Journal of Clinical Geropsychology, 8,* 53–73.

Bourgeois, M. S. (2006). External aids. In D. K. Attix & K. A. Welsh-Bohmer (Eds.), Geriatric neuropsychology: Assessment and intervention (pp. 333–345). New York: Guilford Press.

Bowling, A. (2004). *Measuring health: A review of quality of life measurement scales* (3rd ed.). Berkshire, UK: Open University Press.

Boyle, M. (1989). Reducing phonemic paraphasias in the connected speech of a conduction aphasic subject. In T. E. Prescott (Ed.), *Clinical aphasiology* (Vol. 18, pp. 379–393). Boston: College-Hill/Little, Brown.

Boyle, M. (2004). Semantic feature analysis treatment for anomia in two fluent aphasia syndromes. *American Journal of Speech-Language Pathology, 13,* 236–249.

Boyle, M., & Coelho, C. A. (1995). Application of semantic feature analysis as a treatment for aphasic dysnomia. *American Journal of Speech-Language Pathology, 4*(4), 94–98.

Boyle, M., Coelho, C. A., & Kimbarow, M. L. (1991). Word fluency tasks: A preliminary analysis of variability. *Aphasiology, 5,* 171–182.

Bradley, D. C., Garrett, M. F., & Zurif, E. B. (1980). Syntactic deficits in Broca's aphasia. In D. Caplan (Ed.), *Biological studies of mental processes* (pp. 269–286). Cambridge, MA: MIT Press.

Brady, M., Mackenzie, C., & Armstrong, L. (2003). Topic use following right hemisphere brain damage during three semi-structured conversational discourse samples. *Aphasiology, 17,* 881–904.

Branchereau, L., & Nespoulous, J-L. (1989). Syntactic parsing and the availability of prepositions in agrammatic patients. *Aphasiology, 3,* 411–422.

Breedin, S. D., Saffran, E. M., & Schwartz, M. F. (1998). Semantic factors in verb retrieval: An effect of complexity. *Brain and Language, 63,* 1–31.

Breese, E. L., & Hillis, A. E. (2004). Auditory comprehension: Is muiltiple choice really good enough? *Brain and Language, 89,* 3–8.

Brennan, A. D., Worrall, L. E., & McKenna, K. T. (2005). The relationship between specific features of aphasia-friendly written material and comprehension of written material for people with aphasia: An exploratory study. *Aphasiology, 19,* 693–711.

Brenneise-Sarshad, R., Nicholas, L. E., & Brookshire, R. H. (1991). Effects of apparent listener knowledge and picture stimuli on aphasic and non-brain-damaged speakers' narrative discourse. *Journal of Speech and Hearing Research, 34,* 168–176.

Broca, P. (1960). Remarks on the seat of the faculty of articulate language, followed by an observation of aphemia. In G. von Bonin (Trans.), *Some papers on the cerebral cortex.* Springfield, IL: Charles C. Thomas.

Brodia, H. (1977). Language therapy effects in long term aphasia. *Archives of Physical Medicine and Rehabilitation, 58,* 248–253.

Brooks, N., Campsie, L., Symington, C., Beattie, A., & McKinlay, W. (1986). The five year outcome of severe blunt head injury: A relative's view. *Journal of Neurology, Neurosurgery, and Psychiatry, 49,* 764–770.

Brooks, N., McKinlay, W., Symington, C., Beattie, A., & Campsie, L. (1987). Return to work within the first seven years of severe head injury. *Brain Injury, 1,* 5–19.

Brookshire, R. H. (1967). Speech pathology and the experimental analysis of behavior. *Journal of Speech and Hearing Disorders, 32,* 215–227.

Brookshire, R. H. (1972). Effects of task difficulty on naming by aphasic subjects. *Journal of Speech and Hearing Research, 15,* 551–558.

Brookshire, R. H. (1983). Subject description and generality of results in experiments with aphasic adults. *Journal of Speech and Hearing Disorders, 48,* 342–346.

Brookshire, R. H. (1994). Group studies of treatment for adults with aphasia: Efficacy, effectiveness, and believability. *Special Interest Division 2 Newsletter, 4*(4), 5–14.

Brookshire, R. H. (1997). *Introduction to neurogenic communication disorders* (5th ed.). St. Louis, MO: Mosby.

Brookshire, R. H., & Nicholas, L. E. (1978). Effects of clinician request and feedback behavior on responses of aphasic individuals in speech and language treatment sessions. In R. H. Brookshire (Ed.), *Clinical aphasiology conference proceedings* (pp. 40–48). Minneapolis, MN: BRK.

Brookshire, R. H., & Nicholas, L. E. (1984). Consistency of effects of slow rate and pauses on aphasic listeners' comprehension of spoken sentences. *Journal of Speech and Hearing Research, 27,* 323–328.

Brookshire, R. H., & Nicholas, L. E. (1993). *The Discourse Comprehension Test.* Tucson, AZ: Communication Skill Builders.

Brookshire, R. H., & Nicholas, L. E. (1994). Speech sample size and test-retest stability of connected speech measures for adults with aphasia. *Journal of Speech and Hearing Research, 37,* 399–407.

Brookshire, R. H., Nicholas, L. E., Krueger, K. M., & Redmond, K. J. (1978). The clinical interaction analysis system: A system for observational recording of aphasia treatment. *Journal of Speech and Hearing Disorders, 43,* 437–447.

Brown, J. I., Bennett, J. M., & Hanna, G. (1981). *The Nelson-Denny reading test.* Chicago: Riverside.

Brown, J. R., & Schuell, H. M. (1950). A preliminary report of a diagnostic test for aphasia. *Journal of Speech and Hearing Disorders, 15,* 21–28.

Brownell, H. H. (1988). The neuropsychology of narrative comprehension. *Aphasiology, 2,* 247–250.

Brownell, H. H., Bihrle, A. M., & Michelow, D. (1986). Basic and subordinate level naming by agrammatic and fluent aphasic patients. *Brain and Language, 28,* 42–52.

Brownell, H. H., Griffin, R., Winner, E., Friedman, O., & Happé, F. (2000). Cerebral lateralization and theory of mind. In S. Baron-Cohen, H. Tager-Flusberg, & D. J. Cohen (Eds.), *Understanding other minds: Perspectives from autism and developmental cognitive neuroscience* (2nd ed., pp. 311–338). Oxford, UK: Oxford University Press.

Brownell, H. H., Michel, D., Powelson, J. A., & Gardner, H. (1983). Surprise but not coherence: Sensitivity to verbal humor in right hemisphere patients. *Brain and Language, 18,* 20–27.

Brownell, H. H., Pincus, D., Blum, A., Rehak, A., & Winner, E. (1997). The effects of right-hemisphere brain-damage on patients' use of terms of personal reference. *Brain and Language, 57,* 60–79.

Brownell, H. H., Potter, H. H., Bihrle, A. M., & Gardner, H. (1986). Inference deficits in right brain-damaged patients. *Brain and Language, 27,* 310–321.

Brownell, H. H., Potter, H. H., Michelow, D., & Gardner, H. (1984). Sensitivity to lexical denotation and connotation in brain-damaged patients: A double dissociation? *Brain and Language, 22,* 253–265.

Brownell, H. H., Simpson, T. L., Bihrle, A. M., Potter, H. H., & Gardner, H. (1990). Appreciation of metaphoric alternative word meanings by left and right brain-damaged patients. *Neuropsychologia, 28,* 375–383.

Bruce, C., & Howard, D. (1988). Why don't Broca's aphasics cue themselves? An investigation of phonemic cueing and tip of the tongue information. *Neuropsychologia, 26,* 253–264.

Brumfitt, S. (1993). Losing your sense of self: What aphasia can do. *Aphasiology, 7,* 569–574.

Brush, J. A., & Camp, C. J. (1998). Using spaced retrieval as an intervention during speech-language therapy. *Clinical Gerontologist, 19,* 51–64.

Bryan, K. L. (1989). Language prosody and the right hemisphere. *Aphasiology, 3*(4), 285–300.

Bryan, K. L. (1995). *The Right Hemisphere Language Battery* (2nd ed.). London: Whurr.

Buchanan, L., McEwen, S., Westbury, C., & Libben, G. (2003). Semantics and semantic errors: Implicit access to semantic information from words and nonwords in deep dyslexia. *Brain and Language, 84,* 65–83.

Buck, R., & Duffy, R. J. (1980). Nonverbal communication of affect in brain-damaged patients. *Cortex, 16,* 351–362.

Buckingham, H. W. (1981). Where do neologisms come from? In J. W. Brown (Ed.), *Jargonaphasia* (pp. 39–62). New York: Academic Press.

Buckingham, H. W. (1987). Phonemic paraphasias and psycholinguistic production models for neologistic jargon. *Aphasiology, 1,* 381–401.

Buckingham, H. W. (1989). Mechanisms underlying aphasic transformations. In A. Ardila & P. Ostrosky-Solis (Eds.), *Brain organization of language and cognitive processes* (pp. 123–145). New York: Plenum.

Buckingham, H. W., & Kertesz, A. (1976). *Neologistic jargon aphasia.* Amsterdam: Swets and Zeitlinger.

Buckingham, H. W., & Rekart, D. M. (1979). Semantic paraphasia. *Journal of Communication Disorders, 12,* 197–209.

Burchert, F., De Bleser, R., & Sonntag, K. (2003). Does morphology make the difference? Agrammatic sentence comprehension in German. *Brain and Language, 87,* 323–342.

Burchert, F., Swoboda-Moll, M., & De Bleser, R. (2005). Tense and agreement dissociations in German agrammatic speakers: Underspecification vs. hierarchy. *Brain and Language, 94,* 188–199.

Burke, H. L., Yeo, R. A., Delaney, H. D., & Conner, L. (1993). CT scan cerebral hemispheric asymmetries: Predictors of recovery from aphasia. *Journal of Clinical and Experimental Neuropsychology, 15,* 191–204.

Burkhardt, P., Piñango, M. M., & Wong, K. (2003). The role of the anterior left hemisphere in real-time sentence comprehension: Evidence from split intransivity. *Brain and Language, 86,* 9–22.

Busch, C. (1999). Group treatment reimbursement issues. In R. J. Elman (Ed.), *Group treatment of neurogenic communication disorders: The expert clinician's approach* (pp. 31–34). Boston: Butterworth Heinemann.

Busch, C. R. (1993). Functional outcome: Reimbursement issues. In M. L. Lemme (Ed.), *Clinical aphasiology* (Vol. 21, pp. 73–85). Austin, TX: Pro-Ed.

Busch, C. R., Brookshire, R. H., & Nicholas, L. E. (1988). Referential communication by aphasic and nonaphasic adults. *Journal of Speech and Hearing Disorders, 53,* 475–482.

Butfield, E., & Zangwill, O. L. (1946). Reeducation in aphasia: A review of 70 cases. *Journal of Neurology, Neurosurgery, and Psychiatry, 9,* 75–79.

Butler-Hinz, S., Caplan, D., & Waters, G. (1990). Characteristics of syntactic and semantic comprehension deficits following closed head injury versus left cerebrovascular accident. *Journal of Speech and Hearing Research, 33,* 269–280.

Byng, S. (1988). Sentence processing deficits: Theory and therapy. *Cognitive Neuropsychology, 5,* 629–676.

Byng, S., & Black, M. (1989). Some aspects of sentence production in aphasia. *Aphasiology, 3,* 241–263.

Byng, S., Kay, J., Edmundson, A., & Scott, C. (1990). Aphasia tests reconsidered. *Aphasiology, 4,* 67–92.

Byng, S., Nickels, L., & Black, M. (1994). Replicating therapy for mapping deficits in agrammatism: Remapping the deficit? *Aphasiology, 8,* 315–341.

Calvin, W. H., & Ojemann, G. A. (1980). *Inside the brain.* New York: Mentor.

Camp, C. J. (2006). Spaced retrieval: A model for dissemination of a cognitive intervention for persons with dementia. In D. K. Attix & K. A. Welsh-Bohmer (Eds.), *Geriatric neuropsychology: Assessment and intervention* (pp. 275–292). New York: Guilford Press.

Canter, G. J. (1988). Apraxia of speech and phonemic paraphasia. *Aphasiology, 2,* 251–254.

Canter, G. J., Trost, J. E., Burns, M. S. (1985). Contrasting speech patterns in apraxia of speech and phonemic paraphasia. *Brain and Language, 24,* 204–222.

Cao, Y., Vikingstad, E., George, K., Johnson, A., & Welch, K. (1999). Cortical language activation in stroke patients recovering from aphasia with functional MRI. *Stroke, 30,* 2331–2340.

Capitani, E., Laiacona, M., Mahon, B., & Caramazza, A. (2003). What are the facts of semantic category-specific deficits? *Cognitive Neuropsychology, 20,* 213–262.

Caplan, D. (1985). Syntactic and semantic structures in agrammatism. In M-L. Kean (Ed.), *Agrammatism* (pp. 125–151). Orlando, FL: Academic Press.

Caplan, D. (1987). *Neurolinguistics and linguistic aphasiology: An introduction.* Cambridge, UK: Cambridge University Press.

Caplan, D. (1991). Agrammatism is a theoretically coherent aphasic category. *Brain and Language, 40,* 274–281.

Caplan, D. (2002). The neural basis of syntactic processing: A critical look. In A. E. Hillis (Ed.), *The handbook of adult language disorders* (pp. 331–350). New York: Psychology Press.

Caplan, D., Baker, C., & Dehaut, F. (1985). Syntactic determinants of sentence comprehension in aphasia. *Cognition, 21,* 117–175.

Caplan, D., & Futter, C. (1986). Assignment of thematic roles to nouns in sentence comprehension by an agrammatic patient. *Brain and Language, 27,* 117–134.

Caplan, D., & Hildebrandt, N. (1988). Specific deficits in syntactic comprehension. *Aphasiology, 2,* 255–258.

Caplan, D., Matthei, E., & Gigley, H. (1981). Comprehension of gerundive constructions in Broca's aphasia. *Brain and Language, 13,* 145–160.

Caplan, D., & Waters, G. (2003). On-line syntactic processing in aphasia: Studies with auditory moving window presentation. *Brain and Language, 84,* 222–249.

Caplan, D., & Waters, G. S. (1995). Aphasic disorders of syntactic comprehension and working memory capacity. *Cognitive Neuropsychology, 12,* 637–650.

Caplan, D., & Waters, G. S. (1996). Syntactic processing in sentence comprehension under dual-task conditions in aphasic patients. *Language and Cognitive Processes, 11,* 525–551.

Caplan, D., Waters, G. S., & Hildebrandt, N. (1997). Determinants of sentence comprehension in aphasic patients in sentence-picture matching tasks. *Journal of Speech, Language, and Hearing Research, 40,* 542–555.

Cappa, S. F., Cavallotti, G., & Vignolo, L. (1981). Phonemic and lexical errors in fluent aphasia: Correlation with lesion site. *Neuropsychologia, 19,* 171–177.

Cappa, S. F., Papagno, C., & Vallar, G. (1990). Language and verbal memory after right hemispheric stroke: A clinical-CT scan study. *Neuropsychologia, 28,* 503–509.

Cappa, S. F., Perani, D., Grassi, F., Bressi, S., Alberoni, M., et al. (1997). A PET follow-up study of recovery after stroke in acute aphasics. *Brain and Language, 56,* 55–67.

Caramazza, A. (1989). Cognitive neuropsychology and rehabilitation: An unfulfilled promise? In X. Seron & G. Deloche (Eds.), *Cognitive approaches in neuropsychological rehabilitation* (pp. 383–398). Hillsdale, NJ: Lawrence Erlbaum.

Caramazza, A., & Badecker, W. (1991). Clinical syndromes are not God's gift to cognitive neuropsychology: A reply to a rebuttal to an answer to a response to the case against syndrome-based research. *Brain and Cognition, 16,* 211–227.

Caramazza, A., Basili, A., Koller, J. J., & Berndt, R. S. (1981). A investigation of repetition and language processing in a case of conduction aphasia. *Brain and Language, 14,* 235–271.

Caramazza, A., & Berndt, R. D. (1985). A multicomponential deficit view of agrammatic Broca's aphasia. In M-L. Kean (Ed.), *Agrammatism* (pp. 27–63). Orlando, FL: Academic Press.

Caramazza, A., & Berndt, R. S. (1978). Semantic and syntactic processes in aphasia: A review of the literature. *Psychological Bulletin, 85,* 898–918.

Caramazza, A., Capasso, R., Capitani, E., & Miceli, G. (2005). Patterns of comprehension performance in agrammatic Broca's aphasia: A test of the Trace Deletion Hypothesis. *Brain and Language, 94,* 43–53.

Caramazza, A., Capitani, E., Rey, A., & Berndt, R. S. (2001). Agrammatic Broca's aphasia is not associated with a single pattern of comprehension performance. *Brain and Language, 76,* 158–184

Caramazza, A., Papagno, C., & Ruml, W. (2000). The selective impairment of phonological processing in speech production. *Brain and Language, 75,* 428–450.

Caramazza, A., & Zurif, E. B. (1976). Dissociation of alogorithmic and heuristic processes in language comprehension: Evidence from aphasia. *Brain and Language, 3,* 572–582.

Carlesimo, G. A., Fadda, L., & Caltagirone, C. (1993). Basic mechanisms of constructional apraxia in unilateral brain-damaged patients: Role of visuoperceptual and executive disorders. *Journal of Clinical and Experimental Neuropsychology, 15,* 342–358.

Carlomagno, S., Losanno, N., Emanuelli, S., & Casadio, P. (1991). Expressive language recovery or improved communicative skills: Effects of P. A. C. E. therapy on aphasics' referential communication and story retelling. *Aphasiology, 5,* 419–424.

Carlomagno, S., Pandolfi, M., Labruna, L., Colombo, A., & Razzano, C. (2001). Recovery from moderate aphasia in the first year post-stroke: Effect of type of therapy. *Archives of Physical Medicine and Rehabilitation, 82,* 1073–1080.

Carney, N., Chestnut, R. M., Maynard, H., Mann, N. C., Patterson, P., et al. (1999). Effect of cognitive rehabilitation on outcomes for persons with traumatic brain injury. *Journal of Head Trauma Rehabilitation, 14,* 277–307.

Carpenter, R. L., & Rutherford, D. R. (1973). Acoustic cue discrimination in adult aphasia. *Journal of Speech and Hearing Research, 16,* 534–544.

Caza, N., & Moscovitch, M. (2005). Effects of cumulative frequency, but not of frequency trajectory, in lexical decision times of older adults and patients with Alzheimer's disease. *Journal of Memory and Language, 53,* 456–471.

Center for Outcome Measurement in Brain Injury. (n.d.) *Introduction to the MAST.* Retrieved September 20, 2005, from www.tbims.org.

Cermak, L. S., & Moreines, J. (1976). Verbal retention deficits in aphasic and amnesic patients. *Brain and Language, 3,* 16–27.

Chamberlain, M. A., Neumann, V., & Tennant, A. (Eds.). (1995). *Traumatic brain injury rehabilitation: Services, treatments and outcomes.* London: Chapman & Hall Medical.

Channon, S., Pellijeff, A., & Rule, A. (2005). Social cognition after head injury: Sarcasm and theory of mind. *Brain and Language, 93,* 123–134.

Chapey, R. (Ed.). (2001). *Language intervention strategies in adult aphasia and related neurogenic communication disorders* (4th ed.). Philadelphia: Lippincott Williams & Wilkins.

Chapey, R., Rigrodsky, S., & Morrison, E. B. (1977). Aphasia: A divergent semantic interpretation. *Journal of Speech and Hearing Disorders, 42,* 287–295.

Chapman, S. B., & Ulatowska, H. K. (1989). Discourse in aphasia: Integration deficits in processing reference. *Brain and Language, 36,* 651–668.

Chapman, S. B., Weiner, M. F., Rackley, A., Hynan, L. S., & Zientz, J. (2004). Effects of cognitive-communication stimulation for Alzheimer's disease patients treated with Donepezil. *Journal of Speech, Language, and Hearing Research, 47,* 1149–1163.

Chenery, H. J., Ingram, J. C. L., & Murdoch, B. B. (1990). Automatic and volitional semantic processing in aphasia. *Brain and Language, 38,* 215–232.

Cherney, L. R., & Halper, A. S. (1999). Group treatment for patients with right hemisphere damage. In R. J. Elman (Ed.), *Group treatment of neurogenic communication disorders: The expert clinician's approach* (pp. 121–137). Boston: Butterworth Heinemann.

Cherney, L. R., Halper, A. S., Kwasnica, C. M., Harvey, R. L., & Zhang, M. (2001). Recovery of functional status after right hemisphere stroke: Relationship with unilateral neglect. *Archives of Physical Medicine and Rehabilitation, 82,* 322–328.

Chertkow, H., Bub, D., Deaudon, C., & Whitehead, V. (1997). On the status of object concepts in aphasia. *Brain and Language, 58,* 203–232.

Chialant, D., Costa, A., & Caramazza, A. (2002). Models of naming. In A. E. Hillis (Ed.), *The handbook of adult language disorders: Integrating cognitive neuropsychology, neurology, and rehabilitation* (pp. 123–142). New York: Psychology Press.

Christiansen, J. A. (1995a). Coherence violations and propositional usage in the narratives of fluent aphasics. *Brain and Language, 51,* 291–317.

Christiansen, J. A. (1995b). Getting to the point: Relevance in story production and comprehension by aphasic patients [abstract]. *Brain and Language, 51,* 201–204.

Chusid, J. G. (1979). *Correlative neuroanatomy and functional neurology* (17th ed.). Los Altos, CA: Lange Medical Publications.

Cicerone, K. D., & Giacino, J. T. (1992). Remediation of executive function deficits after traumatic brain injury. *Neuropsychological Rehabilitation, 2,* 12–22.

Cicone, M., Wapner, W., & Gardner, H. (1980). Sensitivity to emotional expressions and situations in organic patients. *Cortex, 16,* 145–158.

Cimino-Knight, A. M., Hollingsworth, A. L., & Gonzalez Rothi, L. J. (2005). The transcortical aphasias. In L. L. LaPointe (Ed.), *Aphasia and related neurogenic language disorders* (3rd ed., pp. 169–185). New York: Thieme.

Clare, L., Wilson, B. A., Carter, G., Hodges, J. R., & Adams, M. (2001). Long-term maintenance of treatment gains following a cognitive rehabilitation intervention in early dementia of Alzheimer type: A single case study. *Neuropsychological Rehabilitation, 11,* 477–494.

Clark, A. E., & Flowers, C. R. (1987). The effect of semantic redundancy on auditory comprehension in aphasia. In R. H. Brookshire (Ed.), *Clinical aphasiology* (Vol. 17, pp. 174–179). Minneapolis: BRK.

Clark, C. M., & Ryan, L. (1993). Implications of statistical tests of variance and means. *Journal of Clinical and Experimental Neuropsychology, 15,* 619–622.

Clark, L. W., & Witte, K. (1995). Nature and efficacy of communication management in Alzheimer's disease. In R. Lubinski (Ed.), *Dementia and communication* (pp. 238–256). San Diego, CA: Singular.

Code, C. (2004). Ten years of PALPAring in aphasia. *Aphasiology, 18,* 75–76.

Code, C., & Müller, D. J. (1992). *The Code Müller Protocols: Assessing perceptions of psychosocial adjustment to aphasia and related disorders.* London: Whurr.

Coelho, C. A. (1990). Acquisition and generalization of simple manual sign grammars by aphasic subjects. *Journal of Communication Disorders, 23,* 383–400.

Coelho, C. A. (1991). Manual sign acquisition and use in two aphasic subjects. In T. E. Prescott (Ed.), *Clinical aphasiology* (Vol. 19, pp. 209–218). Austin, TX: Pro-Ed.

Coelho, C. A. (2002). Story narratives of adults with closed head injury and non-brain-injured adults: Influence of socioeconomic status, elicitation task, and executive functioning. *Journal of Speech, Language, and Hearing Research, 45,* 1232–1248.

Coelho, C. A., DeRuyter, F., & Stein, M. (1996). Treatment efficacy: Cognitive-communicative disorders resulting from traumatic brain injury in adults. *Journal of Speech and Hearing Research, 39,* S5–S17.

Coelho, C. A., & Duffy, R. J. (1987). The relationship of the acquisition of manual signs to severity of aphasia: A training study. *Brain and Language, 31,* 328–345.

Coelho, C. A., & Duffy, R. J. (1990). Sign acquisition in two aphasic subjects with limb apraxia. *Aphasiology, 4,* 1–8.

Coelho, C. A., Liles, B. Z., & Duffy, R. J. (1991). Discourse analyses with closed head injured adults: Evidence for differing patterns of deficits. *Archives of Physical Medicine and Rehabilitation, 72,* 465–468.

Coelho, C. A., Liles, B. Z., Duffy, R. J., & Clarkson, J. V. (1993). Conversational patterns of aphasic, closed-head-injured, and normal speakers. In M. L. Lemme (Ed.), *Clinical aphasiology* (Vol. 21, pp. 183–192). Austin, TX: Pro-Ed.

Coelho, C. A., McHugh, R. E., & Boyle, M. (2000). Semantic feature analysis as a treatment for aphasic dysnomia: A replication. *Aphasiology, 14,* 133–142.

Coelho, C. A., Youse, K. M., & Le, K. N. (2002). Conversational discourse in closed-head-injured and non-brain-injured adults. *Aphasiology, 16,* 659–671.

Cohen, R. Kelter, S. & Woll, G. (1980). Analytical competence and language impairment in aphasia. *Brain and Language, 10,* 331–347.

Cole-Virtue, J., & Nickels, L. (2004). Spoken word to picture matching from PALPA: A critique and some new matched sets. *Aphasiology, 18,* 77–101.

Collie, A., Maruff, P., Darby, D., Makdissi, M., McCrory, P., et al. (2006). CogSport. In R. J. Echemendía (Ed.), *Sports neuropsychology: Assessment and management of traumatic brain injury* (pp. 240–262). New York: Guilford Press.

Collins, M. (2005). Global aphasia. In L. L. LaPointe (Ed.), *Aphasia and related neurogenic language disorders* (3rd ed., pp. 186–198). New York: Thieme.

Collins, M. J. (1986). *Diagnosis and treatment of global aphasia.* San Diego: Singular.

Collins, M. J., McNeil, M. R., Lentz, S., Shubitowski, Y., & Rosenbek, J. C. (1984). Word fluency and aphasia: Some linguistic and not-so-linguistic considerations. In R. H. Brookshire (Ed.), *Clinical aphasiology conference proceedings* (pp. 78–84). Minneapolis, MN: BRK.

Conner, L. T., Obler, L. K., Tocco, M., Fitzpatrick, P. M., & Albert, M. L. (2001). Effect of socioeconomic status on aphasia severity and recovery. *Brain and Language, 78,* 254–257.

Cook, L., Smith, D. S., & Truman, G. (1994). Using Functional Independence Measure profiles as an index of outcome in the rehabilitation of brain-injured patients. *Archives of Physical Medicine and Rehabilitation, 75,* 390–393.

Cooper, P. R. (Ed.). (1982). *Head injury.* Baltimore: Williams & Wilkins.

Cooper, W. E., Soares, C., Nicol, J., Michelow, D., & Goloskie, S. (1984). Clausal intonation after unilateral brain damage. *Language and Speech, 27,* 17–24.

Copland, D. A., Chenery, H. J., & Murdoch, B. E. (2002). Hemispheric contributions to lexical ambiguity resolution: Evidence from individuals with complex language impairment following left-hemisphere lesions. *Brain and Language, 81,* 131–143.

Coppens, P., Hungerford, S., Yamaguchi, S., & Yamadori, A. (2002). Crossed aphasia: An analysis of the symptoms, their frequency, and a comparison with left-hemisphere aphasia symptomatology. *Brain and Language, 83,* 425–463.

Corina, D., Kritchevsky, M., & Bellugi, U. (1996). Visual language processing and unilateral neglect: Evidence from American Sign Language. *Cognitive Neuropsychology, 13,* 321–356.

Corina, D. P. (1999). On the nature of left hemisphere specialization for signed language. *Brain and Language, 69,* 230–240.

Cornett, B. S. (2001). Service delivery issues in health care settings. In R. Lubinski & C. M. Frattali (Eds.), *Professional issues in speech-language pathology and audiology* (2nd ed., pp. 229–250). San Diego, CA: Singular.

Craig, H. K., Hinckley, J. J., Winkelseth, M., Carry, L., Walley, J., Bardach, L., Higman, B., Hilfinger, P., Schall, C., & Sheimo, D. (1993). Quantifying connected speech samples of adults with chronic aphasia. *Aphasiology, 7,* 155–164.

Crary, M. A., Haak, N. J., & Malinsky, A. E. (1989). Preliminary psychometric evaluation of an acute aphasia screening protocol. *Aphasiology, 3,* 611–618.

Crary, M. A., & Rothi, L. J. G. (1989). Predicting the Western Aphasia Battery aphasia quotient. *Journal of Speech and Hearing Disorders, 54,* 163–166.

Crary, M. A., Wertz, R. T., & Deal, J. L. (1992). Classifying aphasias: Cluster analysis of Western Aphasia Battery and Boston Diagnostic Aphasia Examination results. *Aphasiology, 6,* 29–36.

Crawford, J. R., Allan, K. M., Stephen, D. W., Parker, D. M., & Besson, J. A. O. (1989). The Wechsler Adult Intelligence Scale–Revised (WAIS-R): Factor structure in a UK sample. *Personality and Individual Differences, 10,* 1209–1212.

Crawford, J. R., Johnson, D. A., Mychalkiw, B., & Moore, J. W. (1997). WAIS-R performance following closed-head injury: A comparison of the clinical utility of summary IQs, factor scores, and subtest scatter indices. *Clinical Neuropsychologist, 11,* 345–355.

Crawford, J. R., Parker, D. M., Stewart, L. E., Besson, J. A. O., & DeLacey, E. (1989). Prediction of WAIS IQ with the National Adult Reading Test: Cross-validation and extension. *British Journal of Clinical Psychology, 28,* 267–273.

Crepeau, F., & Scherzer, P. (1993). Predictors and indicators of work status after traumatic brain injury: A meta-analysis. *Neuropsychological Rehabilitation, 3,* 5–35.

Crimmins, C. (2000). *Where is the Mango Princess?* New York: Vintage Books.

Cripe, L. I. (1987). The neuropsychological assessment and management of closed head injury: General guidelines. *Cognitive Rehabilitation, 5,* 18–22.

Critchley, M. (1960). Jacksonian ideas and the future, with special reference to aphasia. *British Medical Journal, 6,* 6–11.

Croisile, B., Ska, B., Brabant, M. J., Duchene, A., Lepage, Y., Aimard, G., et al. (1996). Comparative study of oral and written picture description in patients with Alzheimer's disease. *Brain and Language, 53,* 1–19.

Croot, K., Patterson, K., & Hodges, J. R. (1998). Single word production in nonfluent progressive aphasia. *Brain and Language, 61,* 226–273.

Crossley, M., D'Arcy, C., & Rawson, N. (1997). Letter and category fluency in community-dwelling Canadian seniors: A comparison of normal participants to those with dementia of the Alzheimer or Vascular type. *Journal of Clinical and Experimental Neuropsychology, 19,* 52–62.

Crosson, M., Moberg, P. J., Boone, J. R., Rothi, L. G., & Raymer, A. (1997). Category-specific naming deficit for medical terms after dominant thalamic/capsular hemorrhage. *Brain and Language, 60,* 407–442.

Croteau, C., Vychytil, A-M., Larfeuil, C., & Le Dorze, G. (2004). "Speaking for" behaviours in spouses of people with aphasia: A descriptive study of six couples in an interview situation. *Aphasiology, 18,* 291–311.

Crowe, S. F. (1992). Dissociation of two frontal lobe syndromes by a test of verbal fluency. *Journal of Clinical and Experimental Neuropsychology, 14,* 327–339.

Cruice, M., Worrall, L., Hickson, L., & Murison, R. (2003). Finding a focus for quality of life with aphasia: Social and emotional health, and psychological well-being. *Aphasiology, 17,* 333–353.

Cruice, M., Worrall, L., Hickson, L., & Murison, R. (2005). Measuring quality of life: Comparing family members' and friends' ratings with those of their aphasic partners. *Aphasiology, 19,* 111–129.

Cubelli, R., & Beschin, N. (2005). The processing of the right-sided accent mark in left neglect dyslexia. *Brain and Language, 95,* 319–326.

Cubelli, R., Foresti, A., & Consolini, T. (1988). Reeducation strategies in conduction aphasia. *Journal of Communication Disorders, 21,* 239–249.

Cuetos, F., Gonzalez-Nosti, M., & Martinez, C. (2005). The picture-naming task in the analysis of cognitive deterioration in Alzheimer's disease. *Aphasiology, 19,* 545–557.

Cullum, C. M., & Bigler, E. D. (1986). Ventricle size, cortical atrophy and the relationship with neuropsychological status in closed-head injury: A quantitative analysis. *Journal of Clinical and Experimental Neuropsychology, 8,* 437–452.

Cunningham, R., & Ward, C. (2003). Evaluation of a training program to facilitate conversation between people with aphasia and their partners. *Aphasiology, 17,* 687–707.

Curran, J. P. (1982). A procedure for the assessment of social skills: The Simulated Social Interaction Test. In J. P. Curran & P. M. Monti (Eds.), *Social skills training: A practical handbook for assessment and treatment* (pp. 348–373). New York: Guilford.

Curtiss, S., Jackson, C. A., Kempler, D., Hanson, W. R., & Metter, E. H. (1986). Length vs. structural complexity in sentence comprehension in aphasia. In R. H. Brookshire (Ed.), *Clinical aphasiology* (Vol. 16, pp. 45–55). Minneapolis: BRW.

Cutting, L. (1978). Study of anosognosia. *Journal of Neurology, Neurosurgery, and Psychiatry, 41,* 548–555.

Cyr-Stafford, C. (1993). The dynamics of speech therapy in aphasia. In D. Lafond, Y. Joanette, J. Ponzio, R. Degiovani, & M. T. Sarno (Eds.), *Living with aphasia: Psychosocial issues* (pp. 103–116). San Diego, CA: Singular.

Dahlberg, C. C., & Jaffe, J. (1977). *Stroke: A doctor's personal story of his recovery.* New York: Norton.

Damasio, H. (2001). Neural basis of language disorders. In R. Chapey (Ed.), *Language intervention strategies in adult aphasia and related neurogenic communication disorders* (4th ed., pp. 18–36). Philadelphia: Lippincott Williams & Wilkins.

Damasio, H. D., & Damasio, A. R. (1980). The anatomical basis of conduction aphasia. *Brain, 103,* 337–350.

Damico, J. S., & Simmons-Mackie, N. N. (2003). Qualitative research and speech-language pathology: A tutorial for the clinical realm. *American Journal of Speech-Language Pathology, 12,* 131–143.

Daniloff, J. K., Fritelli, G., Buckingham, H. W., Hoffman, P. R., & Daniloff, R. G. (1986). Amer-Ind versus ASL: Recognition and imitation in aphasic subjects. *Brain and Language, 28,* 95–113.

Daniloff, J. K., Lloyd, L., & Fristoe, M. (1983). Amer-Ind transparency. *Journal of Speech and Hearing Disorders, 48,* 103–110.

Daniloff, J. K., Noll, J. D., Fristoe, M., & Lloyd, L. L. (1982). Gesture recognition in patients with aphasia. *Journal of Speech and Hearing Disorders, 47,* 43–49.

Darley, F. L. (1982). *Aphasia.* Philadelphia: W. B. Saunders.

Dash, P., & Villemarette-Pittman, N. (2005). *Alzheimer's disease.* New York: American Academy of Neurology Press.

Davidson, B., Worrall, L., & Hickson, L. (2003). Identifying the communication activities of older people with aphasia: Evidence from naturalistic observation. *Aphasiology, 17,* 243–264.

Davis, G. A. (1973). Linguistics and language therapy: The sentence construction board. *Journal of Speech and Hearing Disorders, 38,* 205–214.

Davis, G. A. (1983). *A survey of adult aphasia.* Englewood Cliffs, NJ: Prentice-Hall.

Davis, G. A. (2000). *Aphasiology: Disorders and clinical practice.* Boston: Allyn & Bacon.

Davis, G. A. (2005). PACE revisited. *Aphasiology, 19,* 21–38.

Davis, G. A., & Coelho, C. A. (2004). Referential cohesion and logical coherence of narration after closed head injury. *Brain and Language, 89,* 508–523.

Davis, G. A., & Holland, A. L. (1981). Age in understanding and treating aphasia. In D. S. Beasley & G. A. Davis (Eds.), *Aging: Communication processes and disorders* (pp. 207–228). New York: Grune & Stratton.

Davis, G. A., O'Neil-Pirozzi, T. M., & Coon, M. (1997). Referential cohesion and logical coherence of narration after right hemisphere stroke. *Brain and Language, 56,* 183–210.

Davis, G. A., & Wilcox, M. J. (1985). *Adult aphasia rehabilitation: Applied pragmatics.* San Diego: Singular.

Davis, K. L., Price, C. C., Moore, P., Campea, S., & Grossman, M. (2001). Evaluating the clinical diagnosis of Frontotemporal degeneration: A re-examination of Neary et al., 1998. *Neurology, 56,* A144–A145.

Dawson, D. R., & Chipman, M. (1995). The disablement experienced by traumatically brain-injured adults living in the community. *Brain Injury, 9,* 339–353.

Deal, J. L., & Deal, L. A. (1978). Efficacy of aphasia rehabilitation: Preliminary results. In R. H. Brookshire (Ed.), *Clinical aphasiology conference proceedings* (pp. 66–77). Minneapolis, MN: BRK.

Dean, C. (2004). *The everything Alzheimer's book.* Avon, MA: Adams Media.

DeBaggio, T. (2002). *Losing my mind: An intimate look at life with Alzheimer's.* New York: Free Press.

Dekoskey, S., Heilman, K. M., Bowers, D., & Valenstein, E. (1980). Recognition and discrimination of emotional faces and pictures. *Brain and Language, 9,* 206–214.

Delis, D. C., Wapner, W., Gardner, H., & Moses, J. A., Jr. (1983). The contribution of the right hemisphere to the organization of paragraphs. *Cortex, 19,* 43–50.

Dell, G. S., Lawler, E. N., Harris, H. D., & Gordon, J. K. (2004). Models of errors of omission in aphasic naming. *Cognitive Neuropsychology, 21,* 125–146.

Dell, G. S., & O'Seaghdha, P. G. (1992). Stages of lexical access in language production. *Cognition, 42,* 287–314.

Dell, G. S., Schwartz, M. F., Martin, N., Saffran, E. M., & Gagnon, D. A. (1997). Lexical access in aphasic and nonaphasic speakers. *Psychological Review, 104,* 801–838.

Deloche, G., Hannequin, D., Dordain, M., Perrier, D., Cardebat, D., et al. (1997). Picture written naming: Performance parallels and divergencies between aphasic patients and normal subjects. *Aphasiology, 11,* 219–234.

Deloche, G., & Seron, X. (1981). Sentence understanding and knowledge of the world. Evidences from a sentence-picture matching task performed by aphasic patients. *Brain and Language, 14,* 57–69.

Denes, G., Perazzolo, C., Piani, A., & Piccione, F. (1996). Intensive versus regular speech therapy in global aphasia: A controlled study. *Aphasiology, 10,* 385–394.

de Partz, M-P. (1986). Re-education of a deep dyslexic patient: Rationale of the methods and results. *Cognitive Neuropsychology, 3,* 149–177.

DeRenzi, E. (1979). A shortened version of the Token Test. In F. Boller & M. Dennis (Eds.), *Auditory comprehension: Clinical and experimental studies with the Token Test* (pp. 33–44). New York: Academic Press.

DeRenzi, E., & Faglioni, P. (1978). Normative data and screening power of a shortened version of the Token Test. *Cortex, 14,* 41–49.

DeRenzi, E., Faglioni, P., & Scotti, G. (1969). Impairment of memory for position following brain damage. *Cortex, 5,* 274–284.

DeRenzi, E., & Lucchelli, F. (1988). Ideational apraxia. *Brain, 111,* 1173–1188.

DeRenzi, E., Motti, F., & Nichelli, P. (1980). Imitating gestures: A quantitative approach to ideomotor apraxia. *Archives of Neurology, 37,* 6–10.

DeRenzi, E., & Nichelli, P. (1975). Verbal and non-verbal short-term memory impairment following hemispheric damage. *Cortex, 11,* 341–354.

DeRenzi, E., & Vignolo, L. A. (1962). The Token Test: A sensitive test to detect receptive disturbances in aphasics. *Brain, 85,* 665–678.

de Riesthal, M., & Wertz, R. T. (2004). Prognosis for aphasia: Relationship between selected biographical and behavioural variables and outcome and improvement. *Aphasiology, 18,* 899–915.

de Roo, E., Kolk, H., & Hofstede, B. (2003). Structural properties of syntactically reduced speech: A comparison of normal speakers and Broca's aphasics. *Brain and Language, 86,* 99–115.

Devescovi, A., Bates, E., D'Amico, S., Hernandez, A., Marangolo, P., et al. (1997). An on-line study of grammaticality judgements in normal and aphasic speakers of Italian. *Aphasiology, 11,* 543–579.

Diaz, M., Sailor, K., Cheung, D., & Kuslansky, (2004). Category size effects in semantic and letter fluency in Alzheimer's patients. *Brain and Language, 89,* 108–114.

DiSimoni, F., Keith, R. L., Holt, D. L., & Darley, F. L. (1975). Practicality of shortening the Porch Index of Communicative Ability. *Journal of Speech and Hearing Research, 18,* 491–497.

Dobkin, B. (1995). The economic impact of stroke. *Neurology* (Suppl. 1), 45, S6–S9.

Doesborgh, S. J. C., van de Sandt-Koenderman, M. W. M. E., Dippel, D. W. J., van Harskamp, F., Koudstaal, P. J., et al. (2004). Cues on request: The efficacy of Multicue, a computer program for wordfinding therapy. *Aphasiology, 18,* 213–222.

Doyle, P. J., & Goldstein, H. (1985). Experimental analysis of acquisition and generalization of syntax in Broca's aphasia. In R. H. Brookshire (Ed.), *Clinical aphasiology* (Vol. 15, pp. 205–213). Minneapolis, MN: BRK.

Doyle, P. J., Goldstein, H., & Bourgeois, M. S. (1987). Experimental analysis of syntax training in Broca's aphasia: A generalization and social validation study. *Journal of Speech and Hearing Disorders, 52,* 143–155.

Doyle, P. J., Hula, W. D., McNeil, M. R., Mikolic, J. M., & Matthews, C. (2005). An application of Rasch Analysis to the measurement of communicative functioning. *Journal of Speech, Language, and Hearing Research, 48,* 1412–1428.

Doyle, P. J., McNeil, M. R., Hula, W. D., & Mikolic, J. M. (2003). The Burdon of Stroke Scale (BOSS): Validating patient-reported communication difficulty and associated psychological distress in stroke survivors. *Aphasiology, 17,* 291–304.

Doyle, P. J., McNeil, M. R., Park, G., Goda, A., Rubenstein, E. et al. (2000). Linguistic validation of four parallel forms of a story retelling procedure. *Aphasiology, 15,* 537–549.

Doyle, P. J., Thompson, C. K., Oleyar, K., Wambaugh, J., & Jackson, A. (1994). The effects of setting variables on conversational discourse in normal and aphasic adults. In M. L. Lemme (Ed.), *Clinical aphasiology* (Vol. 22, pp. 135–144). Austin, TX: Pro-Ed.

Doyle, P. J., Tsironas, D., Goda, A. J., & Kalinyak, M. (1996). The relationship between objective measures and listeners' judgments of the communicative informativeness of the connected discourse of adults with aphasia. *American Journal of Speech-Language Pathology, 5*(3), 53–60.

Drew, R., & Thompson, C. K. (1999). Model-based semantic treatment for naming deficits in aphasia. *Journal of Speech, Language, and Hearing Research, 42,* 972–989.

Dudas, R. B., Berrios, G. E., & Hodges, J. R. (2005). The Addenbrooke's Cognitive Examination (ACE) in the differential diagnosis of early dementias versus affective disorder. *American Journal of Geriatric Psychiatry, 13,* 218–226.

Duffy, J. R. (1995). *Motor speech disorders: Substrates, differential diagnosis, and management.* St. Louis, MO: Mosby.

Duffy, J. R., & Coelho, C. A. (2001). Schuell's stimulation approach to rehabilitation. In R. Chapey (Ed.), *Language intervention strategies in adult aphasia and related neurogenic communication disorders* (4th ed., pp. 341–382). Philadelphia: Lippincott Williams & Wilkins.

Duffy, J. R., & Duffy, R. J. (1989). The limb apraxia test: An imitative measure of upper limb apraxia. In T. E. Prescott (Ed.), *Clinical aphasiology* (Vol. 18, pp. 145–160). Boston: College-Hill/Little, Brown.

Duffy, J. R., Keith, R. L., Shane, H., & Podraza, B. L. (1976). Performance of normal (non-brain-injured) adults on the Porch Index of Communicative Ability. In R. H. Brookshire (Ed.), *Clinical aphasiology conference proceedings* (pp. 32–42). Minneapolis, MN: BRK.

Duffy, J. R., & Liles, B. Z. (1979). A translation of Finkelnberg's (1870) lecture on aphasia as "asymbolia" with commentary. *Journal of Speech and Hearing Disorders, 44,* 156–168.

Duffy, J. R., & Myers, P. S. (1991). Group comparisons across neurologic communication disorders: Some methodological issues. In T. E. Prescott (Ed.), *Clinical aphasiology* (Vol. 19, pp. 1–14). Austin, TX: Pro-Ed.

Duffy, R. J., & Duffy, J. R. (1981). Three studies of deficits in pantomimic expression and pantomimic recognition in aphasia. *Journal of Speech and Hearing Research, 24,* 70–84.

Duffy, R. J., & Duffy, J. R. (1984). *Assessment of Nonverbal Communication.* Tigard, OR: C. C. Publications.

Duffy, R. J., Duffy, J. R., & Mercaitis, P. A. (1984). Comparison of the performance of a fluent and a nonfluent aphasic on a pantomimic referential task. *Brain and Language, 21,* 260–273.

Duffy, R. J., Duffy, J. R., & Pearson, K. (1975). Pantomime recognition in aphasia. *Journal of Speech and Hearing Research, 18,* 115–132.

Duffy, R. J., & Ulrich, S. R. (1976). A comparison of impairments in verbal comprehension, speech, reading, and writing in adult aphasics. *Journal of Speech and Hearing Disorders, 41,* 110–119.

Duffy, R. J., Watt, J. H., & Duffy, J. R. (1994). Testing causal theories of pantomimic deficits in aphasia using path analysis. *Aphasiology, 8,* 361–379.

Duke Health (n.d.). The aphasia center. Retrieved December 15, 2005, from http://dukehealth1.org.

Duncan, J. (1986). Disorganisation of behaviour after frontal lobe damage. *Cognitive Neuropsychology, 3,* 271–290.

Duncan, P. W., Wallace, D., Lai, S. M., Johnson, D., Embretson, S., et al. (1999). The stroke impact scale version 2.0: Evaluation of reliability, validity, and sensitivity to change. *Stroke, 30,* 2131–2140.

Duong, A., Giroux, F., Tardif, A., & Ska, B. (2005). The heterogeneity of picture-supported narratives in Alzheimer's disease. *Brain and Language, 93,* 173–184.

Edelman, G. (1987). Global aphasia: The case for treatment. *Aphasiology, 1,* 75–80.

Ehrlich, J. S. (1988). Selective characteristics of narrative discourse in head-injured and normal adults. *Journal of Communication Disorders, 21,* 1–9.

Eisenson, J. (1954). *Examining for aphasia.* New York: The Psychological Corporation.

Eisenson, J. (1962). Language and intellectual findings associated with right cerebral damage. *Language and Speech, 5,* 49–53.

Eisenson, J. (1984). *Adult aphasia* (2nd ed.). Englewood Cliffs, NJ: Prentice-Hall.

Ellis, A. W., Flude, B. M., & Young, A. W. (1987). "Neglect dyslexia" and the early visual processing of letters in words and nonwords. *Cognitive Neuropsychology, 4,* 439–464.

Ellis, A. W., Kay, J., & Franklin, S. (1992). Anomia: Differentiating between semantic and phonological deficits. In D. I. Margolin (Ed.), *Cognitive neuropsychology in clinical practice* (pp. 207–228). New York: Oxford University Press.

Ellis, A. W., & Young, A. W. (1988). *Human cognitive neuropsychology.* London: Erlbaum.

Elman, R. J. (Ed.). (1999). *Group treatment of neurogenic communication disorders: The expert clinician's approach.* Boston: Butterworth Heinemann.

Elman, R. J. (2005). Social and life participation approaches to aphasia intervention. In L. L. LaPointe (Ed.), *Aphasia and related neurogenic language disorders* (3rd ed., pp. 39–50). New York: Thieme.

Elman, R. J., & Bernstein-Ellis, E. (1999). The efficacy of group communication treatment in adults with chronic aphasia. *Journal of Speech, Language, and Hearing Research, 42,* 411–419.

Emmorey, K. D. (1987). The neurological substrates for prosodic aspects of speech. *Brain and Language, 30,* 305–320.

Enderby, P., & Crow, E. (1996). Frenchay Aphasia Screening Test: Validity and comparability. *Disability Rehabilitation, 18,* 238–240.

Enderby, P., Wood, V., & Wade, D. (1997). *Frenchay Aphasia Screening Test.* London: Whurr Publishers.

Engell, B., Hütter, B-O., Willmes, K., & Huber, W. (2003). Quality of life in aphasia: Validation of a pictorial self-rating procedure. *Aphasiology, 17,* 383–396.

England, J. E., O'Neill, J. J., & Simpson, R. K. (1996). Pragmatic assessment of communication in dementia (PAC-D). *American Journal of Alzheimer's Disease, 11,* 7–10.

Erickson, R. J., Goldinger, S. D., & LaPointe, L. L. (1996). Auditory vigilance in aphasic individuals: Detecting nonlinguistic stimuli with full or divided attention. *Brain and Cognition, 30,* 244–253.

European Observatory on Health Care Systems (2000). *Health Care Systems in Transition: Belgium.* Retrieved August 6, 2004, from www.euro.who.int/document/e71203.pdf.

Fabbro, F. (2001). The bilingual brain: Bilingual aphasia. *Brain and Language, 79,* 201–210

Faglioni, P., Spinnler, H., & Vignolo, L. (1969). Contrasting behavior of right and left hemisphere-damaged patients on a discriminative and a semantic task of auditory recognition. *Cortex, 5,* 366–389.

Farias, D., Davis, C., & Harrington, G. (2006). Drawing: Its contribution to naming in aphasia. *Brain and Language, 97,* 53–63.

Faroqi-Shah, Y., & Thompson, C. K. (2003). Effect of lexical cues on the production of active and passive sentences in Broca's and Wernicke's aphasia. *Brain and Language, 85,* 409–426.

Faroqi-Shah, Y., & Thompson, C. K. (2004). Semantic, lexical, and phonological influences on the production of verb inflections in agrammatic aphasia. *Brain and Language, 89,* 484–498.

Ferguson, A. (1994). The influence of aphasia, familiarity and activity on conversational repair. *Aphasiology, 8,* 143–157.

Ferguson, A., & Armstrong, E. (1996). The PALPA: A valid investigation of language? *Aphasiology, 10,* 193–197.

Ferguson, A., Worrall, L., McPhee, J., Buskell, R., Armstrong, E., et al. (2003). Testamentary capacity and aphasia: A descriptive case report with implications for clinical practice. *Aphasiology, 17,* 965–980.

Ferro, J. M. (1992). The influence of infarct location on recovery from global aphasia. *Aphasiology, 6,* 415–430.

Ferro, J. M., & Kertesz, A. (1987). Comparative classification of aphasic disorders. *Journal of Clinical and Experimental Neuropsychology, 9,* 365–375.

Ferro, J. M., Santos, M. E., Castro-Caldas, A., & Mariano, G. (1980). Gesture recognition in aphasia. *Journal of Clinical Neuropsychology, 2,* 277–292.

Feyereisen, P., Barter, D., Goosens, M., & Clarebaut, N. (1988). Gestures and speech referential communication by aphasic subjects: Channel use and efficiency. *Aphasiology, 2,* 21–32.

Feyereisen, P., & Seron, X. (1982). Nonverbal communication and aphasia: A review. I. Comprehension. *Brain and Language, 16,* 191–212.

Fields, R. B. (1998). The dementias. In P. J. Snyder & P. D. Nussbaum (Eds.), *Clinical neuropsychology : A pocket handbook for assessment* (pp. 211–239). Washington, DC: American Psychological Association.

Fillenbaum, S., Jones, L. V., & Wepman, J. M. (1961). Some linguistic features of speech from aphasic patients. *Language and Speech, 4,* 91–108.

Fink, R. B., Brecher, A., Schwartz, M. F., & Robey, R. R. (2002). A computer-implemented protocol for treatment of naming disorders: Evaluation of clinician-guided and partially self-guided instruction. *Aphasiology, 16,* 1061–1086.

Fink, R. B., Brecher, A., Sobel, P., & Schwartz, M. F. (2005). Computer-assisted treatment of word retrieval deficits in aphasia. *Aphasiology, 19,* 943–954.

Fink, R. B., Schwartz, M. F., Rochon, E., Myers, J. L., Socolof, G. S., et al. (1995). Syntax stimulation revisited: An analysis of generalization of treatment effects. *American Journal of Speech-Language Pathology, 4*(4), 99–104.

Fishman, S. (1988). *A bomb in the brain.* New York: Avon.

Fitch West, J., Sands, E. S., & Ross-Swain, D. (1998). *Bedside Evaluation Screening Test* (2nd ed.). Austin, TX: Pro-Ed.

Fletcher, C. R., & Bloom, C. P. (1988). Causal reasoning in the comprehension of simple narrative texts. *Journal of Memory and Language, 27,* 235–244.

Flowers, C. R., & Wyse, M. (1985). Assessing gestural intelligibility of normal and aphasic subjects. In R. H. Brookshire (Ed.), *Clinical aphasiology* (Vol. 15, pp. 64–71). Minneapolis, MN: BRK.

Flude, B. M., Ellis, A. W., & Kay, J. (1989). Face processing and name retrieval in an anomic aphasic: Names are stored separately from semantic information about familiar people. *Brain and Cognition, 11,* 60–72.

Foldi, N. S. (1987). Appreciation of pragmatic interpretations of indirect commands: Comparison of right and left hemisphere brain-damaged patients. *Brain and Language, 31,* 88–108.

Folstein, M. F., Folstein, S. E., & McHugh, P. R. (1975). Mini-mental state. *Journal of Psychiatric Research, 12,* 189–198.

Forde, E. M. E., & Humphreys, G. W. (1999). Category-specific recognition impairments: A review of important case studies and influential theories. *Aphasiology, 13,* 169–193.

Forster, K. I., & Chambers, S. M. (1973). Lexical access and naming time. *Journal of Verbal Learning and Verbal Behavior, 12,* 627–635.

Fortinski, R. H., Granger, C. V., & Selzer, G. B. (1981). The use of functional assessment in understanding home care needs. *Medical Care, 19,* 489–497.

Foygel, D., & Dell, G. S. (2000). Models of impaired lexical access in speech production. *Journal of Memory and Language, 43,* 182–216.

Fraiser, R. T., & Clemmons, D. C. (Eds.). (1999). *Traumatic brain injury rehabilitation: Practical vocational, neuropsychological, and psychotherapy interventions.* London: CRC Press.

Franklin, S. (1989). Dissociations in auditory word comprehension: Evidence from nine fluent aphasic patients. *Aphasiology, 6,* 63–84.

Franklin, S., Howard, D., & Patterson, K. (1995). Abstract word anomia. *Cognitive Neuropsychology, 12,* 549–566.

Franklin, S. E., Buerk, F., & Howard, D. (2002). Generalised improvement in speech production for a subject with reproduction conduction aphasia. *Aphasiology, 16,* 1087–1114.

Frattali, C. M., Thompson, C. M., Holland, A. L., Wohl, C. B., & Ferketic, M. M. (1995). The FACS of life: ASHA FACS—A functional outcome measure for adults. *Asha, 37*(4), 40–46.

Freed, D., Celery, K., & Marshall, R. C. (2004). Effectiveness of personalized and phonological cueing in long-term naming performance by aphasic subjects: A clinical investigation. *Aphasiology, 18,* 743–757.

Fridriksson, J., Holland, A. L. Beeson, P., & Morrow, L. (2005). Spaced retrieval treatment of anomia. *Aphasiology, 19,* 99–109.

Fridriksson, J., Holland, A. L., Coull, B. M., Plante, E., Trouard, T. P., et al. (2002). Aphasia severity: Association with cerebral perfusion and diffusion. *Aphasiology, 16,* 859–871.

Friederici, A. D. (1983). Aphasics' perception of words in sentential context: Some real-time processing evidence. *Neuropsychologia, 21,* 351–358.

Friederici, A. D. (1988). Agrammatic comprehension: Picture of a computational mismatch. *Aphasiology, 2,* 279–284.

Friederici, A. D., & Frazier, L. (1992). Thematic analysis in agrammatic comprehension: Syntactic structures and task demands. *Brain and Language, 42,* 1–29.

Friederici, A. D., Wessels, J. M. I., Emmorey, K., & Bellugi, U. (1992). Sensitivity to inflectional morphology in aphasia: A real-time processing perspective. *Brain and Language, 43,* 747–763.

Friedman, R. B. (2002). Clinical diagnosis and treatment of reading disorders. In A. E. Hillis (Ed.), *The handbook of adult language disorders* (pp. 27–43). New York: Psychology Press.

Friedmann, N. (2002). Question production in agrammatism: The Tree Pruning Hypothesis. *Brain and Language, 80,* 160–187.

Friedmann, N., & Grodzinsky, Y. (1997). Tense and agreement in agrammatic production: Pruning the syntactic tree. *Brain and Language, 56,* 397–425.

Friedmann, N., & Gvion, A. (2003). Sentence comprehension and working memory limitation in aphasia: A dissociation between semantic-syntactic and phonological reactivation. *Brain and Language, 86,* 23–39.

Friedmann, N., & Shapiro, L. P. (2003). Agrammatic comprehension of simple active sentences with moved constituents: Hebrew OSV and OVS structures. *Journal of Speech, Language, and Hearing Research, 46,* 288–297.

Friedrich, F. J., Glenn, C. G., & Marin, O. S. M. (1984). Interruption of phonological coding in conduction aphasia. *Brain and Language, 22,* 266–291.

Friedrich, F. J., Martin, R., & Kemper, S. J. (1985). Consequences of a phonological coding deficit on sentence processing. *Cognitive Neuropsychology, 2,* 385–412.

Fryer, L. J., & Haffey, W. J. (1987). Cognitive rehabilitation and community readaptation: Outcomes from two program models. *Journal of Head Trauma Rehabilitation, 2,* 51–63.

Frymark, T. B., & Mullen, R. C. (2005). Influence of the Prospective Payment System on speech-language pathology services. *American Journal of Physical Medicine and Rehabilitation, 84,* 12–21.

Fukkink, R. (1996). The internal validity of aphasiological single-subject studies. *Aphasiology, 10,* 741–754.

Funnell, E., & Allport, A. (1989). Symbolically speaking: Communicating with Blissymbols in aphasia. *Aphasiology, 3,* 279–300.

Gaddie, A., Naeser, M. A., Palumbo, C. L., & Stiassny-Eder, D. (1989). Recovery of auditory comprehension after one year: A computed tomography scan study. In T. E. Prescott (Ed.), *Clinical aphasiology* (Vol. 18, pp. 463–478). Boston: College-Hill/Little, Brown.

Gagnon, D. A., & Schwartz, M. F. (1997). Serial position effects in aphasics' neologisms [abstract]. *Brain and Language, 60,* 87–89.

Gagnon, L., Goulet, P., Giroux, G., & Joanetter, Y. (2003). Processing of metaphoric and non-metaphoric alternative meanings of words after right- and left-hemispheric stroke. *Brain and Language, 87,* 217–226.

Gainotti, G. (1972). Emotional behavior and hemispheric side of lesion. *Cortex, 8,* 41–55.

Gainotti, G. (1976). The relationship between semantic impairment in comprehension and naming in aphasic patients. *British Journal of Disorders of Communication, 11,* 57–61.

Gainotti, G., Caltagirone, C., & Ibba, A. (1975). Semantic and phonemic aspects of auditory language comprehension in aphasia. *Linguistics, 154/5,* 15–29.

Gainotti, G., Caltagirone, C., & Miceli, G. (1983). Selective impairment of semantic-lexical discrimination in right-brain-damaged patients. In E. Perecman (Ed.). *Cognitive processing in the right hemisphere* (pp. 149–167). New York: Academic Press.

Gainotti, G., Caltagirone, C., Miceli, G., & Masullo, C. (1981). Selective semantic-lexical impairment of language comprehension in right brain-damaged patients. *Brain and Language, 13,* 201–211.

Gainotti, G., Carlomagno, S., Craca, A., & Silveri, M. C. (1986). Disorders of classificatory activity in aphasia. *Brain and Language, 28,* 181–195.

Gainotti, G., & Lemmo, M. A. (1976). Comprehension of symbolic gestures in aphasia. *Brain and Language, 3,* 451–460.

Gainotti, G., & Tiacci, C. (1970). Patterns of drawing disability in right and left hemispheric patients. *Neuropsychologia, 8,* 379–384.

Gallagher, H. L., & Frith, C. D. (2003). Functional imaging of "theory of mind." *Trends in Cognitive Sciences, 7,* 77–83.

Gallagher, T. M. (1998). National initiatives in outcomes measurement. In C. M. Frattali (Ed.), *Measuring outcomes in speech-language pathology* (pp. 527–557). New York: Thieme.

Gallaher, A. J. (1979). Temporal reliability of aphasic performance on the Token Test. *Brain and Language, 7,* 34–41.

Gallaher, A. J., & Canter, G. J. (1982). Reading and listening comprehension in Broca's aphasia: Lexical versus syntactical errors. *Brain and Language, 17,* 183–192.

Galton, C. J., Erzinclioglu, S., Sahakian, B. J., Antoun, N., & Hodges, J. R. (2005). A comparison of the Addenbrooke's Cognitive Examination (ACE), conventional neuropsychological assessment, and simple MRI-based medial temporal lobe evaluation in the early diagnosis of Alzheimer's disease. *Cognitive & Behavioral Neurology, 18,* 144–150.

Gandour, J., & Dardarananda, R. (1982). Voice onset time in aphasia: Thai. I. Perception. *Brain and Language, 17,* 24–33.

Gandour, J., Marshall, R. C., Kim, S. Y., & Neuburger, S. (1991). On the nature of conduction aphasia: A longitudinal case study. *Aphasiology, 5,* 291–306.

Gansler, D. A., Covall, S., McGrath, N., & Oscar-Berman, M. (1996). Measures of prefrontal dysfunction after closed head injury. *Brain and Cognition, 30,* 194–204.

Gardner, H. (1974). *The Shattered Mind.* New York: Vintage Books.

Gardner, H. (1982). Missing the point: Language and the right hemisphere. In H. Gardner, *Art, mind, and brain: A cognitive approach to creativity* (pp. 309–317). New York: Basic Books.

Gardner, H., & Brownell, H. H. (1986). *Right hemisphere communication battery.* Boston: Psychology Service, Veterans Administration Medical Center.

Gardner, H., Brownell, H. H., Wapner, W., & Michelow, D. (1983). Missing the point: The role of the right hemisphere in the processing of complex linguistic materials. In E. Perecman (Ed.), *Cognitive processing in the right hemisphere* (pp. 169–191). New York: Academic Press.

Gardner, H., & Denes, G. (1973). Connotative judgements by aphasic patients on a pictorial adaptation of the semantic differential. *Cortex, 9,* 183–196.

Gardner, H., Denes, G., & Weintraub, S. (1975). Comprehending a word: The influence of speed and redundancy on auditory comprehension in aphasia. *Cortex, 11,* 155–162.

Gardner, H., Ling, P. K., Flamm, L., & Silverman, J. (1975). Comprehension and appreciation of humorous material following brain damage. *Brain, 98,* 399–412.

Gardner, H., Zurif, E. B., Berry, T., & Baker, E. (1976). Visual communication in aphasia. *Neuropsychologia, 14,* 275–292.

Garrard, P., Lambon Ralph, M. A., Patterson, K., Pratt, K. H., & Hodges, J. R. (2005). Semantic feature knowledge and picture naming in dementia of Alzheimer's type: A new approach. *Brain and Language, 93,* 79–94.

Garrett, K. L., & Ellis, G. J. (1999). Group communication therapy for people with long-term aphasia: Scaffolded thematic discourse activities. In R. J. Elman (Ed.), *Group treatment of neurogenic communication disorders: The expert clinician's approach* (pp. 85–96). Boston: Butterworth Heinemann.

Garrett, M. F. (1984). The organization of processing structure for language production: Applications to aphasic speech. In D. Caplan, A. R., Lecours, & A. Smith (Eds.), *Biological perspectives on language* (pp. 172–193). Cambridge, MA: MIT Press.

Gates, W. H. (1978). *Gates-MacGinitie reading tests.* Chicago: Riverside.

Geigenberger, A., & Ziegler, W. (2001). Receptive prosodic processing in aphasia. *Aphasiology, 15,* 1169–1187.

Germani, M. J., & Pierce, R. S. (1995). Semantic attribute knowledge in adults with right and left hemisphere damage. *Aphasiology, 9,* 1–21.

Gernsbacher, M. A. (Ed.). (1994). *Handbook of psycholinguistics.* San Diego, CA: Academic Press.

Gerratt, B., & Jones, D. (1987). Aphasic performance on a lexical decision task: Multiple meanings and word frequency. *Brain and Language, 30,* 106–115.

Geschwind, N. (1965). Disconnexion syndromes in animals and man. *Brain, 88,* 237–294, 585–644.

Geschwind, N. (1967). The varieties of naming errors. *Cortex, 3,* 96–112.

Gibbs, R. W., Jr. (1999). Interpreting what speakers say and implicate. *Brain and Language, 68,* 466–485.

Giles, E., Patterson, K., & Hodges, J. R. (1996). Performance on the Boston Cookie Theft picture description task in patients with early dementia of the Alzheimer's type: Missing information. *Aphasiology, 10,* 395–408.

Gillick, M. R. (1998). *Tangled minds: Understanding Alzheimer's disease and other dementias.* New York: Plume.

Gillis, R. J. (Ed.). (1996). *Traumatic brain injury rehabilitation for speech-language pathologists.* Boston: Butterworth-Heinemann.

Gillis, R. J. (1999a). Cotreatment and community-oriented group treatment for traumatic brain injury. In R. J. Elman (Ed.), *Group treatment of neurogenic communication disorders: The expert clinician's approach* (pp. 153–163). Boston: Butterworth Heinemann.

Gillis, R. J. (1999b). Traumatic brain injury: Cognitive-communicative needs and early intervention. In R. J. Elman (Ed.), *Group treatment of neurogenic communication disorders: The expert clinician's approach* (pp. 141–151). Boston: Butterworth Heinemann.

Glass, A. V., Gazzaniga, M. S., & Premack, D. (1973). Artificial language training in global aphasia. *Neuropsychologia, 11,* 95–103.

Gleason, J. B., Goodglass, H., Green, E., Ackerman, N., & Hyde, M. R. (1975). The retrieval of syntax in Broca's aphasia. *Brain and Language, 2,* 451–471.

Gleason, J. B., Goodglass, H., Obler, L., Green, E., Hyde, M. R., & Weintraub, S. (1980). Narrative strategies of aphasic and normal-speaking subjects. *Journal of Speech and Hearing Research, 23,* 370–382.

Glindemann, R., & Springer, L. (1995). An assessment of PACE therapy. In C. Code & D. J. Müller (Eds.), *The treatment of aphasia: From theory to practice* (pp. 90–107). San Diego, CA: Singular.

Glindemann, R., Willmes, K., Huber, W., & Springer, L. (1991). The efficacy of modeling in PACE-therapy. *Aphasiology, 5,* 425–430.

Glosser, G., & Deser, T. (1991). Patterns of discourse production among neurological patients with fluent language disorders. *Brain and Language, 40,* 67–88.

Glosser, G., Friedman, R. B., Grugan, P. K., Lee, J. H., & Grossman, M. (1998). Lexical semantic and associative priming in Alzheimer's disease. *Neuropsychology, 12,* 218–224.

Glosser, G., Wiener, M., & Kaplan, E. (1986). Communicative gestures in aphasia. *Brain and Language, 27,* 345–359.

Godfrey, C. M., & Douglass, E. (1959). The recovery process in aphasia. *Canadian Medical Association Journal, 80,* 618–624.

Godfrey, H. P. D., Partridge, F. M., Knight, R. G., & Bishara, S. (1993). Course of insight disorder and emotional dysfunction following closed-head injury: A controlled cross-sectional follow-up study. *Journal of Clinical and Experimental Neuropsychology, 15,* 503–515.

Gold, B. T., & Kertesz, A. (2000). Right hemisphere semantic processing of visual words in an aphasic patient: An fMRI study. *Brain and Language, 73,* 456–465.

Gold, B. T., & Kertesz, A. (2001). Phonologically related lexical repetition disorder: A case study. *Brain and Language, 77,* 241–265.

Gold, M., VanDam, D., & Silliman, E. R. (2000). An open-labeled trial of bromocriptine in nonfluent aphasia: A qualitative analysis of word storage and retrieval. *Brain and Language, 74,* 141–156.

Goldberg, E., & Goldfarb, R. (2005). Grammatical category ambiguity in aphasia. *Brain and* Language, 95, 293–304.

Golden, C. J., Hemmeke, T. A., & Purisch, A. D. (1980). *The Luria-Nebraska Neuropsychological Battery.* Los Angeles: Western Psychological Services.

Goldenberg, G., & Spatt, J. (1994). Influence of size and site of cerebral lesions on spontaneous recovery of aphasia and on success of language therapy. *Brain and Language, 47,* 684–698.

Goldstein, K. (1942). *Aftereffects of brain injuries in war.* New York: Grune & Stratton.

Goldstein, L. B. (1998). Potential effects of common drugs on stroke recovery. *Archives of Neurology, 55,* 454–467.

Goodenough, C., Zurif, E. B., Weintraub, S., & Von Stockert, T. (1977). Aphasics' attention to grammatical morphemes. *Language and Speech, 20,* 11–19.

Goodglass, H., Blumstein, S. E., Gleason, J. B., Hyde, M. R., Green, E., et al. (1979). The effect of syntactic encoding on sentence comprehension in aphasia. *Brain and Language, 7,* 201–209.

Goodglass, H., & Kaplan, E. (1983). *The assessment of aphasia and related disorders* (2nd ed.). Philadelphia: Lea & Febiger.

Goodglass, H., Kaplan, E., & Barresi, B. (2001). *The assessment of aphasia and related disorders* (3rd ed.). Philadelphia: Lippincott, Williams & Wilkins.

Goodglass, H., Kaplan, E., Weintraub, S., & Ackerman, N. (1976). The "tip-of-the-tongue" phenomenon in aphasia. *Cortex, 12,* 145–153.

Goodglass, H., & Mayer, J. (1958). Agrammatism in aphasia. *Journal of Speech and Hearing Disorders, 23,* 99–111.

Goodglass, H., & Menn, L. (1985). Is agrammatism a unitary phenomenon? In M-L. Kean (Ed.), *Agrammatism* (pp. 1–26). Orlando, FL: Academic Press.

Goodglass, H., & Stuss, D. T. (1979). Naming to picture versus description in three aphasic subgroups. *Cortex, 15,* 199–211.

Goodglass, H., Wingfield, A., & Ward, S. E. (1997). Judgments of concept similarity by normal and aphasic subjects: Relation to naming and comprehension. *Brain and Language, 56,* 138–158.

Gordon, B., & Caramazza, A. (1983). Closed- and open-class lexical access in agrammatic and fluent aphasics. *Brain and Language, 19,* 335–345.

Gordon, J. K. (2002). Phonological neighborhood effects in aphasic speech errors: Spontaneous and structured contexts. *Brain and Language, 82,* 113–145.

Gow, D. W., & Caplan, D. (1996). An examination of impaired acoustic-phonetic processing in aphasia. *Brain and Language, 52,* 386–407.

Graham, M. A. (1999). Aphasia group therapy in a subacute setting: Using the American Speech-Language-Hearing Association Functional Assessment of Communication Skills. In R. J. Elman (Ed.), *Group treatment of neurogenic communication disorders: The expert clinician's approach* (pp. 37–46). Boston: Butterworth Heinemann.

Granger, C. V., Cotter, A. C., Hamilton, B. B., & Fiedler, R. C. (1993). Functional assessment scales: A study of persons after stroke. *Archives of Physical Medicine and Rehabilitation, 74,* 133–138.

Grant, D. A., & Berg, E. A. (1948). A behavioral analysis of degree of reinforcement and ease of shifting to new responses in a Weigl-type card-sorting problem. *Journal of Experimental Psychology, 38,* 404–411.

Greitemann, G., & Wolf, E. (1991). *Making dynamic use of different modes of expression: The efficacy of the PACE-approach.* Paper presented to the Academy of Aphasia, Rome.

Grice, L. P. (1975). Logic and conversation. In P. Cole & J. L. Morgan (Ed.), *Syntax and semantics: Speech acts* (Vol. 3, pp. 41–58). New York: Academic Press.

Griffiths, K. M., Cook, M. L., & Newcombe, R. L. G. (1988). Cube copying after cerebral damage. *Journal of Clinical and Experimental Neuropsychology, 10,* 800–812.

Grober, E., & Sliwinski, M. (1991). Development and validation of a model for estimating premorbid verbal intelligence in the elderly. *Journal of Clinical and Experimental Neuropsychology, 13,* 933–949.

Grodzinsky, Y. (1984). The syntactic characterization of agrammatism. *Cognition, 16,* 99–120.

Grodzinsky, Y. (1986). Language deficits and the theory of syntax. *Brain and Language, 27,* 135–159.

Grodzinsky, Y. (1989). Agrammatic comprehension of relative clauses. *Brain and Language, 37,* 480–499.

Grodzinsky, Y. (1991). There is an entity called agrammatic aphasia. *Brain and Language, 41,* 555–564.

Grodzinsky, Y., Piñango, M. M., Zurif, E., & Drai, D. (1999). The critical role of group studies in neuropsychology: Comprehension regularities in Broca's aphasia. *Brain and Language, 67,* 134–147.

Grodzinsky, Y., Swinney, D., & Zurif, E. (1985). Agrammatism: Structural deficits and antecedent processing disruptions. In M-L. Kean (Ed.), *Agrammatism* (pp. 65–81). Orlando, FL: Academic Press.

Grosjean, F. (1989). Neurolinguists, beware! The bilingual is not two monolinguals in one person. *Brain and Language, 36,* 3–15.

Grossman, M. (1981). A bird is a bird is a bird: Making reference within and without superordinate categories. *Brain and Language, 12,* 313–331.

Grossman, M. (1988). Drawing deficits in brain-damaged patients' freehand pictures. *Brain and Cognition, 8,* 189–205.

Grossman, M., & Wilson, M. (1987). Stimulus categorization by brain-damaged patients. *Brain and Cognition, 6,* 55–71.

Gruen, A. K., Frankle, B. C., & Schwartz, R. (1990). Word fluency generation skills of head-injured patients in an acute trauma center. *Journal of Communication Disorders, 23,* 163–170.

Gruetzner, H. (2001). *Alzheimer's: A caregiver's guide and sourcebook* (3rd ed.). New York: John Wiley.

Haaland, K. Y., & Flaherty, D. (1984). The different types of limb apraxia errors made by patients with left vs. right hemisphere damage. *Brain and Cognition, 3,* 370–384.

Haarmann, H. J., & Kolk, H. H. J. (1991). Syntactic priming in Broca's aphasics: Evidence for slow activation. *Aphasiology, 5,* 247–264.

Haarmann, H. J., & Kolk, H. H. J. (1994). On-line sensitivity to subject-verb agreement violations in Broca's aphasics: The role of syntactic complexity and time. *Brain and Language, 46,* 493–516.

Haarmann, H. J., Just, M. A., & Carpenter, P. A. (1997). Aphasic sentence comprehension as a resource deficit: A computational approach. *Brain and Language, 59,* 76–120.

Haberlandt, K. F., & Graesser, A. C. (1990). Integration and buffering of new information. In A. C. Graesser & G. H. Bower (Eds.), *Inferences and text comprehension* (pp. 71–88). San Diego: Academic Press.

Hadar, U., Wenkert-Olenik, D., Krauss, R., & Soroker, N. (1998). Gesture and processing of speech: Neuropsychological evidence. *Brain and Language, 62,* 107–126.

Haendiges, A. N., Berndt, R. S., & Mitchum, C. C. (1996). Assessing the elements contributing to a "mapping" deficit: A targeted treatment study. *Brain and Language, 52,* 276–302.

Hageman, C. F., & Folkestad, A. (1986). Performance of aphasic listeners on an expanded Revised Token Test subtest presented verbally and nonverbally. In R. H. Brookshire (Ed.), *Clinical aphasiology* (Vol. 16, pp. 227–233). Minneapolis, MN: BRK.

Hageman, C. F., & Lewis, D. L. (1983). The effects of intrastimulus pause on the quality of auditory comprehension in aphasia. In R. H. Brookshire (Ed.), *Clinical aphasiology conference proceedings* (pp. 177–185). Minneapolis, MN: BRK.

Hagen, C. (1973). Communication abilities in hemiplegia: Effect of speech therapy. *Archives of Physical Medicine and Rehabilitation, 54,* 454–463.

Hagen, C. (1981). Language disorders secondary to closed head injury: Diagnosis and treatment. *Topics in Language Disorders, 1,* 73–87.

Hagiwara, H., & Caplan, D. (1990). Syntactic comprehension in Japanese aphasics: Effects of category and thematic role order. *Brain and Language, 38,* 159–170.

Hagoort, P. (1993). Impairments of lexical-semantic processing in aphasia: Evidence from the processing of lexical ambiguities. *Brain and Language, 45,* 189–232.

Hagoort, P. (1997). Semantic priming in Broca's aphasics at a short SOA: No support for an automatic access deficit. *Brain and Language, 56,* 287–300.

Hall, K. M., & Cope, D. N. (1995). The benefit of rehabilitation in traumatic brain injury: A literature review. *Journal of Head Trauma Rehabilitation, 10,* 1–13.

Hall, K. M., Hamilton, B. B., & Keith, R. A. (1993). Characteristics and comparisons of functional assessment indices: Disability Rating Scale, Functional Independence Measure, and Functional Assessment Measure. *Journal of Head Trauma Rehabilitation, 8,* 60–74.

Halper, A. S., Cherney, L. R., & Burns, M. S. (1996). *Clinical management of right hemisphere dysfunction: Procedural manual* (2nd ed.). Gaithersburg, MD: Aspen.

Halstead, W. C., & Wepman, J. M. (1949). The Halstead-Wepman aphasia screening test. *Journal of Speech and Hearing Disorders, 14,* 9–15.

Hamilton, B. B., Laughlin, J. A., Granger, C. V., & Kayton, R. M. (1991). Interrater agreement of the seven-level Functional Independence Measure (FIM) [abstract]. *Archives of Physical Medicine and Rehabilitation, 72,* 790.

Hanlon, R. E., Brown, J. W., & Gerstman, L. J. (1990). Enhancement of naming in nonfluent aphasia through gesture. *Brain and Language, 38,* 298–314.

Hanna, G., Schell, L. M., & Schriener, R. (1977). *The Nelson reading skills test.* Chicago: Riverside.

Hannay, H. J., & Levin, H. S. (1989). Visual continous recognition memory in normal and closed head-injured adolescents. *Journal of Clinical and Experimental Neuropsychology, 11,* 444–460.

Hanson, W. R., & Cicciarelli, A. W. (1978). The time, amount, and pattern of language improvement in adult aphasics. *British Journal of Disorders of Communication, 13,* 59–63.

Hanson, W. R., Metter, E. J., & Riege, W. H. (1989). The course of chronic aphasia. *Aphasiology, 3,* 19–30.

Haravon, A., Obler, L. K., & Sarno, M. T. (1994). A method for microanalysis of discourse in brain-damaged patients. In R. L. Bloom, L. K. Obler, S. De Santi, & J. S. Ehrlich (Eds.), *Discourse analysis and applications: Studies in adult clinical populations* (pp. 47–80). Hillsdale, NJ: Lawrence Erlbaum.

Harding, D., & Pound, C. (1999). Needs, function, and measurement: Juggling with multiple language impairment. In S. Byng, K., Swinburn, & C. Pound (Eds.), *The aphasia therapy file* (pp. 13–39). Hove, UK: Psychology Press.

Harley, T. A. (2004a). Does cognitive neuropsychology have a future? *Cognitive Neuropsychology, 21,* 3–16.

Harley, T. A. (2004b). Promises, promises. *Cognitive Neuropsychology, 21,* 51–56.

Hartje, W., Kerschensteiner, M., Poeck, K., & Orgass, B. (1973). A cross-validation study on the Token Test. *Neuropsychologia, 11,* 119–121.

Hartley, L. L. (1995). *Cognitive-communicative abilities following brain injury: A functional approach.* San Diego, CA: Singular.

Hartley, L. L., & Levin, H. S. (1990). Linguistic deficits after closed head injury: A current appraisal. *Aphasiology, 4,* 353–370.

Harvey, M., Milner, A. D., & Roberts, R. C. (1995). An investigation of hemispatial neglect using the Landmark Task. *Brain and Cognition, 27,* 59–78.

Hathaway, S. R., & McKinley, J. C. (1951). *The Minnesota Multiphasic Personality Inventory Manual* (Revised). New York: Psychological Corporation.

Haut, M. W., Petros, T. V., Frank, R. G., & Haut, J. S. (1991). Speed of processing within semantic memory following severe closed head injury. *Brain and Cognition, 17,* 31–41.

Hawkins, K. A., & Bender, S. (2002). Norms and the relationship of Boston Naming Test performance to vocabulary and education: A review. *Aphasiology, 16,* 1143–1153.

Hawley, C. A., Taylor, R., Hellawell, D. J., & Pentland, B. (1999). Use of the Functional Assessment Meaure (FIM+FAM) in head injury rehabilitation: A psychometric analysis. *Journal of Neurology, Neurosurgery, and Psychiatry, 67,* 749–754.

Haynes, W. O., & Oratio, A. R. (1978). A study of clients' perceptions of therapeutic effectiveness. *Journal of Speech and Hearing Disorders, 43,* 21–33.

Head, H. (1920). Aphasia and kindred disorders of speech. *Brain, 43,* 87–165.

Heath, R. L., & Blonder, L. X. (2005). Spontaneous humor among right hemisphere stroke survivors. *Brain and Language, 93,* 267–276.

Heeschen, C. (1980). Strategies of decoding actor-object relations by aphasic patients. *Cortex, 16,* 5–19.

Heeschen, C., & Kolk, H. (1988). Agrammatism and paragrammatism. *Aphasiology, 2,* 299–302.

Heeschen, C., & Schegloff, E. A. (1999). Agrammatism, adaptation theory, conversation analysis: On the role of so-called telegraphic style in talk-in-interaction. *Aphasiology, 13,* 365–405.

Heilman, K. M., Bowers, D., Speedie, L., & Coslett, H. B. (1984). Comprehension of affective and non-affective prosody. *Neurology, 34,* 917–921.

Heilman, K. M., Rothi, L., Campanella, D., & Wolfson, S. (1979). Wernicke's and global aphasia without alexia. *Archives of Neurology, 36,* 129–133.

Heilman, K. M., Safran, A., & Geschwind, N. (1971). Closed head trauma and aphasia. *Journal of Neurology, Neurosurgery, and Psychiatry, 34,* 265–269.

Heilman, K. M., & Scholes, R. J. (1976). The nature of comprehension errors in Broca's, conduction and Wernicke's aphasics. *Cortex, 12,* 258–265.

Heilman, K. M., Schwartz, H. D., & Watson, R. T. (1978). Hypoarousal in patients with the neglect syndrome and emotional indifference. *Neurology, 28,* 229–232.

Helm, N. A., & Barresi, B. (1980). Voluntary control of involuntary utterances: A treatment approach for severe aphasia. In R. H. Brookshire (Ed.), *Clinical aphasiology conference proceedings* (pp. 308–315). Minneapolis, MN: BRK.

Helm-Estabrooks, N. (1981). *Helm Elicited Language Program for Syntax Stimulation (HELPSS).* Chicago: Riverside.

Helm-Estabrooks, N. (1991). *Test of Oral and Limb Apraxia (TOLA).* Austin, TX: Pro-Ed.

Helm-Estabrooks, N. (1992). *Aphasia Diagnostic Profiles.* Austin, TX: Pro-Ed.

Helm-Estabrooks, N., & Albert, M. L. (1991). *A manual of aphasia therapy.* Chicago: Riverside.

Helm-Estabrooks, N., & Albert, M. L. (2004). *Manual of aphasia and aphasia therapy* (2nd ed.). Austin, TX: Pro-Ed.

Helm-Estabrooks, N., Fitzpatrick, P. M., & Barresi, B. N. (1981). Response of an agrammatic patient to a syntax stimulation program for aphasia. *Journal of Speech Hearing Disorders, 46,* 422–427.

Helm-Estabrooks, N., Fitzpatrick, P. M., & Barresi, B. N. (1982). Visual action therapy for global aphasia. *Journal of Speech and Hearing Disorders, 47,* 385–389.

Helm-Estabrooks, N., & Hotz, G. (1990). *Brief Test of Head Injury (BTHI)*. Austin, TX: Pro-Ed.

Helm-Estabrooks, N., & Nicholas, M. (2000). *Sentence Production Program for Aphasia*. Austin, TX: Pro-Ed.

Helm-Estabrooks, N., & Ramsberger, G. (1986). Treatment of agrammatism in long-term Broca's aphasia. *British Journal of Disorders of Communication, 21,* 39–45.

Helm-Estabrooks, N., Ramsberger, G., Morgan, A. R., & Nicholas, M. (1989). *Boston Assessment of Severe Aphasia (BASA)*. Austin, TX: Pro-Ed.

Hemsley, G., & Code, C. (1996). Interactions between recovery in aphasia, emotional and psychosocial factors in subjects with aphasia, their significant others, and speech pathologists. *Disability and Rehabilitation, 18,* 567–584.

Henderson, L. W., Frank, E. M., Pigatt, T., Abramson, R. K., & Houston, M. (1998). Race, gender, and educational level effects on Boston Naming Test scores. *Aphasiology, 12,* 901–911.

Hengst, J. A., (2003). Collaborative referencing between individuals with aphasia and routine communication partners. *Journal of Speech, Language, and Hearing Research, 46,* 831–848.

Hengst, J. A., Frame, S. R., Neuman-Stritzel, T., & Gannaway, R. (2005). Using others' words: Conversational use of reported speech by individuals with aphasia and their communication partners. *Journal of Speech, Language, and Hearing Research, 48,* 137–156.

Henley, S., Pettit, S., Todd-Pokropek, A., & Tupper, A. (1985). Who goes home? Predictive factors in stroke recovery. *Journal of Neurology, Neurosurgery, and Psychiatry, 48,* 1–6.

Herrmann, M., Johannsen-Horbach, H., & Wallesch, C-W. (1993). Empathy and aphasia rehabilitation—Are there contradictory requirements of treatment and psychological support? *Aphasiology, 7,* 575–579.

Herrmann, M., Koch, U., Johannsen-Horbach, H., & Wallesch, C-W. (1989). Communicative skills in chronic and severe nonfluent aphasia. *Brain and Language, 37,* 339–352.

Herrmann, M., & Wallesch, C. W. (1989). Psychosocial changes and psychosocial adjustment with chronic and severe nonfluent aphasia. *Aphasiology, 3,* 513–526.

Hersh, N. A., & Treadgold, L. G. (1994). Neuropage: The rehabilitation of memory dysfunction by prosthetic memory and cuing. *Neurorehabilitation, 4,* 187–197.

Hickin, J., Best, W., Herbert, R., Howard, D., & Osborne, F. (2002). Phonological therapy for word-finding difficulties: A re-evaluation. *Aphasiology, 16,* 981–1000.

Hickok, G., Love-Geffen, T., & Klima, E. S. (2002). Role of the left hemisphere in sign language comprehension. *Brain and Language, 82,* 167–178.

Hilari, K., Byng, S., Lamping, D. L., & Smith, S. C. (2003). Stroke and aphasia quality of life scale-39 (SAQOL-39): Evaluation of acceptability, reliability, and validity. *Stroke, 34,* 1944–1950.

Hillis, A. E. (2001). The organization of the lexical system. In B. Rapp (Ed.), *The handbook of cognitive neuropsychology* (pp. 185–210). Philadelphia: Psychology Press.

Hillis, A. E., Barker, P. B., Wityk, R. J., Aldrich, E. M., Restrepo, L., et al. (2004). Variability in subcortical aphasia is due to variable sites of cortical hypoperfusion. *Brain and Language, 89,* 524–530.

Hillis, A. E., & Caramazza, A. (1991). Category-specific naming and comprehension impairment: A double dissociation. *Brain, 114,* 2081–2094.

Hillis, A. E., & Caramazza, A. (1992). The reading process and its disorders. In D. I. Margolin (Ed.), *Cognitive neuropsychology in clinical practice* (pp. 229–261). New York: Oxford University Press.

Hillis, A. E., & Caramazza, A. (1995a). Converging evidence for the interaction of semantic and sublexical phonological information in accessing lexical representations for spoken output. *Cognitive Neuropsychology, 12,* 187–227.

Hillis, A. E., & Caramazza, A. (1995b). Spatially specific deficits in processing graphemic representations in reading and writing. *Brain and Language, 48,* 263–308.

Hillis, A. E., & Heidler, J. (2002). Mechanisms of early aphasia recovery. *Aphasiology, 16,* 885–895.

Hillis, A. E., & Heidler, J. (2005). Contributions and limitations of the cognitive neuropsychological approach to treatment: Illustrations from studies of reading and spelling therapy. *Aphasiology, 19,* 985–993.

Hillis, A. E., Kane, A., Tuffiash, E., Ulatowski, J. A., Barker, P. B. et al. (2001). Reperfusion of specific brain regions by raising blood pressure restores selective language functions in subacute stroke. *Brain and Language, 79,* 495–510.

Hillis, A. E., Newhart, M., Heidler, J., Marsh, E. B., Barker, P., et al. (2005). The neglected role of the right hemisphere in spatial representation of words for meaning. *Aphasiology, 19,* 225–238.

Hillis, A. E., Wang, P., Barker, P., Beauchamp, N., Gordon, B., et al. (2000). Magnetic resonance perfusion imaging: A new method for localizing regions of brain dysfunction associated with specific lexical impairments? *Aphasiology, 14,* 471–483.

Hinckley, J. J., & Carr, T. H. (2005). Comparing the outcomes of intensive and non-intensive context-based aphasia treatment. *Aphasiology, 19,* 965–974.

Hinckley, J. J., Patterson, J. P., & Carr, T. H. (2001). Differential effects of context- and skill-based treatment approaches: Preliminary findings. *Aphasiology, 15,* 463–476.

Hirsch, F. M., & Holland, A. L. (2000). Beyond activity: Measuring participation in society and quality of life.

In L. E. Worrall & C. M. Frattali (Eds.), *Neurogenic communication disorders: A functional approach* (pp. 35–54). New York: Thieme.

Hodges, J. R., & McCarthy, R. A. (1993). Autobiographical amnesia resulting from bilateral paramedian thalamic infarction. *Brain, 116,* 921–940.

Hodges, J. R., Patterson, K., Ward, R., Garrard, P., Bak, T., et al. (1999). The differentiation of semantic dementia and frontal lobe dementia (temporal and frontal variants of frontotemporal dementia) from early Alzheimer's disease: A comparative neuropsychological study. *Neuropsychology, 13,* 31–40.

Hodges, J. R., Salmon, D. P., & Butters, N. (1992). Semantic memory and impairments in Alzheimer's disease. *Neuropsychologia, 30,* 301–314.

Hoen, B., Thelander, M., & Worsley, J. (1997). Improvement in psychological well-being of people with aphasia and their families: Evaluation of a community-based programme. *Aphasiology, 11,* 681–691.

Hoerster, L., Hickey, E., & Bourgeois, M. (2001). Effects of memory aids on conversations between nursing home residents with dementia and nursing assistants. *Neuropsychological Rehabilitation, 11,* 399–427.

Hofstede, B. T. M., & Kolk, H. H. J. (1994). The effects of task variation on the production of grammatical morphology in Broca's aphasia: A multiple case study. *Brain and Language, 46,* 278–328.

Holland, A. L. (1970). Case studies in aphasia rehabilitation using programmed instruction. *Journal of Speech and Hearing Disorders, 35,* 377–390.

Holland, A. L. (1975). *Aphasics as communicators: A model and its implications.* Paper presented to the American Speech and Hearing Association, November, Washington, D.C.

Holland, A. L. (1977). Some practical considerations in aphasia rehabilitation. In M. Sullivan & M. S. Kommers (Eds.), *Rationale for adult aphasia therapy* (pp. 167–180). University of Nebraska Medical Center.

Holland, A. L. (1978). Functional communication in the treatment of aphasia. In L. J. Branford (Ed.), *Communicative disorders: An audio journal for continuing education.* New York: Grune & Stratton.

Holland, A. L. (1980a). *Communicative abilities in daily living.* Baltimore: University Park Press.

Holland, A. L. (1980b). The usefulness of treatment for aphasia: A serendipitous study. In R. H. Brookshire (Ed.), *Clinical aphasiology conference proceedings* (pp. 240–247). Minneapolis, MN: BRK.

Holland, A. L. (1982). When is aphasia aphasia? The problem of closed head injury. In R. H. Brookshire (Ed.), *Clinical aphasiology conference proceedings* (pp. 345–349). Minneapolis, MN: BRK.

Holland, A. L. (1991). Pragmatic aspects of intervention in aphasia. *Journal of Neurolinguistics, 6,* 197–211.

Holland, A. L. (1995). Patient inputs to increasing understanding of communicative drawing. *Aphasiology, 9,* 57–59.

Holland, A. L. (1998). Why can't clinicians talk to aphasic adults? Comments on supported conversation for adults with aphasia: Methods and resources for training conversational partners. *Aphasiology, 12,* 844–846.

Holland, A. L., & Beeson, P. M. (1993). Finding a new sense of self: What the clinician can do to help. *Aphasiology, 7,* 581–584.

Holland, A. L., & Beeson, P. M. (1999). Aphasia groups: The Arizona experience. In R. J. Elman (Ed.), *Group treatment of neurogenic communication disorders: The expert clinician's approach* (pp. 77–84). Boston: Butterworth Heinemann.

Holland, A. L., Frattali, C. M., & Fromm, D. (1999). *Communication activities of daily living* (2nd ed.). Austin, TX: Pro-Ed.

Holland, A. L., & Fridriksson, J. (2001). Aphasia management during the early phases of recovery following stroke. *American Journal of Speech-Language Pathology, 10,* 19–28.

Holland, A. L., Fromm, D. S., DeRuyter, F., & Stein, M. (1996). Treatment efficacy: Aphasia. *Journal of Speech and Hearing Research, 39,* S27–S36.

Holland, A. L., Greenhouse, J., Fromm, D., & Swindell, C. S. (1989). Predictors of language restitution following stroke: A multivariate analysis. *Journal of Speech and Hearing Research, 32,* 232–238.

Holland, A. L., & Harris, A. (1968). Aphasia rehabilitation using programmed instruction: An intensive case history. In H. N. Sloane & B. D. Macaulay (Eds.), *Operant procedures in remedial speech and language training* (pp. 197–218). New York: Houghton Mifflin.

Holland, A. L., & Sonderman, J. C. (1974). Effects of a program based on the Token Test for teaching comprehension skills to aphasics. *Journal of Speech and Hearing Research, 17,* 589–598.

Holland, A. L., Swindell, C. S., & Forbes, M. M. (1985). The evolution of initial global aphasia: Implications for prognosis. In R. H. Brookshire (Ed.), *Clinical aphasiology* (Vol. 15, pp. 169–175). Minneapolis, MN: BRK.

Holtzapple, P., Pohlman, K., LaPointe, L. L., & Graham, L. F. (1989). Does SPICA and PICA? In T. E. Prescott (Ed.), *Clinical aphasiology* (Vol. 18, pp. 131–144). Boston: College-Hill/Little, Brown.

Hom, J., & Reitan, R. M. (1990). Generalized cognitive function after stroke. *Journal of Clinical and Experimental Neuropsychology, 12,* 644–654.

Hopper, T., & Bayles, K. A. (2001). Management of neurogenic communication disorders associated with dementia. In R. Chapey (Ed.), *Language intervention strategies in adult aphasia and related neurogenic communication disorders* (4th ed., pp. 829–846). Philadelphia: Lippincott Williams & Wilkins.

Hopper, T., & Holland, A. L. (1998). Situation-specific training for adults with aphasia: An example. *Aphasiology, 12,* 933–944.

Hopper, T., Holland, A., & Rewega, M. (2002). Conversational coaching: Treatment outcomes and future directions. *Aphasiology, 16,* 745–762.

Horner, J., Dawson, D., Heyman, A., & Fish, A. M. (1992). The usefulness of the Western Aphasia Battery for differential diagnosis of Alzheimer dementia and focal stroke syndromes: Preliminary evidence. *Brain and Language, 42,* 77–88.

Horner, J., & Wheeler, M. (2005, November 8). HIPAA: Impact on research practices. *The ASHA Leader,* 8–9, 26–27.

Hough, M. S. (1989). Category concept generation in aphasia: The influence of context. *Aphasiology, 3,* 553–568.

Hough, M. S. (1990). Narrative comprehension in adults with right and left hemisphere brain-damage: Theme organization. *Brain and Language, 38,* 253–277.

Hough, M. S. (1993). Treatment of Wernicke's aphasia with jargon: A case study. *Journal of Communication Disorders, 26,* 101–111.

Hough, M. S. (2004). Generative word fluency skills in adults with Parkinson's disease. *Aphasiology, 18,* 581–588.

Hough, M. S., & Barrow, I. (2003). Descriptive discourse abilities of traumatic brain-injured adults. *Aphsiology, 17,* 183–191.

Hough, M. S., & Givens, G. D. (2004). Word fluency skills in dementia of the Alzheimer's type for common and goal-directed categories. *Aphasiology, 18,* 357–371.

Howard, D., & Patterson, K. (1992). *Pyramids and Palm Trees.* San Antonio, TX: Harcourt Assessment.

Howard, D., Patterson, K., Franklin, S., Orchard-Lisle, V., & Morton, J. (1985a). The facilitation of picture naming in aphasia. *Cognitive Neuropsychology, 2,* 49–80.

Howard, D., Patterson, K., Franklin, S., Orchard-Lisle, V., & Morton, J. (1985b). Treatment of word retrieval deficits in aphasia. *Brain, 108,* 817–829.

Howe, T. J., Worrall, L. E., & Hickson, L. M. H. (2004). What is an aphasia-friendly environment? *Aphasiology, 18,* 1015–1037.

Howes, D. H. (1964). Application of the word-frequency concept for aphasia. In A. V. S. de Reuck & M. O'Conner (Eds.), *Disorders of the language.* London: Churchill.

Huber, M. (1946). Linguistic problems of brain-injured servicemen. *Journal of Speech and Hearing Disorders, 11,* 143–147.

Huber, W., & Gleber, J. (1982). Linguistic and nonlinguistic processing of narratives in aphasia. *Brain and Language, 16,* 1–18.

Huff, F. J., Collins, C., Corkin, S., & Rosen, J. T. (1986). Equivalent forms of the Boston Naming Test. *Journal of Clinical and Experimental Neuropsychology, 8,* 556–562.

Hughes, C. P., Berg, L., Danziger, W. L., Cohen, L. A., & Martin, R. L. (1982). A new clinical scale for the staging of dementia. *British Journal of Psychiatry, 140,* 566–572.

Hunt, J. (1999). Drawing on the semantic system: The use of drawing as a therapy medium. In Byng, S., Swinburn, K., & Pound, C. (Eds.), *The aphasia therapy file* (pp. 41–60). Hove, UK: Psychology Press.

Hutton, C. (2005). *After a stroke: 300 tips for making life easier.* New York: Demos Medical Publishing.

Illes, J., Metter, E. J., Dennings, R., Jackson, C., Kempler, D., & Hanson, W. R. (1989). Spontaneous language production in mild aphasia: Relationship to left prefrontal glucose hypometabolism. *Aphasiology, 3,* 527–537.

Ip, R. Y., Dornan, J., & Schentag, C. (1995). Traumatic brain injury: Factors predicting return to work or school. *Brain Injury, 9,* 517–532.

Irwin, W. H., Wertz, R. T., & Avent, J. R. (2002). Relationships among language impairment, functional communication, and pragmatic performance in aphasia. *Aphasiology, 16,* 823–835.

Itoh, M., Sasanuma, S., Hirose, H., Yoshioka, H., & Sawashima, M. (1983). Velar movements during speech in two Wernicke aphasic patients. *Brain and Language, 19,* 283–292.

Itoh, M., Sasanuma, S., Tatsumi, I. F., Murakami, S., Fukusako, Y., & Suzuki, T. (1982). Voice onset time characteristics in apraxia of speech. *Brain and Language, 17,* 193–210.

Jacobs, B. J. (2001). Social validity of changes in informativeness and efficiency of aphasic discourse following Linguistic Specific Treatment (LST). *Brain and Language, 78,* 115–127.

Jacobs, B. J., & Thompson, C. K. (2000). Cross-modal generalization effects of training noncanonical sentence comprehension and production in agrammatic aphasia. *Journal of Speech, Language, and Hearing Research, 43,* 5–20.

Jennett, B., & Bond, M. (1975). Assessment of outcome after severe brain damage. *Lancet, 1,* 480–484.

Jennett, B., & Teasdale, G. (1981). *Management of head injuries.* Philadelphia: F. A. Davis.

Joanette, Y., & Ansaldo, A. I. (1999). Clinical note: Acquired pragmatic impairments and aphasia. *Brain and Language, 68,* 529–534.

Joanette, Y., Goulet, P., & Le Dorze, G. (1988). Impaired word naming in right-brain-damaged right-handers:

Error types and time-course analyses. *Brain and Language, 34,* 54–64.

Joanette, Y., Goulet, P., Ska, B., & Nespoulous, J-L. (1986). Informative content of narrative discourse in right-brain-damaged right-handers. *Brain and Language, 29,* 81–105.

Johannsen-Horback, H., Cegla, B., Mager, U., Schempp, B., & Wallesch, C-W. (1985). Treatment of chronic global aphasia with a non-verbal communication system. *Brain and Language, 24,* 74–82.

Johnson, R. (1998). How do people get back to work after severe head injury? A 10 year follow-up study. *Neuropsychological Rehabilitation, 8,* 61–79.

Johnson-Laird, P. N. (1983). *Mental models.* Cambridge, UK: Cambridge University Press.

Johnstone, B., & Stonnington, H. H. (Eds.). (2001). *Rehabilitation of neuropsychological disorders: A practical guide for rehabilitation professionals.* Philadelphia: Psychology Press.

Jonkers, R., & Bastiannse, R. (1998). How selective are selective word class deficits. Two case studies of action and object naming. *Aphasiology, 12,* 245–256.

Junque, C., Vendrell, P., Vendrell-Brucet, J. M., & Tobena, A., (1989). Differential recovery in naming in bilingual aphasics. *Brain and Language, 36,* 16–22.

Just, M. A., Carpenter, P. A., & Keller, T. A. (1996). The capacity theory of comprehension: New frontiers of evidence and arguments. *Psychological Review, 103,* 773–780.

Kaan, E., & Swaab, T. Y. (2003). Electrophysiological evidence for serial sentence processing: A comparison between non-preferred and ungrammatical continuations. *Cognitive Brain Research, 17,* 621–635.

Kagan, A. (1998). Supported conversation for adults with aphasia: Methods and resources for training conversation partners. *Aphasiology, 12,* 816–830.

Kagan, A., Black, S. E., Duchan, J. F., Simmons-Mackie, N., & Square, P. (2001). Training volunteers as conversation partners using "Supported Conversation for Adults with Aphasia" (SCA): A controlled trial. *Journal of Speech, Language, and Hearing Research, 44,* 624–638.

Kagan, A., & Cohen-Schneider, R. (1999). Groups in the introductory program at the Pat Arato Aphasia Centre. In R. J. Elman (Ed.), *Group treatment of neurogenic communication disorders: The expert clinician's approach* (pp. 97–106). Boston: Butterworth Heinemann.

Kahn, H. J., Joanette, Y., Ska, B., & Goulet, P. (1990). Discourse analysis in neuropsychology: Comment on Chapman and Ulatowska. *Brain and Language, 38,* 454–461.

Kaplan, E., Goodglass, H., & Weintraub, (1983). *The Boston Naming Test.* Philadelphia: Lea & Febiger.

Kaplan, J. A., Brownell, H. H., Jacobs, J. R., & Gardner, H. (1990). The effects of right hemisphere damage on the pragmatic interpretation of conversational remarks. *Brain and Language, 38,* 315–333.

Kapur, N. (1994). Remembering Norman Schwarzkopf: Evidence for two distinct long-term fact learning mechanisms. *Cognitive Neuropsychology, 11,* 661–670.

Karbe, H., Thiel, A., Weber-Luxenburger, G., Herholz, K., Kessler, J., & Heiss, W-D. (1998). Brain plasticity in poststroke aphasia: What is the contribution of the right hemisphere? *Brain and Language, 64,* 215–230.

Karow, C. M., Marquardt, T. P., & Marshall, R. C. (2001). Affective processing in left and right hemisphere brain-damaged subjects with and without subcortical involvement. *Aphasiology, 15,* 715–729.

Karzmark, P., Heaton, R. K., Lehman, R. A. W., & Crouch, J. (1985). Utility of the Seashore Tonal Memory Test in neuropsychological assessment. *Journal of Clinical and Experimental Neuropsychology, 7,* 367–374.

Kashiwagi, T., Kashiwagi, A., Kunimori, Y., Yamadori, A., Tanabe, H., & Okuda, J. (1994). Preserved capacity to copy drawings in severe aphasics with little premorbid experience. *Aphasiology, 8,* 427–442.

Katz, R. C. (2001). Computer applications in aphasia treatment. In R. Chapey (Ed.), *Language intervention strategies in adult aphasia and related neurogenic communication disorders* (4th ed., pp. 718–741). Philadelphia: Lippincott Williams & Wilkins.

Katz, W. F. (1988). An investigation of lexical ambiguity in Broca's aphasics using an auditory lexical priming technique. *Neuropsychologia, 26,* 747–752.

Kaufman, A. S., & Lichtenberger, E. (1999). *Essentials of WAIS-III Assessment.* New York: Wiley.

Kay, J., & Ellis, A.W. (1987). A cognitive neuropsychological case study of anomia: Implications for psychological models of word retrieval. *Brain, 110,* 613–629.

Kay, J., Lesser, R., & Coltheart, M. (1992). *PALPA: Psycholinguistic Assessments of Language Processing in Aphasia.* Hove, UK: Lawrence Erlbaum.

Kay, J., Lesser, R., & Coltheart, M. (1996a). Psycholinguistic Assessments of Language Processing in Aphasia (PALPA): An introduction. *Aphasiology, 10,* 159–180.

Kay, J., Lesser, R., & Coltheart, M. (1996b). PALPA: The proof of the pudding is in the eating. *Aphasiology, 10,* 202–215.

Kay, J., & Terry, R. (2004). Ten years on: Lessons learned from published studies that cite the PALPA. *Aphasiology, 18,* 127–151.

Kazdin, A. E. (1982). *Single-case research designs: Methods for clinical and applied settings.* New York: Oxford University Press.

Kazdin, A. E. (Ed.). (1998). *Methodological issues & strategies in clinical research* (2nd ed.). Washington, DC: American Psychological Association.

Kearns, K. P. (1985). Response elaboration training for patient initiated utterances. In R. H. Brookshire (Ed.), *Clinical Aphasiology* (Vol. 15, pp. 196–204). Minneapolis: BRK.

Kearns, K. P. (1986a). Flexibility of single-subject experimental designs. Part II: Design selection and arrangement of experimental phases. *Journal of Speech and Hearing Disorders, 51,* 204–214.

Kearns, K. P. (1986b). Systematic programming of verbal elaboration skills in chronic Broca's aphasia. In R. C. Marshall (Ed.), *Case studies in aphasia rehabilitation: For clinicians by clinicians* (pp. 225–244). Austin, TX: Pro-Ed.

Kearns, K. P. (1989). Methodologies for studying generalization. In L. V. McReynolds & J. Spradlin (Eds.). *Generalization strategies in the treatment of communication disorders* (pp. 13–30). Lewiston, NY: BC Decker.

Kearns, K. P. (2005). Broca's aphasia. In L. L. LaPointe (Ed.), *Aphasia and related neurogenic language disorders* (3rd ed., pp. 117–141). New York: Thieme.

Kearns, K. P., & Elman, R. J. (2001). Group therapy for aphasia: Theoretical and practical considerations. In R. Chapey (Ed.), *Language intervention strategies in adult aphasia and related neurogenic communication disorders* (4th ed., pp. 316–337). Philadelphia: Lippincott Williams & Wilkins.

Kearns, K. P., & Salmon, S. J. (1984). An experimental analysis of auxiliary and copula verb generalization in aphasia. *Journal of Speech and Hearing Disorders, 49,* 152–163.

Kearns, K. P., & Scher, G. P. (1989). The generalization of response elaboration training effects. In T. E. Prescott (Ed.), *Clinical aphasiology* (Vol. 18, pp. 223–246). Boston: College-Hill.

Kearns, K. P., & Yedor, K. (1991). An alternating treatments comparison of loose training and a convergent treatment strategy. In T. E. Prescott (Ed.), *Clinical aphasiology* (Vol. 20, pp. 223–238). Austin, TX: Pro-Ed.

Keefe, K. A. (1995). Applying basic neuroscience to aphasia therapy: What the animals are telling us. *American Journal of Speech-Language Pathology, 4*(4), 88–93.

Keenan, J. S., & Brassell, E. G. (1974). A study of factors related to prognosis for individual aphasic patients. *Journal of Speech and Hearing Disorders, 39,* 257–269.

Keenan, J. S., & Brassell, E. G. (1975). *Aphasia language performance scales.* Murfreesboro, TN: Pinnacle Press.

Kellermann, K., Broetzmann, S., Lim, T., & Kitao, K. (1989). The conversation MOP: Scenes in the stream of discourse. *Discourse Processes, 12,* 27–61.

Kemmerer, D., & Tranel, D. (2000a). Verb retrieval in brain-damaged subjects: 1. Analysis of stimulus, lexical, and conceptual factors. *Brain and Language, 73,* 347–392.

Kemmerer, D., & Tranel, D. (2000b). Verb retrieval in brain-damaged subjects: 2. Analysis of errors. *Brain and Language, 73,* 393–420.

Kempler, D., Curtiss, S., & Jackson, C. (1987). Syntactic preservation in Alzheimer's disease. *Journal of Speech and Hearing Research, 30,* 343–350.

Kendall, D. L., McNeil, M. R., & Small, S. L. (1998). Rule-based treatment for acquired phonological dyslexia. *Aphasiology, 12,* 587–600.

Kenin, M., & Swisher, L. P. (1972). A study of pattern of recovery in aphasia. *Cortex, 8,* 56–68.

Kennedy, M., & Murdoch, B. E. (1991). Patterns of speech and language recovery following left striato-capsular hemorrhage. *Aphasiology, 5,* 489–510.

Kennedy, M., & Murdoch, B. E. (1994). Thalamic aphasia and striato-capsular aphasia as independent aphasic syndromes. *Aphasiology, 8,* 303–313.

Kennedy, M. R. T. (2000). Topic scenes in conversations with adults with right-hemisphere brain damage. *American Journal of Speech-Language Pathology, 9,* 72–86.

Kennedy, M. R. T., & Nawrocki, M. D. (2003). Delayed predictive accuracy of narrative recall after traumatic brain injury: Salience and explicitness. *Journal of Speech, Language, and Hearing Research, 46,* 98–112.

Kerschensteiner, M., Poeck, K., & Brunner, E. (1972). The fluency-nonfluency dimension in the classification of aphasic speech. *Cortex, 8,* 233–247.

Kertesz, A. (1979). *Aphasia and associated disorders: Taxonomy, localization, and recovery.* New York: Grune & Stratton.

Kertesz, A. (1982). *Western Aphasia Battery.* New York: Grune & Stratton.

Kertesz, A. (1985). Recovery and treatment. In K. M. Heilman & E. Valenstein (Eds.), *Clinical neuropsychology* (2nd ed., pp. 481–505). New York: Oxford University Press.

Kertesz, A. (2006). *Western Aphasia Battery-Enhanced.* San Antonio, TX: Harcourt Assessment.

Kertesz, A., & Benson, D. F., (1970). Neologistic jargon—A clinicopatholgical study. *Cortex, 6,* 362–386.

Kertesz, A., Ferro, J. M., & Shewan, C. M. (1984). Apraxia and aphasia: The functional-anatomical basis for their dissociation. *Neurology, 34,* 40–47.

Kertesz, A., Harlock, W., & Coates, R. (1979). Computer topographic localiztion, lesion size and prognosis in aphasia. *Brain and Language, 8,* 34–50.

Kertesz, A., Lau, W. K., & Polk, M. (1993). The structural determinants of recovery in Wernicke's aphasia. *Brain and Language, 44,* 153–165.

Kertesz, A., Lesk, D., & McCabe, P. (1977). Isotope localization of infarcts in aphasia. *Archives of Neurology, 34,* 590–601.

Kertesz, A., & McCabe, P. (1975). Intelligence and aphasia: Performance of aphasics on Raven's Coloured Progressive Matrices (RCPM). *Brain and Language, 2,* 387–395.

Kertesz, A., & McCabe, P. (1977). Recovery patterns and prognosis in aphasia. *Brain, 100,* 1–18.

Kertesz, A., & Munoz, D. G. (1997). Primary progressive aphasia. *Clinical Neuroscience, 4,* 95–102.

Kertesz, A., & Phipps, J. B. (1977). Numerical taxonomy of aphasia. *Brain and Language, 4,* 1–10.

Kertesz, A., & Poole, E. (1974). The aphasia quotient: The taxonomic approach to measurement of aphasic disability. *Canadian Journal of Neurological Sciences, 1,* 7–16.

Kiernan, R. J., Mueller, J., & Langston, J. W., & Van Dyke, C. (1987). The Neurobehavioral Cognitive Status Examination: A brief but quantitative approach to cognitive assessment. *Annals of Internal Medicine, 107,* 481–485.

Kim, M., & Thompson, C. K. (2000). Patterns of comprehension and production of nouns and verbs in agrammatism: Implications for lexical organization. *Brain and Language, 74,* 1–25.

Kim, M., & Thompson, C. K. (2004). Verb deficits in Alzheimer's disease and agrammatism: Implications for lexical organization. *Brain and Language, 88,* 10–20.

Kimmel, D. C. (1974). *Adulthood and aging.* New York: John Wiley.

Kintsch, W. (1994). The psychology of discourse processing. In M. A. Gernsbacher (Ed.), *Handbook of psycholinguistics* (pp. 721–740). San Diego, CA: Academic Press.

Kintsch, W. (1998). *Comprehension: A paradigm for cognition.* Cambridge, UK: Cambridge University Press.

Kiran, S., & Thompson, C. K. (2003a). Effect of typicality on online category verification of animate category exemplars in aphasia. *Brain and Language, 85,* 441–450.

Kiran, S., & Thompson, C. K. (2003b). The role of semantic complexity in treatment of naming deficits: Training semantic categories in fluent aphasia by controlling exemplar typicality. *Journal of Speech, Language, and Hearing Research, 46,* 773–787.

Kirk, A., & Kertesz, A. (1994). Cortical and subcortical aphasias compared. *Aphasiology, 8,* 65–82.

Kirshner, H. S., Casey, P. F., Henson, J., & Heinrich, J. J. (1989). Behavioural features and lesion localization in Wernicke's aphasia. *Aphasiology, 3,* 169–176.

Kirshner, H. S., Webb, W. G., & Duncan, G. W. (1981). Word deafness in Wernicke's aphasia. *Journal of Neurology, Neurosurgery, and Psychiatry, 45,* 197–201.

Klepousniotou, E., & Baum, S. R. (2005). Unilateral brain damage effects on processing homonymous and polysemous words. *Brain and Language, 93,* 308–326.

Klima, E. S., Bellugi, U., & Poizner, H. (1988). Grammar and space in sign aphasiology. *Aphasiology, 2,* 319–328.

Knopman, D. S., Selnes, O. A., Niccum, N., & Rubens, A. B. (1984). Recovery of naming in aphasia: Relationship to fluency, comprehension and CT findings. *Neurology, 34,* 1461–1471.

Koemeda-Lutz, M., Cohen, R., & Meier, E. (1987). Organization of and access to semantic memory in aphasia. *Brain and Language, 30,* 321–337.

Kohn, S. E., & Goodglass, H. (1985). Picture-naming in aphasia. *Brain and Language, 24,* 266–283.

Kohn, S. E., & Smith, K. L. (1990). Between-word speech errors in conduction aphasia. *Cognitive Neuropsychology, 7,* 133–156.

Kohn, S. E., & Smith, K. L. (1995). Serial effects of phonemic planning during word production. *Aphasiology, 9,* 209–222.

Kohn, S. E., Smith, K. L., & Arsenault, J. (1990). The remediation of conduction aphasia via sentence repetition: A case study. *British Journal of Disorders of Communication, 25,* 45.

Kolk, H. H. J., & Heeschen, C. (1990). Adaptation symptoms and impairment symptoms in Broca's aphasia. *Aphasiology, 4,* 221–232.

Kolk, H. H. J., & Heeschen, C. (1992). Agrammatism, paragrammatism and the management of language. *Language and Cognitive Processes, 7,* 89–130.

Kolk, H. H. J., & van Grunsven, M. M. (1985). Agrammatism as a variable phenomenon. *Cognitive Neuropsychology, 2,* 347–384.

Kopelman, M. D., Wilson, B. A., and Baddeley, A. D. (1989). The Autobiographical Memory Interview: A new assessment of personal and autobiographical semantic memory in amnesic patients. *Journal of Clinical and Experimental Neuropsychology, 11,* 724–744.

Koul, R. K., & Lloyd, L. L. (1998). Comparison of graphic symbol learning in individuals with aphasia and right hemisphere brain damage. *Brain and Language, 62,* 398–421.

Koyama, Y., Ishiai, S., Seki, K., & Nakayama, T. (1997). Distinct processes in line bisection according to severity of left unilateral spatial neglect. *Brain and Cognition, 35,* 271–281.

Kudo, T. (1984). The effect of semantic plausibility on sentence comprehension in aphasia. *Brain and Language, 21,* 208–218.

Labourel, D., & Martin, M-M. (1993). The person with aphasia and the family. In D. Lafond, Y. Joanette, J. Ponzio, R. Degiovani, & M. T. Sarno (Eds.), *Living with aphasia: Psychosocial issues* (pp. 151–172). San Diego, CA: Singular.

Laiacona, M., & Caramazza, A. (2004). The noun/verb dissociation in language production: Varieties of causes. *Cognitive Neuropsychology, 21,* 103–124.

Lambier, J. D., & Bradley, D. (1991). The effects of physical similarity on pantomime recognition in aphasia. *Aphasiology, 5,* 23–37.

LaPointe, L. L. (1985). Aphasia therapy: Some principles and strategies for treatment. In D. F. Johns (Ed.), *Clinical management of neurogenic communicative disorders* (pp. 179–241). Boston: Little, Brown.

LaPointe, L. L., & Erickson, R. J. (1991). Auditory vigilance during divided task attention in aphasic individuals. *Aphasiology, 5,* 511–520.

LaPointe, L. L., & Horner, J. (1998). *Reading Comprehension Battery for Aphasia* (rev. ed.). Austin, TX: Pro-Ed.

Lawton, M. P., & Rubinstein, R. L. (Eds.). (2000). *Interventions in dementia care: Toward improving quality of life.* New York: Springer.

Le Dorze, G., Boulay, N., Gaudreau, J., & Brassard, C. (1994). The contrasting effects of a semantic versus a formal-semantic technique for the facilitation of naming in a case of anomia. *Aphasiology, 8,* 127–141.

Le Dorze, G., & Brassard, C. (1995). A description of the consequences of aphasia on aphasic persons and their relatives and friends, based on the WHO model of chronic diseases. *Aphasiology, 9,* 239–255.

Le Dorze, G., & Nespoulous, J-L. (1989). Anomia in moderate aphasia: Problems in accessing the lexical representation. *Brain and Language, 37,* 381–400.

Lee, C., Grossman, M., Morris, J., Stern, M. B., & Hurtig, H. I. (2003). Attentional resource and processing speed limitations during sentence processing in Parkinson's disease. *Brain and Language, 85,* 347–356.

Legg, C., Young, L., & Bryer, A. (2003). Training sixth-year medical students in obtaining case-history information from adults with aphasia. *Aphasiology, 19,* 559–575.

Lehman-Blake, M. T. (2005). Right hemisphere syndrome. In L. L. LaPointe (Ed.), *Aphasia and related neurogenic language disorders* (3rd ed., pp. 213–224). New York: Thieme.

Lehman-Blake, M. T., Duffy, J. R., Myers, P. S., & Tompkins, C. A. (2002). Prevalence and patterns of right hemisphere cognitive/communicative deficits: Retrospective data from an inpatient rehabilitation unit. *Aphasiology, 16,* 537–548.

Lehman-Blake, M. T., Duffy, J. R., Tompkins, C. A., & Myers, P. A. (2003). Right hemisphere syndrome is in the eye of the beholder. *Aphasiology, 17,* 423–432.

Lehman-Blake, M. T., & Lesniewicz, K. S. (2005). Contextual bias and predictive inferencing in adults with and without right hemisphere brain damage. *Aphasiology, 19,* 423–434.

Le May, A., David, R., & Thomas, A. P. (1988). The use of spontaneous gesture by aphasic patients. *Aphasiology, 2,* 137–146.

Lemme, M. L., Hedberg, N. L., & Bottenberg, D. E. (1984). Cohesion in narratives of aphasic adults. In R. H. Brookshire (Ed.), *Clinical aphasiology conference proceedings* (pp. 215–222). Minneapolis: BRK.

Lendrem, W., & Lincoln, N. B. (1985). Spontaneous recovery of language in patients with aphasia between 4 and 34 weeks after stroke. *Journal of Neurology, Neurosurgery, and Psychiatry, 48,* 743–748.

Leon, S. A., Rosenbek, J. C., Crucian, G. P., Hieber, B., Holiway, B., et al. (2005). Active treatments for aprosodia secondary to right hemisphere stroke. *Journal of Rehabilitation Research and Development, 42,* 93–102.

Leonard, C. L., & Baum, S. R. (1997). The influence of phonological and orthographic information on auditory lexical access in brain-damaged patients: A preliminary investigation. *Aphasiology, 11,* 1031–1041.

Leonard, L. L. (1998). *Children with specific language impairment.* Cambridge, MA: MIT Press.

Lesser, R., & Perkins, L. (1999). *Cognitive neuropsychology and conversation analysis in aphasia: An introductory casebook.* London: Whurr.

Levin, H. S., Goldstein, F. C., High, W. M., & Williams, D. (1988). Automatic and effortful processing after severe closed head injury. *Brain and Cognition, 7,* 283–297.

Levin, H. S., Grossman, R. G., & Kelly, P. J. (1976). Aphasic disorders in patients with closed head injury. *Journal of Neurology, Neurosurgery, and Psychiatry, 39,* 1062–1070.

Levin, H. S., Grossman, R. G., Sarwar, M., & Meyers, C. A. (1981). Linguistic recovery after closed head injury. *Brain and Language, 12,* 360–374.

Levin, H. S., O'Donnell, V. M., & Grossman, R. G. (1979). The Galveston orientation and amnesia test: A practical scale to assess cognition after head injury. *Journal of Nervous and Mental Disease, 167,* 675–684.

Levine, D. N., & Sweet, E. (1983). Localization of lesions in Broca's aphasia. In A. Kertesz (Ed.), *Localization in neuropsychology* (pp. 185–208). New York: Academic Press.

Lezak, M. D., Howieson, D. B., Loring, D. W., Hannay, J. J., & Fischer, J. S. (2004). *Neuropsychological assessment* (4th ed.). New York: Oxford University Press.

Lezak, M. D., & O'Brien, K. P. (1988). Longitudinal study of emotional, social, and physical changes after traumatic brain injury. *Journal of Learning Disability, 21,* 456–465.

Li, E. C., Kitselman, K., Dusatko, D., & Spinelli, C. (1988). The efficacy of PACE in the remediation of naming deficits. *Journal of Communication Disorders, 21,* 491–503.

Li, E. C., & Williams, S. E. (1989). The efficacy of two types of cues in aphasic patients. *Aphasiology, 3,* 619–626.

Li, E. C., & Williams, S. E. (1990). The effects of grammatic class and cue type on cueing responsiveness in aphasia. *Brain and Language, 38,* 48–60.

Liles, B. Z., & Brookshire, R. H. (1975). The effects of pause time on auditory comprehension of aphasic subjects. *Journal of Communication Disorders, 8,* 221–236.

Liles, B. Z., Coelho, C. A., Duffy, R. J., & Zalagens, M. R. (1989). Effects of elicitation procedures on the narratives of normal and closed head-injured adults. *Journal of Speech and Hearing Disorders, 54,* 356–366.

Lincoln, N. B., & Ells, P. (1980). A shortened version of the PICA. *British Journal of Disorders of Communication, 15,* 183–187.

Lincoln, N. B., McGuirk, E., Mully, G. P., Lendrem, W., Jones, A. C., & Mitchell, J. R. A. (1984). The effectiveness of speech therapy for aphasic stroke patients: A randomized controlled trial. *Lancet, 1,* 1197–1200.

Linebarger, M. C. (1990). Neuropsychology of sentence parsing. In A. Caramazza (Ed.), *Cognitive neuropsychology and neurolinguistics: Advances in models of cognitive function and impairment* (pp. 55–122). Hillsdale, NJ: Lawrence Erlbaum.

Linebarger, M. C., McCall, D., & Berndt, R. S. (2004). The role of processing support in the remediation of aphasic language production disorders. *Cognitive Neuropsychology, 21,* 267–282.

Linebarger, M. C., & Schwartz, M. F. (2005). AAC for hypothesis testing and treatment of aphasic language production: Lessons from a processing "prosthesis." *Aphasiology, 19,* 930–942.

Linebarger, M. C., Schwartz, M. F., Romania, J. R., Kohn, S. E., & Stephens, D. L. (2000). Grammatical encoding in aphasia: Evidence from a "processing prosthesis." *Brain and Language, 75,* 416–427.

Linebarger, M. C., Schwartz, M. F., & Saffran, E. M. (1983). Sensitivity to grammatical structure in so-called agrammatic aphasics. *Cognition, 13,* 361–392.

Linebaugh, C. W. (1983). Treatment of anomic aphasia. In W. H. Perkins (Ed.), *Language handicaps in adults* (pp. 35–44). New York: Thieme-Stratton.

Linebaugh, C. W., Margulies, C. P., & Mackisack-Morin, E. L. (1984). The effectiveness of comprehension-enhancing strategies employed by spouses of aphasic patients. In R. H. Brookshire (Ed.), *Clinical aphasiology conference proceedings* (pp. 188–197). Minneapolis: BRK.

Lohman, T., Ziggas, D., & Pierce, R. S. (1989). Word fluency performance on common categories by subjects with closed head injuries. *Aphasiology, 3,* 685–694.

Lomas, J., & Kertesz, A. (1978). Patterns of spontaneous recovery in aphasic groups: A study of adult stroke patients. *Brain and Language, 5,* 388–401.

Lomas, J., Pickard, L., Bester, S., Elbard, H., Finlayson, A., et al. (1989). The Communicative Effectiveness Index: Development and psychometric evaluation of a functional communication measure for adult aphasia. *Journal of Speech and Hearing Disorders, 54,* 113–124.

Love, R. J., & Webb, W. J. (1977). The efficacy of cueing techniques in Broca's aphasia. *Journal of Speech and Hearing Disorders, 42,* 170–178.

Love, T., Swinney, D., Wong, E., & Buxton, R. (2002). Perfusion imaging and stroke: A more sensitive measure of the brain bases of cognitive deficits. *Aphasiology, 16,* 873–883.

Lovell, M. R. (2006). Neuropsychological assessment of the professional athlete. In R. J. Echemendía (Ed.), *Sports neuropsychology: Assessment and management of traumatic brain injury* (pp. 176–192). New York: Guilford Press.

Loverso, F. L., Prescott, T. E., & Selinger, M. (1988). Cueing verbs: A treatment strategy for aphasic adults. *Journal of Rehabilitation Research, 25,* 47–60.

Lowell, S., Beeson, P. M., & Holland, A. L. (1995). The efficacy of a semantic cueing procedure on naming performance of adults with aphasia. *American Journal of Speech-Language Pathology, 4*(4), 109–114.

Lubinski, R. (2001). Environmental systems approach to adult aphasia. In R. Chapey (Ed.), *Language intervention strategies in adult aphasia and related neurogenic communication disorders* (4th ed., pp. 269–296). Philadelphia: Lippincott Williams & Wilkins.

Lubinski, R., Duchan, J., & Weitzner-Lin, B. (1980). Analysis of breakdowns and repairs in aphasic adult communication. In R. H. Brookshire (Ed.), *Clinical aphasiology conference proceedings* (pp. 111–116). Minneapolis: BRK.

Lucchelli, F., Muggia, S., & Spinnler, H. (1997). Selective proper name anomia: A case involving only contemporary celebrities. *Cognitive Neuropsychology, 14,* 881–900.

Luria, A. R. (1966). *Higher cortical functions in man.* New York: Basic Books.

Luria, A. R. (1970a). The functional organization of the brain. *Scientific American, 222*(3), 66–78.

Luria, A. R. (1970b). *Traumatic aphasia.* The Hague, Netherlands: Mouton.

Luzzatti, C., Toraldo, A., Guasti, M. T., Ghirardi, G., Lorenzi, L., et al. (2001). Comprehension of reversible active and passive sentences in agrammatism. *Aphasiology, 15,* 419–441.

Luzzatti, C., Willmes, K., Taricco, M., Colombo, C., & Chiesa, G. (1989). Language disturbances after severe head injury: Do neurological or other associated cognitive disorders influence type, severity and evolution of the verbal impairment? A preliminary report. *Aphasiology, 3,* 643–654.

Lyon, J. G. (1992). Communication use and participation in life for adults with aphasia in natural settings: The scope of the problem. *American Journal of Speech-Language Pathology, 1*(3), 7–14.

Lyon, J. G. (1995). Communicative drawing: An augmentative mode of interaction. *Aphasiology, 9,* 84–94.

Lyon, J. G. (1998). *Coping with aphasia.* San Diego, CA: Singular.

Lyon, J. G. (2001). Treating life consequences of aphasia's chronicity. In R. Chapey (Ed.), *Language intervention strategies in adult aphasia and related neurogenic communication disorders* (4th ed., pp. 297–315). Philadelphia: Lippincott Williams & Wilkins.

Lyon, J. G., Cariski, D., Keisler, L., Rosenbek, J., Levine, R., et al. (1997). Communication partners: Enhancing participation in life and communication for adults with aphasia in natural settings. *Aphasiology, 11,* 693–708.

Lyon, J. G., & Sims, E. (1989). Drawing: Its use as a communicative aid with aphasic and normal adults. In T. E. Prescott (Ed.), *Clinical aphasiology* (Vol. 18, pp. 339–355). Boston: College-Hill/Little, Brown.

MacDonald, M. C., Almor, A., Henderson, V. W., Kempler, D., & Andersen, E. S. (2001). Assessing working memory and language comprehension in Alzheimer's disease. *Brain and Language, 78,* 17–42.

Mace, N. L., & Rabins, P. V. (1999). *The 36-hour day* (3rd ed.). Baltimore: Johns Hopkins University Press.

Mack, J. L., & Boller, F. (1979). Components of auditory comprehension: Analysis of errors in a revised Token Test. In F. Boller & M. Dennis (Eds.), *Auditory comprehension: Clinical and experimental studies with the Token Test* (pp. 45–70). New York: Academic Press.

Mackenzie, C., & Paton, G. (2003). Resumption of driving with aphasia following stroke. *Aphasiology, 17,* 107–121.

MacMillan, P. J., Hart, R. P., Martelli, M. F., & Zasler, N. D. (2002). Pre-injury status and adaptation following traumatic brain injury. *Brain Injury, 16,* 41–49.

MacWhinney, B., & Osman-Sagi, J. (1991). Inflectional marking in Hungarian aphasics. *Brain and Language, 41,* 165–183.

MacWhinney, B., Osman-Sagi, J., & Slobin, D. I. (1991). Sentence comprehension in aphasia in two clear case-marking languages. *Brain and Language, 41,* 234–249.

Madden, M. L., Oelschlaeger, M. L., & Damico, J. S. (2002). The conversational value of laughter for a person with aphasia. *Aphasiology, 16,* 1199–1212.

Mahendra, N. (2004). *Modifying the Communicative Abilities of Daily Living (CADL-2) for use with illiterate persons with aphasia: Preliminary results.* Retrieved October 21, 2005, from http://speechpathology.com/articles/pf_arc_disp.asp?id=242.

Mahoney, F. I., & Barthel, D. (1965). Functional evaluation: The Barthel Index. *Maryland Medical Journal, 14,* 56–61.

Mandleberg, I. A., & Brooks, D. N. (1975). Cognitive recovery after severe head injury: 1. Serial testing on the Wechsler Adult Intelligence Scale. *Journal of Neurology, Neurosurgery, and Psychiatry, 38,* 1121–1126.

Mandler, J. M. (1987). On the psychological reality of story structure. *Discourse Processes, 10,* 1–29.

Margolin, D. I., Pate, D. S., & Friedrich, F. J. (1996). Lexical priming by pictures and words in normal aging and in dementia of the Alzheimer's type. *Brain and Language, 54,* 275–301.

Mariner, W. K. (1994). Outcomes assessment in health care reform: Promise and limitations. *American Journal of Law & Medicine, 20,* 36–57.

Marini, A., Carlomagno, S., Caltagirone, C., & Nocentini, U. (2005). The role played by the right hemisphere in the organization of complex textual structures. *Brain and Language, 93,* 46–54.

Marks, M. M., Taylor, M., & Rusk, H. A. (1957). Rehabilitation of the aphasic patient: A survey of three years' experience in a rehabilitation setting. *Neurology, 7,* 837–843.

Marler, J. R. (2005). *Stroke for dummies.* Indianapolis, IN: Wiley.

Marsh, N. V. (1999). Social skill deficits following traumatic brain injury: Assessment and treatment. In S. McDonald, L. Togher, & C. Code (Eds.), *Communication disorders following traumatic brain injury* (pp. 175–210). Hove, UK: Psychology Press.

Marsh, N. V., & Knight, R. G. (1991). Behavioral assessment of social competence following severe head injury. *Journal of Clinical and Experimental Neuropsychology, 13,* 729–740.

Marshall, J. (1996). The PALPA: A commentary and consideration of the clinical implications. *Aphasiology, 10,* 197–202.

Marshall, J. (1999a). Doing something about a verb impairment: Two therapy approaches. In S. Byng, K. Swinburn, & C. Pound (Eds.). *The aphasia therapy file* (pp. 111–130). Hove, UK: Psychology Press.

Marshall, J. (1999b). "Who ends up with the fiver?"—A sentence production therapy. In S. Byng, K. Swinburn, & C. Pound (Eds.). *The aphasia therapy file* (pp. 143–149). Hove, UK: Psychology Press.

Marshall, J., Atkinson, J., Woll, B., & Thacker, A. (2005). Aphasia in a bilingual user of British Sign Language and English: Effects of cross-linguistic cues. *Cognitive Neuropsychology, 22,* 719–736.

Marshall, J., & Cairns, D. (2005). Therapy for sentence processing problems in aphasia: Working on thinking for speaking. *Aphasiology, 19,* 1009–1020.

Marshall, J., Pound, C., White-Thomson, M., & Pring, T. (1990). The use of picture/word matching tasks to assist word retrieval in aphasic patients. *Aphasiology, 4,* 167–184.

Marshall, J., Pring, T., & Chiat, S. (1993). Sentence processing therapy: Working at the level of the event. *Aphasiology, 7,* 177–199.

Marshall, J., Pring, T., & Chiat, S. (1998). Verb retrieval and sentence production in aphasia. *Brain and Language, 63,* 159–183.

Marshall, J., Robson, J., Pring, T., & Chiat, S. (1998). Why does monitoring fail in jargon aphasia? Comprehension, judgment, and therapy evidence. *Brain and Language, 63,* 79–107.

Marshall, R. C. (1987). Reapportioning time for aphasia rehabilitation: A point of view. *Aphasiology, 1,* 59–74.

Marshall, R. C. (1999). A problem-focused group treatment program for clients with mild aphasia. In R. J. Elman (Ed.), *Group treatment of neurogenic communication disorders: The expert clinician's approach* (pp. 57–65). Boston: Butterworth Heinemann.

Martin, I., & McDonald, S. (2003). Weak coherence, no theory of mind, or executive dysfunction: Solving the puzzle of pragmatic language disorders. *Brain and Language, 85,* 451–466.

Martin, I., & McDonald, S. (2005). Evaluating the causes of impaired irony comprehension following traumatic brain injury. *Aphasiology, 19,* 712–730.

Martin, N., & Ayala, J. (2004). Measurements of auditory-verbal STM span in aphasia: Effects of item, task, and lexical impairment. *Brain and Language, 89,* 464–498.

Martin, N., Fink, R., & Laine, M. (2004). Treatment of word retrieval deficits with contextual priming. *Aphasiology, 18,* 457–474.

Martin, N., & Gupta, P. (2004). Exploring the relationship between word processing and verbal short-term memory: Evidence from associations and dissociations. *Cognitive Neuropsychology, 21,* 213–228.

Martin, P., Serrano, J., & Iglesias, J. (1999). Phonological/semantic errors in two Spanish-speaking patients with anomic aphasia. *Aphasiology, 13,* 225–236.

Martin, R. (2001). Sentence comprehension. In B. Rapp (Ed.), *The handbook of cognitive neuropsychology* (pp. 349–373). Philadelphia: Psychology Press.

Martin, R. C., & He, T. (2004). Semantic short-term memory and its role in sentence processing: A replication. *Brain and Language, 89,* 76–82.

Martin, R. C., & Miller, M. (2002). Sentence comprehension deficits: Independence and interaction of syntax, semantics, and working memory. In A. E. Hillis (Ed.), *The handbook of adult language disorders* (pp. 295–310). New York: Psychology Press.

Martin, R. C., Shelton, J. R., & Yaffee, L. S. (1994). Language processing and working memory: Neuropsychological evidence for separate phonological and semantic capacities. *Journal of Memory and Language, 33,* 83–111.

Mason, R. A., Just, M. A., Keller, T. A., & Carpenter, P. A. (2003). Ambiguity in the brain: What brain imaging reveals about the processing of syntactically ambiguous sentences. *Journal of Experimental Psychology: Learning, Memory, and Cognition, 29,* 1319–1338.

Mathuranath, P. S., Nestor, P. J., Berrios, G. E., Rakowicz, W., & Hodges, J. R. (2000). A brief cognitive test battery to differentiate Alzheimer's disease and frontotemporal dementia. *Neurology, 55,* 1613–1620.

Mattis, S. (1988). *Dementia Rating Scale* (DRS). Odessa, FL: Psychological Assessment Resources.

Mauthe, R. W., Haaf, D. C., Hayn, P., & Krall, J. M. (1996). Predicting discharge destination of stroke patients using a mathematical model based on six items from the Functional Independence Measure. *Archives of Physical Medicine and Rehabilitation, 77,* 10–13.

Mazzocchi, F., & Vignolo, L. A. (1979). Localization of lesions in aphasia: Clinical-CT scan correlations in stroke patients. *Cortex, 15,* 627–654.

Mazzoni, M., Vista, M., Pardossi, L., Avila, L., Bianchi, F., et al. (1992). Spontaneous evolution of aphasia after ischaemic stroke. *Aphasiology, 6,* 387–396.

McCarthy, R. A., & Warrington, E. K. (1990). *Cognitive neuropsychology: A clinical introduction.* San Diego, CA: Academic Press.

McCleary, C. (1988). The semantic organization and classification of fourteen words by aphasic patients. *Brain and Language, 34,* 183–202.

McCleary, C., & Hirst, W. (1986). Semantic classification in aphasia: A study of basic, superordinate, and function relations. *Brain and Language, 27,* 199–209.

McCloskey, M. (2004). Does Harley have a point? Comments on Harley's *Does cognitive neuropsychology have a future? Cognitive Neuropsychology, 21,* 37–40.

McCooey, R. T., Toffolo, D., & Code, C. (2000). A socioenvironmental approach to functional communication in hospital in-patients. In L. E. Worrall & C. M. Frattali (Eds.). *Neurogenic communication disorders: A functional approach* (pp. 295–311). New York: Thieme.

McCrae, K., Jared, D., & Seidenberg, M. S. (1990). On the roles of frequency and lexical access in word naming. *Journal of Memory and Language, 29,* 43–65.

McDermott, F. B., Horner, J., & DeLong, E. R. (1996). Evolution of acute aphasia as measured by the Western Aphasia Battery. In M. L. Lemme (Ed.), *Clinical aphasiology* (Vol. 24, pp. 159–172). Austin, TX: Pro-Ed.

McDonald, S. (1993). Viewing the brain sideways? Frontal versus right hemisphere explanations of non-aphasic language disorders. *Aphasiology, 7,* 535–549.

McDonald, S., & Pearce, S. (1996). Clinical insights into pragmatic theory: Frontal lobe deficits and sarcasm. *Brain and Language, 53,* 81–104.

McDonald, S., & Pearce, S. (1998). Requests that overcome listener reluctance: Impairment associated with executive dysfunction in brain injury. *Brain and Language, 61,* 88–104.

McDonald, S., Tate, R. L., & Rigby, J. (1994). Error types in ideomotor apraxia: A qualitative analysis. *Brain and Cognition, 25,* 250–270.

McDonald, S., & van Sommers, P. (1993). Pragmatic language skills after closed head injury: Ability to negotiate requests. *Cognitive Neuropsychology, 10,* 297–315.

McDonald, S., & Wales, R. (1986). An investigation of the ability to process inferences in language following right hemisphere brain damage. *Brain and Language, 29,* 68–80.

McGlinchey-Berroth, R., Milberg, W. P., Verfaellie, M., Alexander, M., & Kilduff, P. T. (1993). Semantic processing in the neglected visual field: Evidence from a lexical decision task. *Cognitive Neuropsychology, 10,* 79–108.

McGlynn, S. M., & Schacter, D. L. (1989). Unawareness of deficits in neuropsychological syndromes. *Journal of Clinical and Experimental Neuropsychology, 11,* 143–205.

McIntosh, K. W., Ramsberger, G., & Prescott, T. E. (1996). Relationships between and among language impairment, communication disability and quality of life outcome assessments in aphasic patients [abstract]. *Brain and Language, 55,* 23–26.

McKeith, J. G., Fairbarn, A. F., Perry, R. H., & Thompson, P. (1994). The clinical diagnosis of senile dementia of Lewy body type (SDLT). *British Journal of Psychiatry, 165,* 324–332.

McKhann, G., Drachman, D., Folstein, M., Katzman, R., Price, D., et al. (1984). Clinical diagnosis of Alzheimer's disease: Report of the NINCDS-ADRDA work group under the auspices of the Department of Health and Human Services Task Force on Alzheimer's disease. *Neurology, 34,* 939–944.

McNeil, M. R., Doyle, P. J., Fossett, T. R. D., Park, G. H., & Goda, A. J. (2001). Reliability and concurrent validity of the information unit scoring metric for the Story Retell Procedure. *Aphasiology, 10/11,* 991–1006.

McNeil, M. R., Doyle, P. J., Park, G. H., Fossett, T. R. D., & Brodsky, M. B. (2002). Increasing the sensitivity of the Story Retell Procedure for the discrimination of normal elderly subjects from persons with aphasia. *Aphasiology, 16,* 815–822.

McNeil, M. R., Hula, W. D., Matthews, C. T., & Doyle, P. J. (2004). Resource theory and aphasia: A fugacious theoretical dismissal. *Aphasiology, 18,* 836–843.

McNeil, M. R., & Kimelman, M. D. Z. (1986). Toward an integrative information-processing structure of auditory comprehension and processing in adult aphasia. *Seminars in Speech and Language, 7,* 123–146.

McNeil, M. R., Odell, K., & Tseng, C-H. (1991). Toward the integration of resource allocation into a general theory of aphasia. In T. E. Prescott (Ed.), *Clinical aphasiology* (Vol. 20, pp. 21–40). Austin, TX: Pro-Ed.

McNeil, M. R., & Prescott, T. E. (1978). *Revised Token Test.* Baltimore, MD: University Park Press.

McReynolds, L. V., & Kearns, K. P. (1983). *Single-subject experimental designs in communicative disorders.* Baltimore: University Park Press.

McReynolds, L. V., & Thompson, C. K. (1986). Flexibility of single-subject experimental designs. Part I: Review of the basics of single-subject designs. *Journal of Speech and Hearing Disorders, 51,* 194–203.

Mendez, M. F., & Benson, D. F. (1985). Atypical conduction aphasia: A disconnection syndrome. *Archives of Neurology, 42,* 886–891.

Menn, L., & Obler, L. K. (1990). Cross-language data and theories of agrammatism. In L. Menn & L. K. Obler (Eds.), *Agrammatic aphasia: A cross-linguistic narrative sourcebook* (pp. 1369–1389). Philadelphia: John Benjamins.

Menn, L., Reilly, K. F., Hayashi, M., Kamio, A., Fujita, I., et al. (1998). The interaction of preserved pragmatics and impaired syntax in Japanese and English aphasic speech. *Brain and Language, 61,* 183–225.

Mentis, M., & Prutting, C. A. (1987). Cohesion in the discourse of normal and head-injured adults. *Journal of Speech and Hearing Research, 30,* 88–98.

Mesulam, M. M. (1982). Slowly progressive aphasia without generalized dementia. *Annals of Neurology, 11,* 592–598.

Metter, E. J. (1985). Feature: Letter. *Asha, 27,* 43.

Mey, J. L. (2001). *Pragmatics: An introduction* (2nd ed.). Malden, MA: Blackwell.

Miceli, G., Amitrano, A., Capasso, R., & Caramazza, A. (1996). The treatment of anomia resulting from output lexical damage: Analysis of two cases. *Brain and Language, 52,* 150–174.

Miceli, G., Gainotti, G., Caltagirone, C., & Masulo, C. (1980). Some aspects of phonological impairment in aphasia. *Brain and Language, 11,* 159–170.

Miceli, G., Silveri, M. C., Romani, C., & Caramazza, A. (1989). Variation in the pattern of omissions and substitutions of grammatical morphemes in the spontaneous speech of so-called agrammatic patients. *Brain and Language, 36,* 447–492.

Miceli, G., Silveri, M. C., Villa, G., & Caramazza, A. (1984). On the basis for the agrammatic's difficulty in producing main verbs. *Cortex, 20,* 207–220.

Michallet, B., Tétreault, S., & Le Dorze, G. (2003). The consequences of severe aphasia on the spouses of aphasia people. *Aphasiology, 17,* 835–859.

Milberg, W., & Blumstein, S. (1981). Lexical decision and aphasia: Evidence for semantic processing. *Brain and Language, 14,* 371–385.

Milberg, W., Blumstein, S. E., & Dworetzky, B. (1987). Processing of lexical ambiguities in aphasia. *Brain and Language, 31,* 151–170.

Milner, B., Corkin, S., & Teuber, H-L. (1968). Further analysis of the hippocampal amnesic syndrome: 14-year follow-up of H. M. *Neuropsychologia, 6,* 215–234.

Milton, S. B., Wertz, R. T., Katz, R. C., & Prutting, C. A. (1981). Stimulus saliency in the sorting behavior of aphasic adults. In R. H. Brookshire (Ed.), *Clinical aphasiology conference proceedings* (pp. 46–54). Minneapolis: BRK.

Misiurski, C., Blumstein, S. E., Rissman, J., & Berman, D. (2005). The role of lexical competition and acoustic-phonetic structure in lexical processing: Evidence from normal subjects and aphasic patients. *Brain and Language, 93,* 64–78.

Mitchum, C. C., Haendiges, A. N., & Berndt, R. S. (1993). Model-guided treatment to improve written sentence production: A case study. *Aphasiology, 7,* 71–109.

Mitchum, C. C., Haendiges, A. N., & Berndt, R. S. (1995). Treatment of thematic mapping in sentence comprehension: Implications for normal processing. *Cognitive Neuropsychology, 12,* 503–547.

Mitchum, C. C., Haendiges, A. N., & Berndt, R. S. (2004). Response strategies in aphasic sentence comprehension: An analysis of two cases. *Aphasiology, 18,* 675–691.

Mitchum, C. C., Ritgert, B., Sandson, J., & Berndt, R. S. (1990). The use of response analysis in confrontation naming. *Aphasiology, 4,* 261–279.

Miyake, A., Carpenter, P. A., & Just, M. A. (1994). A capacity approach to syntactic comprehension disorders: Making normal adults perform like aphasic patients. *Cognitive Neuropsychology, 11,* 671–717.

Miyake, A., Carpenter, P. A., & Just, M. A. (1995). Reduced resources and specific impairments in normal and aphasic sentence comprehension. *Cognitive Neuropsychology, 12,* 651–679.

Mlcoch, A. G., & Metter, E. J. (2001). Medical aspects of stroke rehabilitation. In R. Chapey (Ed.), *Language intervention strategies in adult aphasia and related neurogenic communication disorders* (4th ed., pp. 37–54). Philadelphia: Lippincott Williams & Wilkins.

Mohr, J., Pessin, M., Finkelstein, S., Funkenstein, H., Duncan, G., & Davis, K. (1978). Broca's aphasia: pathologic and clinical. *Neurology, 28,* 311–324.

Mohr, J. P., Weiss, G., Caveness, W. F., Dillon, J. D., Kistler, J. P., Meirowsky, A. M., & Rish, B. L. (1980). Language and motor deficits following penetrating head injury in Vietnam. *Neurology, 30,* 1273–1279.

Moir, A., & Jessel, D. (1991). *Brain sex: The real difference between men and women.* New York: Laurel.

Molrine, C. J., & Pierce, R. S. (2002). Black and white adults' expressive language performance on three tests of aphasia. *American Journal of Speech-Language Pathology, 11,* 139–150.

Monoi, H., Fukusako, Y., Itoh, M., & Sasanuma, S. (1983). Speech sound errors in patients with conduction and Broca's aphasia. *Brain and Language, 20,* 175–194.

Moore, S., Sandman, C. A., McGrady, K., & Kesslak, J. P. (2001). Memory training improves cognitive ability in patients with dementia. *Neuropsychological Rehabilitation, 11,* 245–261.

Moore, W. H. (1989). Language recovery in aphasia: A right hemisphere perspective. *Aphasiology, 3,* 101–110.

Moreaud, O., David, D., Charnallet, A., & Pellat, J. (2001). Are semantic errors actually semantic?: Evidence from Alzheimer's disease. *Brain and Language, 77,* 176–186.

Morgan, A. L. R., & Helm-Estabrooks, N. (1987). Back to the drawing board: A treatment program for nonverbal aphasic patients. In R. H. Brookshire (Ed.), *Clinical aphasiology* (Vol. 17, pp. 64–72). Minneapolis: BRK.

Morgan, G. A., Gliner, J. A., & Harmon, R. J. (2006). *Understanding and evaluating research in applied and clinical settings.* Mahwah, NJ: Lawrence Erlbaum.

Morganstein, S., & Smith, M. C. (2001). Thematic language stimulation therapy. In R. Chapey (Ed.), *Language intervention strategies in adult aphasia and related neurogenic communication disorders* (4th ed., pp. 383–396). Philadelphia: Lippincott Williams & Wilkins.

Morley, G. K., Lundgren, S., & Haxby, J. (1979). Comparison and clinical applicability of auditory comprehension scores on the Behavioral Neurology Deficit Examination, Boston Diagnostic Aphasia Examination, Porch Index of Communicative Ability and Token Test. *Journal of Clinical Neuropsychology, 1,* 249–258.

Morrow, L., Vrtunski, P. B., Kim, Y., & Boller, F. (1981). Arousal responses to emotional stimuli and laterality of lesion. *Neuropsychologia, 19,* 65–71.

Mortley, J., Wade, J., & Enderby, P. (2004). Superhighway to promoting a client-therapist partnership? Using the

Internet to deliver word-retrieval computer therapy, monitored remotely with minimal speech and language therapy input. *Aphasiology, 18,* 193–212.

Mowrer, D. E. (1982). *Methods of modifying speech behaviors: Learning theory in speech pathology* (2nd ed.). Prospect Heights, IL: Waveland Press.

Mullen, R. (2003, August 8). National outcomes measurement system (NOMS): 2003. Retrieved December 7, 2005, from www.speechpathology.com/articles/pf_arc_disp.asp?id=17.

Muñoz, M. L., Marquardt, T. P., & Copeland, G. (1999). A comparison of the codeswitching patterns of aphasic and neurologically normal bilingual speakers of English and Spanish. *Brain and Language, 66,* 249–274.

Murray, L. L., Holland, A. L., & Beeson, P. M. (1997a). Auditory processing in individuals with mild aphasia: A study of resource allocation. *Journal of Speech, Language, and Hearing Research, 40,* 92–809.

Murray, L. L., Holland, A. L., & Beeson, P. M. (1998). Spoken language of individuals with mild fluent aphasia under focused and divided-attention conditions. *Journal of Speech Language and Hearing Research, 41,* 213–227.

Myers, P. S. (1979). Profiles of communication deficits in patients with right cerebral hemisphere damage. In R. H. Brookshire (Ed.), *Clinical aphasiology conference proceedings* (pp. 38–46). Minneapolis, MN: BRK.

Myers, P. S. (1999). *Right hemisphere damage.* San Diego, CA: Singular.

Myers, P. S. (2001a). Communication disorders associated with right hemisphere damage. In R. Chapey (Ed.), *Language intervention strategies in adult aphasia and related neurogenic communication disorders* (4th ed., pp. 809–828). Philadelphia: Lippincott Williams & Wilkins.

Myers, P. S. (2001b). Toward a definition of RHD syndrome. *Aphasiology, 15,* 913–918.

Myers, P. S., & Brookshire, R. H. (1994). The effects of visual and inferential complexity on the picture descriptions of non-brain-damaged and right-hemisphere-damaged adults. In M. L. Lemme (Ed.), *Clinical aphasiology* (Vol. 22, pp. 25–34). Austin, TX: Pro-Ed.

Myers, P. S., Linebaugh, C. W., & Mackisack-Morin, L. (1985). Extracting implicit meaning: Right versus left hemisphere damage. In R. H. Brookshire (Ed.), *Clinical aphasiology* (Vol. 15, pp. 72–82). Minneapolis, MN: BRK.

Nabors, N., Millis, S., & Rosenthal, M. (1997). Use of the Neurobehavioral Cognitive Status Examination (Cognistat) in traumatic brain injury. *Journal of Head Trauma Rehabilitation, 12,* 79–84.

Nadeau, S. E. (2000). Phonology. In S. E. Nadeau, L. J. Gonzalez Rothi, & B. Crosson (Eds.), *Aphasia and language: Theory to practice* (pp. 40–81). New York: Guilford Press.

Nadeau, S. E., & Crosson, B. (1997). Subcortical aphasia. *Brain and Language, 58,* 355–402.

Naeser, M. A. (1988). Some effects of subcortical white matter lesions on language behavior in aphasia. *Aphasiology, 2,* 363–368.

Naeser, M. A. (1994). Neuroimaging and recovery of auditory comprehension and spontaneous speech in aphasia with some implications for treatment of severe aphasia. In A. Kertesz (Ed.), *Localization and neuroimaging in neuropsychology* (pp. 245–296). San Diego, CA: Academic Press.

Naeser, M. A., & Hayward, R. W. (1978). Lesion localization in aphasia with cranial computed tomography and the Boston Diagnostic Aphasia Exam. *Neurology, 28,* 545–551.

Naeser, M. A., Martin, P. I., Nicholas, M., Baker, E. H., Seekins, H., et al. (2005). Improved picture naming in chronic aphasia after TMS to part of the right Broca's area: An open-protocol study. *Brain and Language, 93,* 95–105.

Naeser, M. A., Palumbo, C. L., Prete, M. N., Fitzpatrick, P. M., Mimura, M., Samaraweera, R., & Albert, M. L. (1998). Visible changes in lesion borders on CT scan after five years poststroke, and long-term recovery in aphasia. *Brain and Language, 62,* 1–28.

Nagata, K., Yunoki, K., Kabe, S., Suzuki, A., & Araki, G. (1986). Regional cerebral blood flow correlates of aphasia outcome in cerebral haemorrhage and cerebral infarction. *Stroke, 17,* 417–423.

Nakano, H., & Blumstein, S. E. (2004). Deficits in thematic integration processes in Broca's and Wernicke's aphasia. *Brain and Language, 88,* 96–107.

Needham, L. S., & Swisher, L. P. (1972). A comparison of three tests of auditory comprehension for adult aphasics. *Journal of Speech and Hearing Disorders, 37,* 123–131.

Nelson, E., Wasson, J., Kirk, J., Keller, A., Clark, D., et al. (1987). Assessment of function in routine clinical practice: Description of the COOP Chart method and preliminary findings. *Journal of Chronic Disease, 40,* 55S–63S.

Nelson, H. E., & O'Connell, A. (1978). Dementia: The estimation of premorbid intelligence levels using the New Adult Reading Test. *Cortex, 14,* 234–244.

Nespoulous, J., Dordain, M., Perron, C., Ska, B., Bub, D., et al. (1988). Agrammatism in sentence production without comprehension deficits: Reduced availability of syntactic structures and/or of grammatical morphemes? A case study. *Brain and Language, 33,* 273–295.

Neumann, M. A., & Cohn, R. (1953). Incidence of Alzheimer's disease in a large mental hospital. *Archives of Neurology and Psychiatry, 69,* 615–636.

Newcombe, F. (1969). *Missile wounds to the brain: A study of psychological deficits*. Oxford: Clarendon Press.

Ni, W., Shankweiler, D., Harris, K. S., & Fulbright, R. K. (1997). Production and comprehension of relative clause syntax in nonfluent aphasia: A coordinated study [abstract]. *Brain and Language, 60,* 93–95.

Nicholas, L. E., & Brookshire, R. H. (1987). Error analysis and passage dependency of test items from a standardized test of multiple-sentence reading comprehension for aphasic and non-brain-damaged adults. *Journal of Speech and Hearing Disorders, 52,* 358–366.

Nicholas, L. E., & Brookshire, R. H. (1993). A system for quantifying the informativeness and efficiency of the connected speech of adults with aphasia. *Journal of Speech and Hearing Research, 36,* 338–350.

Nicholas, L. E., & Brookshire, R. H. (1995a). Comprehension of spoken narrative discourse by adults with aphasia, right-hemisphere brain damage, or traumatic brain injury. *American Journal of Speech-Language Pathology, 4*(3), 69–81.

Nicholas, L. E., & Brookshire, R. H. (1995b). Presence, completeness, and accuracy of main concepts in the connected speech of non-brain-damaged adults and adults with aphasia. *Journal of Speech and Hearing Research, 38,* 145–156.

Nicholas, L. E., Brookshire, R. H., MacLennan, D. L., Schumacher, J. G., & Porrazzo, S. A. (1989). Revised administration and scoring procedures for the Boston Naming Test and norms for non-brain-damaged adults. *Aphasiology, 3,* 569–580.

Nicholas, L. E., MacLennan, D. L., & Brookshire, R. H. (1986). Validity of multiple-sentence reading comprehension tests for aphasic adults. *Journal of Speech and Hearing Disorders, 51,* 82–87.

Nicholas, M., Obler, L. K., Au, R., & Albert, M. L. (1996). On the nature of naming errors in aging and dementia: A study of semantic relatedness. *Brain and Language, 54,* 184–195.

Nicholas, M., Sinotte, M. P., & Helm-Estabrooks, N. (2005). Using a computer to communicate: Effect of executive function impairments in people with severe aphasia. *Aphasiology, 19,* 1052–1065.

Nicholas, M. L., Helm-Estabrooks, N., Ward-Lonergan, J., & Morgan, A. R. (1993). Evolution of severe aphasia in first two years post onset. *Archives of Physical Medicine and Rehabilitation, 74,* 830–836.

Nickels, L. (1995). Getting it right? Using aphasic naming errors to evaluate theoretical models of spoken word production. *Language and Cognitive Processes, 10,* 13–45.

Nickels, L. (2001). Spoken word production. In B. Rapp (Ed.), *The handbook of cognitive neuropsychology* (pp. 291–320). Philadelphia: Psychology Press.

Nickels, L. (2002). Therapy for naming disorders: Revisiting, revising, and reviewing. *Aphasiology, 16,* 935–979.

Nickels, L., & Best, W. (1996). Therapy for naming deficits (part II): Specifics, surprises and suggestions. *Aphasiology, 10,* 109–136.

Nickels, L., & Howard, D. (1995). Phonological errors in aphasic naming: Comprehension, monitoring and lexicality. *Cortex, 31,* 209–237.

Nickels, L., & Howard, D. (2004). Dissociating effects of number of phonemes, number of syllables, and syllabic complexity on word production in aphasia: It's the number of phonemes that counts. *Cognitive Neuropsychology, 21,* 57–78.

Nicol, J. L., Jakubowicz, & Goldblum, M-C. (1996). Sensitivity to grammatical marking in English-speaking and French-speaking non-fluent aphasics. *Aphasiology, 10,* 593–622.

Noll, J. D., & Randolf, S. R. (1978). Auditory semantic, syntactic, and retention errors made by aphasic subjects on the Token Test. *Journal of Communication Disorders, 11,* 543–553.

Norman, D. A., & Shallice, T. (1986). Attention to action: Willed and automatic control of behavior. In R. J. Davidson, G. E. Schwarts, & D. Shapiro (Eds.). *Consciousness and self-regulation: Advances in research and therapy* (pp. 1–18). New York: Plenum.

Nyffeler, T., Gutbrod, K., Pflugshaupt, T., von Wartburg, R., Hess, C. W., et al. (2005). Allocentric and egocentric spatial impairments in a case of topographical disorientation. *Cortex, 41,* 133–143.

Ober, B. A., & Shenaut, G. K. (1995). Semantic priming in Alzheimer's disease: Meta-analysis and theoretical evaluation. In P. A. Allen & T. R. Bashore (Eds.), *Age differences in word and language processing* (pp. 247–271). Amsterdam: Elsevier.

Obler, L. K., & Albert, M. L. (1977). Influence of aging on recovery from aphasia in polyglots. *Brain and Language, 4,* 460–463.

Obler, L. K., Goral, M., & Albert, M. L. (1995). Variability in aphasia research: Aphasia subject selection in group studies. *Brain and Language, 48,* 341–350.

Oczkowski, W. J., & Barreca, S. (1993). The Functional Independence Measure: Its use to identify rehabilitation needs in stroke survivors. *Archives of Physical Medicine and Rehabilitation, 74,* 1291–1294.

Odell, K. H., Wollack, J. A., & Flynn, M. (2005). Functional outcomes in patients with right hemisphere brain damage. *Aphasiology, 19,* 807–830.

Oelschlaeger, M. L., & Damico, J. S. (1998). Spontaneous verbal repetition: A social strategy in aphasic conversation. *Aphasiology, 12,* 971–988.

Oelschlaeger, M. L., & Thorne, J. C. (1999). Application of the correct information unit analysis to the naturally occurring conversation of a person with aphasia.

Journal of Speech, Language, and Hearing Research, 42, 636–648.

O'Grady, W., & Lee, M. (2005). A mapping theory of agrammatic comprehension deficits. *Brain and Language, 92,* 91–100.

Oleyar, K. S., Doyle, P. J., Keefe, K., & Goldstein, H. (1991). The effects of a time-delay procedure on comprehension of verb-noun commands in severe aphasia. In T. E. Prescott (Ed.), *Clinical aphasiology* (Vol. 20, pp. 271–284). Austin, TX: Pro-Ed.

Osborne, C. L. (1998). *Over my head: A doctor's own story of head injury from the inside looking out.* Kansas City, MO: Andrews McMeel.

Ostrin, R. K., & Schwartz, M. F. (1986). Reconstructing from a degraded trace: A study of sentence repetition in agrammatism. *Brain and Language, 28,* 328–345.

Ostrin, R. K., & Tyler, L. K. (1993). Automatic access to lexical semantics in aphasia: Evidence from semantic and associative priming. *Brain and Language, 45,* 147–159.

Ousset, P. J., Viallard, G., Puel, M., Celsis, P., Démonet, J. F., et al. (2002). Lexical therapy and episodic word learning in dementia of the Alzheimer type. *Brain and Language, 80,* 14–20.

Paradis, M. (1977). Bilingualism and aphasia. In H. Whitaker & H. A. Whitaker (Eds.), *Studies in neurolinguistics* (Vol. 3, pp. 65–122). New York: Academic Press.

Paradis, M. (1998). Aphasia in bilinguals: How atypical is it? In P. Coppens, Y. Lebrun, & Basso, A. (Eds.), *Aphasia in atypical populations* (pp. 35–66). Mahwah, NJ: Lawrence Erlbaum.

Paradis, M., Goldblum, M-C., & Abidi, R. (1982). Alternate antagonism with paradoxical translation behavior in two bilingual aphasic patients. *Brain and Language, 15,* 55–69.

Paradis, M., & Goldblum, M-C. (1989). Selective crossed aphasia in a trilingual aphasic patient followed by reciprocal antagonism. *Brain and Language, 36,* 62–75.

Paradis, M., & Libben, G. (1997). *The assessment of bilingual aphasia.* Hillsdale, NJ: Lawrence Erlbaum.

Park, G. H., McNeil, M. R., & Tompkins, C. A. (2000). Reliability of the five-item Revised Token Test for individuals with aphasia. *Aphasiology, 14,* 527–535.

Parr, S. (1994). Coping with aphasia: Conversations with 20 aphasic people. *Aphasiology, 8,* 457–466.

Pashek, G. V., & Holland, A. L. (1988). Evolution of aphasia in the first year post-stroke. *Cortex, 24,* 411–423.

Pashek, G. V., & Tompkins, C. A. (2002). Context and word class influences on lexical retrieval in aphasia. *Aphasiology, 16,* 261–286.

Patronas, N. J., Deveikis, J. P., & Schellinger, D. (1987). The use of computed tomography in studying the brain. In H. G. Mueller & V. C. Geoffrey (Eds.), *Communication disorders in aging: Assessment and management* (pp. 107–134). Washington, DC: Gallaudet University Press.

Patterson, K. E., & Wilson, B. (1990). A ROSE is a ROSE or a NOSE: A deficit in initial letter identification. *Cognitive Neuropsychology, 7,* 447–478.

Patterson, M. B., & Mack, J. L. (1985). Neuropsychological analysis of a case of reduplicative paramnesia. *Journal of Clinical and Experimental Neuropsychology, 7,* 111–121.

Paul, D. R., Frattali, C. M., Holland, A. L., Thompson, C. K., Caperton, C. J., et al. (2004). *Quality of Communication Life Scale* (ASHA QCL). Rockville, MD: American Speech-Language-Hearing Association.

Peach, R. K. (1987). A short-term memory treatment approach to the repetition deficit in conduction aphasia. In R. H. Brookshire (Ed.), *Clinical aphasiology* (Vol. 17, pp. 35–45). Minneapolis: BRK.

Peach, R. K. (1996). Treatment for aphasic phonological output planning deficits. In M. L. Lemme (Ed.), *Clinical aphasiology* (Vol. 24, pp. 109–120). Austin, TX: Pro-Ed.

Peach, R. K. (2001). Clinical intervention for global aphasia. In R. Chapey (Ed.), *Language intervention strategies in adult aphasia and related neurogenic communication disorders* (4th ed., pp. 487–512). Philadelphia: Lippincott Williams & Wilkins.

Peach, R. K., Canter, G. J., & Gallaher, A. J. (1988). Comprehension of sentence structure in anomic and conduction aphasia. *Brain and Language, 35,* 119–137.

Peach, R. K., Rubin, S. S., & Newhoff, M. (1994). A topographic event-related potential analysis of the attention deficit for auditory processing in aphasia. In M. L. Lemme (Ed.), *Clinical aphasiology* (Vol. 22, pp. 81–96). Austin, TX: Pro-Ed.

Pease, D. M., & Goodglass, H. (1978). The effects of cuing on picture naming in aphasia. *Cortex, 14,* 178–189.

Pell, M. D. (2006). Cerebral mechanisms for understanding emotional prosody in speech. *Brain and Language, 96,* 221–234.

Pell, M. D., & Baum, S. R. (1997). Unilateral brain damage, prosodic comprehension deficits, and the acoustic cues to prosody. *Brain and Language, 57,* 195–214.

Pendleton, M. G., Heaton, R. K., Lehman, R. A. W., & Hulihan, D. (1982). Diagnostic utility of the Thurstone Word Fluency Test in neuropsychological evaluations. *Journal of Clinical Neuropsychology, 4,* 307–318.

Pendley, A., & Ramsberger, G. (1996). Self-awareness in patients with right hemisphere damage. In M. L. Lemme (Ed.), *Clinical aphasiology* (Vol. 24, pp. 243–253). Austin, TX: Pro-Ed.

Penfield, W., & Perot, P. (1963). The brain's record of visual and auditory experience: A final summary and discussion. *Brain, 86,* 595–696.

Penn, C. (2005). Who's tired of the WHO? A commentary on Ross and Wertz, "Advancing appraisal: Aphasia and the WHO." *Aphasiology, 19,* 875–879.

Penn, C., & Jones, D. (2000). Functional communication and the workplace: A neglected domain. In L. E. Worrall & C. M. Frattali (Eds.). *Neurogenic communication disorders: A functional approach* (pp. 103–124). New York: Thieme.

Perani, D., Cappa, S. F., Tettamanti, M., Rosa, M., Scifo, P., et al. (2003). A fMRI study of word retrieval in aphasia. *Brain and Language, 85,* 357–368.

Perecman, E. (1984). Spontaneous translation and language mixing in a polyglot aphasic. *Brain and Language, 23,* 43–63.

Peretz, I. (2001). Music perception and recognition. In B. Rapp (Ed.), *The handbook of cognitive neuropsychology* (pp. 519–540). Philadelphia: Psychology Press.

Perfetti, C. A., Beverly, S., Bell, L., Rodgers, K., & Faux, R. (1987). Comprehending newspaper headlines. *Journal of Memory and Language, 26,* 692–713.

Perkins, L., Crisp, J., & Walshaw, D. (1999). Exploring conversation analysis as an assessment tool for aphasia: The issue of reliability. *Aphasiology, 13,* 259–281.

Perkins, L., Whitworth, A., & Lesser, R. (1997). *Conversation analysis profile for people with cognitive impairment.* Chichester, UK: Whurr Publishers.

Petersen, R. (2002). *Mayo Clinic on Alzheimer's disease.* Rochester, MN: Mayo Clinic Health Information.

Petersen, R. C., Smith, G. E., Tangalos, E. G., Kokmen, E., & Ivnik, R. J. (1993). Longitudinal outcome of patients with a mild cognitive impairment. *Annals of Neurology, 34,* 294–295.

Peterson, L. N., & Kirshner, H. S. (1981). Gestural impairment and gestural ability in aphasia: A review. *Brain and Language, 14,* 333–348.

Petocz, A., & Oliphant, G. (1988). Closed-class words as first syllables do interfere with lexical decisions for nonwords: Implications for theories of agrammatism. *Brain and Language, 34,* 127–146.

Phillips, P. P., & Halpin, G. (1978). Language impairment evaluation in aphasic patients. *Archives of Physical Medicine and Rehabilitation, 59,* 327–329.

Pickersgill, M. J., & Lincoln, N. B. (1983). Prognostic indicators and the pattern of recovery of communication in aphasic stroke patients. *Journal of Neurology, Neurosurgery, and Psychiatry, 46,* 130–139.

Pierce, R. S., & Beekman, L. A. (1985). Effects of linguistic and extralinguistic context on semantic and syntactic processing in aphasia. *Journal of Speech and Hearing Research, 28,* 250–254.

Pierce, R. S., & Wagner, C. M. (1985). The role of context in facilitating syntactic decoding in aphasia. *Journal of Communication Disorders, 18,* 203–219.

Pimental, P. A., & Knight, J. A. (2000). *The Mini Inventory of Right Brain Injury* (MIRBI-2). Austin, TX: Pro-Ed.

Pizzamiglio, L., & Appicciafuoco, A. (1971). Semantic comprehension in aphasia. *Journal of Communication Disorders, 3,* 280–288.

Pizzamiglio, L., Mammucari, A., & Razzano, C. (1985). Evidence for sex differences in brain organization in recovery in aphasia. *Brain and Language, 25,* 213–223.

Plourde, G., Joanette, Y., Fontaine, F. S., Laplante, L., & Renaseau-Leclerc, C. (1993). The severity of visual hemineglect follows a bimodal frequency distribution. *Brain and Cognition, 21,* 131–139.

Poeck, K., & Hartje, W. (1979). Performance of aphasic patients in visual versus auditory presentation of the Token Test: Demonstration of a supramodal deficit. In F. Boller & M. Dennis (Eds.), *Auditory comprehension: Clinical and experimental studies with the Token Test* (pp. 107–116). New York: Academic Press.

Poeck, K., Huber, W., & Willmes, K. (1989). Outcome of intensive language treatment in aphasia. *Journal of Speech and Hearing Disorders, 54,* 471–478.

Poeck, K., & Pietron, H. (1981). The influence of stretched speech presentation on Token Test performance of aphasic and right brain damaged patients. *Neuropsychologia, 19,* 133–136.

Poizner, H., Klima, E. S., & Bellugi, U. (1987). *What the hands reveal about the brain.* Cambridge, MA: MIT Press.

Ponsford, J., & Kinsella, G. (1992). Attentional deficits following closed-head injury. *Journal of Clinical and Experimental Neuropsychology, 14,* 822–838.

Ponsford, J., Olver, J., Nelms, R., Curran, C., & Ponsford, M. (1999). Outcome measurement in an inpatient and outpatient traumatic brain injury rehabilitation program. *Neuropsychological Rehabilitation, 9,* 517–534.

Ponsford, J., Sloan, S., & Snow, P. (1995). *Traumatic brain injury: Rehabilitation for everyday adaptive living.* Hove, UK: Psychology Press.

Ponzio, J., & Degiovani, R. (1993). Typical behavior of persons with aphasia and their families. In D. Lafond, Y. Joanette, J. Ponzio, R. Degiovani, & M. T. Sarno (Eds.), *Living with aphasia: Psychosocial issues* (pp. 117–128). San Diego, CA: Singular.

Porch, B. E. (1967). *Porch Index of Communicative Ability, Volume I: Theory and development.* Palo Alto, CA: Consulting Psychologists Press.

Porch, B. E. (1981). *Porch Index of Communicative Ability, Volume II: Administration, scoring, and interpretation* (3rd ed.). Palo Alto, CA: Consulting Psychologists Press.

Porch, B. E., Collins, M., Wertz, R. T., & Friden, T. P. (1980). Statistical prediction of change in aphasia. *Journal of Speech and Hearing Research, 23,* 312–321.

Porch, B. E., & Palmer, P. M. (1986). Right hemisphere PICA percentiles revised. In R. H. Brookshire (Ed.),

Clinical aphasiology (Vol 16, pp. 275–280). Minneapolis: BRK.

Porch, B. E., & Porec, J. P. (1977). Medical-legal application of PICA results. In R. H. Brookshire (Ed.), *Clinical aphasiology conference proceedings* (pp. 302–309). Minneapolis: BRK.

Porec, J. P., & Porch, B. E. (1977). The behavioral characteristics of "simulated" aphasia. In R. H. Brookshire (Ed.), *Clinical aphasiology conference proceedings* (pp. 297–301). Minneapolis: BRK.

Porter, J. L., & Dabul, B. (1977). The application of transactional analysis to therapy with wives of adult aphasic patients. *Asha, 19,* 244–248.

Posner, M. I., Walker, J. A., Friedrich, F. J., & Rafal, R. D. (1984). Effects of parietal lobe injury on covert orienting of visual attention. *Journal of Neuroscience, 4,* 1863–1874.

Posner, M. I., Walker, J. A., Friedrich, F. J., & Rafal, R. D. (1987). How do the parietal lobes direct covert attention. *Neuropsychologia, 25,* 135–146.

Prather, P. A., Love, T., Finkel, L., & Zurif, E. B. (1994). Effects of slowed processing on lexical activation: Automaticity without encapsulation [abstract]. *Brain and Language, 47,* 326–329.

Price, C. C., & Grossman, M. (2005). Verb agreements during on-line sentence processing in Alzheimer's disease and frontotemporal dementia. *Brain and Language, 94,* 217–232.

Prigatano, G. P. (1999). *Principles of neuropsychological rehabilitation.* New York: Oxford University Press.

Prigatano, G. P., & Klonoff, P. S. (1998). A clinician's rating scale for evaluating impaired self-awareness and denial of disability after brain injury. *Clinical Neuropsychologist, 12,* 56–67.

Pring, T., Hamilton, A., Harwood, A., & Macbride, L. (1993). Generalization of naming after picture/word matching tasks: Only items appearing in therapy benefit. *Aphasiology, 7,* 383–394.

Prins, R. S., Snow, C. E., & Wagenaar, E. (1978). Recovery from aphasia: Spontaneous speech versus language comprehension. *Brain and Language, 6,* 192–211.

Prior, M., Kinsella, G., & Giese, J. (1990). Assessment of musical processing in brain-damaged patients: Implications for laterality of music. *Journal of Clinical and Experimental Neuropsychology, 12,* 301–312.

Prutting, C. A., & Kirchner, D. M. (1987). A clinical appraisal of the pragmatic aspects of language. *Journal of Speech and Hearing Disorders, 52,* 105–119.

Pulvermüller, F., Neininger, B., Elbert, T., Mohr, B., Rockstroh, B., et al. (2001). Constraint-induced therapy of chronic aphasia after stroke. *Stroke, 32,* 1621–1626.

Purdy, M., & Hindenlang, J. (2005). Educating and training caregivers of persons with aphasia. *Aphasiology, 19,* 377–387.

Purdy, M. H., Duffy, R. J., & Coelho, C. A. (1994). An investigation of the communicative use of trained symbols following multimodality training. In M. L. Lemme (Ed.), *Clinical aphasiology* (Vol. 22, pp. 345–356). Austin, TX: Pro-Ed.

Radanovic, M., & Scaff, M. (2003). Speech and language disturbances due to subcortical lesions. *Brain and Language, 84,* 337–352.

Radin, L., & Radin, G. (2003). *What if it's not Alzheimer's?* Amherst, NY: Prometheus.

Rao, P. R. (1995). Drawing conclusions on the efficacy of 'drawing' as a treatment for persons with severe aphasia. *Aphasiology, 9,* 59–62.

Rapp, B. (Ed.). (2001). *The handbook of cognitive neuropsychology.* Philadelphia: Psychology Press.

Rapp, B., Folk, J. R., & Tainturier, M-J. (2001). Word reading. In B. Rapp (Ed.), *The handbook of cognitive neuropsychology* (pp. 233–262). Philadelphia: Psychology Press.

Rappaport, M., Hall, K. M., Hopkins, K., Belieza, T., & Cope, D. N. (1982). Disability Rating Scale for severe head trauma: Coma to community. *Archives of Physical Medicine and Rehabilitation, 63,* 118–123.

Rappaport, M., Herrero-Backe, C., Rappaport, M. L., & Winterfield, K. M. (1989). Head injury outcome up to ten years later. *Archives of Physical Medicine and Rehabilitation, 70,* 885–892.

Raskin, S. A., & Sohlberg, M. M. (1996). The efficacy of prospective memory training in two adults with brain injury. *Journal of Head Trauma Rehabilitation, 11,* 32–51.

Raven, J. C. (1938/1965). *Progressive Matrices.* New York: Psychological Corporation.

Raymer, A. M. (2005). Naming and word-retrieval problems. In L. L. LaPointe (Ed.), *Aphasia and related neurogenic language disorders* (3rd ed., pp. 68–82). New York: Thieme.

Raymer, A. M., & Ellsworth, T. A. (2002). Response to contrasting verb retrieval treatments: A case study. *Aphasiology, 16,* 1031–1045.

Raymer, A. M., Maher, L. M., Foundas, A. L., Heilman, K. M., & Rothi, L. J. G. (1997). The significance of body part as tool errors in limb apraxia. *Brain and Cognition, 34,* 287–292.

Raymer, A. M., Moberg, P., Crosson, B., Nadeau, S., & Rothi, L. J. (1997). Lexical-semantic deficits in two patients with dominant thalamic infarction. *Neuropsychologia, 35,* 211–219.

Raymer, A. M., Rowland, L., Haley, M., & Crosson, B. (2002). Nonsymbolic movement training to improve sentence generation in transcortical motor aphasia: A case study. *Aphasiology, 16,* 493–506.

Raymer, A. M., Thompson, C. K., Jacobs, B., & Le Grand, H. R. (1993). Phonological treatment of naming deficits in aphasia: Model-based generalization analysis. *Aphasiology, 7,* 27–53.

Reed, V. A. (2005). *An introduction to children with language disorders* (3rd ed.). Boston: Pearson Education.

Reisberg, B., Ferris, S. H., de Leon, M. J., & Crook, T. (1982). The Global Deterioration Scale for assessment of primary degenerative dementia. *American Journal of Psychiatry, 139,* 1136–1139.

Reisberg, B., Ferris, S. H., & Franssen, E. (1985). An ordinal functional assessment tool for Alzheimer's type dementia. *Hospital and Cummunity Psychiatry, 36,* 939–944.

Reitan, R. M., & Wolfson, D. (1993). *The Halstead-Reitan Neuropsychological Test Battery: Theory and clinical interpretation.* Tucson, AZ: Neuropsychology Press.

Reitan, R. M., & Wolfson, D. (1995). Category Test and Trail Making Test as measures of frontal lobe functions. *Clinical Neuropsychologist, 9,* 50–55.

Richardson, J. T. E. (2000). *Clinical and neuropsychological aspects of closed head injury* (2nd ed.). Hove, UK: Psychology Press.

Riddoch, M. J., Humphreys, G. W., Cleton, P., & Ferry, P. (1990). Interaction of attentional and lexical processes in neglect dyslexia. *Cognitive Neuropsychology, 7,* 479–518.

Riedel, K., & Studdert-Kennedy, M. (1985). Extending formant transitions may not improve aphasics' perception of stop consonant place of articulation. *Brain and Language, 24,* 223–232.

Riege, W. H., Metter, E. J., & Hanson, W. R. (1980). Verbal and nonverbal recognition memory in aphasic and nonaphasic stroke patients. *Brain and Language, 10,* 60–70.

Rimel, R. W., & Jane, J. A. (1983). Characteristics of the head-injured patient. In M. Rosenthal, E. R. Griffith, M. R. Bond, & J. D. Miller (Eds.), *Rehabilitation of the head injured adult* (pp. 9–22). Philadelphia: F. A. Davis.

Rinnert, C., & Whitaker, H. A. (1973). Semantic confusions by aphasic patients. *Cortex, 9,* 56–81.

Ripich, D. N. (1996). *Alzheimer's disease communication guide: The FOCUSED program for caregivers.* San Antonio, TX: The Psychological Corporation.

Ripich, D. N., Ziol, E., & Lee, M. M. (1998). Longitudinal effects of communication training on caregivers of persons with Alzheimer's disease. *Clinical Gerontologist, 19,* 37–55.

Rispens, J., Bastiaanse, R., van Zonneveld, R., Jarema, G., & Edwards, S. (1997). Negation in agrammatism: A crosslinguistic comparison [abstract]. *Brain and Language, 60,* 75–78.

Rivers, D. L., & Love, R. J. (1980). Language performance on visual processing tasks in right hemisphere lesion cases. *Brain and Language, 10,* 348–366.

Roach, A., Schwartz, M. F., Martin, N., Grewal, R. S., & Brecher, A. (1996). The Philadelphia Naming Test: Scoring and rationale. In M. L. Lemme (Ed.), *Clinical aphasiology* (Vol. 24, pp. 121–134). Austin, TX: Pro-Ed.

Roberts, J. A., & Wertz, R. T. (1989). Comparison of spontaneous and elicited oral-expressive language in aphasia. In T. E. Prescott (Ed.), *Clinical aphasiology* (Vol. 18, pp. 479–488). Boston: College-Hill/Little, Brown.

Roberts, P. M., Code, C., & McNeil, M. R. (2003). Describing participants in aphasia research: Part 1. Audit of current practice. *Aphasiology, 17,* 911–932.

Robertson, I. H., Ward, T., Ridgeway, V., & Nimmo-Smith, I. (1994). *Test of Everyday Attention* (TEA). Oxford, UK: Harcourt Assessment.

Robertson, I. H., Ward, T., Ridgeway, V., & Nimmo-Smith, I. (1996). The structure of normal human attention: The Test of Everyday Attention. *Journal of the International Neuropsychological Society, 2,* 525–534.

Robey, R. R. (1998). A meta-analysis of clinical outcomes in the treatment of aphasia. *Journal of Speech, Language, and Hearing Research, 41,* 172–187.

Robey, R. R., & Dalebout, S. D. (1998). A tutorial on conducting meta-analyses of clinical outcome research. *Journal of Speech Language and Hearing Research, 41,* 1227–1241.

Robey, R. R., Schultz, M. C., Crawford, A. B., & Sinner, C. A. (1999). Single-subject clinical-outcome research: Designs, data, effect sizes, and analyses. *Aphasiology, 13,* 445–473.

Robin, D. A., & Schienberg, S. (1990). Subcortical lesions and aphasia. *Journal of Speech and Hearing Disorders, 55,* 90–100.

Robinson, R. G., Kubos, K. L., Starr, L. B., Rao, K., & Price, T. R. (1984). Mood disorders in stroke patients: Importance of location of lesion. *Brain, 107,* 81–93.

Robson, J., Marshall, J., Pring, T., Montagu, A., & Chiat, S. (2004). Processing proper nouns in aphasia: Evidence from assessment and therapy. *Aphasiology, 18,* 917–935.

Robson, J., Pring, T., Marshall, J., & Chiat, S. (2003). Phoneme frequency effects in jargon aphasia: A phonological investigation of nonword errors. *Brain and Language, 85,* 109–124.

Rochon, E., Saffran, E. M., Berndt, R. S., & Schwartz, M. F. (2000). Quantitative analysis of aphasic sentence production: Further development and new data. *Brain and Language, 72,* 193–218.

Rochon, E., Waters, G. S., & Caplan, D. (1994). Sentence comprehension in patients with Alzheimer's disease. *Brain and Language, 46,* 329–349.

Rogers, C. R. (1951). *Client-centered therapy.* Boston: Houghton Mifflin.

Rolak, L. A. (Ed.). (1993). *Neurology secrets.* Philadelphia: Hanley & Belfus.

Rollin, W. J. (1987). *The psychology of communication disorders in individuals and their families.* Englewood Cliffs, NJ: Prentice-Hall.

Roman, M., Brownell, H. H., Potter, Seibold, M. S., & Gardner, H. (1987). Script knowledge in right hemisphere-damaged and in normal elderly adults. *Brain and Language, 31,* 151–170.

Rose, S. (1989). *The conscious brain* (rev. ed.). New York: Paragon.

Rose, T., Worrall, L., & McKenna, K. (2003). The effectiveness of aphasia-friendly principles for printed health education materials for people with aphasia following stroke. *Aphasiology, 17,* 947–963.

Rosen, W. G., Mohs, R. C., & Davis, K. L. (1984). A new rating scale for Alzheimer's disease. *American Journal of Psychiatry, 141,* 1356–1364.

Rosenbek, J. C., LaPointe, L. L., & Wertz, R. T. (1989). *Aphasia: A clinical approach.* San Diego: Singular.

Rosenberg, B., Zurif, E., Brownell, H., Garrett, M., & Bradley, D. (1985). Grammatical class effects in relation to normal and aphasic sentence processing. *Brain and Language, 26,* 287–303.

Ross, E. D. (1981). The aprosodias: Functional-anatomic organization of the affective components of language in the right hemisphere. *Archives of Neurology, 38,* 561–569.

Ross, E. D., & Mesulam, M. (1979). Dominant language functions of the right hemisphere? Prosody and emotional gesturing. *Archives of Neurology, 36,* 144–148.

Ross, K. B., & Wertz, R. T. (1999). Comparison of impairment and disability measures for assessing severity of, and improvement in, aphasia. *Aphasiology, 13,* 113–124.

Ross, K. B., & Wertz, R. T. (2002). Relationships between language-based disability and quality of life in chronically aphasic adults. *Aphasiology, 16,* 791–800.

Ross, K. B., & Wertz, R. T. (2003). Quality of life with and without aphasia. *Aphasiology, 17,* 355–364.

Ross, K. B., & Wertz, R. T. (2004). Accuracy of formal tests for diagnosing mild aphasia: An application of evidence-based medicine. *Aphasiology, 18,* 337–355.

Ross, K. B., & Wertz, R. T. (2005). Advancing appraisal: Aphasia and the WHO. *Aphasiology, 19,* 860–870.

Rothi, L. J. G., Mack, L., Verfaellie, M., Brown, P., & Heilman, K. M. (1988). Ideomotor apraxia: Error pattern analysis. *Aphasiology, 2,* 381–388.

Rubens, A. B. (1977a). The role of changes within the central nervous system during recovery from aphasia. In M. Sullivan & M. S. Kommers (Eds.), *Rationale for adult aphasia therapy* (pp. 28–43). University of Nebraska Medical Center.

Rubens, A. B. (1977b). What neurologists expect of clinical aphasiologists. In R. H. Brookshire (Ed.), *Clinical aphasiology conference proceedings* (pp. 1–4). Minneapolis: BRK.

Ruff, R. M., Marshall, L. F., Crouch, J., & Klauber, M. R. (1993). Predictors of outcome following severe head trauma: Follow-up data from the Traumatic Coma Data Bank. *Brain Injury, 7,* 101–111.

Ruml, W., Caramazza, A., Shelton, J. R., & Chialant, D. (2000). Testing assumptions in computational theories of aphasia. *Journal of Memory and Language, 43,* 217–248.

Russell, W. R., & Espir, M. L. E. (1961). *Traumatic aphasia.* London: Oxford University Press.

Ryff, C. D. (1989). Happiness is everything, or is it? Explorations on the meaning of well-being. *Journal of Personality and Social Psychology, 57,* 1069–1081.

Sabbagh, M. A. (1999). Communicative intentions and language: Evidence from right-hemisphere damage and autism. *Brain and Language, 70,* 29–69.

Sacks, O. (1985). *The man who mistook his wife for a hat and other clinical tales.* New York: Summit.

Saffran, E. M., Schwartz, M. F., & Linebarger, M. C. (1998). Semantic influences on thematic role assignment: Evidence from normals and aphasics. *Brain and Language, 62,* 255–297.

Saffran, E. M., Schwartz, M. F., & Marin, O. S. M. (1980). The word order problem in agrammatism. II. Production. *Brain and Language, 10,* 263–280.

Salvatore, A. P. (1985). Experimental analysis of acquisition and generalization of syntax in Broca's aphasia. In R. H. Brookshire (Ed.), *Clinical aphasiology* (Vol. 15, pp. 214–221). Minneapolis: BRK.

Samples, J. M., & Lane, V. W. (1980). Language gains in global aphasia over a three-year period: Case study. *Journal of Communication Disorders, 13,* 49–57.

Sanders, S. B., & Davis, G. A. (1978). A comparison of the Porch Index of Communicative Ability and the Western Aphasia Battery. In R. H. Brookshire (Ed.), *Clinical aphasiology conference proceedings* (pp. 117–126). Minneapolis: BRK.

Sanders, S. B., Hamby, E. I., & Nelson, M. (1984). *You are not alone: Organizing your local stroke club.* Nashville, Tennessee Affiliate of the American Heart Association.

Sands, E., Sarno, M. T., & Shankweiler, D. (1969). Long-term assessment of language function in aphasia due to stroke. *Archives of Physical Medicine and Rehabilitation, 50,* 202–207.

Santo Pietro, M. J., & Boczko, R. (1997). The Breakfast Club and related programs. In B. Shadden & M. A. Toner (Eds.). *Aging and communication* (pp. 341–359). Austin, TX: Pro-Ed.

Santo Pietro, M. J., & Boczko, F. (1998). The Breakfast Club: Results of a study examining the effectiveness of a multi-modality group communication treatment. *American Journal of Alzheimer's Disease, 13,* 146–158.

Sarno, J. E., Sarno, M. T., & Levita, E. (1971). Evaluating language improvement after completed stroke. *Archives of Physical Medicine and Rehabilitation, 52,* 73–78.

Sarno, M. T. (1969). *The functional communication profile manual of directions.* Rehabilitation Monograph *42,* New York University Medical Center.

Sarno, M. T. (1980). The nature of verbal impairment after closed head injury. *Journal of Nervous and Mental Disease, 168,* 685–692.

Sarno, M. T. (1993). Aphasia rehabilitation: Psychosocial and ethical considerations. *Aphasiology, 7,* 321–334.

Sarno, M. T., Buonaguro, A., & Levita, E. (1987). Aphasia in closed head injury and stroke. *Aphasiology, 1,* 331–338.

Sarno, M. T., & Levita, E. (1971). Natural course of recovery in severe aphasia. *Archives of Physical Medicine and Rehabilitation, 52,* 175–178.

Sarno, M. T., & Levita, E. (1979). Recovery in treated aphasia during the first year post-stroke. *Stroke, 10,* 663–670.

Sarno, M. T., & Levita, E. (1981). Some observations on the nature of recovery in global aphasia after stroke. *Brain and Language, 13,* 1–12.

Sarno, M. T., Silverman, M., & Sands, E. (1970). Speech therapy and language recovery in severe aphasia. *Journal of Speech and Hearing Research, 13,* 607–623.

Schacter, D. L. (1996). *Searching for memory: The brain, the mind, and the past.* New York: BasicBooks.

Schacter, D. L., & Graf, P. (1986). Preserved learning in amnesic patients: Perspectives from research on direct priming. *Journal of Clinical and Experimental Neuropsychology, 8,* 727–743.

Scheinberg, S., & Holland, A. (1980). Conversational turn-taking in Wernicke's aphasia. In R. Brookshire (Ed.), *Clinical aphasiology conference proceedings* (pp. 106–110). Minneapolis: BRK.

Scherzer, E. (1992). Functional assessment: A clinical perspective. *Aphasiology, 6,* 101–104.

Schiffrin, D. (1994). *Approaches to discourse.* Malden, MA: Blackwell.

Schlanger, B. B., Schlanger, P., & Gerstman, L. J. (1976). The perception of emotionally toned sentences by right hemisphere-damaged and aphasic subjects. *Brain and Language, 3,* 396–403.

Schlanger, P. H., & Schlanger, B. B. (1970). Adapting role playing activities with aphasic patients. *Journal of Speech and Hearing Disorders, 35,* 229–235.

Schmitter-Edgecombe, M. E., Marks, W., Fahy, J. F., & Long, C. J. (1992). Effects of severe closed-head injury on three stages of information processing. *Journal of Clinical and Experimental Neuropsychology, 14,* 717–737.

Schmitzer, A. B., Strauss, M., & DeMarco, S. (1998). Contextual influences on comprehension of multiple-meaning words by right hemisphere brain-damaged and non-brain damaged adults. *Aphasiology, 11,* 447–460.

Schneider, S. L., & Thompson, C. K. (2003). Verb production in agrammatic aphasia: The influence of semantic class and argument structure properties on generalization. *Aphasiology, 17,* 213–241.

Schnitzer, M. L. (1978). Toward a neurolinguistic theory of language. *Brain and Language, 6,* 342–361.

Schretlin, D. Bobholz, J. H., & Brandt, J. (1996). Development and psychometric properties of the Brief Test of Attention. *Clinical Neuropsychologist, 10,* 80–89.

Schriefers, H., Meyer, A. S., & Levelt, W. J. M. (1990). Exploring the time course of lexical access in language production: Picture-word interference studies. *Journal of Memory and Language, 29,* 86–102.

Schuell, H. M. (1966). A re-evaluation of the short examination for aphasia. *Journal of Speech and Hearing Disorders, 31,* 137–147.

Schuell, H. M. (1969). *Aphasia in adults. In Human communication and its disorders—an overview.* Bethesda, MD: U.S. Department of Health, Education, and Welfare.

Schuell, H. M. (1973). *Differential diagnosis of aphasia with the Minnesota test* (2nd ed., revised by Sefer, J. W.). Minneapolis: University of Minnesota Press.

Schuell, H. M., & Jenkins, J. J. (1961). Reduction of vocabulary in aphasia. *Brain, 84,* 243–261.

Schuell, H. M., Jenkins, J. J., & Jimenez-Pabon, E. (1964). *Aphasia in adults.* New York: Harper and Row.

Schulz, R. (2000). *Handbook on dementia caregiving.* New York: Springer.

Schwartz, M. F. (1987). Patterns of speech production deficit within and across aphasia syndromes: Application of a psycholinguistic model. In M. Coltheart, G. Sartori, & R. Job (Eds.). *The cognitive neuropsychology of language* (pp. 163–199). London: Erlbaum.

Schwartz, M. F., Linebarger, M. C., & Saffran, E. M. (1985). The status of the syntactic deficit theory of agrammatism. In M-L. Kean (Ed.), *Agrammatism* (pp. 83–124). Orlando, FL: Academic Press.

Schwartz, M. F., Saffran, E. M., Fink, R., Myers, J., & Martin, N. (1994). Mapping therapy: A treatment programme for agrammatism. *Aphasiology, 8,* 19–54.

Schwartz, M. F., Saffran, E. M., & Marin, O. S. M. (1980). The word order problem in agrammatism. I. Comprehension. *Brain and Language, 10,* 249–262.

Schwartz, M. F., Wilshire, C. E., Gagnon, D. A., & Polansky, M. (2004). Origins of nonword phonological errors in aphasic picture naming. *Cognitive Neuropsychology, 21,* 159–186.

Schwartz-Cowley, R., & Stepanik, M. J. (1989). Communication disorders and treatment in the acute trauma center setting. *Topics in language disorders, 9,* 1–14.

Scott, C., & Byng, S. (1989). Computer assisted remediation of a homophone comprehension disorder in surface dyslexia. *Aphasiology, 3,* 301–320.

Searle, J. R. (1969). *Speech acts.* London: Cambridge University Press.

Seddoh, S. A. (2002). How discrete or independent are "affective prosody" and "linguistic prosody"? *Aphasiology, 16,* 683–692.

Seddoh, S., Robin, D., Sim, H., Hageman, C., Moon, J., et al. (1996). Speech timing in apraxia of speech versus conduction aphasia. *Journal of Speech, Language, and Hearing Research, 39,* 590–603.

Seidenberg, M. S., Tanenhaus, M. K., Leiman, J. M., & Bienkowski, M. (1982). Automatic access of the meanings of ambiguous words in context: Some limitations of knowledge-based processing. *Cognitive Psychology, 14,* 489–537.

Senelick, R. C., Rossi, P. W., & Dougherty, K. (1994). *Living with stroke: A guide for families.* Chicago: Contemporary Books.

Seron, X., & de Partz, M-P. (1993). The re-education of aphasics: Between theory and practice. In A. L. Holland & M. M. Forbes (Eds.), *Aphasia treatment: World perspectives* (pp. 131–144). San Diego, CA: Singular.

Seron, X., Van Der Kaa, M., Remitz, A., & Van Der Linden, M. (1979). Pantomime interpretation and aphasia. *Neuropsychologia, 17,* 661–668.

Shallice, T. (1988). *From neuropsychology to mental structure.* Cambridge, UK: Cambridge University Press.

Shallice, T., & Warrington, E. K. (1977). Auditory-verbal short-term memory impairment and spontaneous speech. *Brain and Language, 4,* 479–491.

Shankweiler, D., Crain, S., Gorrell, P., & Tuller, B. (1989). Reception of language in Broca's aphasia. *Language and Cognitive Processes, 4,* 1–34.

Shankweiler, D., & Harris, K. S. (1966). An experimental approach to the problem of articulation in aphasia. *Cortex, 2,* 277–292.

Shapiro, B. E., & Danly, M. (1985). The role of the right hemisphere in the control of speech prosody in propositional and affective contexts. *Brain and Language, 25,* 19–36.

Shapiro, B. E., Grossman, M., & Gardner, H. (1981). Selective musical processing deficits in brain damaged populations. *Neuropsychologia, 19,* 161–169.

Shapiro, K., & Caramazza, A. (2001a). Language is more than its parts: A reply to Bird, Howard, and Franklin (2001). *Brain and Language, 78,* 397–401

Shapiro, K., & Caramazza, A. (2001b). Sometimes a noun is just a noun: Comments on Bird, Howard, and Franklin (2000). *Brain and Language, 76,* 202–212.

Shapiro, L. P. (1997). Tutorial: An introduction to syntax. *Journal of Speech and Hearing Research, 40,* 254–272.

Shapiro, L. P., Gordon, B., Hack, N., & Killackey, J. (1993). Verb-argument structure processing in complex sentences in Broca's and Wernicke's aphasia. *Brain and Language, 45,* 423–447.

Shapiro, L. P., & Levine, B. A. (1990). Verb processing during sentence comprehension in aphasia. *Brain and Language, 38,* 21–47.

Shapiro, L. P., Swinney, D., & Borsky, S. (1998). Online examination of language performance in normal and neurologically impaired adults. *American Journal of Speech-Language Pathology, 7,* 49–60.

Sheehan, V. M. (1946). Rehabilitation of aphasics in an army hospital. *Journal of Speech and Hearing Disorders, 11,* 149–157.

Sheehy, L. M., & Haines, M. E. (2004). Crossed Wernicke's aphasia: A case report. *Brain and Language, 89,* 203–206.

Shelton, J. R., & Caramazza, A. (2001). The organization of semantic memory. In B. Rapp (Ed.), *The handbook of cognitive neuropsychology* (pp. 423–443). Philadelphia: Psychology Press.

Shelton, J. R., Weinrich, M., McCall, D., & Cox, D. M. (1996). Differentiating globally aphasic patients: Data from in-depth language assessments and production training using C-VIC. *Aphasiology, 10,* 319–342.

Shenaut, G. K., & Ober, B. A. (1996). Methodological control of semantic priming in Alzheimer's disease. *Psychology and Aging, 11,* 443–448.

Shenk, D. (2002). *The forgetting: Alzheimer's: Protrait of an epidemic.* New York: Anchor Books.

Shephard, J. M., & Kosslyn, S. M. (2005). The Minicog Rapid Assessment Battery: Developing a "blood pressure cuff for the mind." *Aviation, Space & Environmental Medicine, 76,* B192–197.

Sherer, M., Parsons, O. A., Nixon, S. J., & Adams, R. L. (1991). Clinical validity of the Speech-Sounds Perception Test and the Seashore Rhythm Test. *Journal of Clinical and Experimental Neuropsychology, 13,* 741–751.

Sherer, M., Sander, A. M., Nick, T. G., High, Jr., W. M., Males, J. F., et al. (2002). Early cognitive status and productivity outcome after traumatic brain injury: Findings from the TBI Model Systems. *Archives of Physical Medicine and Rehabilitation, 83,* 183–192.

Shewan, C. M. (1979). *Auditory Comprehension Test for Sentences.* Chicago: Biolinguistics Clinical Institutes.

Shewan, C. M. (1982). To hear is not to understand: Auditory processing deficits and factors influencing performance in aphasic individuals. In N. J. Lass (Ed.), *Speech and language: Advances in basic research and practice* (Vol. 7, pp. 1–70). New York: Academic Press.

Shewan, C. M. (1988). The Shewan Spontaneous Language Analysis (SSLA) system for aphasic adults: Description, reliability, and validity. *Journal of Communication Disorders, 21,* 103–138.

Shewan, C. M., & Bandur, D. L. (1986). *Treatment of aphasia: A language-oriented approach.* San Diego: Singular.

Shewan, C. M., & Canter, G. J. (1971). Effects of Vocabulary, syntax, and sentence legnth on auditory comprehension in aphasic patients. *Cortex, 7,* 209–226.

Shewan, C. M., & Kertesz, A. (1980). Reliability and validity characteristics of the Western Aphasia Battery (WAB). *Journal of Speech and Hearing Disorders, 45,* 308–324.

Shewan, C. M., & Kertesz, A. (1984). Effects of speech and language treatment on recovery from aphasia. *Brain and Language, 23,* 272–299.

Shisler, R. J., Baylis, G. C., & Frank, E. M. (2000). Pharmacological approaches to the treatment and prevention of aphasia. *Aphasiology, 14,* 1163–1186.

Shuster, L. I. (2004). Resource theory and aphasia reconsidered: Why alternative theories can better guide our research. *Aphasiology, 18,* 811–830.

Shuster, L. I., & Thompson, J. C. (2004). Resource theory: Here, there, and everywhere. *Aphasiology, 18,* 850–854.

Sidtis, J. J., & Volpe, B. T. (1988). Selective loss of complex-pitch or speech discrimination after unilateral lesion. *Brain and Language, 34,* 235–245.

Sies, L. F. (Ed.). (1974). *Aphasia theory and therapy: Selected lectures and papers of Hildred Schuell.* Baltimore: University Park Press.

Silberman, E. K., & Weingartner, H. (1986). Hemispheric lateralization of functions related to emotion. *Brain and Cognition, 5,* 322–354.

Simmons, N. N., Kearns, K. P., & Potechin, G. (1987). Treatment of aphasia through family member training. In R. H. Brookshire (ed.), *Clinical aphasiology* (Vol. 17, pp. 106–116). Minneapolis: BRK.

Simmons-Mackie, N. (2005). Conduction aphasia. In L. L. LaPointe (Ed.), *Aphasia and related neurogenic language disorders* (3rd ed., pp. 155–168). New York: Thieme.

Simmons-Mackie, N. N. (2000). Social approaches to the management of aphasia. In L. E. Worrall & C. M. Frattali (Eds.). *Neurogenic communication disorders: A functional approach* (pp. 162–187). New York: Thieme.

Simmons-Mackie, N. N. (2001). Social approaches to aphasia intervention. In R. Chapey (Ed.), *Language intervention strategies in adult aphasia and related neurogenic communication disorders* (4th ed.,

pp. 246–268). Philadelphia: Lippincott Williams & Wilkins.

Simmons-Mackie, N. N., & Damico, J. S. (1996). The contribution of discourse markers to communicative competence in aphasia. *American Journal of Speech-Language Pathology, 5,* 37–43.

Simmons-Mackie, N. N., & Damico, J. S. (1997). Reformulating the definition of compensatory strategies in aphasia. *Aphasiology, 11,* 761–781.

Simmons-Mackie, N. N., & Kagan, A. (1999). Communication strategies used by 'good' versus 'poor' speaking partners of individuals with aphasia. *Aphasiology, 13,* 807–820.

Simpson, G. B., & Burgess, C. (1985). Activation and selection processes in the recognition of ambiguous words. *Journal of Experimental Psychology: Human Perception and Performance, 11,* 28–39.

Skelly, M. (1975). Aphasic patients talk back. *American Journal of Nursing, 75,* 1140–1142.

Skelly, M. (1979). *Amer-Ind gestural code based on universal American Indian hand talk.* New York: Elsevier.

Skilbeck, C. E., Wade, D. T., Hewer, R. L., & Wood, V. A. (1983). Recovery after stroke. *Journal of Neurology, Neurosurgery, and Psychiatry, 46,* 5–8.

Skotko, B. G., Andrews, E., & Einstein, G. (2005). Language and the medial temporal lobe: Evidence from H. M.'s spontaneous discourse. *Journal of Memory and Language, 53,* 397–415.

Small, J. A., Gutman, G., Makela, S., & Hillhouse, B. (2003). Effectiveness of communication strategies used by caregivers of persons with Alzheimer's disease during activities of daily living. *Journal of Speech, Language, and Hearing Research, 46,* 353–367.

Small, J. A., Kemper, S., & Lyons, K. (2000). Sentence repetition and processing resources in Alzheimer's disease. *Brain and Language, 75,* 232–258.

Small, J. A., & Perry, J. (2005). Do you remember? How caregivers question their spouses who have Alzheimer's disease and the impact on communication. *Journal of Speech, Language, and Hearing Research, 48,* 125–136.

Small, S. L. (1994). Pharmacotherapy of aphasia: A critical review. *Stroke, 25,* 1282–1289.

Small, S. L. (2002). Biological approaches to the treatment of aphasia. In A. E. Hillis (Ed.), *The handbook of adult language disorders* (pp. 397–411). New York: Psychology Press.

Small, S. L. (2004). A biological model of aphasia rehabilitation: Pharmacological perspectives. *Aphasiology, 18,* 476–491.

Smith, F. (1982). *Understanding reading: A psycholinguistic analysis of reading and learning to read* (3rd ed.). New York: Holt, Rinehart and Winston.

Smith, P. B., Kenan, M. M., & Kunik, M. E. (2004). *Alzheimer's for dummies.* Hoboken, NJ: Wiley.

Smith, S. D., & Bates, E. (1987). Accessibility of case and gender contrasts for agent-object assignment in Broca's aphasics and fluent anomics. *Brain and Language, 30,* 8–32.

Smith, S. D., & Mimica, I. (1984). Agrammatism in a case-inflected language: Comprehension of agent-object relations. *Brain and Language, 21,* 274–290.

Snow, P., Douglas, J., & Ponsford, J. (1995). Discourse assessment following traumatic brain injury: A pilot study examining some demographic and methodological issues. *Aphasiology, 9,* 365–380.

Snowden, J. S., Neary, D., & Mann, D. A. (2002). Frontotemporal dementia. *British Journal of Psychiatry, 180,* 140–143.

Snyder, P. J., & Nussbaum, P. D. (Eds.). (1998). *Clinical neuropsychology: A pocket handbook for assessment.* Washington, D.C.: American Psychological Association.

Sohlberg, M. M., & Mateer, C. A. (1987). Effectiveness of an attention training program. *Journal of Clinical and Experimental Neuropsychology, 9,* 117–130.

Sohlberg, M. M., & Mateer, C. A. (1989). Training use of compensatory memory books: A three-stage behavioral approach. *Journal of Clinical and Experimental Neuropsychology, 11,* 871–891.

Sohlberg, M. M., & Mateer, C. A. (2001). *Cognitive rehabilitation: An integrative neuropsychological approach.* New York: Guilford Press.

Sohlberg, M. M., McLaughlin, K., Pavese, A., Heidrich, A., & Posner, M. (2000). Evaluation of attention process training and brain injury education in persons with aquired brain injury. *Journal of Clinical and Experimental Neuropsychology, 22,* 656–676.

Sohlberg, M. M., White, O., Evans, E., & Mateer, C. A. (1992). An investigation into the effects of prospective memory training. *Brain Injury, 6,* 139–154.

Solin, D. (1989). The systematic misrepresentation of bilingual-crossed aphasia data and its consequences. *Brain and Language, 36,* 92–116.

Solso, R. L. (1988). *Cognitive psychology* (2nd ed.). Boston: Allyn & Bacon.

Solso, R. L. (1991). *Cognitive psychology* (3rd ed.). Boston: Allyn & Bacon.

Sparks, R. W. (1978). Parastandardized examination guidelines for adult aphasia. *British Journal of Disorders of Communication, 13,* 135–146.

Sparks, R. W., Helm, N. A., & Albert, M. L. (1974). Aphasia rehabilitation resulting from melodic intonation therapy. *Cortex, 10,* 303–316.

Sparks, R. W., & Holland, A. L. (1976). Method: Melodic intonation therapy for aphasia. *Journal of Speech and Hearing Disorders, 41,* 287–297.

Spector, A., Orrell, M., Davies, S., & Woods, B. (2001). Can reality orientation be rehabilitated? Development and piloting of an evidence-based programme of cognition-based therapies for people with dementia. *Neuropsychological Rehabilitation, 11,* 377–397.

Spellacy, F. J., & Spreen, O. (1969). A short form of the Token Test. *Cortex, 5,* 390–397.

Sperber, D., & Wilson, D. (1986). *Relevance: Communication and cognition.* Cambridge, MA: Harvard University Press.

Spinnler, H., & Vignolo, L. (1966). Impaired recognition of meaningful sounds in aphasia. *Cortex, 2,* 337–348.

Spreen, O., & Benton, A. L. (1977). *Neurosensory center comprehensive examination for aphasia* (NCCEA) (Revised). Victoria, British Columbia: Neuropsychology Laboratory, University of Victoria.

Springer, L., Glindemann, R., Huber, W., & Willmes, K. (1991). How efficacious is PACE-therapy when "Language Systematic Training" is incorporated? *Aphasiology, 5,* 391–399.

Springer, S. P., & Deutsch, G. (1998). *Left brain, right brain* (5th ed.). New York: W. H. Freeman.

Squire, L. R. (1987). *Memory and brain.* New York: Oxford University Press.

Stambrook, M., Moore, A. D., Peters, L. C., Zubek, E., McBeath, S., & Friesen, I. C. (1991). Head injury and spinal cord injury: Differential effects on psychosocial functioning. *Journal of Clinical and Experimental Neuropsychology, 13,* 521–530.

Starch, S., & Falltrick, E. (1990). The importance of a home evaluation for brain injured clients: A team approach. *Cognitive Rehabilitation, 8*(6), 28–32.

Starkstein, S. E., & Robinson, R. G. (1988). Aphasia and depression. *Aphasiology, 2,* 1–20.

State University of New York at Buffalo. (1990). *Guide for use of the uniform data set for medical rehabilitation.* Buffalo, NY: Research Foundation.

Stein, J. (2004). *Stroke and the family: A new guide.* Cambridge, MA: Harvard University Press.

Stein, N. L., & Glenn, C. G. (1979). An analysis of story comprehension in elementary school children. In R. O. Freedle (Ed.), *New directions in discourse processes* (pp. 53–120). Norwood, NJ: Ablex.

Stern, B. H. (1995, June). The neuropsychologist in a mild traumatic brain injury case: How to conduct the direct examination. *Trial,* 66–73.

Sternberg, S. (1975). Memory scanning: New findings and current controversies. In D. Deutsch & J. A. Deutsch (Eds.), *Short-term memory.* New York: Academic Press.

Stemmer, B., Giroux, F., & Joanette, Y. (1994). Production and evaluation of requests by right hemisphere brain-damaged individuals. *Brain and Language, 47,* 1–31.

Stimley, M. A., & Noll, J. D. (1991). The effects of semantic and phonemic prestimulation cues on picture naming in aphasia. *Brain and Language, 41,* 496–509.

Stoler, D. R., & Hill, B. A. (1998). *Coping with mild traumatic brain injury: A guide to living with the challenges associated with concussion/brain injury.* New York: Avery.

Strand, E. A. (1995). Ethical issues related to progressive disease. *Special Interest Division 2 Newsletter, 5*(3), 3–8.

Stubbs, M. (1983). *Discourse analysis: The sociolinguistic analysis of natural language.* Chicago: University of Chicago Press.

Sullivan, M. P., Fisher, B., & Marshall, R. C. (1986). Treating the repetition deficit in conduction aphasia. In R. H. Brookshire (Ed.), *Clinical aphasiology* (Vol. 16, pp. 172–180). Minneapolis: BRK.

Sunderland, A., Harris, J. E., & Baddeley, A. D. (1983). Do laboratory tests predict everyday memory? A neuropsychological study. *Journal of Verbal Learning and Verbal Behavior, 22,* 341–357.

Sundet, K. (1986). Sex differences in cognitive impairment following unilateral brain damage. *Journal of Clinical and Experimental Neuropsychology, 8,* 51–61.

Swaab, T. Y., Brown, C., & Hagoort, P. (1998). Understanding ambiguous words in sentence contexts: Electrophysiological evidence for delayed contextual selection in Broca's aphasia. *Neuropsychologia, 36,* 737–761.

Swindell, C. S., Holland, A. L., & Fromm, D. (1984). Classification of aphasia: WAB type versus clinical impression. In R. H. Brookshire (Ed.), *Clinical aphasiology conference proceedings* (pp. 48–54). Minneapolis: BRK.

Swindell, C. S., Holland, A. L., Fromm, D., & Greenhouse, J. B. (1988). Characteristics of recovery of drawing ability in left and right brain-damaged subjects. *Brain and Cognition, 7,* 16–30.

Swinney, D. A. (1979). Lexical access during sentence comprehension: (Re)consideration of context effects. *Journal of Verbal Learning and Verbal Behavior, 20,* 645–660.

Swinney, D. A., & Zurif, E. (1995). Syntactic processing in aphasia. *Brain and Language, 50,* 225–239.

Swinney, D. A., Zurif, E., & Cutler, A. (1980). Effects of sentential stress and word class upon comprehension in Broca's aphasics. *Brain and Language, 10,* 132–144.

Swinney, D. A., Zurif, E., & Nicol, J. (1989). The effects of focal brain damage on sentence processing: An examination of the neurological organization of a mental module. *Journal of Cognitive Neuroscience, 1,* 25–37.

Swisher, L., & Hirsh, I. J. (1972). Brain damage and the ordering of two temporally successive stimuli. *Neuropsychologia, 10,* 137–152.

Swisher, L. P., & Sarno, M. T. (1969). Token Test scores of three matched patient groups: Left brain-damaged with aphasia; right brain-damaged without aphasia, non-brain damaged. *Cortex, 5,* 264–273.

Szelies, B., Mielke, R., Kessler, J., & Heiss, W-D. (2002). Prognostic relevance of quantitative topographical EEG in patients with poststroke aphasia. *Brain and Language, 82,* 87–94.

Taft, M. (1990). Lexical processing of functionally constrained words. *Journal of Memory and Language, 29,* 245–257.

Tanner, D. C., & Culbertson, W. (1999). *Quick Assessment for Aphasia.* Oceanside, CA: Academic Communication Associates.

Tanner, D. C., & Gerstenberger, D. L. (1988). The grief response in neuropathologies of speech and language. *Aphasiology, 2,* 79–84.

Tanridag, O., Kirshner, H. S., & Casey, P. F. (1987). Memory functions in aphasic and non-aphasic stroke patients. *Aphasiology, 1,* 201–214.

Taylor, M. L., & Marks, M. M. (1959). *Aphasia rehabilitation manual and therapy kit.* New York: McGraw-Hill.

Terman, L. M., & Merrill, M. A. (1937). *Measuring intelligence.* Boston: Houghton Mifflin.

Tesak, J., & Niemi, J. (1997). Telegraphese and agrammatism: A cross-linguistic study. *Aphasiology, 11,* 145–155.

Thompson, C. K. (1989). Generalization research in aphasia: A review of the literature. In T. E. Prescott (Ed). *Clinical aphasiology* (Vol. 18, pp. 195–222). Austin, TX: Pro-Ed.

Thompson, C. K. (2001). Treatment of underlying forms: A linguistic specific approach to sentence production deficits in agrammatic aphasia. In R. Chapey (Ed.), *Language intervention strategies in adult aphasia and related neurogenic communication disorders* (4th ed., pp. 605–628). Philadelphia: Lippincott Williams & Wilkins.

Thompson, C. K. (2005). Functional neuroimaging: Applications for studying aphasia. In L. L. LaPointe (Ed.), *Aphasia and related neurogenic language disorders* (3rd ed., pp. 19–38). New York: Thieme.

Thompson, C. K. and Byrne, M. E. (1984). Across setting generalization of social conventions in aphasia: An experimental analysis of "loose training." In R. H. Brookshire (Ed.), *Clinical aphasiology conference proceedings* (pp. 132–144). Minneapolis: BRK.

Thompson, C. K., & Johnson, N. (2006). Language interventions in dementia. In D. K. Attix & K. A. Welsh-Bohmer (Eds.), *Geriatric neuropsychology: Assessment and intervention* (pp. 315–332). New York: Guilford Press.

Thompson, C. K., & Kearns, K. P. (1981). An experimental analysis of acquisition, generalization, and maintenance of naming behavior in a patient with anomia. In R. H.

Brookshire (Ed.), *Clinical aphasiology conference proceedings* (pp. 35–45). Minneapolis, MN: BRK.

Thompson, C. K., Lange, K. L., Schneider, S. L., & Shapiro, L. P. (1997). Agrammatic and non-brain-damaged subjects' verb and verb argument structure production. *Aphasiology, 11,* 473–490.

Thompson, C. K., & McReynolds, L. V. (1986). Wh-interrogative production in agrammatic aphasia: An experimental analysis of auditory-visual stimulation and direct-production treatment. *Journal of Speech and Hearing Research, 29,* 193–206.

Thompson, C. K., & Shapiro, L. P. (1994). A linguistic-specific approach to treatment of sentence production deficits in aphasia. In M. L. Lemme (Ed.), *Clinical aphasiology* (Vol. 22, pp. 307–324). Austin, TX: Pro-Ed.

Thompson, C. K., & Shapiro, L. P. (2005). Treating agrammatic aphasia within a linguistic framework: Treatment of Underlying Forms. *Aphasiology, 19,* 1021–1036.

Thompson, C. K., Shapiro, L. P., Ballard, K. J., Jacobs, B. J., Schneider, S. S., et al. (1997). Training and generalized production of wh- and NP-movement structures in agrammatic aphasia. *Journal of Speech, Language, and Hearing Research, 40,* 228–244.

Thompson, C. K., Shapiro, L. P., Kiran, S., & Sobecks, J. (2003). The role of syntactic complexity in treatment of sentence deficits in agrammatic aphasia: The complexity account of treatment efficacy (CATE). *Journal of Speech, Language, and Hearing Research, 46,* 591–607.

Thompson, C. K., Shapiro, L. P., Tait, M. E., Jacobs, B. J., & Schneider, S. L. (1996). Training Wh-question production in agrammatic aphasia: Analysis of argument and adjunct movement. *Brain and Language, 52,* 175–228.

Thompson, C. K., Shapiro, L. P., Tait, M. E., Jacobs, B. J., Schneider, S. L., et al. (1995). A system for the linguistic analysis of agrammatic language production [abstract]. *Brain and Language, 51,* 124–129.

Thompson, J., & Enderby, P. (1979). Is all your Schuell really necessary? *British Journal of Disorders of Communication, 14,* 195–201.

Thomson, A. M., Taylor, R., Fraser, D., & Whittle, I. R. (1997a). Stereotactic biopsy of nonpolar tumors in the dominant hemisphere: A prospective study of effects on language functions. *Journal of Neurosurgery, 86,* 923–926.

Thomson, A. M., Taylor, R., Fraser, D., & Whittle, I. R. (1997b). The utility of the Right Hemisphere Language Battery in patients with brain tumours. *European Journal of Disorders of Communication, 32,* 325–332.

Thorndyke, P. W. (1977). Cognitive structures in comprehension and memory of narrative discourse. *Cognitive Psychology, 9,* 77–110.

Thurlborn, K. R., Carpenter, P., & Just, M. A. (1999). Plasticity of language-related brain function during recovery from stroke. *Stroke, 30,* 749–754.

Tirassa, M. (1999). Communicative competence and the architecture of the mind/brain. *Brain and Language, 68,* 419–441.

Togher, L., Hand, L., & Code, C. (1997). Measuring service encounters with the traumatic brain injury population. *Aphasiology, 11,* 491–504.

Togher, L., McDonald, S., Code, C., & Grant, S. (2004). Training communication partners of people with traumatic brain injury: A randomized controlled trial. *Aphasiology, 18,* 313–335.

Tompkins, C. A. (1990). Knowledge and strategies for processing lexical metaphor after right or left hemisphere brain damage. *Journal of Speech and Hearing Research, 33,* 307–316.

Tompkins, C. A. (1995). *Right hemisphere communication disorders: Theory and management.* San Diego, CA: Singular.

Tompkins, C. A., Baumgaertner, A., Lehman-Blake, M. T., & Fassbinder, W. (2000). Mechanisms of discourse comprehension impairment after right hemisphere brain damage: Suppression and enhancement in lexical ambiguity resolution. *Journal of Speech, Language, and Hearing Research, 43,* 62–78.

Tompkins, C. A., Bloise, C. G. R., Timko, M. L., & Baumgaertner, A. (1994). Working memory and inference revision in brain-damaged and normally aging adults. *Journal of Speech and Hearing Research, 37,* 896–912.

Tompkins, C. A., Fassbinder, W., Blake, M. L., Baumgaertner, A., & Jayaram, N. (2004). Inference generation during text comprehension by adults with right hemisphere brain damage: Activation failure versus multiple activation. *Journal of Speech, Language, and Hearing Research, 47,* 1380–1395.

Tompkins, C. A., Jackson, S. T., & Schulz, R. (1990). On prognostic research in adult neurologic disorders. *Journal of Speech and Hearing Research, 33,* 398–401.

Tompkins, C. A., Lehman-Blake, M. T., Baumgaertner, A., & Fassbinder, W. (2002). Characterising comprehension difficulties after right brain damage: Attention demands of suppression function. *Aphasiology, 16,* 559–572.

Tonkovich, J. D., & Loverso, F. (1982). A training matrix approach for gestural acquisition by the agrammatic patient. In R. H. Brookshire (Ed.), *Clinical aphasiology conference proceedings* (pp. 283–288). Minneapolis, MN: BRK.

Tree, J. J., Kay, J., & Perfect, T. J. (2005). "Deep" language disorders in nonfluent progressive aphasia: An evaluation of the "summation" account of semantic errors across language production tasks. *Cognitive Neuropsychology, 22,* 643–660.

Trexler, L. E., & Zappala, G. (1988). Neuropathological determinants of acquired attention disorders in traumatic brain injury. *Brain and Cognition, 8,* 291–302.

Trueblood, W., & Schmidt, M. (1993). Malingering and other validity considerations in the neuropsychological evaluation of mild head injury. *Journal of Clinical and Experimental Neuropsychology, 15,* 578–590.

Trupe, E. H. (1984). Reliability of rating spontaneous speech in the Western Aphasia Battery: Implications for classification. In R. H. Brookshire (Ed.), *Clinical aphasiology conference proceedings* (pp. 55–69). Minneapolis: BRK.

Trupe, E. H., & Hillis, A. (1985). Paucity vs. verbosity: Another analysis of right hemisphere communication deficits. In R. H. Brookshire (Ed.) *Clinical Aphasiology* (Vol. 15, pp. 83–96). Minneapolis: BRK.

Tseng, C-H., McNeil, M. R., & Milenkovic, P. (1993). An investigation of attention allocation deficits in aphasia. *Brain and Language, 45,* 276–296.

Tucker, D. M., Watson, R. T., & Heilman, K. M. (1977). Discrimination and evocation of affectively intoned speech in patients with right parietal disease. *Neurology, 27,* 947–950.

Tulving, E. (1972). Episodic and semantic memory. In E. Tulving & W. Donaldson (Eds.), *Organization of memory* (pp. 382–403). New York: Academic Press.

Tyler, L. K. (1985). Real-time comprehension processes in agrammatism: A case study. *Brain and Language, 26,* 259–275.

Tyler, L. K. (1987). Spoken language comprehension in aphasia: A real-time processing perspective. In M. Coltheart, G. Sartori, & R. Job (Eds.), *The cognitive neuropsychology of language* (pp. 145–162). London: Erlbaum.

Tyler, L. K. (1988). Spoken language comprehension in a fluent aphasic patient. *Cognitive Neuropsychology, 5,* 375–400.

Tyler, L. K. (1989). Syntactic deficits and the construction of local phrases in spoken language comprehension. *Cognitive Neuropsychology, 6,* 333–355.

Tyler, L. K., & Cobb, H. (1987). Processing bound grammatical morphemes in context: The case of an aphasic patient. *Language and Cognitive Processes, 2,* 245–262.

Tyler, L. K., & Moss, H. E. (1997). Imageability and category-specificity. *Cognitive Neuropsychology, 14,* 293–318.

Tyler, L. K., Ostrin, R. K., Cooke, M., & Moss, E. (1995). Automatic access of lexical information in Broca's aphasics: Against the automaticity hypothesis. *Brain and Language, 48,* 131–162.

Udell, R., Sullivan, R. A., & Schlanger, P. H. (1980). Legal competency of aphasic patients: Role of speech-language pathologists. *Archives of Physical Medicine and Rehabilitation, 61,* 374–375.

Ulatowska, H. K., Allard, L., Reyes, B. A., Ford, J., & Chapman, S. (1992). Conversational discourse in aphasia. *Aphasiology, 6,* 325–330.

Ulatowska, H. K., Freedman-Stern, R., Doyel, A. W., Macaluso-Haynes, S., & North, A. J. (1983). Production of narrative discourse in aphasia. *Brain and Language, 19,* 317–334.

Uryase, D., Duffy, R. J., & Liles, B. Z. (1990). Analysis and description of narrative discourse in right-hemisphere-damaged adults: A comparison to neurologically normal and left-hemisphere-damaged aphasic adults. In T. E. Prescott (Ed.), *Clinical aphasiology* (Vol. 19). Austin, TX: Pro-Ed.

U.S. National Institutes of Health. (n.d.). An investigation of constraint induced language therapy for aphasia. Retrieved March 30, 2006, from www.clinicaltrials.gov/ct/show/NCT00223847.

Vallar, G., & Baddeley, A. D. (1984). Fractionation of working memory: Neuropsychological evidence for a phonological short-term store. *Journal of Verbal Learning and Verbal Behavior, 23,* 151–161.

Vallar, G., & Baddeley, A. D. (1987). Phonological short-term store and sentence processing. *Cognitive Neuropsychology, 4,* 417–438.

Van Allen, M. W., Benton, A. L., & Gordon, M. C. (1966). Temporal discrimination in brain-damaged patients. *Neuropsychologia, 4,* 159–167.

Van Demark, A. A., Lemmer, E. C., & Drake, M. L. (1982). Measurement of reading comprehension in aphasia with the RCBA. *Journal of Speech and Hearing Disorders, 47,* 288–291.

Van der Linden, M., Brédart, S., Depoorter, N., & Coyette, F. (1996). Semantic memory and amnesia: A case study. *Cognitive Neuropsychology, 13,* 391–414.

Van der Linden, M., Coyette, F., & Seron, X. (1992). Selective impairment of the "central executive" component of working memory: A single case study. *Cognitive Neuropsychology, 9,* 301–326.

Van Eeckhout, P. (1993). Aphasia and artistic creation. In D. Lafond, Y. Joanette, R. Ponzio, R. Degiovani, & M. T. Sarno (Eds.), *Living with aphasia: Psychosocial issues* (pp. 87–102). San Diego, CA: Singular.

van Gompel, R. P. G., Pickering, M. J., Pearson, J., & Liversedge, S. P. (2005). Evidence against competition during syntactic ambiguity resolution. *Journal of Memory and Language, 52,* 284–307.

Van Lancker, D. R., & Kempler, D. (1987). Comprehension of familiar phrases by left- but not by right-hemisphere damaged patients. *Brain and Language, 32,* 265–277.

Van Lancker, D. R., Kreiman, J., & Cummings, J. (1989). Voice perception deficits: Neuroanatomical correlates of phonagnosia. *Journal of Clinical and Experimental Neuropsychology, 11,* 665–674.

Varney, N. R. (1980). Sound recognition in relation to aural language comprehension in aphasia. *Journal of Neurology, Neurosurgery, and Psychiatry, 43,* 71–75.

Varney, N. R. (1982). Pantomime recognition defect in aphasia: Implications for the concept of asymbolia. *Brain and Language, 15,* 32–39.

Varney, N. R. (1984). Phonemic imperception in aphasia. *Brain and Language, 21,* 85–94.

Vignolo, L. A., Boccardi, E., & Caverni, L. (1986). Unexpected CT-scan findings in global aphasia. *Cortex, 22,* 55–69.

Visch-Brink, E. G., van Harskamp, F., Van Amerongen, N. M., Wielaert, S. M., & van de Sandt-Koenderman, M. E. (1993). A multidisciplinary approach to aphasia therapy. In A. L. Holland & M. M. Forbes (Eds.), *Aphasia treatment: World perspectives* (pp. 227–262). San Diego, CA: Singular.

Vogel, D., & Costello, R. M. (1986). Bilingual aphasic adults: Measures of word retrieval. In R. H. Brookshire (Ed.). *Clinical aphasiology* (Vol. 16, pp. 80–86). Minneapolis: BRK.

Walker, J. P., Daigle, T., & Buzzard, M. (2002). Hemispheric specialization in processing prosodic structures: Revisited. *Aphasiology, 16,* 1155–1172.

Walker-Batson, D., Barton, M. M., Wendt, J. S., & Reynolds, S. (1987). Symbolic and affective non-verbal deficits in left- and right-hemisphere injured adults. *Aphasiology, 1,* 257–262.

Walker-Batson, D., Curtis, S., Smith, P., & Ford, S. (1999). An alternative model for the treatment of aphasia: The LifeLink© approach. In R. J. Elman (Ed.), *Group treatment of neurogenic communication disorders: The expert clinician's approach* (pp. 67–75). Boston: Butterworth Heinemann.

Wallace, G. L., & Canter, G. J. (1985). Effects of personally relevant language materials on the performance of severely aphasic individuals. *Journal of Speech and Hearing Disorders, 50,* 385–390.

Wallander, J. L., Conger, A. J., & Conger, J. C. (1985). Development and evaluation of a behaviorally referenced rating system for heterosocial skills. *Behavioral Assessment, 7,* 137–153.

Wallesch, C-W., Bak, T., & Schulte-Mönting, J. (1992). Acute aphasia—Patterns and prognosis. *Aphasiology, 6,* 373–385.

Wallesch, C-W., & Johannsen-Horbach, H. (2004). Computers in aphasia therapy: Effects and side-effects. *Aphasiology, 18,* 223–228.

Wambaugh, J. L., Cameron, R., Kalinyak-Fliszar, M., Nessler, C., & Wright, S. (2004). Retrieval of action names in aphasia: Effects of two cueing treatments. *Aphasiology, 18,* 979–1004.

Wambaugh, J. L., & Martinez, A. L. (2000). Effects of modified Response Elaboration Training with apraxic and aphasic speakers. *Aphasiology, 15,* 603–617.

Wambaugh, J. L., Martinez, A. L., & Alegre, M. N. (2001). Qualitative changes following application of modified response elaboration training with apraxic-aphasic speakers. *Aphasiology, 15,* 965–976.

Wang, L., & Goodglass, H. (1992). Pantomime, praxis, and aphasia. *Brain and Language, 42,* 402–418.

Warrington, E. K. (1991). Right neglect dyslexia: A single case study. *Cognitive Neuropsychology, 8,* 193–212.

Warrington, E. K., & Shallice, T. (1984). Category-specific semantic impairments. *Brain, 107,* 829–854.

Waters, G. S., & Caplan, D. (1996). The capacity theory of sentence comprehension: Critique of Just and Carpenter (1992). *Psychological Review, 103,* 761–772.

Waters, G. S., Caplan, D., & Hildebrandt, N. (1991). On the structure of verbal short-term memory and its functional role in sentence comprehension: Evidence from neuropsychology. *Cognitive Neuropsychology, 8,* 81–126.

Waters, G. S., Caplan, D., & Rochon, E. (1995). Processing capacity and sentence comprehension in patients with Alzheimer's disease. *Cognitive Neuropsychology, 12,* 1–30.

Waters, G. S., Rochon, E., & Caplan, D. (1998). Task demands and sentence comprehension in patients with dementia of Alzheimer's type. *Brain and Language, 62,* 361–397.

Watson, C. M., Chenery, H. J., & Carter, M. S. (1999). An analysis of trouble and repair in the natural conversations of people with dementia of the Alzheimer's type. *Aphasiology, 13,* 195–218.

Webb, W. G. (2005). Acquired dyslexias: Reading disorders associated with aphasia. In L. L. LaPointe (Ed.), *Aphasia and related neurogenic language disorders* (3rd ed., pp. 83–96). New York: Thieme.

Webster, J., Franklin, S., & Howard, D. (2001). An investigation of the interaction between thematic and phrasal structure in nonfluent agrammatic subjects. *Brain and Language, 78,* 197–211.

Webster, J., Morris, J., & Franklin, S. (2005). Effects of therapy targeted at verb retrieval and the realization of the predicate argument structure: A case study. *Aphasiology, 19,* 748–764

Webster, J. S., Cottam, G., Gouvier, W. D., Blanton, P., Beissel, G. F., et al. (1988). Wheelchair obstacle course performance in right cerebral vascular accident victims. *Journal of Clinical and Experimental Neuropsychology, 11,* 295–310.

Webster, J. S., Godlewski, M. C., Hanley, G. L., & Sowa, M. V. (1992). A scoring method for logical memory that is sensitive to right-hemisphere dysfunction. *Journal of Clinical and Experimental Neuropsychology, 14,* 222–238.

Wechsler, D. (1945). A standardized memory scale for clinical use. *Journal of Psychology, 19,* 87–95.

Wechsler, D. (1997a). *Wechsler Adult Intelligence Scale—Third Edition (WAIS III).* San Antonio, TX: Psychological Corporation.

Wechsler, D. (1997b). *Wechsler Memory Scale—Third Edition (WMS III).* San Antonio, TX: Psychological Corporation.

Weddell, R. A. (1989) Recognition memory for emotional facial expressions in patients with focal cerebral lesions. *Brain and Cognition, 11,* 1–17.

Weekes, B., & Coltheart, M. (1996). Surface dyslexia and surface dysgraphia: Treatment studies and their theoretical implications. *Cognitive Neuropsychology, 13,* 277–315.

Wehman, P., Bricout, J., & Targett, P. (1999). Supported employment for persons with traumatic brain injury: A guide for implementation. In R. T. Fraiser & D. C. Clemmons (1999). (Eds.), *Traumatic brain injury rehabilitation: Practical vocational, neuropsychological, and psychotherapy interventions.* London: CRC Press.

Weiller, C., Isensee, C., Rijntjes, M., Huber, W., Muller, S., et al. (1995). Recovery from Wernicke's aphasia: A positron emission tomographic study. *Annals of Neurology, 37,* 723–732.

Weinrich, M., McCall, D., Weber, C., Thomas, K., & Thornburg, L. (1995). Training on an iconic communication system for severe aphasia can improve natural language production. *Aphasiology, 9,* 343–364.

Weinrich, M., Shelton., J. R., Cox, D. M., & McCall, D. (1997). Remediating production of tense morphology improves verb retrieval in chronic aphasia. *Brain and Language, 58,* 23–45.

Weisenburg, T. H., & McBride, K. E. (1935). *Aphasia.* New York: Commonwealth Fund.

Weiss, H. D. (1982). Neoplasms. In M. A. Samuels (Ed.), *Manual of Neurologic Therapeutics with Essentials of Diagnosis* (2nd ed.). Boston: Little, Brown.

Welland, R. J., Lubinski, R., & Higginbotham, D. J. (2002). Discourse Comprehension Test performance of elders with dementia of Alzheimer type. *Journal of Speech, Language, and Hearing Research, 45,* 1175–1187.

Wenzlaff, M., & Clahsen, H. (2005). Finiteness and verb-second in German agrammatism. *Brain and Language, 92,* 33–44.

Wepman, J. M. (1951). *Recovery from aphasia.* New York: Ronald Press.

Wepman, J. M. (1968). Aphasia therapy: Some "relative" comments and some purely personal prejudices. In J. W. Black & E. G. Jancosek (Eds.), *Proceedings of the conference on language retraining for aphasics* (pp. 95–107). Columbus, OH: Ohio State University.

Wepman, J. M. (1972). Aphasia therapy: A new look. *Journal of Speech and Hearing Disorders, 37,* 203–214.

Wepman, J. M., & Jones, L. V. (1961). *Studies in aphasia: An approach to testing.* Chicago: Education-Industry Service.

Wepman, J. M., & Van Pelt, D. (1955). A theory of cerebral language disorders based on therapy. *Folia Phoniatrica, 7,* 223–235.

Wernicke, C. (1977). The aphasia symptom complex: A psychological study on an anatomic basis. In G. H. Eggert (Trans.), *Wernicke's works on aphasia: A sourcebook and review.* The Hague, Netherlands: Mouton.

Wertz, R. T. (1983). Classifying the aphasias: Commodious or chimerical? In R. H. Brookshire (Ed.), *Clinical aphasiology conference proceedings* (pp. 296–303). Minneapolis: BRK.

Wertz, R. T. (1985). Neuropathologies of speech and language: An introduction to patient management. In D. F. Johns (Ed.), *Clinical management of neurogenic communicative disorders* (2nd ed., pp. 1–96). Boston: Little, Brown.

Wertz, R. T. (1996). The PALPA's proof is in the predicting. *Aphasiology, 10,* 180–190.

Wertz, R. T., Auther, L. L., & Ross, K. B. (1997). Aphasia in African-Americans and Caucasians: Severity, improvement, and rate of improvement. *Aphasiology, 11,* 533–542.

Wertz, R. T., Collins, M. J., Weiss, D. G., Kurtzke, J. F., Friden, T., et al. (1981). Veterans Administration cooperative study on aphasia: A comparison of individual and group treatment. *Journal of Speech and Hearing Research, 24,* 580–594.

Wertz, R. T., Deal, J. L., Holland, A. L., Kurtzke, J. F., & Weiss, D. G. (1986). Comments on an uncontrolled aphasia no treatment trial. *Asha, 28,* 31.

Wertz, R. T., Deal, J. L., & Robinson, A. J. (1984). Classifying the aphasias: A comparison of the Boston Diagnostic Aphasia Examination and the Western Aphasia Battery. In R. H. Brookshire (Ed.), *Clinical aphasiology conference proceedings* (pp. 40–47). Minneapolis: BRK.

Wertz, R. T., Deal, L. M., & Deal, J. L. (1980). Prognosis in aphasia: Investigation of the High-Overall Predition (HOAP) method and the Short-Direct or HOAP-Slope method to predict change in PICA performance. In R. H. Brookshire (Ed.), *Clinical aphasiology conference proceedings* (pp. 164–173). Minneapolis: BR

Wertz, R. T., & Dronkers, N. F. (1994). PICA performance following left or right hemisphere brain damage: Influence of side and severity. M. L. Lemme (Ed.), *Clinical aphasiology* (Vol. 22, pp. 157–164).

Wertz, R. T., Dronkers, N. F., & Shubitowski, Y. (1986). Discriminant function analysis of performance by normals and left hemisphere, right hemisphere, and bilaterally brain damaged patients on a word fluency measure. In R. H. Brookshire (Ed.), *Clinical aphasiology* (Vol. 16, pp. 257–266). Minneapolis: BRK.

Wertz, R. T., & Katz, R. C. (2004). Outcomes of computer-provided treatment for aphasia. *Aphasiology, 18,* 229–244.

Wertz, R. T., Weiss, D. G., Aten, J. L., Brookshire, R. H., Garcia-Bunuel, L., et al. (1986). Comparison of clinic, home, and deferred language treatment for aphasia: A Veterans Administration cooperative study. *Archives of Neurology, 43,* 653–658.

Westbury, C., & Bub, D. (1997). Primary progressive aphasia: A review of 112 cases. *Brain and Language, 60,* 381–406.

Westmacott, R., Freedman, M., Black, S. E., Stokes, K. A., & Moscovitch, M. (2004). Temporally graded semantic memory loss in Alzheimer's disease: Cross-sectional and longitudinal studies. *Cognitive Neuropsychology, 21,* 353–378.

Weylman, S. T., Brownell, H. H., Roman, M., & Gardner, H. (1989). Appreciation of indirect requests by left- and right-brain-damaged patients: The effects of verbal context and conventionality of wording. *Brain and Language, 36,* 580–591.

Whatmough, C., Chertkow, H., Murtha, S., Templeman, D., Babins, L., et al. (2003). The semantic category effect increases with worsening anomia in Alzheimer's type dementia. *Brain and Language, 84,* 134–147.

Wheeler, B. M. (2001). *Close to me, but far away: Living with Alzheimer's.* Columbia, MO: University of Missouri Press.

WHOQOL Group (1998). Development of the World Health Organization WHOQOL-BREF quality of life assessment. *Psychological Medicine, 28,* 551–558.

Wilcox, M. J., Davis, G. A., & Leonard, L. L. (1978). Aphasics' comprehension of contextually conveyed meaning. *Brain and Language, 6,* 362–377.

Williams, L. S., Weinberger, M., Harris, L. E., Clark, D. O., & Biller, J. (1999). Development of a stroke-specific quality of life scale. *Stroke, 30,* 1362–1369.

Williams, S. E., & Canter, G. J. (1982). The influence of situational context on naming performance in aphasic syndromes. *Brain and Language, 17,* 92–106.

Williams, S. E., & Canter, G. J. (1987). Action-naming performance in four syndromes of aphasia. *Brain and Language, 32,* 124–136.

Williams, S. E., & Seaver, E. J. (1986). A comparison of speech sound durations in three syndromes of aphasia. *Brain and Language, 29,* 171–182.

Willmes, K. (1990). Statistical methods for a single-case study approach to aphasia therapy research. *Aphasiology, 4,* 415–436.

Willmes, K. (1995). Aphasia therapy research: Some psychometric considerations and statistical methods for the single-case study approach. In C. Code & D. J.

Müller (Eds.), *The treatment of aphasia: From theory to practice* (pp. 286–308). San Diego, CA: Singular.

Wilshire, C. E. (2002). Where do aphasic phonological errors come from? Evidence from phoneme movement errors in picture naming. *Aphasiology, 16,* 169–197.

Wilshire, C. E., & Fisher, C. A. (2004). "Phonological" dysphasia: A cross-modal phonological impairment affecting repetition, production, and comprehension. *Cognitive Neuropsychology, 21,* 187–210.

Wilson, B. A. (1987). *Rehabilitation of memory.* New York: Guilford Press.

Wilson, B. A., Alderman, N., Burgess, P. W., Emslie, H. C., & Evans, J. J. (1996). *The Behavioural Assessment of the Dysexecutive Syndrome.* Reading, UK: Thames Valley Test Company.

Wilson, B. A., Baddeley, A. D., Cockburn, J., & Hiorns, R. (1989). The development and validation of a test battery for detecting and monitoring everyday memory problems. *Journal of Clinical and Experimental Neuropsychology, 11,* 855–870.

Wilson, B. A., Cockburn, J., & Baddeley, A. D. (1985). *The Rivermead Behavioural Memory Test.* Reading, UK: Thames Valley Test Company.

Wilson, B. A., Shannon, M. T., & Stang, C. L. (2006). *Prentice Hall nurse's drug guide 2006.* Upper Saddle River, NJ: Pearson Education.

Winner, E., Brownell, H., Happé, F., Blum, A., & Pincus, D. (1998). Distinguishing lies from jokes: Theory of mind deficits and discourse interpretation in right hemisphere brain-damaged patients. *Brain and Language, 62,* 89–106.

Winner, E., & Gardner, H. (1977). Comprehension of metaphor in brain damaged patients. *Brain, 100,* 717–729.

Winner, E., & von Karolyi, C. (1998). Artistry and aphasia. In M. T. Sarno (Ed.), *Acquired aphasia* (3rd ed., pp. 375–411). New York: Academic Press.

World Health Organization (WHO). (1997). *ICIDH-2 International classification of impairments, activities, and participation.* Geneva, Switzerland: World Health Organization.

World Health Organization (WHO). (2001). *International classification for functioning, disability and health* (ICF). Geneva, Switzerland: World Health Organization.

Worrall, L., & Cruice, M. (2005). Why the WHO ICF and QOL constructs do not lend themselves to programmatic appraisal for planning therapy for aphasia: A commentary on Ross and Wertz, "Advancing appraisal: Aphasia and the WHO." *Aphasiology, 19,* 885–893.

Worrall, L. E. (2000). The influence of professional values on the functional communication approach in aphasia. In L. E. Worrall & C. M. Frattali (Eds.). *Neurogenic communication disorders: A functional approach* (pp. 191–205). New York: Thieme.

Worrall, L. E., Rose, T., Howe, T., Brennan, A., Egan, J., et al. (2005). Access to information for people with aphasia. *Aphasiology, 19,* 923–929.

Worrall, L. E., & Yiu, E. (2000). Forging partnerships with volunteers. In L. E. Worrall & C. M. Frattali (Eds.). *Neurogenic communication disorders: A functional approach* (pp. 125–136). New York: Thieme.

Wright, H. H., & Newhoff, M. (2004). Inference revision processing in adults with and without aphasia. *Brain and Language, 89,* 450–463.

Wright, H. H., & Shisler, R. J. (2005). Working memory in aphasia: Theory, measures, and clinical implications. *American Journal of Speech-Language Pathology, 14,* 107–118

Wulf, H. H. (1979). *My world alone.* Detroit: Wayne State University Press.

Wulfeck, B., Bates, E., & Capasso, R. (1991). A cross-linguistic study of grammaticality judgments in Broca's aphasia. *Brain and Language, 41,* 311–336.

Wunderlich, A., Ziegler, W., & Geigenberger, A. (2003). Implicit processing of prosodic information in patients with left and right hemisphere stroke. *Aphasiology, 17,* 861–880.

Yedor, K. E., Conlon, C. P., & Kearns, K. P. (1993). Measurements predictive of generalization of response elaboration training. In M. L. Lemme (Ed.), *Clinical aphasiology* (Vol. 21, pp. 213–223). Austin, TX: Pro-Ed.

Yesavage, J. A., Brink, T. L., Rose, T. L., Lum, O., Huang, V., et al. (1982). Development and validation of a geriatric depression screening scale: A preliminary report. *Journal of Psychiatric Research, 17,* 37–49.

Yiu, E. M-L., & Worrall, L. E. (1996). Sentence production ability of a bilingual Cantonese/English agrammatic speaker. *Aphasiology, 10,* 505–522.

Ylvisaker, M., Szekeres, S. F., & Feeney, T. (2001). Communication disorders associated with traumatic brain injury. In R. Chapey (Ed.), *Language intervention strategies in adult aphasia and related neurogenic communication disorders* (4th ed., pp. 745–808). Philadelphia: Lippincott Williams & Wilkins.

Yorkston, K. M., & Beukelman, D. R. (1980). An analysis of connected speech samples of aphasic and normal speakers. *Journal of Speech and Hearing Disorders, 45,* 27–36.

Youmans, G., Holland, A., Munoz, M. L., & Bourgeois, M. (2005). Script training and automaticity in two individuals with aphasia. *Aphasiology, 19,* 435–449.

Young, A. W., Newcombe, F., & Ellis, A. W. (1991). Different impairments contribute to neglect dyslexia. *Cognitive Neuropsychology, 8,* 177–192.

Youse, K. M., Coelho, C. A., Mozeiko, J. L., & Feinn, R. (2005). Discourse characteristics of closed-head-injured and non-brain-injured adults misclassified by discriminant function analyses. *Aphasiology, 19,* 297–313.

Zaidel, E., Kasher, A., Soroker, N., & Batori, G. (2002). Effects of right and left hemisphere damage on performance of the "Right hemisphere communication battery." *Brain and Language, 80,* 510–535.

Zanetti, O., Zanieri, G., Di Giovanni, G., De Vreese, L. P., Pezzini, A., et al. (2001). Effectiveness of procedural memory stimulation in mild Alzheimer's disease patients: A controlled study. *Neuropsychological Rehabilitation, 11,* 263–272.

Zanini, S., Bryan, K., De Luca, G., & Bava, A. (2005). The effects of age and education on pragmatic features of verbal communication: Evidence from the Italian version of the Right Hemisphere Language Battery (IRHLB). *Aphasiology, 19,* 1107–1133.

Zatorre, R. J. (1989). On the representation of multiple languages in the brain: Old problems and new directions. *Brain and Language, 36,* 127–147.

Zevin, J. D., & Seidenberg, M. S. (2002). Age of acquisition effects in word reading and other tasks. *Journal of Memory and Language, 47,* 1–29.

Zingeser, L. B., & Berndt, R. S. (1990). Retrieval of nouns and verbs in agrammatism and anomia. *Brain and Language, 39,* 14–32.

Zoccolotti, P., Scabini, D., & Violani, C. (1982). Electrodermal responses in patients with unilateral brain damage. *Journal of Clinical Neuropsychology, 4,* 143–150.

Zraick, R. I., & Boone, D. R. (1991). Spouse attitudes toward the person with aphasia. *Journal of Speech and Hearing Research, 34,* 123–128.

Zurif, E. B., Swinney, D., Prather, P., Soloman, J., & Bushell, C. (1993). An on-line analysis of syntactic processing in Broca's and Wernicke's aphasia. *Brain and Language, 45,* 448–464.

SUBJECT INDEX